MUSCLE DISORDERS IN CHILDHOOD

SECOND EDITION

MUSCLE DISORDERS IN CHILDHOOD

SECOND EDITION

Victor Dubowitz, MD, PhD, FRCP, DCH

Professor of Paediatrics
Royal Postgraduate Medical School
University of London
Consultant Paediatrician
Hammersmith Hospital
Medical Director, Neuromuscular Unit
Hammersmith Hospital, London

W.B. SAUNDERS COMPANY LTD
London · Philadelphia · Toronto · Sydney · Tokyo

W.B. Saunders Company Ltd   24–28 Oval Road
London NW1 7DX

The Curtis Center
Independence Square West
Philadelphia, PA 19106–3399, USA

Harcourt Brace Company
55 Horner Avenue
Toronto, Ontario M8Z 4X6, Canada

Harcourt Brace Company, Australia
30–52 Smidmore Street
Marrickville, NSW 2204, Australia

Harcourt Brace Company, Japan
Ichibancho Central Building, 22–1 Ichibancho
Chiyoda-ku, Tokyo, 102, Japan

A catalogue record for this book is available from the British Library.

ISBN 0 7020 1437 0

Editorial and Production Services by Fisher Duncan
10 Barley Mow Passage, London W4 4PH

Typeset by Preset Graphics, Derby
Printed in Great Britain by the Bath Press, Lower Bristol Road, Bath

Preface

We live in momentous times. The whole neuromuscular world has been turned on its head. The first edition of this book antedated the molecular genetic revolution. Some ten years later saw the discovery of the gene and the protein for Duchenne muscular dystrophy, the first example of the application of reverse genetics, where a previously unknown protein was identified via the location of the gene and its subsequent cloning and sequencing. The flood of new knowledge has continued unabated, and hardly a month passes without some exciting new addition. This is graphically illustrated by the state-of-the-art gene table I included in the first issue of the new journal, *Neuromuscular Disorders*, I launched in 1990; it comfortably filled one page of generously spaced print. In the latest issue, 5 years on, it occupies three full, closely compressed, pages, with half as much again being added by the mitochondrial genome.

In many ways it would have been much easier to start over again and write a completely new book. However, in some ways there proved to be advantages in retaining the core of the first edition. It has certainly helped me to keep my feet firmly on the ground and not to get entirely lost in the molecular clouds. Notwithstanding all the exciting new revelations, the clinician still needs to diagnose the clinical disorders, and the molecular geneticist still needs an accurate clinical diagnosis in order to pursue any rational research in relation to a particular genetic disorder. Throughout the writing of this book, I have had the clinician firmly in my sights, and I hope I have succeeded in providing an intelligible and reasonably digestible presentation, in trying to give an up-to-date appraisal of all the scientific advances in the context of the clinical syndromes. At the same time I hope the book will provide a clinical perspective for the dedicated scientist, ensconced in the isolation of his laboratory.

I dedicated the first edition of my book to David Smith (1943–1959), an extremely bright and courageous young boy with Duchenne dystrophy, whom I came to know on the muscular dystrophy ward at Queen Mary's Hospital for Children. I would like to dedicate this second edition to the fighting spirit of all the children with muscular dystrophy, spinal muscular atrophy, or other neuromuscular disorders, who have taught me so much, in so many ways, over the years.

Victor Dubowitz

Acknowledgements

As always, one is dependent on, and eternally grateful to, many people for helping to bring a work such as this to fruition. In addition to having to come to terms with the molecular genetic world, with its totally new jargon and impossible acronyms, I was also faced with the transition from the traditional, hand-written manuscript to the electronic age, and I am still not sure which was the more daunting. My attitude to the personal computer was much like my attitude to downhill skiing – if you've missed the critical period for learning the skill, you might as well stick to cross country. I am grateful to my son Michael, my computer guru, for coming to my rescue on so many occasions when the system crashed, which always seemed to be between the hours of two and four in the morning. At the end of the day, the survival of this book was entirely due to my one-time secretary, Valerie Botten, who had nursed me through the first edition, and came to my rescue at the eleventh hour, so that I could get on with the writing, while she looked after the rest.

I am indebted to Dr John Heckmatt, and latterly Dr Francesco Muntoni, Nattrass Memorial lecturers, who have been actively involved in the running of the Muscle Unit, and to Dr Caroline Sewry, who has ensured that all our muscle biopsies have benefited from the most up-to-date immunocytochemical techniques.

I am also appreciative of the contribution we have had over the years from a succession of highly motivated and enthusiastic trainee clinical fellows, supported by the Muscular Dystrophy Group of Great Britain; the late Christine Saunders (who developed a special interest in juvenile dermatomyositis, and helped to establish our special dermatomyositis clinic as well as the parents' support group); Nathan Hasson, Dina El Melhedgy, Neil Friedman, Alison Sansome, Joanne Philpot, Rudi Rapisarda and Fiona Goodwin; and from a series of distinguished clinical research fellows, both home-grown and from abroad. These have included, amongst others, Allie Moosa, Shirley Hodgson, Michel Vanasse, Hans Neville, Gwilym Hosking, Basil Thompson, Geoffrey Miller, Helen Skouteli, Nathaniel Pier, Stephanie Robb, Thomas Voit, Rivka Regev, Janet Hislop, Neil Thomas, Eliana Rodillo, Adnan Manzur, Antonella Pini, Akira Okuno, Haluk Topaloglu, Zamir Shorer and Eugenio Mercuri.

I have also benefited considerably from the stimulating discussions I have had over the years with a number of colleagues and fellow-travellers; in particular Gerta Vrbova, who has provided an interesting interface between experimental neurobiology and clinical neuromuscular disorders, Martin Bobrow and Kay Davies, who have provided a continuing interface with the advances in molecular genetics, and Barry Cooper, who has provided me with direct access to his veterinary patients. There surely cannot be many physicians who can quote their personal experience, not only with countless cases of Duchenne and Becker muscular dystrophy, but also with all the known animal models with a mutation in this gene, including the dystrophic mouse, the dystrophic dog, both Golden Retriever and Rotweiler, and the dystrophic cat.

I am also indebted to George Bentley, who has added an expert orthopaedic dimension to our rehabilitation programme, and also wish to acknowledge the expertise and support we have had from our physiotherapy department, and in particular the former director, Mrs Sylvia Hyde, in the rehabilitation of our neuromuscular patients, and the orthotic expertise of Mr John Florence.

I have always looked upon clinical photography as an extension of the clinical documentation and record of the patient, and am indebted to Karen Davison for the consistently high standard she has achieved. In the first edition of this book we prided ourselves in being able to illustrate fully the book with our own photographic material; we all but achieved this again for the second edition, except for a few special syndromes such as Bethlem myopathy and Schwartz–Jampel, for which I am grateful to Drs Luciano Merlini and Haluk Topaloglu, respectively. I am also grateful to a number of colleagues, and in particular Dr Billi Di Mauro and Drs Lou Kunkel and Andy Ahn, for their permission to reproduce a number of charts and diagrams, which I have acknowledged individually in the respective legends. I am also extremely grateful to Drs Jean-Claude Kaplan and Bertrand Fontaine, keepers of the gene table in *Neuromuscular Disorders*, for their permission for me to poach liberally from the tables for the new chapter on genetics I have introduced in this edition, and likewise to Dr Serenella Servidei for her recently compiled table on the mitochondrial genome. I also wish to thank Fiona Foley, Publishing Director at Mosby-Wolfe, for her agreement for me to include some of the illustrative cases from my *Colour Atlas of Muscle Disorders in Childhood*.

I owe a particular debt to Seán Duggan, Editor-in-Chief at W.B. Saunders, for his long-suffering support and faith in seeing this book to fruition, often I suspect against his better judgement and patience, and for his inspired decision to invite Jane Duncan of Fisher Duncan to provide the editorial and production expertise and back-up, which enabled me to achieve something practically unique for an author, to be completely satisfied and content with his publisher. Jane's meticulous eye for perfection in the layout of text and illustrations has even surpassed the obsession of Val Botten and myself. What better accolade?

My clinical and research activities have been continuously supported for over thirty-five years by the Muscular Dystrophy Group of Great Britain, since their first modest grant in 1958 to pursue my histochemical studies of normal and diseased muscle. This provided the basis for my continued interest in the clinical and pathological aspects of muscle diseases ever since, and I am pleased to take this opportunity of acknowledging this support.

Victor Dubowitz

Preface
to the First Edition

The past few years have seen an avalanche of interest in muscle disorders, coming from various directions – clinicians, pathologists, biochemists, geneticists, cell biologists, physiologists and a host of other scientists. Although we still remain ignorant of the cause of most of the major genetic disorders of the neuromuscular system, important strides have been made in various areas of study. It thus seemed timely to try and bring together the clinical and associated advances.

My interest in muscle disorders began in 1957 during a residency at Queen Mary's Hospital for Children in Carshalton, Surrey. Part of my duties entailed an occasional call to the Muscular Dystrophy Ward to treat a child who had pneumonia or other severe illness. Having never heard of muscular dystrophy, let alone seen a case, my curiosity was fired and from this clinical beginning grew an interest in investigating this mysterious condition. This led me to the laboratory of Professor Everson Pearse at the Royal Postgraduate Medical School at Hammersmith Hospital, where I spent many an interesting evening (or night) applying the then relatively new techniques of histochemistry to the biopsies I had taken from the patients.

My fruitful association with Queen Mary's Hospital for Children and the Royal Postgraduate Medical School reinforced my view that the clinician's place is not only at the bedside but also in the laboratory, in order to get a comprehensive overview of the patient and his investigations and not try to draw conclusions from either alone. This combined interest in the patient as well as the biopsy has continued throughout my period in Sheffield and latterly at the Hammersmith Hospital.

In our book, *Muscle Biopsy: A Modern Approach*, Dr Michael Brooke and I reviewed the advances in techniques of processing and interpreting the muscle biopsy, against a background of the various clinical syndromes. In this book I have tried to bring together all the clinical syndromes, both old and new, against a background of the muscle biopsy. The two are interdependent and the days are long past when the clinician, however astute, could make a definitive diagnosis on clinical grounds alone, and stand unchallenged.

Any work of this nature is dependent on the help and goodwill of many people; to name them all would entail another chapter to this book. I would like particularly to mention the following: Dr David Lawson at Queen Mary's Hospital for Children for his encouragement and the facilities he placed at my disposal in the early years; Mr Bob Reynolds, Head Physiotherapist at Queen Mary's, who first drew my attention to many of the problems of patients with muscular dystrophy, and Miss Mary Pugh for her excellent photographic documentation of those cases; Professor Peter Daniel at the Institute of Psychiatry, The Maudsley Hospital, who taught me the rudiments of muscle pathology; Professor Everson Pearse at the Hammersmith who provided me with instant bench space and access to the one and only prototype cryostat ('wheezy') then being developed in his laboratory, and fired my interest in histochemistry, and the many colleagues from all corners of the world who converged on his laboratory and were my constant mentors; the late Professor John Cumings who provided facilities for continuation of this work during my tenure of a lectureship in his department of Clinical Pathology at the National Hospital for Nervous Diseases; Professor Ronald Illingworth for the encouragement and autonomy to pursue my interests during my 11 years at the Children's Hospital in Sheffield; Mr Alan Tunstill for the excellent clinical photography and his continued interest and enthusiasm in this work throughout that period; Mr David Hawtin for the clinical photography at Hammersmith; a succession of superb technicians including Joan Wingfield, Julie Franks (née Binns) and in particular Christine Hutson (née Heinzmann) who has emigrated from her native Yorkshire to London with me; my clinical research associates, Allie Moosa, Mary Cunningham and Gwilym Hosking, and all the short-term research fellows who have been attached to my unit; Charles Galasko, and latterly Sean Hughes, for their interest in the orthopaedic problems; and finally the many paediatric colleagues who referred their patients – without them this book would never have been possible.

Writing a book always seems to start as a challenge and invariably ends up as an intimate love-hate relationship, and I am surely not the first author to be accused by his wife of bigamy. One always owes a particular debt to one's family for their tolerance and understanding during this time of split loyalties.

Throughout the preparation of this book my task has been considerably lightened by the outstanding secretarial expertise of Mrs Valerie Chalk. I would also like to record my thanks to Mr Bill Schmitt and Miss Patricia Terry at W. B. Saunders for their help and enthusiasm.

Much of my research over the years has been generously supported by the Muscular Dystrophy Group of Great Britain. I also wish to acknowledge additional grants from the Medical Research Council, Action Research for the Crippled Child and the Coxen Trust, as well as the munificent grant from the Muscular Dystrophy Association of America in 1975 to establish the Jerry Lewis Muscle Research Centre at Hammersmith Hospital.

Victor Dubowitz
London, 1978

Contents

Preface   v

Acknowledgements   vi

Preface to the First Edition   viii

1   Diagnosis and Classification of the Neuromuscular Disorders   1

2   The Muscular Dystrophies   34

3   The Congenital Myopathies   134

4   Metabolic Myopathies I: Glycogenoses   177

5   Metabolic Myopathies II: Lipid Disorders   Mitochondrial Disorders   211

6   Metabolic Myopathies III: Ion Channel Disorders   266

7   Endocrine Myopathies   315

8   Disorders of the Lower Motor Neurone: The Spinal Muscular Atrophies   325

9   Disorders of the Lower Motor Neurone: Hereditary Motor Neuropathies   370

10   Myasthenia   398

11   Inflammatory Myopathies   422

12   The Floppy Infant Syndrome   457

13   Disorders with Muscle Contracture and Joint Rigidity   473

14   Disorders of Movement   497

15   Genetics   509

Index   529

CHAPTER 1

Diagnosis and Classification of the Neuromuscular Disorders

INTRODUCTION

The traditional approach to the classification of neuromuscular disorders has aimed at distinguishing primary disorders of muscle (myopathies) from disorders affecting peripheral nerve (neuropathies). The myopathies have included muscular dystrophies, congenital myopathies, metabolic myopathies and a few more general disorders affecting primarily, or predominantly muscle. It has also been realized that some conditions, such as myotonic dystrophy, are multisystem disorders and that skeletal muscle, as well as the cardiac muscle and smooth muscle components are but part of a wide-ranging multisystem complex of features. The same applies to mitochondrial disorders, which are essentially cytopathies involving many different cells and tissues.

Moreover, even traditional muscle disorders such as Duchenne dystrophy have a central nervous system component, with the associated intellectual deficit, and we now know that the gene product in this Xp21 disorder, dystrophin, is expressed in the nervous system as well as in skeletal and cardiac muscle.

In congenital muscular dystrophy there is also associated central nervous system involvement, which can take the form of severe structural and developmental abnormalities in the brain, with associated severe intellectual retardation at one extreme, pure muscular dystrophy with no clinical or other evidence of central nervous system involvement at the other extreme, and in between cases of muscle involvement, with no intellectual or other clinical evidence of neurological involvement but striking changes in the brain white matter on cerebral imaging.

Some biochemical advances, such as recognition of ion channel disorders, have also cut across traditional syndrome boundaries and brought together some anticipated and some less likely bedfellows, with an abnormality in common in the same ion channel, for example the sodium channel.

Molecular genetic advances have pinpointed specific genes for some neuromuscular disorders and once again helped to prove the anticipated common factor basis for phenotypically divergent disorders such as Duchenne and Becker dystrophy or the wide-ranging clinical phenotypes of childhood spinal muscular atrophy from the severe infantile Werdnig-Hoffmann to the mild ambulant Kugelberg-Welander. They have also helped to identify some of the deviant phenotypes, such as 'quadriceps myopathy' or cases with cramps on exercise, or myoglobinuria, and no apparent clinical weakness, as variants of Becker dystrophy, and other cases with a clinical dystrophy as manifesting carriers of this gene mutation.

Where do we go from here? The laboratory buffs would probably wish us to categorize collectively all the 'Xp21 myopathies', or all the 'dystrophinopathies', but this does not help the clinician who has to deal with the patient or his family to discuss the nature of the disease, its clinical implications and its course and prognosis. There is a world of difference between the boy with Duchenne muscular dystrophy who will be unable to walk by the time he is 12 years old and the 60-year-old man with Becker dystrophy who is still ambulant, although they both have in common an Xp21 myopathy or a dystrophinopathy. It is much easier for the patient (and possibly also the clinician) to relate to a specific named disorder, even if eponymous, which defines a clearly described clinical syndrome than to its biochemistry or its molecular genetics. Patients find comfort and some security in specific labels, even if they relate to serious disorders, rather than being left insecure without a conclusive decision.

With the dramatic changes in the whole neuromuscular world, I have naturally faced a considerable dilemma in how to fully update this book, the first edition of which dates to the pre-molecular era. I have decided not to capitulate completely to new technology and for the present I propose to stick to the traditional approach of trying to define and identify the various clinical syndromes in relation to neuromuscular disorders and to review our current knowledge in relation to molecular genetics, biochemistry and pathogenesis in this context. To me this is still logical, as the patient presents with his clinical phenotype, and it is up to the clinician to assess how the various investigative results fit in with, or deviate from, a specific clinical diagnosis.

CLINICAL CLASSIFICATION

Muscle disorders can be broadly subdivided into myopathies, in which the pathology is confined to the muscle itself, with no associated structural abnormality in the peripheral nerve, and neuropathies or neurogenic atrophies, in which muscle weakness is secondary to an abnormality along the course of the peripheral nerve, from the anterior horn cell to the neuromuscular junction. Both myopathies and neuropathies can be further subdivided into hereditary syndromes and acquired syndromes, and into acute and chronic disorders. In trying to classify the various syndromes it is helpful to follow the anatomical route of the lower motor neurone (Figure 1-1).

Further categorization is based on the characteristic pattern of particular disorders. Thus the term muscular dystrophy is used for the genetically determined, progressive, degenerative myopathies, and these are subdivided on the basis of clinical distribution and severity of weakness and mode of inheritance (see Chapter 2, Table 2-1). Similarly, spinal muscular atrophies and neuropathies are neurogenic disorders in which the lesion is in the anterior horn cell or the peripheral nerve and these are further characterized on the basis of clinical features, mode of inheritance and structural changes (see Chapters 8 and 9).

The so-called congenital myopathies are a new generation of genetically determined muscle disorders whose clinical presentation may be somewhat similar to the muscular dystrophies or neurogenic atrophies, but in which specific structural abnormalities have beeen recognized in the muscle.

The metabolic myopathies comprise those syndromes in which a specific metabolic abnormality has been identified or presumed, and include glyco-

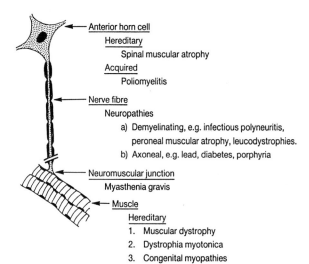

Anterior horn cell
  Hereditary
    Spinal muscular atrophy
  Acquired
    Poliomyelitis

Nerve fibre
  Neuropathies
    a) Demyelinating, e.g. infectious polyneuritis, peroneal muscular atrophy, leucodystrophies.
    b) Axoneal, e.g. lead, diabetes, porphyria

Neuromuscular junction
  Myasthenia gravis

Muscle
  Hereditary
  1. Muscular dystrophy
  2. Dystrophia myotonica
  3. Congenital myopathies
  4. Metabolic myopathies, e.g. glycogenoses types II and V, malignant hyperpyrexia.

  Aquired
  1. Dermatomyositis/polymyositis
  2. Endocrine myopathies, e.g. thyrotoxic
  3. Iatrogenic, e.g. steroid myopathy

Figure 1-1 Disorders of the lower motor neurone. Anatomical approach. (Courtesy of Dr A. Moosa.)

genoses, mitochondrial myopathies, disorders of lipid metabolism, and ion channel disorders.

The myotonic and myasthenic disorders have been recognized on the basis of their specific features, both clinically and on electrodiagnostic investigation. It is now known that myotonias are ion channel disorders, whereas myasthenic syndromes may have an immunological basis.

The various acquired muscle disorders include sundry inflammatory, endocrine and toxic conditions affecting either the peripheral nerve or the muscle itself.

The floppy or hypotonic infant presents a diagnostic problem unto itself and may reflect either a neuromuscular disorder or be associated with a primary disorder in another system, particularly the central nervous system, in which the hypotonia is an incidental feature.

Accurate diagnosis in this wide array of disorders is dependent on a careful clinical assessment followed by the appropriate investigations.

EPIDEMIOLOGY

Muscle disorders are ubiquitous and affect all races. The apparent high incidence of some disorders in particular countries, such as congenital muscular dystrophy in Finland and Japan, Werdnig–Hoffmann disease in Saudi Arabia, and limb girdle muscular dystrophy in Reunion Island and parts of North Africa, may reflect inbreeding in isolated communities increasing the incidence of relatively uncommon recessive disorders.

Statistics on the incidence of various muscle disorders are not readily available and estimates vary widely. The estimated incidence of Duchenne muscular dystrophy, the commonest neuromuscular disorder in childhood, based on a number of population studies and on data from screening programmes, is about 1 in 3500 male births. Spinal muscular atrophies in childhood, inherited through an autosomal recessive mechanism, may be equally prevalent, with an estimated incidence of 1 in 6–10 000 births, second only to cystic fibrosis amongst the recessive disorders. Emery (1991) has recently completed a monumental survey of the world literature on the population frequencies of the more common neuromuscular disorders, covering both the *prevalence* (the number of affected individuals in a population at a given time in relation to the total number of individuals who are at risk) and the *incidence* (the number of individuals born during a particular period who will develop the disease in relation to the number of live births over the same period). In the case of X-linked conditions the reference population will be only males, in the autosomal conditions the total population (Table 1-1).

Table 1.1 Estimated overall prevalences ($\times 10^{-6}$) of the commoner inherited neuromuscular diseases in the general population. The figure for Becker muscular dystrophy is an underestimate and that for limb girdle muscular dystrophy an overestimate

Muscular dystrophies	
Duchenne	32
Duchenne-like	5
Becker	>7
Facioscapulohumeral	20
Limb girdle	<40
Myotonic dystrophy	50
Congenital myotonias	10
Spinal muscular atrophies	
(II + III)	12
Hereditary motor and sensory	
neuropathies	100
Familial motor neurone	
disease and myasthenia gravis	10
Total	286

From Emery (1991) *Neuromuscular Disorders* **1**: 19–29, by kind permission of the author and Pergamon Press.

CLINICAL ASSESSMENT OF MUSCLE PROBLEMS IN CHILDHOOD

HISTORY

A careful clinical history may often give the clue to the particular disorder that the child has. Common presenting symptoms of muscle disorders in childhood include delay in motor milestones, an abnormal gait, tendency to fall, overt muscle weakness, floppiness or hypotonia, muscle cramps or muscle stiffness.

It is always worth starting with an open question to the parents such as, 'What have you noticed wrong?' and allowing them to give a detailed description of their observations before asking direct questions. This presenting story may at times be so perceptive and precise as to allow a fairly confident diagnosis. Thus I was able to diagnose myotonia congenita in a child whose father gave the presenting complaint as, 'It's like this doctor. When we travel on the tube [subway] train between Neasden and Wembley, which is only one stop, she becomes so stiff that she practically stumbles off the train and has to be helped, but after a short while she loosens up and becomes normal again.' Often the description the parents have for a particular gait or the way in which a child manages a particular activity such as getting up from the floor or climbing stairs may also give a very good idea of the extent of the child's disability.

In addition to the presenting features one should routinely ask about other associated features suggestive of muscle disorder (see the Questionnaire in the Appendix at the end of this chapter). It is also worth routinely asking as a direct question whether the particular disability or weakness is becoming better, becoming worse, or remaining static. At times one may hear a history of weakness being static over 6 or 12 months or more in progressive disorders such as Duchenne dystrophy, which highlights the importance of assessing the progression of a chronic muscle disorder over relatively long periods. One may also at times hear a history of apparent improvement in Duchenne dystrophy because the child has achieved a new activity, such as riding a tricycle. It is important in such instances to obtain a history as to whether certain specific activities the child had difficulty with, such as climbing stairs, getting up from the floor, running, hopping or skipping, have shown improvement or deterioration. In other conditions, such as spinal muscular atrophy, which are relatively static, one may hear a history of stability over a number of years and then a sudden deterioration. This may coincide with a growth spurt of the child without any measurable loss of power.

From the type of problem the child has one can often get an idea as to whether the weakness is proximal or distal or generalized. One should also enquire about any associated difficulty with chewing and swallowing or associated respiratory deficit.

The parents should be questioned as to any variability in the muscle weakness from day to day or from one time of the day to another, or whether there is fatigue on effort and improvement with rest (suggesting myasthenia) or increased disability with inactivity and improvement with activity (suggesting myotonia).

Any change in the appearance of particular muscles, suggesting either an increase in prominence (such as the enlarged calves in Duchenne and other forms of dystrophy) or wasting, should be noted.

If the patient presents with cramps in the muscles one should particularly ask whether these are related to exercise or not. Cramps occurring at rest are usually not of muscle origin and in most cases do not warrant any further neuromuscular investigations. These are the commonest cramps occurring in childhood. Cramps related to exercise and relieved by rest usually point to a muscle disorder (see Table 1-2). They are a presenting feature of some of the more benign and chronic forms of muscular dystrophy such as the Becker and limb girdle varieties (see Chapter 2). There is usually associated weakness, together with changes in serum enzyme levels and on muscle biopsy. Cramps on exertion are also a presenting feature in some of the rare metabolic myopathies, such as the glycogenoses associated with phosphorylase and phosphofructokinase deficiency and the disorders of lipid metabolism associated with deficiency of the enzyme carnitine palmitoyl transferase. An additional enquiry of possible associated myoglobinuria should be made in all these cases. The muscle power of these patients may be normal. Muscle cramps are also an associated feature of other myoglobinuric syndromes (see Chapter 6).

If the patient presents with recurrent episodes of muscle weakness one should think of one of the syndromes with periodic weakness (Table 1-3) and investigate appropriately. Patients presenting with stiffness of muscle, without evidence of myotonia, may still have an abnormality of the ion channels.

FAMILY HISTORY

A detailed family history and pedigree chart is essential in every case in order to establish a possible genetic mechanism. In X-linked conditions one should find out as much detail as possible, particularly of male relatives on the maternal side, and it is also worth noting female relatives who may be

Table 1-2 Cause of muscle cramps

A. Occurring at rest. Usually not muscle disorder.

B. Occurring with exertion. Relieved by rest. May be associated myoglobinuria.

   1. Benign and low-grade muscular dystrophy (limb girdle or Becker type)

   2. Metabolic disorders

     (a) Glycogenoses:

       type V (phosphorylase deficiency)
       type VII (phosphofructokinase deficiency)

     (b) Lipid metabolism disorders:

       carnitine palmityl transferase deficiency

   3. Other myoglobinuric syndromes

Table 1-3 Causes of episodic weakness

1. Periodic paralysis

2. Relapsing polyneuropathy

3. Dermatomyositis; polymyositis

4. Myasthenia gravis

5. Rhabdomyolysis

available for investigation to establish possible carrier status.

In autosomal recessive conditions the earlier generations may be normal and the parents of affected siblings are presumptive heterozygotes. Consanguinity of the parents will increase the chances of carrying the same genes.

Before giving genetic counselling in any family it is also essential first to establish as accurately as possible the diagnosis in the index case.

CLINICAL EXAMINATION

One can often acquire much more information on the degree and localization of muscle weakness in a small child by observing some of his spontaneous activities before trying to do a formal assessment along the lines of the traditional 'adult' neurological examination. Attempts to undress and forcibly restrain a child in a supine position on an examination couch are likely to end up with a thoroughly uncooperative and irritable child and an equally irritable and frustrated examiner.

The child should be carefully observed from the time he comes into the consulting room and throughout the period that the history is being obtained from the parents. His gait should be noted and his posture in the standing position. If he is not ambulant, note his general activity or lack of it. The face as well as the limbs should be observed.

A number of assessments can be done while the child is still clothed. These include: a detailed assessment of his gait, whether he walks on a wide or narrow base, on his toes or on flat fleet, whether the feet are excessively everted, and whether he can walk on his heels or along a straight line heel to toe; his ability to get up from a chair, to sit up from the supine, or go down on to and to get up from the floor, to go up and down two or three steps, to jump with both legs, to stand on one leg and to hop on one leg.

A small infant can be engaged in play activity and given small cubes to handle and to place on top of each other. This will help assess his co-ordination as well as his ability to raise the arms against gravity. Ocular movements can be assessed by his ability to follow an object of interest to him.

These general assessments will help to decide if there is any obvious weakness present and also whether its location is proximal, distal or generalized. The child who is able to hop on one leg and to get up from the floor without any difficulty and without supporting a hand on the knee is unlikely to have any significant weakness in the lower limbs. The examination can then be followed by a more detailed assessment of individual muscle groups after the child is undressed.

Motor milestones

In each age group there are milestones of motor development which are helpful in assessing the integrity of the neuromuscular system. The clinical examination should thus be geared to the age of the child (Table 1-4).

In the neonatal period and in very young infants one can observe general mobility of face and limbs (Figure 1-2). If the limbs are not being moved spontaneously one can observe the response to a stimulus such as stroking the soles, or the ability to sustain a passively elevated arm or leg. The control of the head and limbs in ventral suspension and with traction on the hands while lying supine will give a good general idea of abilities and disabilities. Even in

Table 1-4 Some motor milestones in normal development (average)

Birth:
  Flexed posture of limbs, able to sustain head in line with body in ventral suspension and supine.

3 months:
  Momentary sitting posture, flexed forward.

6 months:
  Sits leaning forward on hands. Lifts head spontaneously in supine. Takes weight on legs well.

9 months:
  Sits. Pivots. Pulls to standing position.

1 year:
  Walks with help. Cruises.

15 months:
  Walks unaided. Creeps up stairs.

18 months:
  Walks without falling. Runs. Climbs stairs unaided.

2 years:
  Able to run well. Kicks a ball. Goes up and down stairs.

3 years:
  Stands on one leg. Jumps off a step.

4 years:
  Hops on one foot (just).

5 years:
  Good ability to hop on either leg.

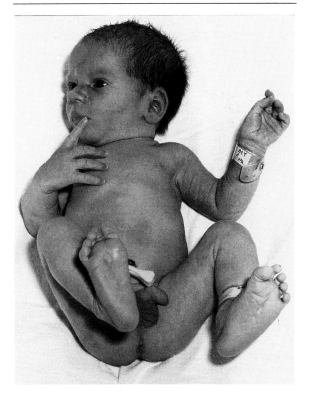

Figure 1-2 Newborn infant showing flexed posture of limbs and ability to maintain arms and legs against gravity. Note expressive face and closed mouth.

the immediate newborn period a full-term infant should be able to keep the head in line with the body in both the prone and supine postures and should also have a good degree of flexor tone in the limbs in ventral suspension (Figures 1-3 and 1-4). These manoeuvres can be used throughout the first three months, and one should again look for the degree of head control and the mobility of the limbs.

From the age of 3 months onwards one can also note the child's ability to reach out for objects, his ability to support weight on the legs when held

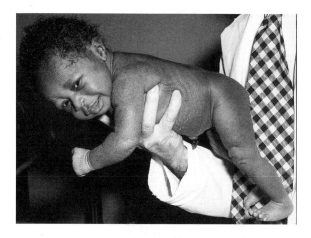

Figure 1-3 Newborn infant. Ventral suspension showing ability to maintain head in line with body. Note flexed posture of limbs.

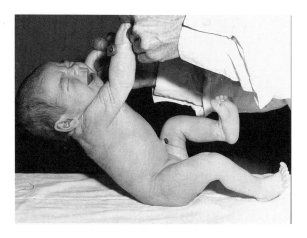

Figure 1-4 Newborn infant showing ability to maintain head in line with body in supine posture with traction on hands. Note sustained elevation of leg against gravity.

vertically and bounced on his feet, and his head control in the vertical, prone and supine positions.

Later milestones such as sitting without support, pivoting, and standing with and without support are useful (Figure 1-5). In addition to observing the weight-bearing ability of the legs, one can also assess the mobility of the arms in the 'parachute' response when the child pushes out his hands when he is inverted and moved head-first towards the floor (Figure 1-6). This is usually well developed by about 9 months of age. The power in the arms and shoulder girdle muscles can be assessed in the 'wheelbarrow' posture by his being kept suspended with his head down and made to 'walk' on his hands (Figure 1-7).

Once he starts walking one can observe his ability to get up from a sitting, prone or supine position on the floor, and his ability to go up and down steps (a simple two-step wooden construction with non-slip rubber sheeting on the steps is useful for outpatient purposes).

After the age of 3 years he should be able to stand on one leg; from the age of 4 to jump on both legs and after the age of 5 to hop on one leg. From the age of 3 onwards one can usually get the co-operation of the child in attempting various manoeuvres, as long as one can make it interesting to him and win his attention.

In assessing the shoulder girdle one should also note, in addition to any weakness and difficulty with movements, the upward and forward riding of the scapulae with abduction of the arms, giving a very typical terraced appearance in the facioscapulo-humeral syndromes (see Chapter 2).

The face can be assessed by noting its appearance at rest, the presence of an open drooping or tent-shaped mouth, and whether there is lack of movement and expression. The power can be assessed by getting the child to screw his eyes tightly closed – normally he should be able to bury his eyelashes completely (Figure 1-8). In the presence of weakness, even of mild degree, the eyelashes will remain out. The lower face can be assessed by getting the child to show his teeth, smile, puff out his cheeks and pout his lips, and to blow or whistle.

Once a general appraisal has been made in this way one can go on to more detailed quantitative assessment of individual muscle groups. The standard Medical Research Council (MRC) classification (1943) provides a useful baseline (Table 1-5). This is a rough but practical clinical guide, originally developed during World War II for the assessment of peripheral nerve injuries, and designates five categories ranging from zero movement in the muscle (0) to full strength (5) and antigravity power in between (3). Grade 1 denotes a flicker of movements only, grade 2 contraction short of antigravity power, and grade 4 power more than antigravity but not full.

Table 1-5   MRC scale for evaluation of muscle power

(0)	No contraction
(1)	Flicker or trace of contraction
(2)	Active movement, with gravity eliminated
(3)	Active movement against gravity
(4)	Active movement against gravity and resistance
(5)	Normal power

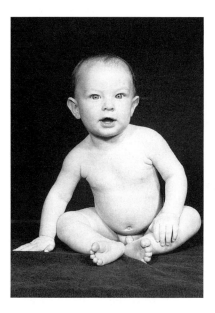
(a)

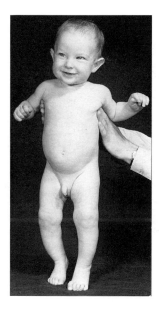
(b)

Figure 1-5a,b   Infant, 7 months old, showing ability (a) to sit steadily without support and (b) to sustain weight of body on legs, when held.

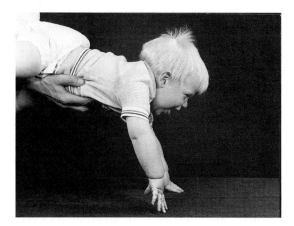

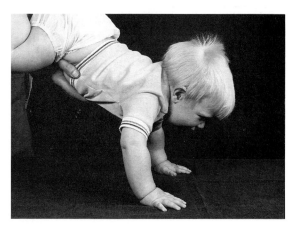

Figure 1-6   'Parachute' response showing outstretching of arms when held in a head-down position.

Figure 1-7   'Wheelbarrow' posture. Ability to take weight of body and locomote with hands. (Same infant as Figure 1-6.)

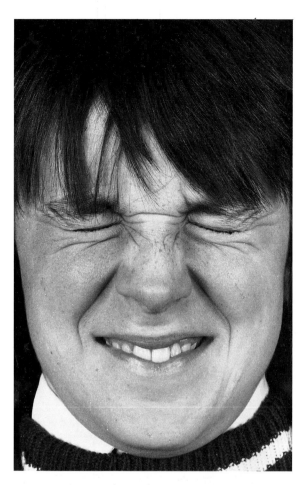

Figure 1-8 Ability to screw up eyes tightly and bury the eyelashes completely. Note also the symmetrical facial movement with showing of teeth.

do so, and (1) partial ability with help. One can thus assess the severity of a child's functional deficit by relating the score to the maximum of 40 (Scott *et al.*, 1982; see Table 1-6).

Table 1-6   Assessment of motor ability

1. Lifts head
2. Supine to prone over right
3. Supine to prone over left
4. Prone to supine over right
5. Prone to supine over left
6. Gets to sitting
7. Sitting
8. Gets to standing
9. Standing
10. Standing on heels
11. Standing on toes
12. Stands on right leg
13. Stands on left leg
14. Hops on right leg
15. Hops on left leg
16. Gets off chair
17. Climbing step right leg
18. Descending step right leg
19. Climbing step left leg
20. Descending step left leg

Score [a]
2 for every completed movement
1 for help and/or reinforcement
0 if unable to achieve the movement
Total possible score = 40

[a]All movements are attempted and scored
From Scott *et al.* (1982) *Muscle and Nerve* **5**: 291–301, by kind permission of the author and J. Wiley and Sons Ltd

Attempts have been made to quantify muscle function and muscle power or force. As an extension of the MRC score on individual muscles, one can obtain a global assessment of the muscle function of the child by scoring several muscle groups, adding up the scores and expressing the total as a percentage of the maximum score. Thus:

$$\% \text{ MRC Score} = \frac{\text{Total score} \times 100}{\text{No. of muscles tested} \times 5}$$

One may also glean useful information from timing various activities such as walking a set distance, going up a series of steps, getting up from the floor and so forth. These activities can be measured longitudinally in assessing the progression of a disease or the response to treatment. A Motor Ability Score has also been developed in our physiotherapy department, based on 20 sequential activities, each scored on a 3-point scale, with (2) being full ability to perform the task, (0) inability to

The development of a sensitive handheld myometer by Edwards and McDonnell (1974) (Figure 1-9) provided a more objective measurement of the actual force exerted by a particular group of muscles. We found this myometer to be practical in the childhood period as well, although different grades of force and calibration were necessary in weaker cases (Hosking *et al*, 1976). It is of particular value in assessing the progress of weak muscles but can also provide a useful index of the degree of weakness in a particular muscle in comparison with the normal for the age, or with other children of equivalent age with the same disorder such as Duchenne dystrophy.

The subsequent development of an electronic instrument, with the help of the father of one of our Duchenne boys, had the advantage of a wider range of sensitivity to different forces and was particularly useful in very weak children (Scott *et al.*, 1982)

(Figure 1-10). This myometer can be used to assess various muscle groups, but the technique needs to be carefully standardized, so that in the assessment of a particular movement, e.g. flexion of the elbow, the myometer is always placed at a constant distance from the fulcrum (the elbow). (This myometer is available commercially from Penny & Giles, Dorset, England.)

Associated features

In addition to the assessment of muscle weakness, other signs may be helpful in the identification of particular muscle syndromes.

Muscle enlargement. Prominence of various muscles is a common feature in Duchenne dystrophy, the so-called, 'pseudohypertrophy'. It is symmetrical and commonly affects the calves, but may affect various other upper and lower limb muscles and may at times be fairly universal. It is not specific to Duchenne dystrophy, but also occurs in the Becker variety and in other forms of dystrophy and also occasionally in neurogenic syndromes. In Duchenne carriers there may be asymmetrical enlargement of one calf. Focal hypertrophy may also occur in association with disc lesions or focal radiculitis of the lumbosacral cord.

In addition to its association with neuromuscular disorders, muscle hypertrophy may be an isolated feature, and patients may present with generalized

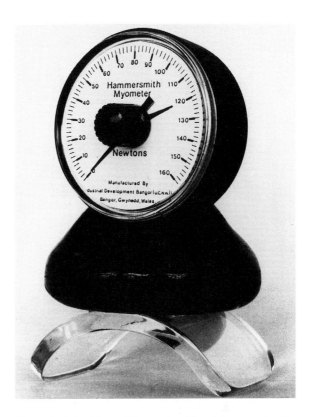

Figure 1-9 The 'Hammersmith Myometer' for measuring force of muscle (Edwards and McDonnell, 1974). (Courtesy Professor R.H.T. Edwards.)

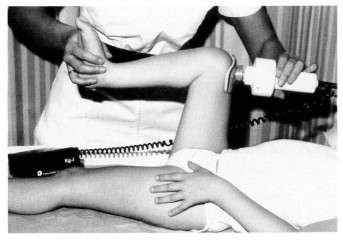

Figure 1-10 Electronic myometer being used with patients.

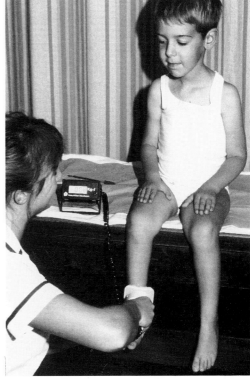

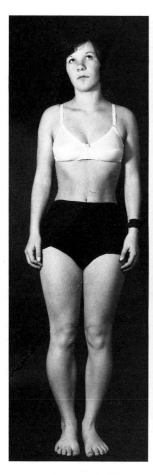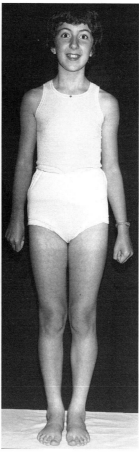

Figure 1-11 Focal hypertrophy. Two girls, aged 14 and 10 respectively, each presenting with progressive enlargement of one calf. No associated symptoms. No clinical weakness. CK and EMG normal. Muscle biopsy not done.

muscle hypertrophy (a feature of myotonia congenita), hemihypertrophy or focal hypertrophy (Figure 1-11). In cases of hemihypertrophy careful observation is necessary to exclude an associated neoplasm, usually nephroblastoma.

Muscle atrophy. Selective atrophy of some muscles may also relate to specific disorders. Thus in facioscapulohumeral dystrophy there may be selective wasting of the deltoids, in Emery-Dreifuss dystrophy of the humeral muscles, particularly the biceps, and of the distal leg muscles such as tibialis anterior and gastrocnemius, and in myotonic dystrophy of the temporalis and sternomastoids.

The *tendon reflexes* are usually depressed in the spinal muscular atrophies and neurogenic syndromes. In severe infantile muscular atrophy they are invariably absent. The presence of easily elicited tendon jerks in a hypotonic infant excludes a severe spinal muscular atrophy and the presence of brisk jerks and particularly ankle clonus should raise the possibility of a central nervous system disorder rather than a neuromuscular one. However, it is not completely exclusive and one may occasionally see brisk reflexes in the newborn infant or in older children in the presence of various neuromuscular disorders, other than spinal muscular atrophy.

In Duchenne dystrophy the tendon reflexes in the upper limbs as well as the knee jerks are lost early, whereas the ankle jerks are often retained and may even be brisk until late in the disease. The same distribution is found in the limb girdle and Becker forms of dystrophy but the upper limb and knee jerks may be less depressed. In congenital myopathies and other neuromuscular disorders the reflexes are variable and not diagnostically helpful.

The presence of *fasciculation*, particularly of the tongue and less frequently of peripheral muscles, is a useful diagnostic sign in spinal muscular atrophies. A coarse *tremor* of the hands is another common feature both in spinal atrophies and occasionally in motor neuropathies.

Table 1-7 Some causes of toe-gait

---

1. Normal feature in early stages of walking.

2. Muscular dystrophies:
   Duchenne
   Mild limb girdle form
   Emery-Dreifuss

3. Motor neuropathies; HMSN; Charcot-Marie-Tooth

4. Spastic syndromes:
   Cerebral diplegia
   Spastic paraparesis

A *toe-gait* is a common feature in many different neuromuscular disorders (Table 1-7). It may be observed in Duchenne as well as in milder types of muscular dystrophy, especially Emery-Dreifuss, and in the motor neuropathies, particularly of the peroneal muscular atrophy type, with their associated footdrop. In all these situations there is a progressive tightening of the tendo Achillis. Toe-gait is also a feature of spastic conditions such as cerebral diplegia and this diagnosis will be suspected if there is a general increase in tone in the legs and the presence of ankle clonus, brisk reflexes and an extensor plantar response. Toe-gait is also a transitory phenomenon in many normal children, particularly in the early stages of independent walking.

In the spinal muscular atrophies the feet are often in an everted, hypotonic, position, so that the child stands with a marked flat-footed posture rather than a cavus or equinus one.

Joint abnormalities are a common feature of locomotor disorders. In the floppy infant syndrome laxity of ligaments in isolation or in association with a general connective tissue disorder may account for all the clinical features. Limitation of joint movements as a result of permanent shortening (contractures) of various muscles is a common complication of many of the dystrophies and also other myopathies and neurogenic syndromes, particularly in the non-ambulant child. They usually take the form of flexion contractures of the hips, knees and other joints and relate to the habitual posture of the joint. Much can be done for the prevention of these deformities by passive movements and by maintaining neutral postures in the early phases. Early onset of contractures may be a major component of congenital muscular dystrophy and also some of the congenital myopathies.

Scoliosis is a common complication occurring in various muscle disorders with loss of ambulation. It is also a common feature of intermediate severity spinal muscular atrophy; sufferers are able to sit unsupported but not to stand or walk (see Chapter 8). Early diagnosis and adequate efforts to combat the progression are important.

After the clinical assessment it should be possible to decide whether the child has a neuromuscular problem or whether his presenting symptoms are due to a disorder outside the neuromuscular system. One can then proceed to the special investigations to try to confirm and further identify the nature of the muscle disease, or to help exclude its presence.

SPECIAL INVESTIGATIONS

The three traditional investigations in the differential diagnosis of muscle disorders are serum enzymes, electrophysiological procedures and muscle biopsy. Of these the serum enzymes and electrodiagnosis can be looked upon as screening procedures, and the muscle biopsy as a definitive procedure likely to give a more exact and definitive diagnosis. All have their pitfalls and limitations and the results should always be analysed in conjunction with the clinical picture.

Over the past few years ultrasound imaging has proved to be a very useful screening technique for recognizing normal or pathological muscle and has already largely superceded electromyography in our own clinic as a screening procedure. It has the distinct advantage of being non-invasive and readily acceptable to children. One can thus rapidly screen several different muscle groups and obtain information on the distribution of pathological change and even the presence of selective involvement of different components within the quadriceps or other muscle groups. It also has the advantage over other imaging techniques, such as computerized tomography and magnetic resonance imaging, of being portable and thus readily available in the setting of the outpatient clinic.

SERUM ENZYMES

Historically, the first serum enzymes found to be elevated in muscular dystrophy were the transaminases (aminotransferases) and subsequently aldolase, but the most consistent and reliable one has proved to be creatine kinase (CK). This enzyme catalyses the release of high energy phosphate from creatine phosphate and occurs mainly in muscle, so that in any degenerative disorder of muscle it is likely to leak into the serum in large amounts. It is important to check the CK in any patient found to have unsuspected high transaminase levels, to avoid the blunder (which still occurs these days) of proceeding to a liver biopsy.

In some conditions, such as Duchenne dystrophy and Becker dystrophy, the elevation in CK is gross, with levels up to 50 times the normal in the early stages. This means that the test is of value not only in the diagnosis of early Duchenne dystrophy but also in excluding it in the presence of a normal or only moderately elevated level. Other forms of dystrophy such as Emery–Dreifuss may have a more modest elevation, with levels in the hundreds rather than thousands of units, and with a wide variability from case to case.

Other conditions with degeneration of muscle fibres also give elevation of serum CK, but of variable degree. In some, such as acute rhabdomyolysis or malignant hyperpyrexia, it may also run into several thousand units, but in others the elevation is more modest.

In many of the congenital myopathies with structural abnormalities, such as central core disease or nemaline myopathy, the serum CK is likely to be normal or only slightly elevated. In congenital muscular dystrophy it is usually moderately elevated, but is extremely variable and can range from normal to a fairly marked elevation.

In spinal muscular atrophies and other neurogenic syndromes, the levels are usually normal, although some cases of the more benign varieties of spinal atrophy (Kugelberg–Welander syndrome) may have moderate elevation and associated focal degenerative fibres on biopsy. Cases that have been documented as spinal muscular atrophy with grossly elevated levels have proved to be misjudged cases of Becker dystrophy.

Where serum CK is used to detect milder degrees of elevation, such as in some of the non-dystrophic myopathies, or in carrier detection in Duchenne dystrophy, or subclinical malignant hyperpyrexia, it is essential that the laboratory uses a reliable method, produces its own normal range and carries out regular control checks. It is also important not to depend on a single isolated CK level for such important decisions as genetic counselling but always to repeat the estimation on separate occasions.

In a child with muscle weakness a normal CK does not exclude a myopathy, and a very high CK does not necessarily imply a severe myopathy, since very high levels, comparable with those in Duchenne dystrophy, can also be obtained in the milder Becker type dystrophy and is no reflection of severity. Normal CK levels are also common in the acute active phase of childhood dermatomyositis even in the presence of severe weakness and this correlates with the frequent absence of any degenerative changes in the muscle fibres at biopsy. Normal levels are also the rule in many of the congenital myopathies, even those with marked clinical weakness.

IMAGING OF MUSCLE

ULTRASOUND IMAGING

Realtime ultrasound imaging is a useful and practical tool in the screening of muscle for pathological change (Heckmatt *et al.*, 1980, 1982, 1988; Heckmatt and Dubowitz, 1987; Fischer *et al.*, 1988; Topalogu *et al.*, 1992). The machine is portable and can be brought to the patient, unlike the more complex facilities required for computerized tomography or magnetic resonance imaging. It can be used as a routine procedure in the outpatient clinic, is non-invasive, several different muscles can rapidly be assessed, and it is readily acceptable to children (Figure 1-12). Any interface between tissues of different structure or consistency gives a strong echo. Thus in assessing the ultrasound image of the thigh one can identify the skin, the outer sheath over the quadriceps and a strong echo from the underlying bone (Figure 1-13a). One can get an idea of the bulk of the muscle by measuring the depth of the subcutaneous tissue from skin to muscle sheath and of the muscle from sheath to bone. The muscle usually comprises about 60% or more of the distance from skin to bone. The muscle itself is relatively free of echo, although there may be some echogenic

streaks within the muscle due to fascial or tendinous intersections.

In various pathological conditions there will be an increase in echo from the muscle (Figure 1-13b-d). Thus in Duchenne dystrophy changes can already be detected at an early stage of the disease. In congenital muscular dystrophy there is often a particularly bright echo with loss of the bone echo. The muscle bulk in the dystrophies is retained despite the extensive changes within the muscle.

In the spinal muscular atrophies there is also an increase in the echo from the muscle, but the bulk of the muscle is strikingly reduced and the depth of the muscle may be less than 50% of the distance from skin to bone, with corresponding increase in the depth of the subcutaneous tissue.

Ultrasound imaging is also helpful in picking out selective involvement of some muscles compared with others and may help in deciding which muscle to biopsy (Figure 1-14).

As in the case of other investigations of muscle, a normal echogenicity does not exclude the possibility of an underlying muscle disorder. Thus a normal pattern may be found in some of the metabolic myopathies without structural changes in the muscle, such as the glycogenoses and mitochondrial myopathies, or in severe infantile spinal muscular atrophy. Some congenital myopathies, such as central core disease, may show a striking increase in echogenicity.

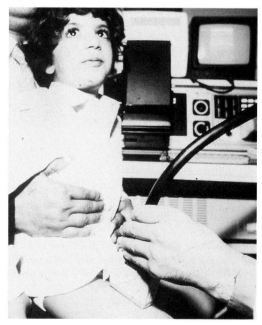

Figure 1-12 Ultrasound imaging has proved a useful screening technique for detection of muscle pathology. It can be used as a routine procedure in the outpatient clinic, is non-invasive, several different muscles can rapidly be assessed, and it is readily acceptable to children.

Transverse ultrasound scans of the thigh

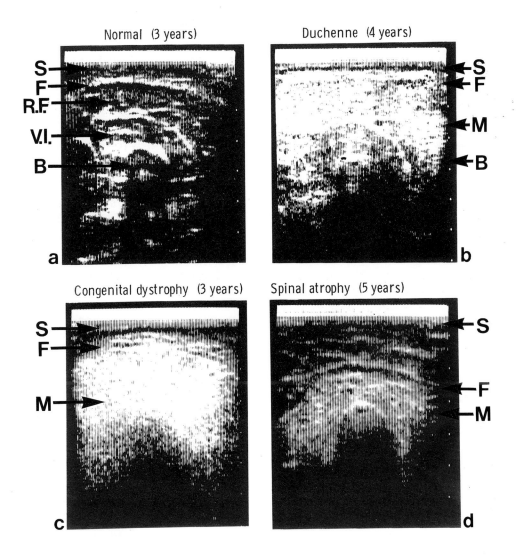

Figure 1-13a–d Ultrasound imaging of normal and diseased muscle. Normal muscle (a), being a fairly homogeneous tissue, is relatively echo-free. Bright echoes are produced by the skin (S), the fascial planes (F) around and between muscle bellies, tendinous intersections within muscle and by the underlying bone (B).

In the muscular dystrophies there is a diffuse increase in echo throughout the muscle which correlates with the degree of pathological change and particularly the proliferation of fat or connective tissue (b, Duchenne muscular dystrophy 4 years). It is particularly striking in congenital muscular dystrophy where there is often marked adipose replacement and the bone echo may be lost (c, congenital muscular dystrophy 3 years). The thickness of the muscle is retained in the dystrophies.

In spinal muscular atrophies there is increased echogenicity in the muscle and, in addition, marked atrophy of the muscle with reduction in the muscle depth to 50% or less of the skin to bone distance (d, mild spinal muscular atrophy 5 years).

(RF = rectus femoris; VI = vastus intermedius; M = muscle.)

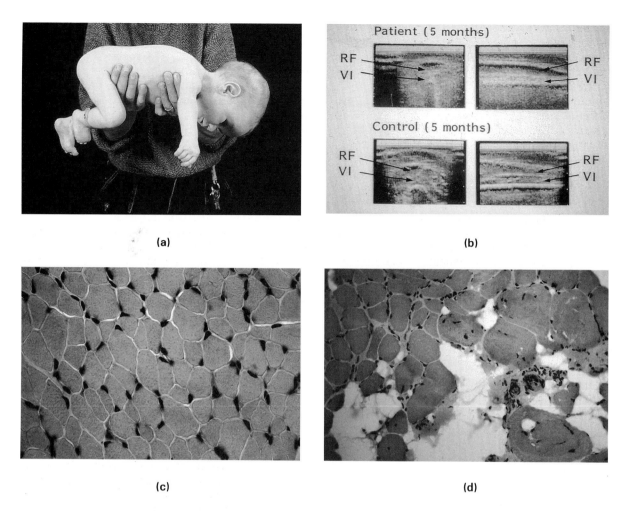

Figure 1-14a–d Congenital muscular dystrophy (differential involvement). This 5-month-old floppy infant presented with delay in motor milestones (a). Ultrasonography of the quadriceps showed a striking differential involvement with sparing of rectus femoris and involvement of vasti (b). Selective needle biopsy of both components through the same incision confirmed this with an essentially normal picture in the rectus (c) and a striking dystrophic picture in the vastus lateralis (d). The pathology would have been completely missed by a standard open biopsy of the rectus.

In dermatomyositis the muscle may show normal echogenicity when the probe is held in the usual vertical position, but may show increased echo when the probe is angulated obliquely in the long axis of the muscle, presumably reflecting the perifascicular atrophy.

COMPUTERIZED TOMOGRAPHY

A number of studies in the early 1980s established the value of computerized tomography (CT) imaging in the detection of pathological change in muscle (Bulcke and Baert, 1982; Bulcke and Herpels, 1983; Jiddane *et al.*, 1983; Hawley *et al.*, 1984; Calo *et al.*, 1986; Fischer *et al.*, 1988). The technique allows the possibility of assessing changes in either muscle size

or density within about 150 muscles using five standard 'cuts' of the body taken at the level of shoulder, lumbar spine, hip, thigh and calf (Bulcke and Baert, 1982) (Figures 1-15 to 1-17). Density changes observed on CT scans are particularly helpful in assessing progression and may be useful in clinical trials. In individuals with focal, unusual, or asymptomatic myopathy, muscle-CT allows a better recognition of the extent and distribution of muscle involvement. Also CT localizes lesions in deeply seated muscles, and may be helpful in selecting the site for a muscle biopsy.

MAGNETIC RESONANCE IMAGING

Magnetic resonance imaging (MRI) may be valuable

as a supplementary tool for assessing the distribution and severity of muscle pathology and also for following the course of a disease or the response to treatment (Murphy *et al.*, 1986; Kaiser *et al.*, 1986; Schreiber *et al.*, 1987; Shabas *et al.*, 1987; Lamminen, 1990; Wallgren-Pettersson *et al.*, 1990; Udd *et al.*, 1991; Åhlberg *et al.*, 1994). Experience with this technique is not as extensive as with CT scanning, and the facility is not as readily available at all centres.

Both CT scanning and MRI are specialized and expensive techniques and should be looked upon as supplementary to the basic investigation of the neuromuscular patient, in contrast to ultrasound imaging which is a useful and practical tool for the routine screening, by a clinician or specialized ultrasonographer, of all muscle patients in an outpatient clinic environment.

ELECTROPHYSIOLOGICAL INVESTIGATIONS

Nerve conduction velocity

Measurement of motor nerve conduction velocity is a relatively simple technique which can be performed with surface electrodes and little objection from the patient. We have found small strips of lead foil very practical and reliable as electrodes (Figures 1-18 and 1-19). The commercially available stimulating pads are also effective. This investigation frequently gives useful information on the state of normality or otherwise of the lower motor neurone.

The conduction velocity is dependent on the diameter and the degree of myelination of the neurone. In the newborn infant the velocity is only about half the adult level and does not reach the adult level until about 3–5 years of age, or later, varying with different nerves. This has to be taken into account when assessing infants (Moosa and Dubowitz, 1971a).

In diseases affecting the peripheral nerve the pathology may be primarily in the axon itself ('axonal' or 'neuronal' neuropathy) or in the supporting Schwann cells, giving a segmental demyelination (demyelinating neuropathy). In the demyelinating neuropathies the motor nerve conduction velocity is markedly slowed to half the normal rate or less. In the axonal neuropathies the conduction velocity may be normal or only slightly depressed.

Demyelinating neuropathies may occur in isolation or in association with central nervous system disorders. Among the isolated peripheral neuropathies are the so-called hereditary motor and sensory neuropathies (HMSN) (Charcot–Marie–Tooth disease), a genetically heterogeneous group (see Chapter 9). It is always important in these cases to estimate the nerve conduction velocities of the

parents and siblings as well, since subclinical cases commonly occur. Demyelinating neuropathy may also be found in post-infective polyneuritis (Guillain–Barré syndrome).

Demyelinating neuropathies in association with central nervous system involvement include the leucodystrophies such as metachromatic leucodystrophy and Krabbe's disease; a slow motor nerve conduction velocity in a case presenting with hypotonia and motor retardation is a useful diagnostic sign. A similar demyelinating neuropathy has been demonstrated in Cockayne's syndrome (Moosa and Dubowitz, 1970) and in some cases of Leigh's syndrome (Dunn and Dolman, 1969).

A slow nerve conduction velocity has also been found in congenital hypothyroidism (Moosa and Dubowitz, 1971b), presumably reflecting the generalized delay in myelination. The conduction velocity increases to normal after treatment.

Slow motor nerve conduction in infantile spinal muscular atrophy seems to correlate directly with the clinical severity of the condition and suggests a selective loss of faster neurones in the more severe forms (Moosa and Dubowitz, 1976).

Sensory conduction velocity is also a useful diagnostic tool, particularly in relation to the mixed neuropathies such as HMSN and Friedreich's ataxia. The technique is more difficult and requires more sophisticated equipment but can be used with infants and children.

Nerve conduction velocity studies can also be of value in the study of latent peripheral neuropathies in conditions such as diabetes.

In myasthenia gravis the fatiguability of the muscle can be demonstrated by the fall-off in the size of the muscle action potential following repetitive stimulation of the nerve (Figure 1-20).

Electromyography

This is a valuable tool in deciding whether a particular muscle is normal or abnormal and whether the abnormality is of a 'myopathic' or 'neuropathic' form.

The amount of information one receives is directly proportional to the amount of co-operation one can obtain from the child, and a few minutes spent patiently playing with the child initially and gaining his confidence will pay dividends. The small child is often best assessed on his mother's lap, and once the child has reached an age of understanding he will usually be fascinated by the 'television' display on the oscilloscope (Figure 1-21).

The muscle selected for study should be appropriate to the distribution of weakness. For most proximal muscle syndromes the deltoid or quadriceps is most convenient.

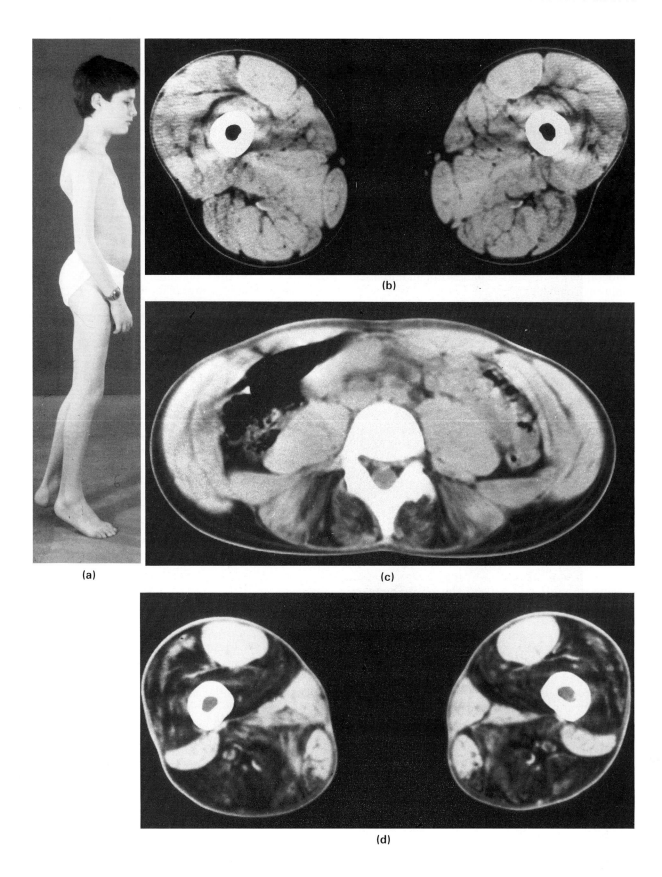

(a)

(b)

(c)

(d)

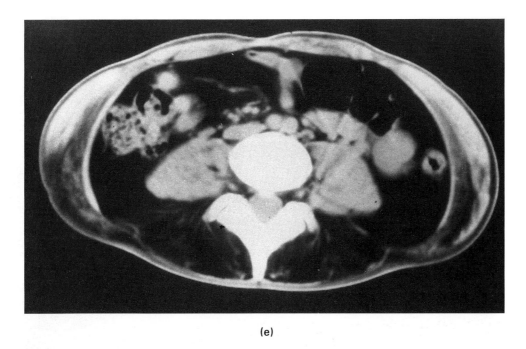

(e)

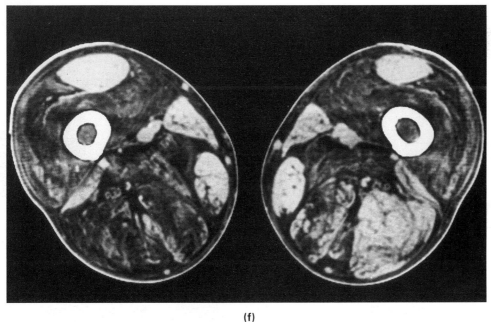

(f)

Figure 1-15a-f Muscle CT is very helpful in defining the pattern of muscle involvement in unusual neuromuscular disorders, as in this family with possible autosomal dominant Emery–Dreifuss muscular dystrophy. This index case (a) presented with toe walking, mild humeroperoneal wasting and weakness, flexion of the elbows and rigid spine. Muscle CT (b) taken when he was 15 shows a diffuse decrease in density in the muscle of the thigh apart from the rectus which is well preserved, while lumbar scan (c) shows a clear involvement of paravertebral muscles. His mother, aged 34, has a diffuse muscle wasting and weakness with humeroperoneal muscles more involved, flexion of the elbows and marked rigidity of the spine and frequent supraventricular ectopic tachycardia. CT shows a complete low density fat and connective tissue substitution of the thigh muscles with preservation of rectus femoris, sartorius, gracilis and caput brevis of biceps femoris (d) and of the paravertebral muscles at the lumbar level (e). Her father, aged 64, who had a milder muscle wasting weakness and had a pacemaker inserted at the age of 57, showed a similar CT pattern of thigh muscle involvement (f) but less involvement in the lumbar level. (Courtesy Professor L. Merlini.)

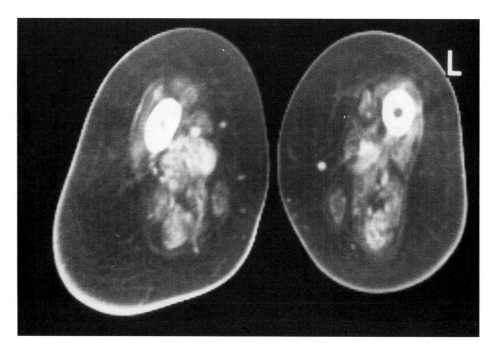

(a)

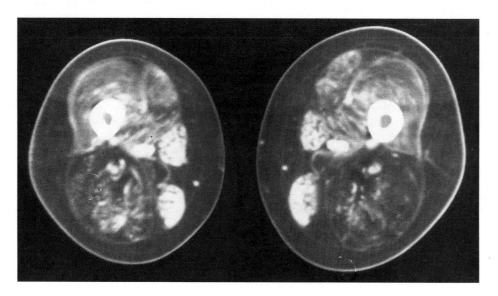

(b)

Figure 1-16a,b Muscle CT may help to differentiate spinal muscle atrophy from muscular dystrophy. (a): Muscle CT in a 15-year-old boy with mild SMA shows marked muscle atrophy with diffusely spread low-density changes in all muscles. (b): In this 17-year-old boy with Becker muscular dystrophy there is preservation of muscle bulk with differential involvement of muscles, relative sparing of gracilis and sartorius, severe replacement of muscle by fat or connective tissue in the hamstrings and diffuse involvement of quadriceps. (Courtesy Professor L. Merlini.)

The responses one is looking for are the irritability of the muscle on insertion of the needle, the state of the muscle at complete rest and the pattern of the potentials with slight, moderate and maximal activity of the muscle.

A normal muscle at rest shows electrical silence, but with activity motor unit potentials are generated. Each potential is produced by groups of fibres responding to a single motor neurone. The motor unit potential is usually triphasic with an amplitude of 1–5mV and a duration of 1–5 ms. As the muscle increases its activity the individual action potentials become summated and confluent, to give the so-called interference pattern, and the baseline disappears (Figure 1-22).

By looking for deviations from this basic normal pattern one may be able to localize a lesion to the anterior horn cell, peripheral nerve or the muscle itself.

Denervation. Spontaneous fibrillation potentials occur at rest. These are 'sharp' biphasic, short duration, low amplitude potentials of about 100μV (Figure 1-23). They may be picked up acoustically on the amplifying system of the recorder as isolated single short sounds. They are probably produced by isolated single and small groups of denervated muscle fibres.

Fasciculation potentials are high amplitude polyphasic (more than three phases) potentials of long duration occurring at rest and produced mainly by lesions of the anterior horn cell, such as spinal muscular atrophy and motor neurone disease (Figure 1-24).

In denervation there is a reduced interference pattern on full activity so that part of the baseline of the electromyograph (EMG) becomes visible. Individual motor unit potentials are either normal or of large amplitude, long duration and polyphasic. These are characteristically seen in spinal muscular atrophies but also in some of the polyneuropathies (Figure 1-24). They indicate collateral reinnervation by surviving neurones and thus increase the territory of the motor neurone. In severe infantile spinal muscular atrophy the motor unit potentials are usually normal but fibrillation potentials are present at rest (Figure 1-23).

Myopathies. In various myopathies, both hereditary and acquired, there is random loss of muscle fibres resulting in a characteristic EMG pattern of low amplitude, polyphasic, potentials of short duration (Figure 1-25). This produces a characteristic 'crackling' sound on the acoustic amplification and is as readily picked up 'by ear' as on the oscilloscope display.

There is no clearcut correlation between the pattern of the EMG and the severity of the myopathy or dystrophy.

Occasional fibrillation potentials are seen in longstanding muscular dystrophies. If they occur with any frequency in association with the myopathic EMG the possibility of dermatomyositis should be considered.

Myotonia. The classical myotonic pattern on EMG is a very striking one. It consists of spontaneous bursts of potentials in rapid succession (up to 100 per second or more) with waxing and gradual waning (Figure 1-26). The acoustic pattern is equally striking and resembles the sound of a divebomber (pre-jet era) or of a motorbike taking off at speed and fading into the distance.

The myotonic bursts may be provoked by tapping the muscle adjacent to the needle or by moving the needle. In infants with congenital myotonic dystrophy the myotonia is not present in the early hypotonic phase but comes on later (after about two years). In the affected mother with mild features of myotonic dystrophy the myotonia may not be apparent in the proximal muscles one usually tests and should also be looked for in a distal muscle such as the first dorsal interosseous of the hand.

'Pseudomyotonia' is the term that has been applied to bursts of activity seen in other neuromuscular disorders without clinical myotonia, such as type II glycogenosis. The repetitive potentials do not show the characteristic waning of true myotonia. In continuous muscle fibre activity there is no myotonia but continuous normal potentials.

MUSCLE BIOPSY

A muscle biopsy is essential for establishing a definitive diagnosis in any patient with a suspected neuromuscular disorder. This basically means any child with muscle weakness, or with any other symptoms suggesting an underlying neuromuscular disorder, such as cramps or fatigue on exercise.

It may be argued that in some instances where the diagnosis is obvious and apparently unequivocal muscle biopsy may be unnecessary, but even in the case of an apparently typical infantile spinal muscular atrophy (Werdnig–Hoffmann) a very similar clinical picture may be produced by a type II glycogenosis, a myotubular myopathy or a congenital fibre type disproportion, with a correspondingly different prognostic outlook. Similarly, a clinical picture like a Duchenne dystrophy may be presented by the more benign Becker type or by one of the congenital myopathies. In addition, recent advances at the molecular level have helped to more accurately define the changes in the muscle.

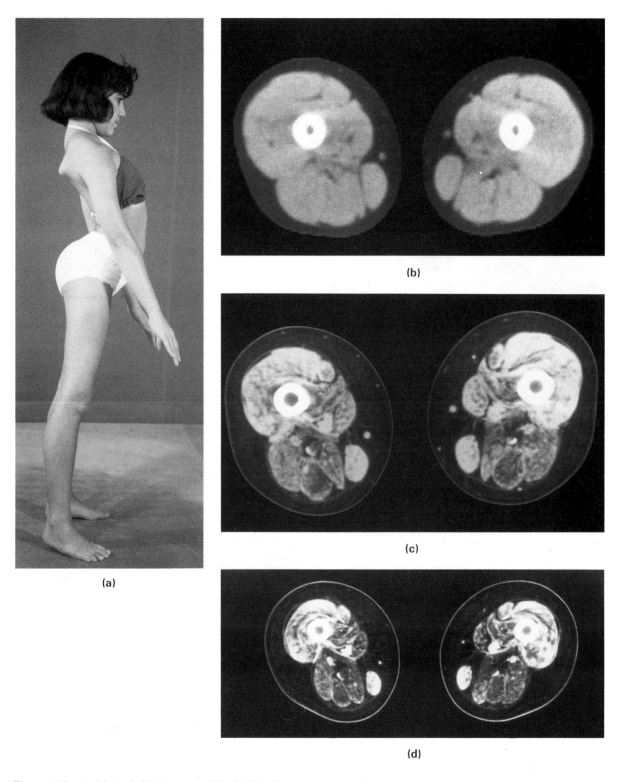

(a)

(b)

(c)

(d)

Figure 1-17a-d   Limb girdle dystrophy (SCARMD). The progression of the disease with time is very well illustrated in this girl, with childhood onset of limb girdle muscle wasting and weakness, marked elevation of CK (more than 50 times normal), followed between the age of 8 and 14 years; (a) shows the girl at the age of 14 with marked lordosis and winging of the scapula (lateral view); (b), (c) and (d) are CT scans of the thighs at 8, 12 and 14 years showing the progressive loss of muscle tissue and replacement by low density fat and connective tissue.

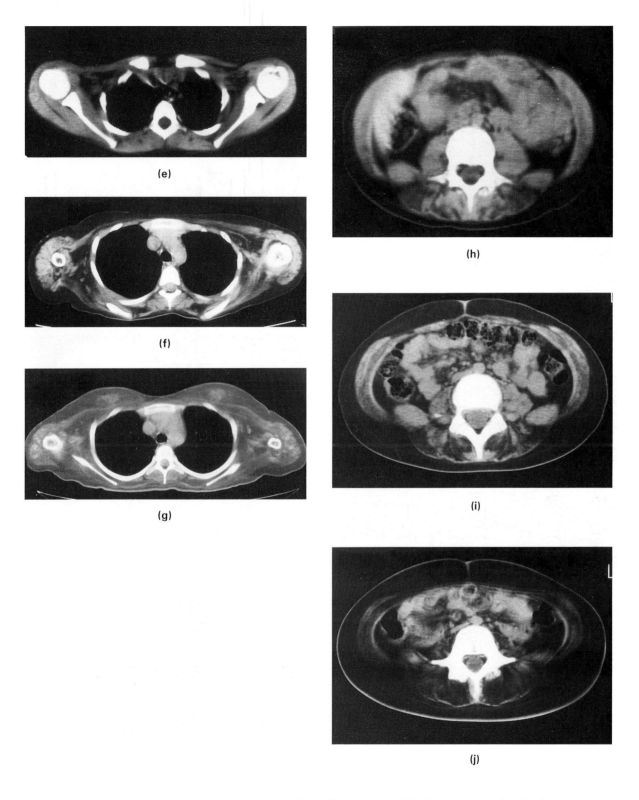

Figure 1-17e-j   (e), (f) and (g) are CT scans of the shoulder girdle at the age of 8, 12 and 14 years showing the progressive wasting of muscle. (h), (i) and (j) are CT scans of the lumbar level at the age of 8, 12 and 14 years showing the progressive replacement of paravertebral and abdominal muscles by low density connective tissue and fat. (Courtesy of Professor L. Merlini.)

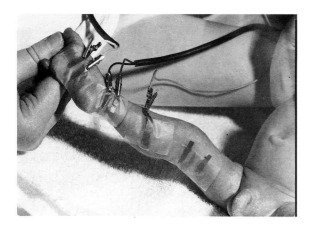

Figure 1-18 Measurement of motor nerve conduction velocity in a small infant, using surface electrodes. The two recording electrodes are on the sole of the foot and the stimulating electrodes along the course of the posterior tibial nerve at the ankle and behind the knee. The single central electrode (mid-calf) is an earth.

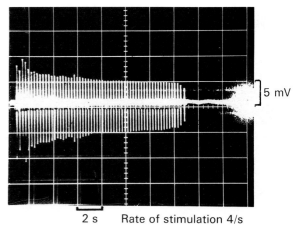

2 s   Rate of stimulation 4/s

Figure 1-20 Myasthenia gravis. Shows waning of size of motor potential on repetitive stimulation of the nerve.

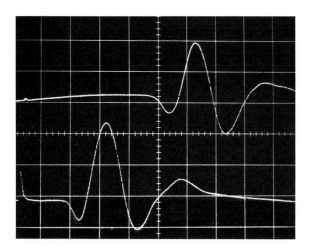

Figure 1-19 The motor potentials produced by stimulation of the nerve. Note the difference in latency in upper and lower traces due to stimulation at two different sites along the course of the nerve.

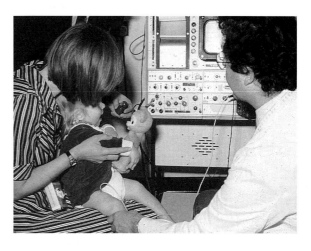

Figure 1-21 Clinical picture of EMG.

Figure 1-22 Concentric needle electromyogram of deltoid in a normal child. Upper trace shows normal 'interference pattern' due to summation of motor unit potentials on voluntary contraction. The baseline is obliterated. The potentials are about 1–2 mV in amplitude. Lower trace shows a normal single triphasic motor unit potential. (Note faster time scale.)

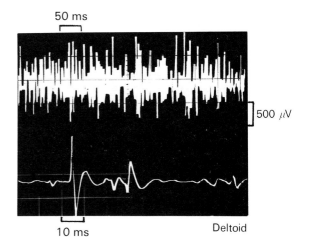

50 ms

500 μV

10 ms   Deltoid

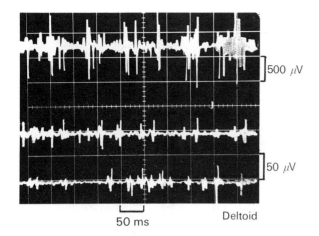

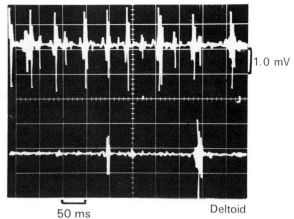

Figure 1-23 EMG of deltoid in infant with severe spinal muscular atrophy (Werdnig–Hoffmann disease). Note fairly normal sized potentials in upper trace, but reduced interference pattern and baseline visible between potentials. Lower trace shows spontaneous biphasic small (about 50–100 μV) potentials at rest (fibrillation potentials) indicative of denervation.

Figure 1-24 EMG of deltoid in child with intermediate severity spinal muscle atrophy. Upper trace shows reduced interference pattern and large amplitude (3mV or more) polyphasic potentials (note that scale is twice that of Figure 1-22). Lower trace shows spontaneous large amplitude polyphasic potentials at rest (fasciculation potential) characteristic of chronic anterior horn cell degeneration.

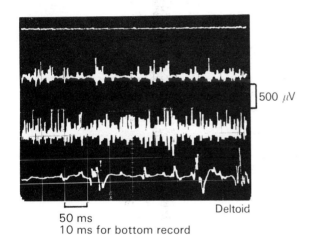

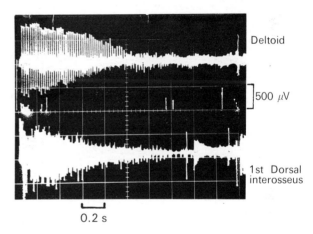

Figure 1-26 EMG of 4-year-old child with congenital myotonic dystrophy (upper trace) and his mother (lower trace). Note the characteristic burst of spontaneous repetitive motor unit potentials with gradual waning.

Figure 1-25 EMG of deltoid in boy with Duchenne dystrophy. Upper trace shows electrical silence and no spontaneous activity at rest (as in normal muscle). Second and third traces at moderate and full muscle contraction show typical myopathic pattern with full interference pattern and low amplitude, short duration, polyphasic potentials. Lower trace (at higher speed) shows individual polyphasic potentials.

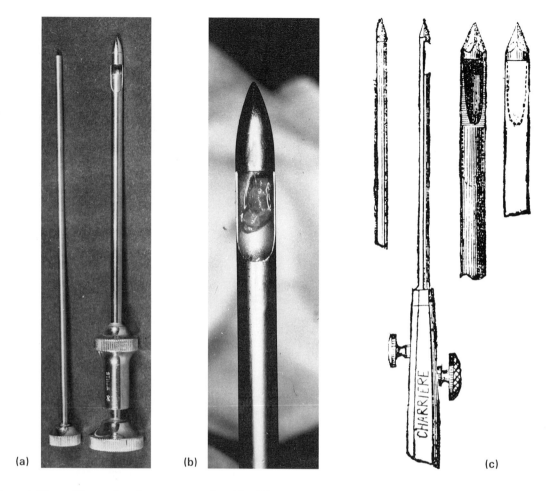

(a)   (b)   (c)

Figure 1-27a-c The modern Bergstrom needle with sliding trochar with cutting blade, which moves in a cannula (a,b) is very similar to Duchenne's original 'emporte pièce histologique', the first biopsy needle ever (c). (b) shows the muscle sample within the cannula.

In floppy infants where the serum enzymes, nerve conduction and EMG are normal and the hypotonia is the predominant feature rather than muscle weakness, the diagnosis should be sought in systems other than the neuromuscular, and muscle biopsy can accordingly be deferred.

The procedure itself is a relatively simple one, yet it is frequently poorly done. The pathologist who receives from the surgeon a small fragment of an unnamed muscle coiled into a disoriented ball in a pot of formalin is unlikely to produce any meaningful information. Certain guidelines are thus worth following when planning a biopsy.

Selection of the muscle should be based on the distribution of muscle weakness, as assessed clinically. The muscle should not be so severely affected that it is largely replaced by connective tissue or fat with little residual evidence of the underlying muscle disorder, or so little affected that it does not reflect the changes. In most proximal disorders of muscle weakness the quadriceps or the biceps provides a readily accessible muscle which also has the advantage of longitudinally running fibres, allowing easy orientation of the specimen. One should avoid undertaking a biopsy in an area that has been subjected to needling for EMG as this may produce local cellular changes.

TECHNIQUE OF BIOPSY

There are two ways of obtaining a muscle sample: needle biopsy or the more traditional open biopsy. Either procedure should be performed under local anaesthesia; it is unnecessary, and indeed contraindicated, to subject a patient with neuromuscular disorder, and possible compromised respiratory function, to a general anaesthetic. In addition to the well-recognized risk of general anaesthetic in malignant hyperthermia, and the increased sensitivity to muscle relaxants as well as anaesthetics and analgesics in myotonic dystrophy, there have also been several reports of reactions to anaesthesia in cases of Duchenne dystrophy and recently also in Becker dystrophy (Bush and Dubowitz, 1991) (see Chapter 6).

In children between 6 months and 10 years we usually give a sedative such as oral chloral hydrate (80 mg/kg). In infants under 6 months and in older children and adolescents who are able to cooperate we have generally found the sedation to be unnecessary.

Needle biopsy

More than a century after Duchenne devised his famous muscle biopsy needle, the forerunner of all biopsy needles (Duchenne, 1861), there has in recent years been renewed enthusiasm for its use. Bergstrom (1962) introduced a percutaneous needle, with features somewhat similar to those of Duchenne's (Figure 1-27), mainly for the study of normal muscle in relation to various physiological changes. Edwards *et al.* (1973) applied the Bergstrom needle for routine muscle biopsy, mainly in adult patients, and subsequently reviewed their experience over a 10-year period in some 1000 cases (Edwards *et al.*, 1983). We followed a similar approach in our paediatric practice, and over the past 15 years have exclusively done needle biopsies, using the Bergstrom needle. We documented our early experience in 670 mainly childhood cases (Heckmatt *et al.*, 1984). Although the needle biopsy technique is being widely used in many European centres, there has been a remarkable reluctance to adopt it in most American units, although there has been some change of heart in a few centres in recent years.

The major advantages of the needle biopsy procedure over open biopsy are its simplicity, its speed and the fact that it can readily be done by physicians as an outpatient procedure in a clinic without any special theatre facilities. From the patient's point of view it is relatively atraumatic and leaves a practically invisible scar. It also has the distinct advantage of being a practical procedure in the newborn infant, even while severely ill and on a ventilator, with practically no disturbance to the infant.

The procedure. Most of our biopsies have been from the quadriceps (vastus lateralis) (see Figures 1-28 to 1-36) The skin is prepared in the usual way with antiseptic and draped. The skin and the subcutaneous tissues down to the muscle sheath are infiltrated with 1% lignocaine. A small stab incision is made with a pointed scalpel blade down into the muscle sheath, at approximately mid-thigh level in the midline. Pressure is applied with a swab until any bleeding has completely stopped. The needle with

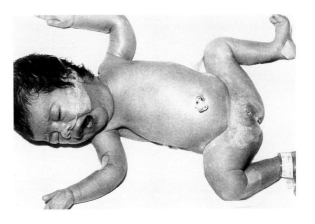

Figure 1-28 Needle muscle biopsy in a 1-week-old floppy infant with congenital muscular dystrophy (plus a fracture at birth of the right femur).

the sliding cannula assembled is then inserted into the muscle while the other hand steadies the thigh and squeezes the muscle towards the window of the needle to ensure a reasonably sized sample. After a few quick to-and-fro movements of the cannula with the palm of the hand the needle is withdrawn and the muscle sample removed. The needle can be reinserted and multiple samples obtained through the same incision.

If selective involvement of muscles has been noted on ultrasound scanning, samples can be obtained from contiguous muscles such as rectus femoris and vastus lateralis through the same incision.

After completion of the biopsy, firm finger pressure is applied to the site for a few minutes. This prevents any haematoma formation and associated complications. A butterfly dressing is then applied to approximate the skin edges. No sutures are necessary.

After removal, the biopsy specimens should be kept moist on a piece of gauze lightly moistened with isotonic saline prior to further processing. Multiple samples can be mounted collectively on a slice of cork and oriented in a transverse plane under a dissecting microscope. In this way about 1000 fibres per single section can be obtained for detailed assessment.

A separate sample of muscle can be fixed for electron microscopy and, where indicated, additional samples can be taken for biochemical analysis. It is worth fixing a specimen from every biopsy for possible electron microscopy but, because of the time involved in processing, one has to be selective in the choice of samples for examination in the electron microscope, depending on the results of the light microscopic observations.

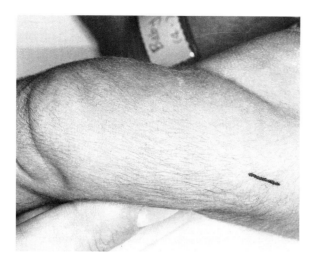

Figure 1-29   The site for biopsy over the middle of the left thigh is marked.

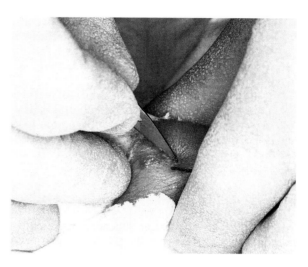

Figure 1-31   A small incision is made in the skin with a pointed scalpel blade.

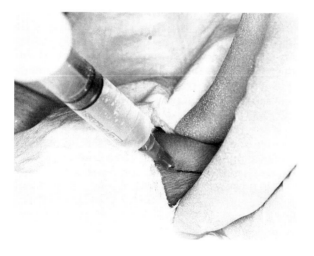

Figure 1-30   After appropriate cleansing and draping, the site is infiltrated with local anaesthetic.

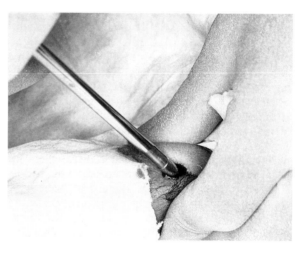

Figure 1-32   The biopsy needle (with cannula in) is inserted.

The same technique can also be used for other muscles such as gastrocnemius, deltoid and biceps, but particular care is necessary to keep clear of any vital structures such as major vessels or nerves.

An alternative type of needle is the conchotome or alligator forceps (Henriksson, 1979). It needs a slightly larger incision and obtains a somewhat larger sample. Disposable needles of the type used for renal or liver biopsy are not satisfactory for muscle biopsy. A spring-load, automatic release, version of the Bergstrom needle has also been designed. A suction system attached to the Bergstrom needle has been used to obtain larger samples but we have found it somewhat cumbersome in practice and it has not found general appeal.

Preparation of the specimen. In order to obtain satisfactory results, care needs to be taken with the

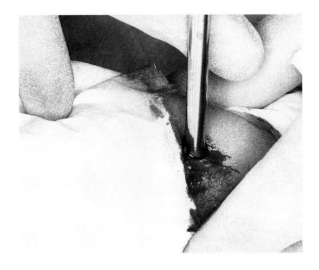

Figure 1-33 The needle is advanced into the muscle.

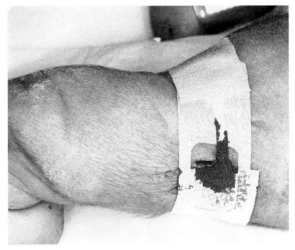

Figure 1-35 After withdrawal of the needle, and firm pressure on the site for 5 minutes, the wound edges are approximated with a butterfly dressing. No sutures are needed.

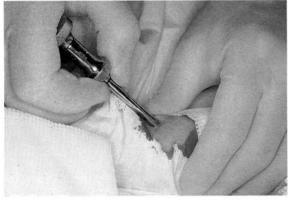

Figure 1-34 The cutting cannula is moved in and out a few times by the palm of the operator's hand, while the left hand holds the thigh steady and squeezes the muscle towards the needle.

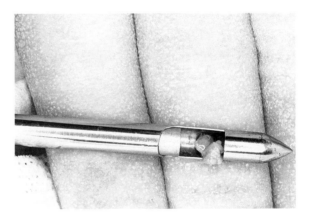

Figure 1-36 The biopsy sample is removed from the needle.

preparation of the specimen. Transverse sections yield much more information than longitudinal and it is an advantage to prepare multiple samples from the same area since muscle pathology can at times be focal.

After orientation of the specimen in the appropriate transverse plane, using a dissecting microscope, it can be held in position by gently pipetting Tissue-Tek® around the base. It is then rapidly frozen in Arcton 12 cooled in liquid nitrogen (Figures 1-37 to 1-40). This rapid freezing preserves the architecture as well as the enzymes. The specimen is then ready for cutting of frozen sections in a cold microtome (cryostat) and can be stored at −70°C until required. All the histological, histochemical and immunocytochemical studies can be done on frozen sections. For further details on methodology see Dubowitz (1985).

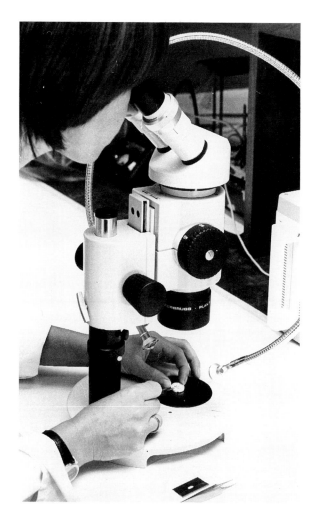

Figure 1-37 The sample(s) is placed on a slice of cork and oriented into a transverse plane under a dissecting microscope, using a cold fibreoptic light source to prevent drying.

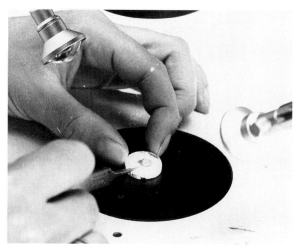

Figure 1-38 Close-up view of two samples being oriented alongside each other.

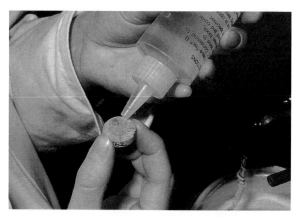

Figure 1-39 The specimens are kept in position by Tissue-Tek® pipetted gently around the base.

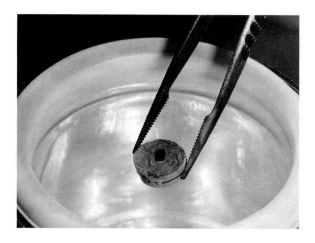

Figure 1-40 The specimen is rapidly frozen by submersion in Arcton 12 cooled in liquid nitrogen (−160°C).

Histology/histochemistry

Several histological and histochemical stains are done routinely on every biopsy and usually provide adequate diagnostic information (Dubowitz, 1985). In selected cases, for example where a specific enzyme deficiency may be present, further preparations can be made. The stains found most useful for routine screening are haematoxylin and eosin (H & E), Verhoeff–van Gieson, Gomori trichrome, PAS for glycogen, and Oil red O for lipid. The histochemical reactions include NADH-tetrazolium re-

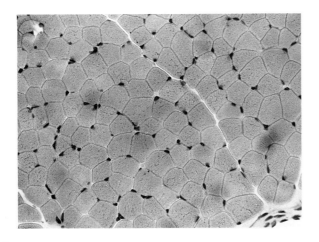

Figure 1-41 Transverse section of normal muscle from 2-year-old boy showing polygonal shaped fibres, closely approximated to each other, with peripherally placed nuclei (under sarcolemma) and only slight variation in fibre size. (H & E × 200.)

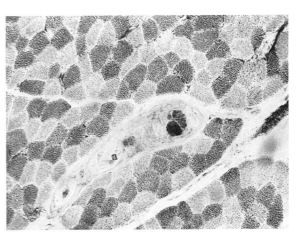

Figure 1-42 Same muscle as in Figure 1-41, showing checkerboard of different fibre types. Note muscle spindle with intrafusal fibres in centre of picture. Oxidative enzyme reaction. (NADH-TR × 200.)

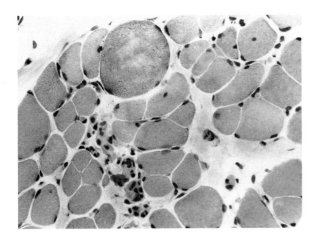

Figure 1-43 Dystrophic picture (Duchenne dystrophy) showing diffuse abnormality throughout section, with variation in fibre size, internal nuclei, degenerating fibres undergoing phagocytosis (lower left), splitting of fibres and separation of fibres from each other by proliferating connective tissue (lighter areas). (H & E × 200.)

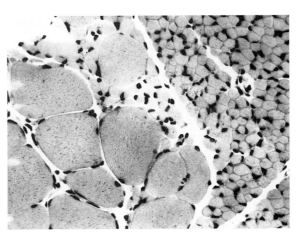

Figure 1-44 Denervation pattern (spinal muscular atrophy) showing group atrophy with a large group of uniformly atrophic fibres on right of picture and normal looking or enlarged fibres (which are probably reinnervated fibres) to the left (H & E × 200.)

ductase (NADH-TR), cytochrome oxidase, succinate dehydrogenase (oxidative activity), adenosine triphosphatase (ATPase) with preincubation at pH 9.4, 4.6 and 4.3, and acid phosphatase. Other enzyme reactions such as cytochrome oxidase or phosphorylase can be done selectively in cases where deficiency is suspected, such as fatigue or cramps on exercise or a floppy infant.

This approach provides information not only on the general histological pattern of the muscle and whether there is pathological change or not, but also information on the individual fibre types as defined histochemically by the ATPase reaction, and their distribution and selective involvement (Figures 1-41 to 1-45). The oxidative enzyme reaction shows up structural abnormalities such as central cores,

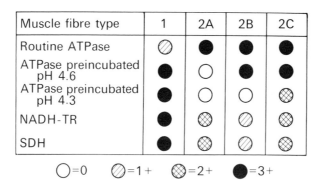

Muscle fibre type	1	2A	2B	2C
Routine ATPase	◨	●	●	●
ATPase preincubated pH 4.6	●	○	●	●
ATPase preincubated pH 4.3	●	○	○	⊗
NADH-TR	●	⊗	◨	⊗
SDH	●	⊗	◨	⊗

○ = 0   ◨ = 1+   ⊗ = 2+   ● = 3+

Figure 1-45 Fibre types in human muscle based on the ATPase reaction, and the corresponding activities of other enzymes in these individual fibre types. (From Dubowitz and Brooke, 1973.)

disruption of the intermyofibrillar network pattern ('moth-eaten fibres') and mitochochondrial abnormalities. The glycogen and lipid stains will show up excess of either of these, and the acid phosphatase and RNA stain help to pinpoint focal degenerative or regenerative fibres.

Immunocytochemistry

Major advances in recent years in the preparation of monoclonal or polyclonal antibodies to specific proteins, and the application of these antibodies to the study of tissue sections by fluorescence and other labelling techniques, have considerably widened the horizons of the muscle biopsy. For example, the development of antibodies to the different forms of myosin – fetal, neonatal, slow and fast – has provided a powerful tool for studying the process of maturation in muscle, both in relation to the development of normal and diseased muscle and in the context of special situations, such as the process of regeneration in normal and diseased muscle. It also provides an alternative means of fibre typing based on the presence of slow and/or fast myosins in the individual fibres. (For a review see Sewry and Dubowitz, 1994).

These new techniques have also made possible the localization at tissue level of dystrophin, the protein gene product involved in Duchenne/Becker muscular dystrophy, and proved a research as well as a clinical diagnostic tool (see Chapter 2). The same has now happened with the second wave of dystrophin-associated glycoproteins (see Chapter 2) and no doubt other diseases will in time follow suit once their molecular genetic basis is unravelled, and muscle immunocytochemistry will become an everyday routine for muscle biopsies, much as enzyme histochemistry did in the 1970s (Dubowitz and Brooke, 1973).

APPENDIX:
QUESTIONNAIRE FOR CASES OF MUSCLE DISORDER

A. Pregnancy

1. Was there anything unusual about the pregnancy?
2. Did you have any illness during pregnancy?
3. Were the movements normal, more than normal, less than normal?
4. Was an X-ray taken?
5. Did you take any drugs during pregnancy?
6. Was there excessive or a reduced amount of liquor, or premature rupture of the membranes?

B. Labour

1. Was the labour normal, prolonged, very short?
2. Were instruments used? Or Caesarean section?
3. Were there any complications?
4. Was the child normal at birth?
5. Did he cry normally?
6. Did he need oxygen?
7. What was the birthweight?
8. Was he breast fed? How long?
9. Did he suck normally?
10. Was he an active child?
11. Was there anything unusual about his appearance?

C. Milestones

At what age did he:
1. Maintain a sitting posture on the floor?
2. Stand on his own without holding on?
3. Crawl?
4. Walk without support?
5. Say sentences (two to three words) with meaning?

D. Illness

What was the first abnormality you observed? Describe in detail. Give age.
1. Was there anything unusual about his mode of walking?
2. Did he walk on his toes? At what age?
3. Was he able to run normally? Climb up stairs normally?
4. Did he tend to fall? From what age?
5. Was he able to get up after falling?
6. Did he do this in a normal manner?
7. Did you note enlargement or wasting of any muscles? Specify which muscles. At what age?
8. Did he complain of pain in his muscles?
9. Did he tire readily?
10. Has the weakness got worse?
11. If not walking, at what age did he go off his feet? Did any illness or episode cause this?

12. Did you observe any weakness of his
    - arms?　　At age of:
    - face?　　At age of:
    - neck?　　At age of:
    - back?　　At age of:
13. Have you noted any abnormality of his tongue?
14. Has there been any difficulty with chewing or swallowing?
15. Has he gained or lost weight? From age of
16. Has he ever had a squint or double vision?
17. Has he ever had a persistent skin rash?
18. Has his mental development been normal?
19. At what age was the diagnosis first made? By whom?
20. What type of school does he attend?
21. Have you noted a tremor of his hands?
22. Was there any twitching of any muscle?
23. How is his general health?
24. Is he prone to chest infections?

E. Past illnesses

1. Give age of previous illnesses (including childhood illnesses)
   operations
   fractures of bones
2. Did any of these affect his muscular weakness?

F. Family history

1. Give ages of his parents, brothers and sisters
2. Were there any stillbirths or miscarriages?
3. Has any other member of the family on either side had a similar illness? Describe in detail
4. If father and mother married previously, give details of children
5. Do any relatives have mental illness, epilepsy, nervous disease, diabetes, or other illness of note?
6. Are the parents related? Give details.
7. Have there been any marriages between cousins, or near relatives in the family at any time?
8. Tabulate brothers and sisters of his mother and father from eldest to youngest, and give details of children of each, stating sex and age.

Father: Brothers and Sisters

Children (Sex and Age)

Mother: Brothers and Sisters

Children (Sex and Age)

REFERENCES

Åhlberg, G., Jakobsson, F., Fransson, A. *et al.* (1994) Distribution of muscle degeneration in Welander distal myopathy: a magnetic resonance imaging and muscle biopsy study. *Neuromuscular Disorders* **4**: 55–62.

Bergström, J. (1962) Muscle electrolytes in man determined by neutron activation analysis on needle biopsy specimen: a study in normal subjects, kidney patients, and patients with chronic diarrhoea. *Scandinavian Journal of Clinical and Laboratory Investigation*, **14** (Suppl 68): 1–110.

Bush, A. and Dubowitz, V. (1991) Fatal rhabdomyolysis complicating general anaesthesia in a child with Becker muscular dystrophy. *Neuromuscular Disorders* **1**: 201–204.

Bulcke, J.A.L. and Baert, A.L. (1982) *Clinical and Radiological Aspects of Myopathies.* Berlin: Springer.

Bulcke, J.A.L. and Herpels, V. (1982) Diagnostic value of CT scanning in neuromuscular diseases. *Radiologie* **23**: 523–528.

Calo, M., Crisi, G., Martinelli, C. *et al.* (1986) CT and the diagnosis of myopathies. *Neuroradiology*, **28**: 53–57.

Dubowitz, V. (1985) *Muscle Biopsy: A Practical Approach* 2nd edn. London: Bailliere Tindall.

Dubowitz, V. and Brooke, M.H. (1973) *Muscle Biopsy: A Modern Approach.* London and Philadelphia: W.B. Saunders.

Duchenne, G.-B. (1861) *De l'électrisation localisée et son application à la pathologie et à la thérapeutique.* 2nd edn. Paris: Bailliere et Fils.

Dunn, H.G. and Dolman, C.L. (1969) Necrotizing encephalomyelopathy. Report of a case with relapsing polyneuropathy and hyperalaninemia and with manifestations resembling Friedreich's ataxia. *Neurology*, **19**: 536.

Edwards, R.H.T. and McDonnell, M. (1974) Hand-held dynamometer for evaluating voluntary muscle function. *Lancet* **ii**: 757.

Edwards, R.H.T., Maunder, C., Lewis, P.D. and Pearse, A.G.E. (1973) Percutaneous needle biopsy in the diagnosis of muscle diseases. *Lancet* **ii**: 1070–1071.

Edwards, R.H.T., Round, J.M. and Jones, D.A. (1983) Needle biopsy of skeletal muscle: a review of 10 years' experience. *Muscle and Nerve* **6**: 676–683.

Emery, A.E.H. (1991) Population frequencies of inherited neuromuscular diseases – a world survey. *Neuromuscular Disorders*, **1**: 19–29.

Fischer, A.Q., Carpenter, D.W., Hartlage, P.L. *et al.* (1988) Muscle imaging in neuromuscular disease using computerized real-time sonography. *Muscle and Nerve* **11**: 270–275.

Hawley, R.J., Schellinger, D. and O'Doherty, D.S. (1984) Computed tomographic patterns of muscles in neuromuscular diseases. *Archives of Neurology* **41**: 383–387.

Heckmatt, J.Z. and Dubowitz, V. (1987) Ultrasound imaging and directed needle biopsy in the diagnosis of selective involvement in neuromuscular disease. *Journal of Child Neurology* **2**: 205–213.

Heckmatt, J.Z., Dubowitz, V. and Leeman, S. (1980) Detection of pathological change in dystrophic muscle with B-scan ultrasound imaging. *Lancet*, **i**: 1389–1390.

Heckmatt, J.Z., Leeman, S. and Dubowitz, V. (1982) Ultrasound imaging in the diagnosis of muscle disease. *Journal of Pediatrics* **101**: 656–660.

Heckmatt, J.Z., Pier, N. and Dubowitz, V. (1988) Real-time ultrasound imaging of muscles. *Muscle and Nerve* **11**: 56–65.

Heckmatt, J.Z., Moosa, A., Hutson, C., Maunder-Sewry, C.A. and Dubowitz, V. (1984) Diagnostic needle muscle biopsy: a practical and reliable alternative to open biopsy. *Archives of Disease in Childhood* **59**: 528–532.

Henriksson, K.G. (1979) 'Semi-open' muscle biopsy technique: a simple outpatient procedure. *Acta Neurologica Scandinavica* **59**: 317–323.

Hosking, G.P., Bhat, U.S., Dubowitz, V. and Edwards, R.H.T. (1976) Measurements of muscle strength and performance in children with normal and diseased muscle. *Archives of Disease in Childhood* **51**: 957–963.

Jiddane, M., Gastaut, J.L., Pellissier, J.F. *et al.* (1983) CT of primary muscle diseases. *American Journal of Neuroradiology* **4**: 773–776.

Kaiser, W.A., Scalke, B.C. and Rohkamm, R. (1986) Nuclear magnetic resonance tomography in the diagnosis of muscular diseases. *ROFO Fortschritte auf dem Gebiete der Rontgenstrahlen und der Neuen Bildgebenden Verfahren* **145**: 199–205.

Lamminen, A.E. (1990) Magnetic resonance imaging of primary skeletal muscle diseases: patterns of distribution and severity of involvement. *British Journal of Radiology* **63**: 946–950.

Medical Research Council (1943) Aids to the investigation of peripheral nerve injuries. *War Memorandum* (revised 2nd edn).

Moosa, A. and Dubowitz, V. (1970) Peripheral neuropathy in Cockayne's syndrome. *Archives of Disease in Childhood* **45**: 674–677.

Moosa, A. and Dubowitz, V. (1971a) Postnatal maturation of peripheral nerves in preterm and full-term infants. *Journal of Pediatrics* **79**: 915–922.

Moosa, A. and Dubowitz, V. (1971b) Slow nerve conduction velocity in cretins. *Archives of Disease in Childhood* **46**: 852–854.

Moosa, A. and Dubowitz, V. (1976) Motor nerve conduction velocity in spinal muscular atrophy of childhood. *Archives of Disease in Childhood* **51**: 974–977.

Murphy, W.A., Totty, W.G. and Carroll, J.E. (1986) MRI of normal and pathologic skeletal muscle. *American Journal of Roentgenology* **146**: 565–574.

Schreiber, A., Smith, W., Ionassescu, V. *et al.* (1987) Magnetic resonance imaging of children with Duchenne muscular dystrophy. *Pediatric Radiology* **17**: 495–497.

Scott, O.M., Hyde, S.A., Goddard, C. *et al.* (1982) Quantitation of muscle function in children: a prospective study in Duchenne muscular dystrophy. *Muscle and Nerve* **5**: 291–301.

Sewry, C.A. and Dubowitz, V. (1994) Histochemical and immunocytochemical studies in neuromuscular diseases. In: Walton, J.N. and Karpati, G. eds, *Disorders of Voluntary Muscle* 5th edn. Edinburgh: Churchill Livingstone, pp. 261–318.

Shabas, D., Gerard, G. and Rossi, D. (1987) Magnetic resonance imaging examination of denervated muscle. *Computerized Radiology* **11**: 9–13.

Topalogu, H., Gucuyener, K., Yalaz, K. *et al.* (1992) Selective involvement of the quadriceps muscle in congenital muscular dystrophies: an ultrasono-graphic study. *Brain and Development* **14**: 84–87.

Udd, B., Lamminen, A. and Somers, H. (1991) Imaging methods reveal unexpected patchy lesions in late onset distal myopathy. *Neuromuscular Disorders* **1**: 279–285.

Wallgren-Pettersson, C., Kivisaari, L., Jaskelainen, J. *et al.* (1990) Ultrasonography, CT, and MRI of muscles in congenital nemaline myopathy. *Pediatric Neurology* **6**: 20–28.

CHAPTER 2

The Muscular Dystrophies

Our forebears in the last century laid a firm foundation of clinical descriptions of diseases, and this was continued into the first half of this century. The advent of new techniques such as histochemistry and electron microscopy for the investigation of muscle biopsies in the 1950s led to the recognition of many new disorders. The advent of the new genetics and the application of recombinant DNA techniques in the 1970s has brought a new revolution, with the location of genes and their subsequent isolation and sequencing and recognition of their specific protein products. This has resulted in the definition of diseases not only on clinical grounds but in terms of their gene mutations and the abnormality in the protein product.

The muscular dystrophies have traditionally been defined as a group of genetically determined disorders with progressive degeneration of skeletal muscle and no associated structural abnormality in the central or peripheral nervous system, and have been subdivided into various types on the basis of the clinical distribution and severity of muscle weakness and pattern of inheritance (Table 2-1). The situation has been compounded by the fact that the same clinical phenotype may have different modes of inheritance and presumably different genes and different gene products.

The majority of muscular dystrophies show a progressive clinical course but this is not absolute and patients with some of the milder forms such as facioscapulohumeral dystrophy may be relatively static and others such as congenital dystrophy may even show functional improvement. Moreover, some dystrophies, such as facioscapulohumeral dystrophy, may not show a typically dystrophic pattern in the muscle and one may question whether this condition is appropriately categorized as a dystrophy. Furthermore, some cases of congenital muscular dystrophy may have associated involve-

ment of the nervous system, with structural changes in the brain.

We may be heading eventually for a redefining and a renaming of the dystrophies on the basis of their particular type of abnormality rather than on their general pathological appearance. Thus Duchenne and Becker (clinical phenotype) dystrophy (pathology) may end up being classified as disorders of the muscle membrane ('membranopathy'?) due to a genetically determined (Xp21) absence or abnormality of the protein dystrophin ('dystrophinopathy'?). It was anticipated that some of the other dystrophies, such as the autosomal recessive limb girdle dystrophy with a similar clinical phenotype and pathological pattern to Duchenne muscular dystrophy (DMD), might be due to an abnormality of an autosomally inherited, dystrophin-like or dystrophin-related protein ('DRP'; utrophin) (Love et al., 1989) or possibly a protein closely linked with dystrophin, such as the dystrophin-associated glycoproteins identified by Campbell and Kahl (1989), and this has now been shown for one specific clinical form of limb girdle dystrophy (see below).

Until this whole field is more adequately resolved, it would be wise, for the present, to stick to the categories based on clinical phenotype, pathology and inheritance. The patient and his family will still need information on the nature of the disease and its course and management and appropriate genetic counselling. A definitive and recognizable clinical label is also important for the patient, and I anticipate that some of the well-entrenched names such as Duchenne and Becker dystrophy will persist in clinical practice, rather than Xp21 dystrophy or dystrophinopathy, although the scientists may argue that these new terms have particular advantages for accurate designation from a scientific point of view.

Table 2-1 The muscular dystrophies

Disease/phenotype (eponym; acronym)	Mode of inheritance	Gene location	Gene symbol (Gene product/protein abnormality)
Duchenne muscular dystrophy (DMD)	XLR	Xp21	DYS (Dystrophin)
Becker muscular dystrophy (BMD)	XLR	Xp21	DYS (Dystrophin)
Limb girdle muscular dystrophy (LGMD)			
(SCARMD)[a] (adhalin[b] deficient)	AR	13q12	
(SCARMD) (adhalin deficient)	AR	17q12-q21	(adhalin)
(SCARMD) (adhalin normal)	AR	?	
LGMD	AR	15q	
LGMD	AR	2p	
LGMD	AD	5q	
LGMD	AD	?	
Congenital muscular dystrophy (CMD)			
CMD (merosin deficient)	AR	6q	(α2 laminin; merosin)
CMD (merosin normal)	AR	?	
CMD + CNS Abnormality			
Fukuyama CMD	AR	9q31-33	FCMD
Walker–Warburg	AR	?	
Muscle–Eye–Brain (Santavuori)	AR	?	
?Other			
Distal muscular dystrophy			
(Welander)	AD		
(Miyoshi)	AR	2p12-14	
(Nonaka)	AR		
Tibial (Udd)	AD		
Bethlem myopathy	AD		
Emery–Dreifuss muscular dystrophy	XLR	Xq28	EMD (emerin)
Facioscapulohumeral dystrophy	AD	4q35	FSHD
Scapulohumeral dystrophy	AD		

[a]SCARMD: Severe Childhood Autosomal Recessive Muscular Dystrophy.
[b]adhalin = 50 kD Dystrophin Associated Glycoprotein.
For gene update and recent references see Chapter 15.

HISTORICAL

It is logical for any historical review of muscular dystrophy to start with the name of Duchenne, whom we associate with the childhood or Duchenne type of muscular dystrophy. Duchenne was a somewhat unusual physician who practised most of his life in Boulogne before moving to Paris. Although he had no formal appointment to any of the Paris hospitals he was allowed to visit the outpatient clinics and to apply faradism, from the mysterious box he always carried with him, to the muscles of patients with a wide range of chronic neurological disorders (Figure 2-1). When he died he was held in such high esteem that Charcot himself is said to have kept vigil at his deathbed (Emery, 1993a).

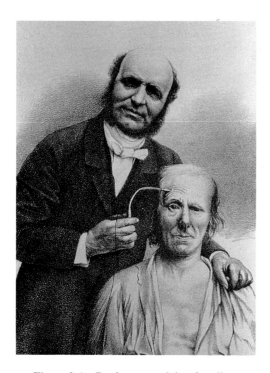

Figure 2-1 Duchenne applying faradism.

Duchenne is the father of the application of electricity to medicine, both diagnostic and therapeutic, and this work formed the basis of his famous book, *De l'électrisation localisée et son application à la pathologie et à la thérapeutique*, which ran to three editions (1855, 1861 and 1872). He was also the inventor of a biopsy needle for muscle biopsies, the forerunner of all subsequent biopsy needles (see Chapter 1).

Duchenne described his first case of muscular dystrophy in the second edition of his book (Duchenne, 1861) under the name 'paraplégie hypertrophique de l'enfance de cause cérébrale'. Because of the associated intellectual impairment of the child he suggested the condition might have a cerebral origin. This was followed by a spate of case reports in the German and French literature, and subsequently also from England, America, Australia and Denmark (Dubowitz, 1978).

In 1868 Duchenne gave a comprehensive account of the disease based on a study of 13 cases. He defined it as a condition of childhood or adolescence, occurring more frequently in males and characterized by (1) progressive weakness of movements, initially affecting the muscles of the lower limbs and lumbar spine, gradually getting worse and spreading to the upper limbs; (2) enlargement of some of the paralysed muscles and in some cases of almost all; and (3) hyperplasia of interstitial connective tissue in the paralysed muscle with production of abundant fibrous and adipose tissue in the final stages. He suggested the alternative names 'paralysie musculaire pseudohypertrophique' to draw attention to the unusual muscle enlargement with the weakness, and 'paralysie myosclérosique' to highlight the extreme fibrosis in the muscle. Duchenne was also a pioneer in the annals of photography, and illustrated several of his muscle cases in his book, 'Album de Photographies Pathologiques', published in 1862. He was probably one of the first clinicians to use photography as a means of recording clinical disorders.

In 1879 Gowers gave five clinical lectures on 'pseudohypertrophic muscular paralysis' and described with masterly clarity and colour the features of 21 personal cases, and reviewed 139 cases of previous authors (Gowers, 1879a, b). His poetic and almost photographic word pictures of the disease have never been equalled:

> The disease is one of the most interesting,
> and at the same time most sad,
> of all those with which we have to deal;
> interesting on account of its peculiar features
> and mysterious nature;
> sad on account of our powerlessness
> to influence its course,
> except in a very slight degree,
> and on account of the conditions in which it occurs.
> It is a disease of early life and of early growth.
> Manifesting itself commonly at the transition from infancy to childhood,
> it develops with the child's development, grows with his growth —
> so that every increase in stature means an increase in weakness, and each year takes him a step further on the road to a helpless infirmity, and in most cases to an early and inevitable death.

Gowers 1879

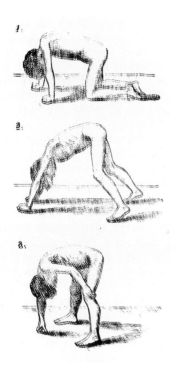

Figure 2-2   Gowers' sign or manoeuvre. (From Gowers, 1879b.)

Gowers also observed (and illustrated in his paper) the unusual way in which these boys get up from the floor by climbing up their legs – the Gowers' manoeuvre (Figure 2-2).

Although Gowers took up the term 'pseudo-hypertrophic', coined by Duchenne, we came to realize in the 1960s that this feature is not specific to childhood muscular dystrophy but may occur in other forms of dystrophy and indeed even in some of the neurogenic syndromes. We thus preferred the eponymous title Duchenne dystrophy.

It seems inevitable that if someone's name is attached to a disease he turns out to be the second person to have described it. Muscular dystrophy is no exception. Pride of place for the first accurate and detailed description should probably go to a London physician, Meryon, who in 1852, some 10 years before Duchenne, described in lucid detail a family in which four boys were affected with the condition (Meryon, 1852). He pointed out the striking pathological changes within the muscle and, in a necropsy on one of the cases, noted the apparent normality of the central nervous system. Like Gowers, he also had a flair for clinical description: 'In May 1847, when nearly 9 years of age, he walked from Bruton Street to Westminster Bridge, but in November 1848, he could neither walk nor stand, and in 1850 his arms were fast losing power.' Meryon (1864) subsequently wrote a comprehensive mono-graph on muscular dystrophy and other forms of muscle paralysis. Emery has recently traced back the family of Meryon, who were Huguenots who fled from France to England in the sixteenth century (Emery, 1993b), and has provided a detailed account of Meryon's perceptive contribution to our knowledge on Duchenne dystrophy, including the nature of the pathological changes in the muscle, a suggestion that the sarcolemma was principally at fault, the genetic transmission through females and affecting only males, and the normality of the central nervous system.

There is a possible earlier reference to Duchenne muscular dystrophy. Schmidt (1839) quoted the report of Coste and Gioja on two brothers with progressive weakness of the lower limbs, starting at the age of 10 years, and later becoming generalized and associated with striking enlargement of several muscles. However, my search through all the volumes prior to 1839 of the journal quoted (*Annali Clinici dell'Ospedale degl'Incurabili (Napoli)*), in the reading room of the British Museum, failed to reveal the paper by these authors. A paper I tracked down by Conte and Gioja on Scrofula musculorum I wrongly presumed to be tuberculosis (Conte and Gioja, 1836). During a meeting in Naples in 1981 I visited the Ospedale degl'Incurabili and Professor Nigro subsequently researched the paper of Conte and Gioja and showed that this was indeed an early clinical description of Duchenne dystrophy (Nigro, 1986). This led to the foundation of the Gaetano Conte Academy in the University of Naples to honour the contribution of Conte to myology and to stake a claim for the contribution from Italy in the history of muscular dystrophy. Surely Meryon deserves a similar accolade?

OTHER FORMS OF DYSTROPHY

Although the literature prior to 1852 contains no further records of the childhood form of progressive muscular dystrophy, adolescent and adult forms of progressive muscular paralysis were already well documented, but these early authors did not distinguish between those forms of muscular atrophy associated with diseases of the nervous system and those without neurological abnormality. In 1879 Möbius commented on the similarity between the atrophic pelvifemoral form of muscle weakness described by Leyden (1876) and the pseudohypertrophic muscular paralysis of Duchenne. This formed the basis of the Leyden–Möbius, or limb girdle, muscular dystrophy.

Erb (1884) described (at great length) a 'juvenile form' of progressive muscular atrophy which he considered distinct from those previously recorded. Although the muscles of the back, shoulders and upper arms were usually more severely affected, some showed marked involvement of the pelvic girdle and lower limbs. He also commented on the similarity between the various clinical types of progressive muscular atrophies without neural involvement, and proposed the name 'dystrophia muscularum progressiva' to cover the whole group. In 1891 he gave a comprehensive account of the histological features of dystrophic muscle.

Landouzy and Déjerine (1884) drew attention to a progressive muscular atrophy affecting the scapulo-humeral muscles and associated with weakness of the facial musculature. In some cases the facial weakness presented in early childhood as the first manifestation of the disease, whereas in others it appeared only later. In the third edition of his book, some years ahead of Landouzy and Déjerine, Duchenne (1872) had already described nine cases of this facioscapulohumeral muscular paralysis.

These early descriptions formed the basis for the clinical classifications that evolved in the 1950s (Levison, 1951; Stevenson, 1953; Walton and Nattrass, 1954). Numerous contributions in the literature over the years helped to identify the various patterns of inheritance of the different clinical varieties. The wider use of serum enzymes and electromyography to separate the dystrophies from neurogenic syndromes and the advent of more sophisticated techniques, such as histochemistry and electron microscopy in the 1950s and 1960s for study of muscle biopsies, subsequently led to the recognition of a large number of neuromuscular disorders which are indistinguishable from the various dystrophies on clinical grounds alone. 'All that waddles is not dystrophy'. Thus, for example, a large proportion of the cases which in the past were labelled as limb girdle dystrophy were found to be due to spinal muscular atrophy (Kugelberg–Welander syndrome) or to some of the rarer congenital myopathies. Similarly, cases with facioscapulohumeral, scapulo-humeral, distal and ocular distribution of weakness, which in the past have been categorized as dystrophies, may have various different forms of underlying pathology. This brought in its path a different problem, namely the same genetic disorder (such as FSH syndrome) having a variable pathological picture and thus causing confusion in the minds of clinicians wishing to split syndromes into tightly defined subcompartments. These problems and their resolution will be discussed in more detail in the appropriate clinical sections.

NOMENCLATURE

For the present it is probably still useful to categorize cases clinically by their distribution of muscle weakness (Table 2-1). I have preferred to reserve the term limb girdle dystrophy for those cases with a pelvifemoral weakness and to designate those with scapulohumeral weakness as scapulohumeral dystrophy, rather than to use limb girdle as an all-embracing term for both the scapular and the pelvic girdles (Walton and Nattrass, 1954; Walton and Gardner–Medwin, 1974). Similarly, other unusual combinations of weakness, such as scapuloperoneal, are best having a descriptive label based on anatomical distribution rather than trying to place them under one or other girdle nomenclature. In other instances an eponymous title is more practical and less cumbersome for a distinctive form of dystrophy with a consistent inheritance and distribution of muscle involvement, such as Emery–Dreifuss muscular dystrophy with its humero-peroneal distribution of weakness and wasting and its associated contractures of the spinal extensors, elbow flexors and ankle plantar flexors. The situation is, however, compounded by the occurrence of the same phenotype with a dominant inheritance, and also occasionally with a different underlying pathology. With the recent developments in molecular genetics, these individual syndromes and their range of clinical phenotype are gradually being clarified, as has already happened with Duchenne and Becker dystrophy.

Once a particular structural or metabolic abnormality is revealed by investigation it is customary to label the disease accordingly, irrespective of the distribution of weakness, e.g. central core disease, type V glycogenosis (phosphorylase deficiency glycogenosis; McArdle's syndrome), mitochondrial myopathy, carnitine deficiency myopathy.

The advent of molecular genetics has now helped to resolve many of these semantic conflicts and to clarify whether a particular clinical variant conforms to the same gene or not. This will undoubtedly help to identify some of the aberrant presentations of individual disorders, as has already occurred in the Duchenne/Becker phenotype.

DUCHENNE MUSCULAR DYSTROPHY

This is a well-defined form of muscular dystrophy and the term Duchenne muscular dystrophy is preferable to such earlier alternatives as 'childhood muscular dystrophy', since some of the milder forms may also start in childhood; or 'pseudohypertrophic muscular dystrophy', since pseudohypertrophy may be absent in otherwise typical cases and may also occur in other forms of neuromuscular disorder. For the present at least, I think the eponymous title is also still preferable to the latter-day, forward-

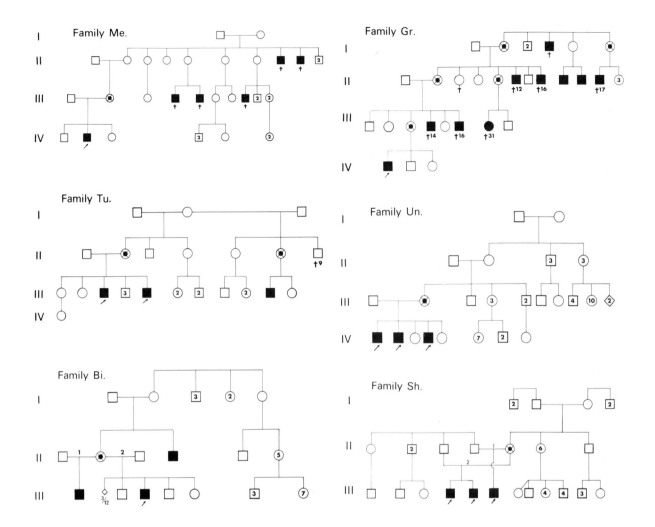

Figure 2-3 Pedigree charts showing X-linked pattern of inheritance in Duchenne dystrophy. In family Un. previous generations were unaffected but the mother of the three affected boys (III,2) must be a definite carrier. The disease may have started as a new mutation in her. The same applies to II,5 in family Sh. Creatine (CK) studies may help to reveal female carriers in the earlier generations of families such as these and the new techniques of molecular genetics have helped to confirm or exclude this. In family Gr. the female affected by muscular dystrophy (III,7) was a presumptive case of Turner syndrome, although chromosome studies were not done.

looking titles such as Xp21 dystrophy or dystrophinopathy, as will be discussed later.

Following the recent advances in molecular genetics we can now define Duchenne dystrophy as an X-linked disorder characterized by progressive weakness of skeletal muscle, with associated pathological changes in the muscle, due to deficiency of protein dystrophin.

INCIDENCE AND INHERITANCE

The incidence of Duchenne dystrophy based on a number of population studies as well as neonatal screening has been estimated to be around 1 in 3500 male births (Emery, 1991). There is also a very high mutation rate and it has been estimated that a third of isolated cases are due to new mutations, which is considerably higher than any other X-linked condition. This may well relate to the gigantic size of the gene which makes it more susceptible to mutations.

CLINICAL FEATURES

The onset

The parents are usually unaware of any abnormality until the child starts walking. Because of the

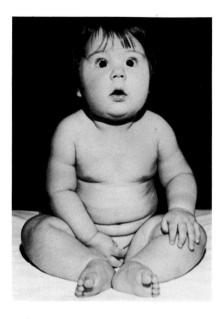
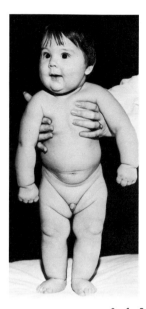

Figure 2-4 Preclinical Duchenne dystrophy in a 7-month-old boy with completely normal motor milestones, able to sit without support and to stand with support. He has an affected brother. CK 2500 iu/litre.

insidious nature of the onset it is often difficult to pinpoint with accuracy the exact age of onset. Moreover, in the past, before the advent of serum enzymes, there was often a long delay before the diagnosis was made. In a family with a previously affected child the mother would often suspect involvement of a subsequent child much earlier, even prior to any abnormal clinical features being apparent to a medical observer.

With the advent of serum enzyme estimations we are now able to diagnose muscular dystrophy with confidence before it is clinically apparent (Figures 2-3, 2-4), and also to exclude it with certainty in cases where it may have seemed clinically likely.

The three landmarks that most clearly define the overall clinical course of a case of muscular dystrophy are the age at onset of symptoms, the age at loss of ambulation and the age at death.

The clinical course in a personal series of 65 cases of Duchenne type dystrophy (Dubowitz, 1960a) is illustrated in Figure 2-5. This shows the variability in the age of onset based on the first observed presenting symptom. In 47 (74%) the onset was before the age of 4 years, and in 13 of these it was before the age of 2 years. The apparent additional peak at 5 years of age probably reflects an increasing awareness of the problem when starting school.

The most frequent presenting symptoms in this series were an abnormal gait (24 cases), frequent falls (17 cases) and difficulty in climbing steps (6 cases).

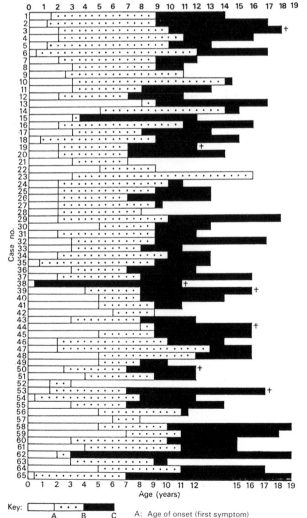

Key:

A: Age of onset (first symptom)
B: Age of inability to walk
C: Present age or age at death (†)

Figure 2-5 Clinical course of disease in 65 cases of Duchenne dystrophy.

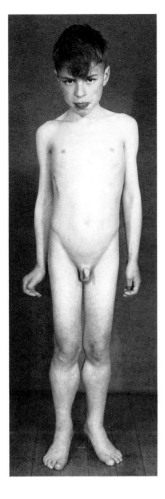
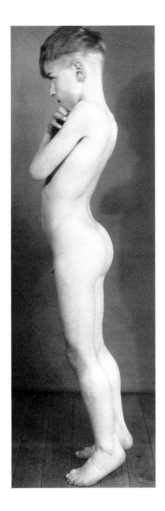
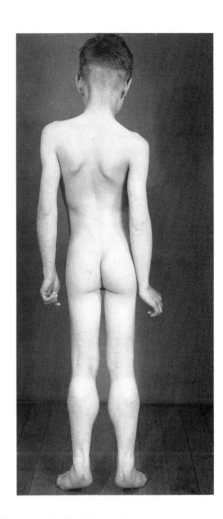

Figure 2-6   Duchenne dystrophy showing prominence of calves, toe-gait, forward tilt of pelvis and compensatory lordosis.

Other presenting symptoms included an apparent deterioration in walking in cases with previous poliomyelitis (3 cases), reluctance to walk (3), delayed walking (2), floppy infant (2), walking on toes (2), difficulty in getting up (1), difficulty in crawling (1), 'sluggish' infant (1), delay in holding head up (1), stiff feet (1) and excessive fatigue (1).

Where abnormality of gait was not the initial presenting symptom, it still occurred at an early stage of the disease. Descriptive terms used by the parents included 'waddling', 'swaying', 'like a crab', 'like a duck', 'as if he had a stone in his shoe', 'like a penguin'. A waddling gait is the most generally applied description in medical circles.

Motor milestones

Parents can usually recall the age at which a child started to walk but may have more difficulty with the

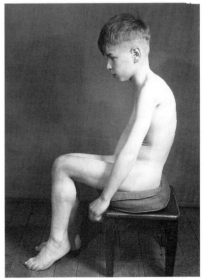

Figure 2-7   Same child as in Figure 2-6 showing disappearance of lordosis in sitting posture.

age of standing unsupported or maintaining a sitting posture without support. In the above series of 65 cases the motor milestones were analysed on the basis of an upper limit for normal sitting, standing and walking of 9, 14 and 18 months respectively. On this basis, 26 children were late in walking and one or both additional milestones, while a further eight were delayed in walking alone or delayed in the other two milestones but walking by 18 months. This high incidence of delay in motor milestones may be due to the underlying involvement of the muscle itself or may reflect the associated intellectual impairment in a proportion of children with Duchenne dystrophy, since in some instances the delay in intellectual development is clinically apparent before any evidence of muscle weakness (Dubowitz, 1965).

Other early features

The characteristic waddling gait, on a wide base, is usually associated with a lumbar lordosis and a tendency to walk on the toes. Owing to the early weakness of the gluteus medius and minimus muscles the child is unable to support the weight of his body when raising one leg. He accordingly inclines towards the other leg to bring the centre of gravity of the body over that leg. When he moves forward on to the other leg the same action is repeated. This accounts for the waddle and the broad, more stable, base. The weakness of the hip extensors leads to a forward tilt of the pelvis and a compensatory lumbar lordosis to maintain an up-right posture (Figure 2-6). The lordosis disappears with sitting (Figure 2-7). It is easier to maintain this vertical posture standing on the toes than on the flat feet. There is also usually some weakness of the dorsiflexors of the feet, but toe-walking will often occur before any fixed shortening of the tendo Achillis.

These children may be able to stand on one leg (after the age of 3 years) but are never able to hop or to run in a normal manner. Any attempt at running accentuates the waddling gait and makes it more ungainly.

Difficulty in negotiating steps is an early feature and even climbing on to the kerb or a bus can present a particular problem. There is a tendency to fall frequently, often without any tripping or stumbling, with a description by parents of the child apparently just seizing up or slumping to the floor as if his legs were swept out from under him. There is progress-ively more difficulty in getting up from the floor, which the child does by the manoeuvre so vividly described by Gowers (1879a,b). Initially he may simply have to push one hand on to a knee in getting erect. A normal child can get up from a sitting position on the floor in under one second; a child with Duchenne will invariably take over two

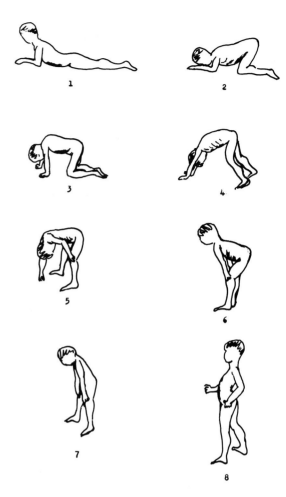

Figure 2-8 The Gowers' manoeuvre showing sequence of postures used in getting up from the ground: 1, lying prone; 2,3, getting on to hands and knees; 4, legs and arms extended and legs brought as close as possible to arms; 5, hand placed on knee; 6, both hands on knees, knees extended; 7, hands move alternately up thighs 'climbing up himself'; 8, erect posture.

seconds. Later the Duchenne boy goes through the whole Gowers' sequence (Figure 2-8). In order to rise from a supine posture he first has to go into the prone, then into a knee–elbow position, followed by extension of the knees and elbows to raise the body, then gradually to bring the hands and feet as close as possible together so that the centre of gravity of the body is brought over the legs. He is then able to let go one hand at a time and support it on the knee. He may also be too weak to extend the hips and spine, and has to achieve this by placing the hands on the knees and gradually ascending the thighs by alternative steps with the hands ('climbing up himself'). Gowers' manoeuvre is a characteristic feature of Duchenne dystrophy but not patho-gnomonic, since it will also occur in other forms of neuromuscular disease with a similar distribution of muscle weakness.

Pain in the muscles, especially the calves, is a fairly common symptom (22 of 65 in the above series) and is usually associated with exercise. At times the calf muscles may appear to go into a state of spasm and the heels be raised off the ground at the time of the pain. It is not usually a presenting symptom though, as it may be in the milder Becker type (see below).

Enlargement of muscles, particularly the calves (see Figure 2-6), is a common feature and was observed by the parents in 41 of the above 65 cases. It may increase while the child is still ambulant but tends to become less after loss of ambulation. Other muscles such as the deltoids and serrati anterior may also be prominent and some cases may show a fairly universal prominence of their muscles (Figures 2-9 a,b) (the 'infant Hercules' already illustrated by Duchenne). The tongue is also frequently enlarged and this was fairly gross in 21 of the 65 cases studied. There is also commonly an associated wide arch to the mandible and maxilla with separation of the teeth, presumably secondary to the macroglossia. This may partly account for the fairly typical facies in Duchenne dystrophy.

Weakness of the arms is not a common symptom in the early stages but may be found in the proximal muscles on clinical examination. As the disease progresses the patient becomes aware of proximal and later also of more distal weakness of the arm muscles. The weakness in the legs as well as the arms is always symmetrical.

Sphincter control is usually unaffected and there is also no difficulty with chewing and swallowing.

The weakness progresses steadily but the rate is very variable. Some children show a smooth steady decline whereas others may appear to be static for periods up to a year or more, and some show periods of fairly rapid deterioration over short periods of time. On quantitative assessment, however, all will show a downward trend. Immobilization for any reason can lead to a marked and often precipitous decline in muscle power and ability.

The age of loss of ability to walk is variable but in the majority it occurs between 7 and 13 years of age (see Figure 2-5). Occasionally, sufferers may lose ambulation as early as 6 years, with no apparent precipitating factor, whereas others may remain ambulant beyond the age of 12, which should always raise the suspicion of a milder form of muscular dystrophy such as the Becker or limb girdle variety. In order to try and separate the Duchenne from the Becker phenotype I have used a dividing line of loss of ambulation before the 13th birthday to categorize the Duchenne phenotype, ambulant beyond 16 years to characterize the Becker, and classified those with loss of ambulation between 13 and 16 years as

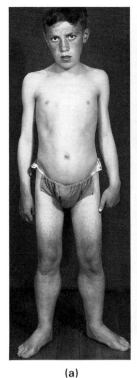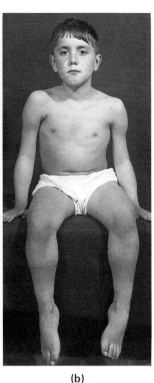

(a)   (b)

Figure 2-9a,b Two half-brothers (Cases 14 and 15 in Figure 2-5) showing fairly general prominence of muscles. The older brother (a) remained ambulant until 14 years; the younger (b) lost ambulation at 3½ years.

intermediate between Duchenne and Becker phenotypes (Dubowitz, 1989). This also helps to stress the continuity in phenotype between the Duchenne and Becker, and the variability within each, so that all borders are arbitrary but nevertheless useful for clinical assessment and prognostication. Loss of ambulation may be precipitated by immobilization even for trivial reasons over short periods and was a factor in 13 of the 65 cases studied above.

Some cases in the above series were atypical (see Figure 2-5). Subjects 56 and 57 were females with a Duchenne-like dystrophy and presumably represent a severe limb girdle dystrophy with autosomal recessive inheritance (Dubowitz, 1960b). Subject 38 was never able to walk and almost certainly had a congenital dystrophy and not Duchenne dystrophy. He died at 12 years but autopsy permission was refused. Subject 15 had a clinical onset at the age of 3, with reluctance to walk, and stopped walking 3 months later. When seen at 11 years of age he looked like a typical Duchenne dystrophy patient (Figure 2-9b). His older half-brother (by the same mother but a different father) (Subject 14) had a more typical course but was in fact ambulant unusually long, until about 14 years of age (Figure 2-9a). This

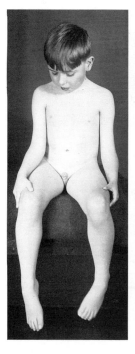
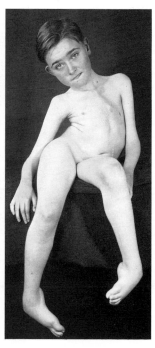

Figure 2-10 Rapid development of scoliosis and equinovarus deformities within 3 years of loss of ambulation.

illustrates an unusual variability within the same family, more commonly seen in limb girdle than Duchenne dystrophy. Subject 23 was still ambulant at 16 years and would now be more appropriately classified as a Becker dystrophy patient. Subject 62 lost the ability to walk at the age of 3 years after a period of 2 weeks' immobilization with measles.

Emery (1993a) compiled centile charts from his own data and the published data of a number of authors in relation to the course of the disease. The 50th percentile for loss of ambulation in his series of 120 boys was 8.5 years, the 95th percentile 11.9 and the 99th 13.2 years. The mean age of loss of ambulation in various published series ranged from 9 to 10.8 years. The 50th percentile for age at death in Emery's series of 129 boys was 15.5, the 95th 20.5 and the 99th 23.5. The mean age of death in various published series ranged mainly between 16 and 18 years.

Of some importance from the diagnostic point of view is the fact that about half of all boys with Duchenne dystrophy do not achieve independent walking till after 18 months of age. A serum creatine kinase should be included as a diagnostic screen in any child presenting with delay in walking beyond this age.

Deformities

While still ambulant these children do not tend to develop skeletal deformities. There may, however, be early tightness of the hip flexors, the tendo Achillis and to a lesser extent the knee flexors. There may also be an incipient scoliosis if they have an asymmetrical stance, usually associated with asymmetrical contractures of the tendo achilles. Once they stop walking they very rapidly tend to develop fixed deformities which are related to their habitual posture (Figure 2-10). As a result of spending most of their time in a sitting position in a wheelchair they develop contractures of the flexors of the hips and knees and a tendency to equinovarus deformity of the feet. There is also a tendency for contractures of the flexors of the elbows and pronators of the forearms. A high proportion of these children also develop progressive scoliosis from this time onwards. Much can be done to slow the progression of the contractures by active exercises, and to prevent the scoliosis and talipes equinovarus by attention to posture and special supports to hold the back or feet in an optimal position (Figure 2-11). These aspects of management will be dealt with in more detail later in this chapter.

With the progression of the disease some patients retain their muscle bulk in spite of the progressive weakness, presumably due to fat and connective tissue replacement of the muscle itself, whereas others become very thin and atrophic. This is illustrated by the three affected siblings in two separate families in Figures 2-12 and 2-13.

In the earlier stages there may be selective symmetrical wasting of particular muscles, such as the sternal head of the pectoralis major, but gradually other muscles also become atrophic and distal muscles also are affected by the disease process. The facial muscles and external ocular muscles do not show overt weakness, although some facial weakness may be present in the late stages of the disease.

The tendon reflexes show an unusual but fairly consistent pattern. Reflexes in the upper limbs, and the knee jerks, are almost invariably absent from early on in the disease whereas the ankle jerks are often preserved even in the late stages. Thus ankle jerks were present in 40 of the 65 cases analysed above, and were unusually brisk in 25, with sustained clonus in three cases. A tap on the front of the tibia will also elicit an ankle jerk in many of these cases, but not in normal children. The plantar response is flexor.

Course and prognosis

The majority of sufferers die before the age of 20 but

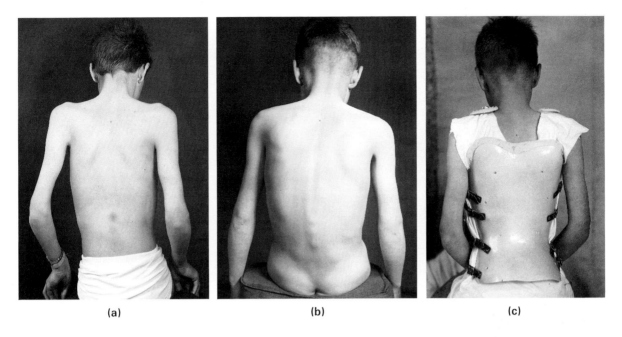

(a) **(b)** **(c)**

Figure 2-11a-c Same subject as in Figure 2-6 showing (a) prevention of scoliosis (age 15) by (b and c) fitting of spinal brace at time of loss of ambulation (11 years).

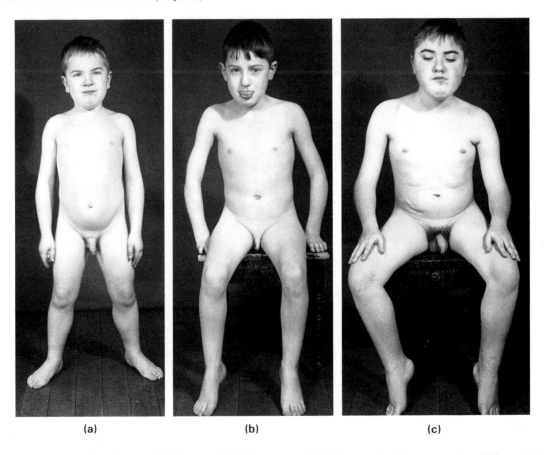

(a) **(b)** **(c)**

Figure 2-12a-c Three brothers aged (a) 8 years, (b) 9½ years, and (c) 13 years, showing progression of disease but not striking wasting. (Cases 26-28 in Figure 2-5.)

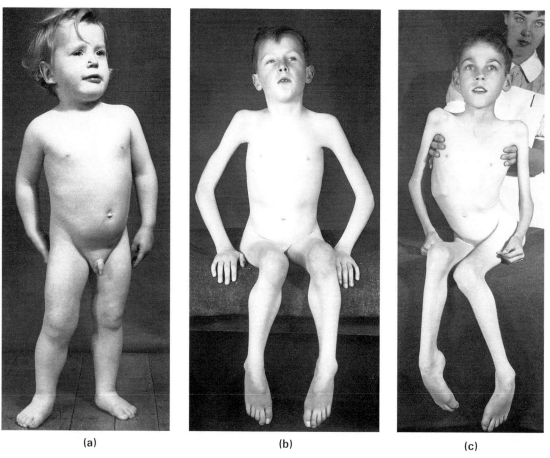

(a)   (b)   (c)

Figure 2-13a-c   Three brothers aged (a) 2 years, (b) 10 years and (c) 12 years, showing progression of disease and striking wasting of muscles and loss of subcutaneous fat. (Cases 50–52 in Figure 2-5.)

some do survive into their 20s. Death usually results from a respiratory infection which may progress extremely rapidly after initially being rather trivial. Some subjects die quite suddenly in an apparent shock-like state in the course of a mild respiratory infection and this may be due to acute myocardial insufficiency, since cardiac involvement is a common, possibly invariable, feature in Duchenne dystrophy. Others develop nocturnal hypoventilation in their late teens/early 20s and lapse into respiratory failure.

Respiratory deficit

The respiratory problems in Duchenne dystrophy are mainly the result of the restrictive defect resulting from the weak intercostal and associated muscles. In the early years the vital capacity in these children continues to increase with age and growth, but in their early teens it tends to plateau and then to show a steady decline. This may pose a particular problem if surgery for scoliosis is contemplated in their late

teens and the respiratory function measurements have fallen to around 25% or less of the expected level for the age or body size, and the anaesthetist may be reluctant to administer an anaesthetic for fear of being unable to wean the patient from supportive ventilation postoperatively. It is thus important to monitor the respiratory function on a regular basis, by such simple techniques as vital capacity, to anticipate these problems. These children may be precipitated into respiratory failure by an intercurrent infection. If a patient's underlying respiratory function is still reasonable it should be possible to tide him over a crisis with intensive therapy with antibiotics and supportive physiotherapy. If the respiratory function is already severely compromised the need for assisted ventilation may arise and this will need to be carefully assessed in each individual case.

Respiratory failure

In the later stages of the disease, usually in the late

teens or early 20s, respiratory failure may occur as a result of increasing nocturnal hypoventilation and hypoxia. This is often insidious in its development but a careful history will usually reveal the tell-tale symptoms, such as morning drowsiness, headache or confusion, daytime somnolence, and night-time restlessness, with an increased need to be turned. The sleep hypoventilation is easily confirmed by overnight oximetry, which often shows precipitous falls in the oxygen saturation. Concomitant cardiac monitoring may show associated cardiac arrhythmia which can be life threatening (Smith *et al.*, 1989; Carroll *et al.*, 1991). The patients often show a dramatic improvement with assisted night-time ventilation, with rapid disappearance of their early morning symptoms and a considerable improvement in their daytime wellbeing. The development of mask ventilation, together with light-weight, portable and relatively silent ventilators, has revolutionized the management of these patients and largely replaced the need for tracheostomy or cuirass ventilation (Heckmatt *et al.*, 1990). Things may remain stable for a considerable time, but in due course the respiratory function may decline, with the need for supportive ventilation during periods of the day as well as at night.

Night-time oximetry studies in asymptomatic teenage boys with Duchenne dystrophy have shown significant, usually short-duration, dips in oxygen saturation (Smith *et al.*, 1988; Manni *et al.*, 1989; Khan and Heckmatt, 1994). This raises the question of the potential benefit, as well as the feasibility, of prophylactic night-time mask ventilation in the prevention or delay of respiratory failure in Duchenne dystrophy and whether this would have any advantage over waiting for symptoms before treatment. The same argument applies to the possible benefit of any respiratory exercises in relation to the falling respiratory function with time. There has been enthusiasm for such efforts over several years, including the recent introduction of computerized video games (DiMarco *et al.*, 1985; Estrup *et al.*, 1986; Rodillo *et al.*, 1989; Stern *et al.*, 1989; Vilozni *et al.*, 1994). These questions will be difficult to answer without long-term controlled studies.

Cardiac involvement

Symptoms and signs of cardiomyopathy are usually not apparent clinically, but ECG abnormalities are often present, even in the early stages of the disease. These typically show evidence of right ventricular strain, with tall R waves over the right ventricular leads and deep Q waves in the left praecordial and limb leads; T-wave inversion over the praecordial

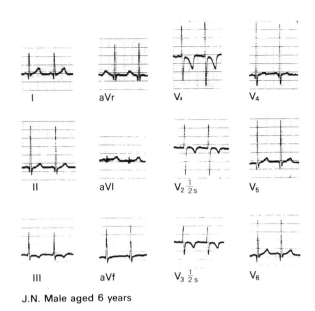

J.N. Male aged 6 years

Figure 2-14 ECG from patient, aged 6 years, with Duchenne dystrophy showing tall R waves and inverted T waves over R praecordial leads (V_{1-3}) and deep Q waves over left ($V_{5,6}$).

leads, especially the right, is also common (Figure 2-14). In 56 cases analysed in my original series of 65 cases, only 10 patients did not show some evidence of abnormality. The main changes observed were abnormal Q waves over leads V 4-7 and leads II and III; prominent R waves in V 1; evidence of right ventricular hypertrophy; depression or elevation of ST segment and flattening or inversion of T waves; and prominent U waves especially over leads V 1-3. Two cases showed changes suggestive of recent infarction and on serial examination 18 months later showed some evidence of improvement. It is thus possible that there may be acute episodes of myocardial insufficiency with subsequent improvement.

In an autopsy study of five of these patients there were macroscopic areas of fibrosis in the left ventricular wall in three and microscopic evidence of plaques of collagen and extensive fibrosis in all five. One had a plaque of atheroma in the right main coronary artery; in the rest the vessels appeared normal.

In a subsequent analysis of the ECGs of 29 cases of Duchenne dystrophy, only three showed a normal pattern; the remainder showed the typical changes as above. Emery (1972) found that in addition to the frequent prominence of the R waves in V 1 the algebraic sum of the R and S waves in this lead gave a useful measure of the abnormality in 80% of affected boys.

The application of new techniques has thrown further light on the nature of the cardiac involvement in Duchenne dystrophy. Perloff *et al.* (1967) suggested that the ECG changes reflect selective scarring of the posterobasal portion of the left ventricle, with lateral extension, and an autopsy study in two cases showed focal changes in this area. Kovick *et al.* (1975) studied the movement of the posterior left ventricular wall by echocardiography in a series of patients with various forms of muscular dystrophy, including three Duchenne patients, in whom they found a reduction in the maximal diastolic endocardial velocity, suggesting impaired myocardial relaxation due to the dystrophic involvement. In a similar study of 13 children with Duchenne muscular dystrophy (Ahmad *et al.*, 1977), we also found a reduction in the maximal diastolic endocardial velocity but other indices were normal, including all the systolic phase indices. Some patients with marked ECG changes still had normal function on echocardiography, suggesting that myocardial function is well preserved in Duchenne muscular dystrophy despite the ECG changes. In a further study with two dimensional echocardiography, Goldberg *et al.* (1982) documented abnormalities in the contraction of the left ventricle in most patients, which is first noted in the posterior free wall behind the mitral valve.

Utsunomiya *et al.* (1990) undertook serial studies of cardiac function in 34 cases of Duchenne dystrophy over periods ranging from 2 to 12 years, by assessing systolic time intervals and echocardiography. They showed a steady decline in left ventricular function, which correlated with the rate of deterioration in skeletal muscle function in only about a half of the patients, and recommended that cardiac function needs to be assessed independently of the stage of physical dysfunction in Duchenne dystrophy.

Smooth muscle involvement

Since dystrophin is also expressed in smooth muscle, one might have anticipated dysfunction of smooth muscle in Duchenne dystrophy. There is, however, no firm clinical evidence of smooth muscle involvement in Duchenne dystrophy. Derangement of bladder or bowel function or loss of sphincter control are not a part of the clinical picture. These children have a tendency to constipation after they lose the ability to walk, but this may not be any different from similar problems in immobile children with other neuromuscular disorders and weak abdominal muscles. There have been occasional case reports of acute dilation of the stomach but this has usually been a terminal event. There have been a number of autopsy studies that documented changes in the smooth muscle of the bowel wall (Huvos and Pruzanski, 1967; Leon *et al.*, 1986) and a recent clinical study suggested delayed emptying of the stomach (Barohn *et al.*, 1988).

Intellectual impairment

The association of intellectual impairment with Duchenne dystrophy has long been recognized but there was a tendency in the 1950s to ascribe it to lack of educational opportunity or other factors associated with the physical disability (Morrow and Cohen, 1954; Walton and Nattrass, 1954; Truitt, 1955). Since then there have been several detailed psychometric studies of children with Duchenne dystrophy showing a fairly consistent pattern of lowered IQ (Table 2-2). The mean IQ in most of these series is in the region of 85, compared with a mean for a normal population of about 105, using the Wechsler scale. The range of IQ seems to follow a normal distribution curve, perhaps with some skewing to the left. If one takes a cut-off point of 75

Table 2-2   IQ in Duchenne dystrophy

Authors	No. of subjects	Age of subjects (years)	Mean IQ	Range of IQ	% Below IQ 75
Allen and Rodgin (1960)	30	2–23	82	14–117	30
Worden and Vignos (1962)	38	4–17	83	46–134	29
Murphy *et al.* (1964)	87	(not given)	83	40–119	41[a]
Dubowitz (1965)	27	8–16	68	42–118	70[b]
Zellweger and Niedermeyer (1965)	42	3–16	83	42–131	33
Zellweger and Hanson (1968)	38	2–18	83	48–127	31
Prosser *et al.* (1969)	52	2–18	87	51–113	30
Kozicka *et al.* (1971)	52	3–17	76	35–114	40
Marsh and Munsat (1974)	34	5–15	89	63–118	20
Florek and Karolak (1977)	129	4–15	79	30–127	21
Leibowitz and Dubowitz (1981)	54	4–13	86	47–132	18

[a] IQ < 80.

[b] Series of long-term inpatients which may account for higher proportion with low IQ.

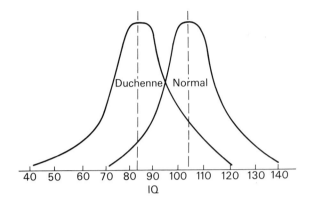

Figure 2-15 Stylized distribution curve of IQ in Duchenne dystrophy showing normal bell-shape but a shift to the left.

as the lower limit for the normal range, about 30% of children with Duchenne dystrophy will fall below this level, compared with about 5% in the normal population. Similarly, a smaller proportion of Duchenne patients will be found in the upper IQ range above 110 than would be expected for a normal population. The easiest way to explain the apparent intellectual retardation in association with Duchenne dystrophy was on the basis of a single gene which is pleiotrophic and accounts for the involvement not only of the skeletal muscle but also the myocardium and the central nervous system, perhaps on the basis of a single biochemical abnormality. One could then look upon Duchenne dystrophy as having a consistent intellectual impairment with a small shift to the left at all levels across the IQ range (Figure 2-15).

Several studies have shown that the intellectual retardation in Duchenne dystrophy is non-progressive and that there is no correlation of IQ either with the age of the patient or with the duration or severity of the disease (Worden and Vignos, 1962; Zellweger and Hanson, 1968; Prosser *et al.*, 1969). This suggests that damage to the nervous system may occur at an early vulnerable stage of development. The physical handicap is unlikely to be an important factor in the IQ level since children with spinal muscular atrophy with equivalent or more severe handicap do not have any lowering of their IQ (Worden and Vignos, 1962; Dubowitz, 1965).

A number of studies have shown a greater reduction in the verbal than the performance IQ, by about 7 or 8 points (Zellweger and Niedermeyer, 1965; Marsh and Munsat, 1974; Karagan and Zellweger, 1978; Leibowitz and Dubowitz, 1981). Some depression of verbal IQ has also been found in Becker muscular dystrophy (Karagan and Sorensen, 1981). In our detailed study of 57 cases of Duchenne

dystrophy (Leibowitz and Dubowitz, 1981), we also documented the associated emotional disturbances, which seemed to have a higher incidence than in other physically handicapped children without cerebral involvement. The unimodal distribution of the IQ in boys with Duchenne dystrophy, the concordance of intellectual impairment of affected subjects within a family, the normal intellect of siblings and the lack of correlation with any variation in clinical severity all pointed to the intellectual impairment being a manifestation of the Duchenne gene. This has now been further supported by the recent demonstration of dystrophin in brain and the presence of subtle differences between brain and muscle in the transcript of the Duchenne gene and the amino terminal end of the encoded protein (Nudel *et al.*, 1989). We were unable to show any correlation between the presence or absence of intellectual impairment and the occurrence and location of deletions, using a series of cDNA probes, in an analysis of 287 cases of Duchenne and Becker muscular dystrophy (Hodgson *et al.*, 1989).

The absence of any structural changes in the central nervous system was already noted by the early authors (Meryon, 1852, 1864; Eulenburg and Cohnheim, 1866), but more recently Rosman and Kakulas (1966) reported significant changes in the brains of patients in a retrospective series of cases of Duchenne dystrophy and myotonic dystrophy from the archives of the Massachusetts General Hospital in Boston. In a prospective study of 21 patients with Duchenne dystrophy who subsequently died, Dubowitz and Crome (1969) were unable to identify any consistent abnormality in the nervous system.

INVESTIGATIONS ————————————————

Serum enzymes

Several serum enzymes are raised in muscular dystrophy, as well as in other muscle disorders. These include the aminotransferases (transaminases), aldolase, lactate dehydrogenase and creatine kinase. Creatine kinase (CK) is by far the most sensitive of these and has the added advantage that it is not influenced by haemolysis of the blood sample owing to its insignificant level in red blood cells, or by hepatic dysfunction, which may cause elevation of the other enzymes, especially the aminotransferases. Many a Duchenne boy has ended up with a liver biopsy as a result of an overenthusiastic investigation of an 'unexplained' elevation of transaminases, perhaps in the course of a routine screening investigation.

In Duchenne dystrophy there is *gross* elevation of CK, particularly in the early stages of the disease.

Levels as high as 50–100 times normal may be found and, depending on the upper limit of the method used, one would anticipate a level well over 5000 iu/litre in the preclinical stages of the disease. Levels lower than 1000 iu/litre should be queried, as they may represent other forms of myopathy rather than Duchenne dystrophy, and in the first weeks of life may reflect the normal rise following the trauma of birth.

The level of itself is, however, no index of severity since equally high levels may also be present in the milder Becker type dystrophy. It is thus important to correlate the clinical picture with the serum enzyme levels and other investigations. In the course of the disease the serum CK gradually falls but even in the late stages still remains above normal. The high CK represents a leakage of enzyme from the muscle cell and the decline with time may simply reflect the loss of muscle tissue with the progression of the disease.

Screening for Duchenne dystrophy. Zellweger and Antonik (1975) introduced a new micromethod for CK, applicable to a drop of blood dried on filter paper. It was based on the amount of light released by the ATP of the reaction process on luciferin-luciferase present. The luciferase is obtained from fireflies. The test can be done on the same blood spot used for the Guthrie screen for phenylketonuria. Zellweger and Antonik recommended application for routine screening of normal populations of newborns on the grounds that early diagnosis of muscular dystrophy might prevent second affected subjects in a family by appropriate genetic counselling and also allow earlier institution of supportive therapy. It seemed unlikely at the time that such a screening programme would find wide appeal under circumstances where no specific therapy was available for Duchenne dystrophy, and some 20 years later the introduction of universal screening for Duchenne dystrophy has still not found enthusiastic support, mainly because of the absence yet of any specific therapy for the disease, and to date only a small number of fairly local pilot studies have been undertaken. With the remarkable advances in the molecular genetics over the past few years, and the current enthusiasm and some optimism for gene or cell therapy, the climate may well change and screening could be introduced in the hope of an early breakthrough in treatment. The development of new techniques for the measurement of CK which are less costly and more readily available (Adriaenssens and Vermeiren, 1980; Orfanos and Naylor, 1984; Moser, 1984) will also be helpful. A positive CK result can now be followed up by accurate confirmation with DNA and dystrophin studies. A recent workshop has critically reviewed all aspects in relation to the introduction of screening programmes for Duchenne dystrophy and concluded that, whilst the time may be approaching for the introduction of such schemes on a large scale, caution and constraint are still necessary in order to ensure that this is done on a voluntary basis, of either opting in or opting out, and that the public are adequately prepared for the implications of such testing (van Ommen and Scheuerbrandt, 1993).

Antenatal diagnosis. A female carrier of the Duchenne gene would have a 50% risk of giving birth to an affected male and until comparatively recently the only option for preventing this was selective abortion of all male fetuses. This of course meant that half of the fetuses aborted were potentially normal, and also that a female infant carried a 50% risk of being a carrier. What was needed was a reliable means of detecting an affected male fetus. With the high CK already present in the neonatal period it seemed reasonable to assume that this elevation might already be present prenatally. Coupled with the technical advances in obtaining fetal blood samples by direct fetoscopy (Hobbins and Mahoney, 1974), a number of centres with the availability of the sophisticated obstetrical expertise used this approach in trying to predict an affected or unaffected fetus. Two major problems with this approach were first to obtain reliable control values from fetuses not at risk of muscular dystrophy obtained by the same method at the same gestation (around 16–18 weeks), and secondly to obtain reliable information as to whether indeed the CK was already elevated in the Duchenne fetus at this gestation. Following the report, however, by Golbus *et al.* (1979), of two false negative results with an apparently normal CK level in a dystrophic fetus, the initial enthusiasm was somewhat dampened and the method was shelved.

The recent advent of DNA technology has now placed antenatal diagnosis on a much firmer footing. Fetal DNA can be extracted from amniotic fluid cells at 16–18 weeks gestation, but even this has now been largely superseded by using chorionic villus sampling, which is also of fetal origin and has the advantage of being done much earlier in pregnancy, at around 10 weeks (see below).

Electromyography

This shows the characteristic pattern of low amplitude, short-duration polyphasic motor unit action potentials. This is non-specific and occurs in all forms of myopathy. It is thus helpful in supporting the clinical diagnosis of a myopathic process and differentiating it from a normal or a denervating pattern.

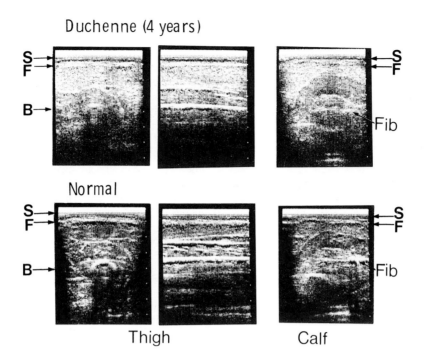

Duchenne (4 years)

Normal

Thigh   Calf

Figure 2-16 Ultrasound scan of thigh and calf in a 4-year-old boy with Duchenne dystrophy showing uniform increase in echo in the muscle compared with control of same age. On the transverse scan of the thigh (left) the bone echo of the femur is reduced from a semi-circle to a short line as a result of attenuation of the ultrasound beam by the dystrophic muscle, and it is also reduced in the longitudinal image (centre). (S = Skin; F = Fascia; B = Bone; Fib = Fibula.)

In the early preclinical phases of Duchenne dystrophy the EMG may appear normal, although CK is already grossly elevated and focal changes may be present on a muscle biopsy. There hardly seems a place any more for use of the EMG in the diagnosis of Duchenne dystrophy, particularly since ultrasound imaging (see below) has proved a more useful and paediatrically more acceptable, non-invasive, screening tool.

Ultrasound imaging

The introduction of ultrasound imaging as a screening procedure for muscular dystrophy (Heckmatt *et al.*, 1982) has proved very useful in clinical practice and has largely replaced electromyography in our clinic. From an early stage of the disease it will already show an increase in echogenicity in some muscles, with a corresponding reduction in the underlying bone echo (Figure 2-16).

It has the advantage that it is non-invasive and readily acceptable to children and one can compare different muscles and also the sequential progression of the pathological process. It also has a potential place in monitoring changes in therapeutic trials.

Muscle biopsy

This remains the definitive means of confirming the tissue diagnosis, although some of the molecular geneticists might now argue that with a positive result for a deletion with cDNA probes this is sufficient confirmation of an Xp21 myopathy. The histological changes will depend on the stage of the disease and to some extent on the muscle selected. The pattern of change in the muscle with progression of the disease is illustrated in Figures 2-17 to 2-21.

In the early preclinical stages the changes may be minimal and consist mainly of variation in fibre size together with focal areas of degenerating or

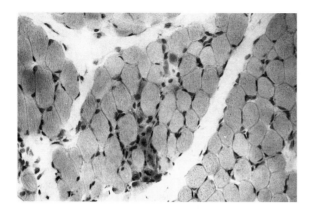

Figure 2-17 Histological changes in Duchenne dystrophy. Early preclinical stage (biopsy at 3 months) showing reasonably normal-looking muscle, but with unequivocal pathological change consisting of abnormal variation in fibre size and focal areas of necrosis and regenerating fibres (lower centre, basophilic (darker) small fibres). Rectus femoris. (H & E × 200.)

Figure 2-18 More advanced stage of Duchenne dystrophy. Fibres still in bundles but more widely separated from each other by proliferating endomysial connective tissue. Note the marked variation in fibre size, the presence of round dark-staining fibres, the internal nuclei and the small cluster (centre) of dark-staining (basophilic) small regenerating fibres. Gastrocnemius. (H & E × 190.)

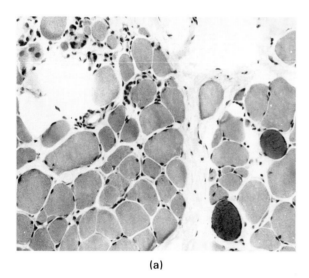

(a)

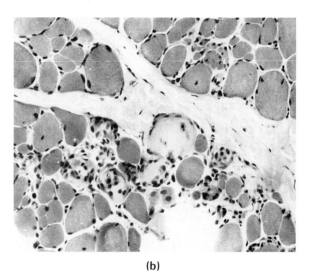

(b)

Figure 2-19a,b Duchenne muscular dystrophy. Two areas from same biopsy showing proliferation of adipose tissue (clear areas), (a) presence of rounded dark-staining opaque fibres and (b) clusters of necrotic fibres undergoing phagocytosis. Bundle architecture still maintained. Note marked variation in fibre size and numerous clusters of very small fibres. Gastrocnemius. (H & E × 140.)

regenerating fibres (Figure 2-17). In the later preclinical phase changes are more pronounced, with more marked variation in fibre size, degeneration and regeneration, and also the presence of rounded opaque fibres, internal nuclei, splitting of fibres and proliferation of connective tissue and adipose tissue (Figure 2-18).

With further progression of the disease there is less marked regenerative activity and gradual loss of fibres and replacement by connective tissue and later adipose tissue (Figures 2-19, 2-20). In the terminal stages of the disease the muscle may be largely replaced by adipose tissue with residual islets of muscle fibres in a sea of fat (Figure 2-21).

Histochemically the most consistent features are a predominance of type 1 fibres and relative loss of clear-cut differentiation into the fibre types with the standard ATPase reaction (at pH 9.4). Electron

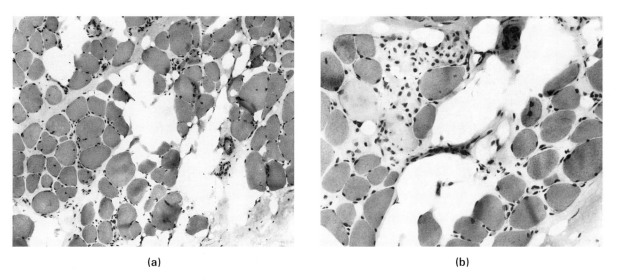

(a)   (b)

Figure 2-20a,b Duchenne muscular dystrophy. Two areas from same biopsy. Further proliferation of adipose tissue (clear areas) resulting in break up of bundle architecture. Note (b) large cluster of necrotic (pale-staining) fibres (upper left) undergoing phagocytosis. Gastrocnemius. (a, H & E × 90; b, H & E × 140.)

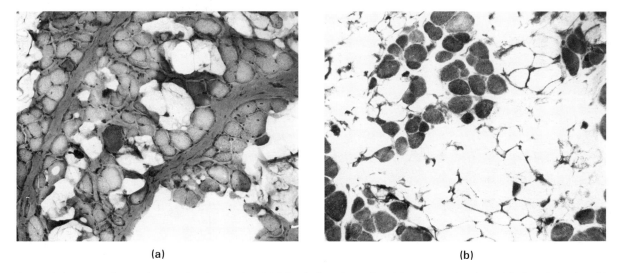

(a)   (b)

Figure 2-21a,b Advanced muscular dystrophy. (a) Muscle largely replaced by connective tissue (dark-staining bands) and adipose tissue (clear areas). (b) Histochemical preparation shows more clearly the isolated clusters of residual muscle fibres and extensive adipose tissue replacement. Gastrocnemius. (a) Verhoeff-van Gieson stain × 95; (b) NADH-TR × 95.)

microscopy shows non-specific changes of degeneration of fibres. Immunocytochemical techniques have shown the persistence of fetal and slow myosin in many of these fibres, even after they acquire fast myosin.

The term 'dystrophic' as applied to a muscle biopsy is a summation of the various changes described above. The degree of change varies from patient to patient and does not always correlate closely with the clinical picture. Any attempt at accurate diagnosis and prognosis, and particularly at trying to differentiate Duchenne type dystrophy from the milder Becker or limb girdle varieties, should be based on a combined appraisal of the clinical severity relative to the patient's age, together with the muscle biopsy and other special investigations.

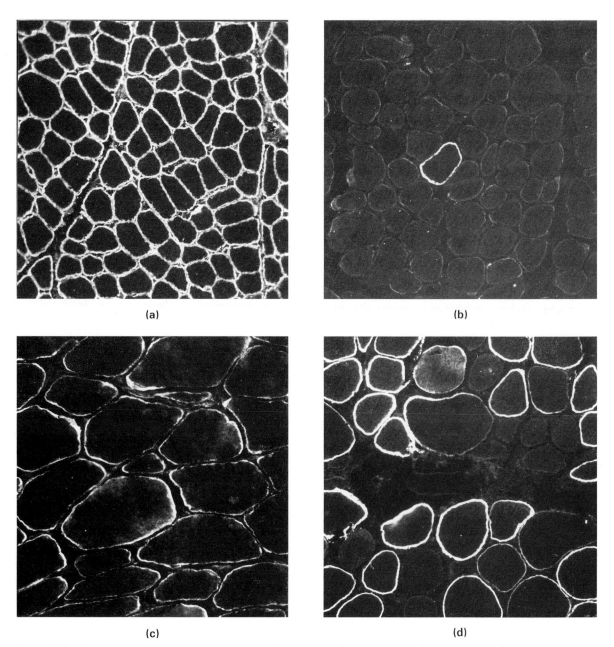

(a)

(b)

(c)

(d)

Figure 2-22a-d Immunocytochemical staining for dystrophin using an immunofluorescence antibody technique. (a) Normal muscle showing localization to the sarcolemma. (b) Duchenne dystrophy showing complete absence of dystrophin, apart from occasional positive ('revertant') fibre (centre). (c) Becker dystrophy showing irregular, patchy staining of dystrophin. (d) Manifesting Duchenne carrier showing mosaic of normal and negative or partly deficient fibres.

Dystrophin

With the recognition of the protein that is specific to Duchenne dystrophy, the assessment of dystrophin in the muscle biopsy has become an essential part of the examination (Figures 2-22, 2-23). Immunocytochemical staining of sections is a very sensitive way for assessing the presence and distribution of dystrophin. For assessing molecular size or quantity of dystrophin, Western blot is necessary, using similar antibodies. Absence of dystrophin confirms the diagnosis; presence of normal levels of dystrophin is incompatible with a diagnosis of Duchenne dystrophy and suggests an alternative diagnosis of an autosomal recessive, Duchenne-like dystrophy. The presence of altered size or abundance suggests a milder form of the Xp21 dystrophy

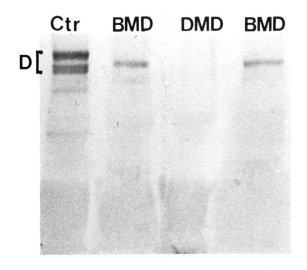

Figure 2-23 Western blot showing presence of normal dystrophin bands (230 kD) in control muscle (lane 1), absence of dystrophin in Duchenne muscle (lane 3), and dystrophin of reduced amount and size in Becker dystrophy (lanes 2 & 4).

and usually conforms to the clinical picture of the Becker type or an intermediate severity. Carriers usually show a normal pattern on immunocytochemical staining of muscle sections, but young carriers or manifesting carriers may show a mosaic pattern.

Certain regions of the massive Duchenne gene (over two million base pairs) have been found to be hot spots for deletions, and most of the Becker deletions have been confined to an area between exons 40 and 55 (see below).

MANAGEMENT

As long as the child with Duchenne dystrophy is ambulant, he can usually lead a reasonably independent existence and cope with most of his daily activities. These children can usually manage at an ordinary school while ambulant and should be encouraged to do so.

Once the child loses ambulation he loses much of his independence too, and is also prone to various complications in the way of muscle contractures and deformities. Efforts should thus be directed at maintenance of ambulation for as long as possible and at prevention of deformity.

While ambulant there is little tendency to deformity apart from fixed equinus of the feet and flexion contractures at the hips as a result of the tendency to forward tilting of the pelvis and toe

walking. These contractures can be prevented or slowed in their progression by regular passive exercises, which take the joints through a full range of movement, and by encouraging the child to spend part of his time lying prone on the floor when reading or watching television. This will keep the hips extended. Night splints to support the ankles in a neutral position (90°) are also useful.

The patient should be encouraged to remain ambulant under all circumstances, since even short periods of immobility in association with minor illness or trauma can lead to marked deterioration in muscle power and loss of ambulation.

Rehabilitation after loss of ambulation

Spencer and Vignos (1962) introduced the concept of prolonging the period of active walking in Duchenne dystrophy by the fitting of leg braces at the stage when the child is losing the ability to get around independently. In this way ambulation may continue for up to a further 3 years or so. Any contractures at the hip, knees or ankles present at the time of fitting of callipers have to be released by tenotomy, in order to get the patient into a functional position for fitting the callipers. Although this approach has not found universal appeal, perhaps because of the combined team effort required from the orthopaedic surgeon, the physician and the physiotherapist to achieve any degree of success, those centres that have adopted it have usually been enthusiastic about the results, as have the patients and their families.

It is important to get the child mobile rapidly after any surgical procedure, which usually means standing in his plaster casts within 24 hours of surgery. The use of percutaneous tenotomy has shortened the postoperative period and also means less extensive incisions (Siegel *et al.*, 1968). Tenotomy for release of contractures in Duchenne dystrophy is of practical value *only* in the context of fitting these orthoses and has no place in isolation in the management of muscular dystrophy.

These children usually co-operate well with the fitting of callipers and can also be readily mobilized in their plaster casts within 24 hours postoperatively (Figures 2-24 and 2-25). The casts can then be bivalved the following day to allow for measurements for the orthoses. In some boys where the fixed equinovarus deformity of the feet is not too marked it is possible to take a mould for preparation of the orthoses prior to the tenotomy and to antipate the position of the ankle, and thus go straight into the orthoses postoperatively. This enables one to dispense with the somewhat cumbersome provision of the plaster casts in between, which always need to be well moulded and well padded around the ankles to avoid any pressure sores.

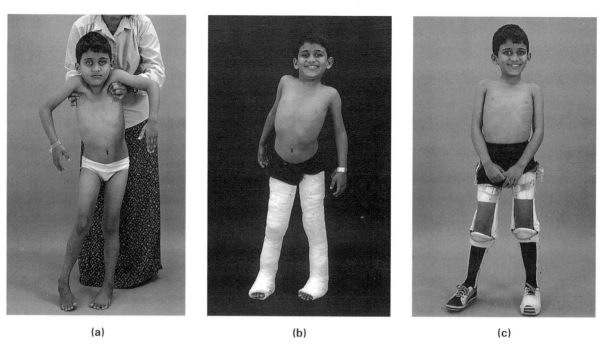

(a)   (b)   (c)

Figure 2-24a-c Duchenne muscular dystrophy. An 8-year-old boy with loss of ability to stand or walk. Note fixed equinovarus deformity particularly affecting the right foot (a); (b) the same boy 12 days later after percutaneous tenotomy of tendo Achilles bilaterally, and ambulant postoperatively in plaster casts and (c) subsequently 2 weeks later fully ambulant in lightweight polypropylene orthoses.

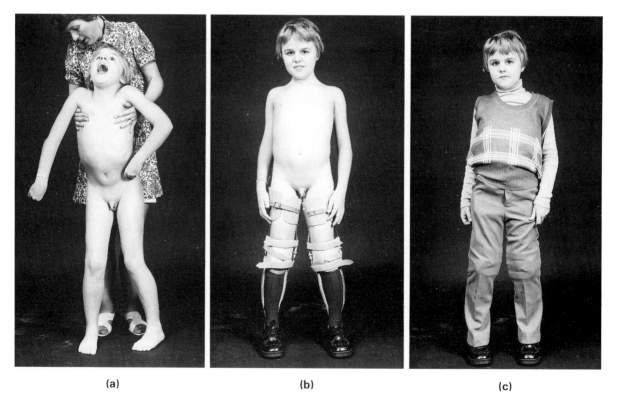

(a)   (b)   (c)

Figure 2-25a-c Duchenne dystrophy in an 11-year-old boy who had been off his feet for 3 months and unable to stand (a), remobilized (b) and (c) within a week of fitting lightweight moulded polypropylene callipers.

The use of lightweight polyethylene, ischial weightbearing orthoses, which can be closely moulded to the contour of the legs, instead of the more traditional metal ones ('leg irons'), has distinct advantages of being lighter in weight and being more cosmetic, as well as more functional. It allows the use of ordinary trousers and light-weight shoes, and the child can usually be mobilized much more speedily (Siegel, 1977) (Figures 2-24, 2-25).

It has been our policy to provide these orthoses only at the stage that the child has lost functional walking and is at the stage that he is still able to stand independently but not able to take more than a few steps. There does not seem to be any advantage in intervening at an earlier stage, when the boy is still independently ambulant. It is also important to monitor the patient regularly at this phase of difficulty in ambulation, in order to anticipate and plan the intervention and not to have to face the additional problem of having lost ambulation some weeks or even months earlier with increase in contractures, loss of power and more difficulty with achieving rehabilitation. In general we have not found associated intellectual retardation to be a contraindication to rehabilitation, as long as the child and his parents have been reasonably motivated to go ahead.

In our experience, percutaneous tenotomy of the tendo Achillis by itself is usually sufficient to achieve a good posture of the legs in the orthoses and additional release of the hip flexors is unnecessary. In a review of our initial 57 consecutive cases (Heckmatt *et al.*, 1985), including early failures due to delay in supply of orthoses, 47 achieved independent ambulation, and in the 27 who had subsequently already lost ambulation, we obtained on average a period of further ambulation in callipers of 22 months, with a range from 6 to 48 months.

One additional bonus is that these children, while continuing ambulation, do not develop scoliosis, which is a major problem of the non-ambulant child, and in addition when they do subsequently stop walking and become chairbound, particularly if after the age of 12, the rate of progression of scoliosis is much slower than those going directly into wheelchairs at an earlier age (Rodillo *et al.*, 1988).

Early surgical intervention

In an effort to avoid the need for orthoses, Rideau (1984) tried to stabilize ambulation, in boys approaching a stage of increasing difficulty, by transferring various tendons around the hips or ankles in an effort to balance the selective weakness of the hip extensors or ankle dorsiflexors. When this

proved unsuccessful, he tried to intervene surgically at an earlier stage and eventually found that early surgical procedures at around 4–6 years of age, when muscle power was still good but early contractures already present, could be beneficial (Rideau *et al.*, 1986). He recommended percutaneous lengthening of the tendo Achillis, plus percutaneous release, as appropriate, of any tight superficial muscles at the hip or knee flexors, together with bilateral resection of the whole fascia lata. He claimed that this improved the quality of the motor funtion by normalizing the gait, allowing some of the children to achieve the ability to run, and also improving the ability to get up from the floor with a quicker Gowers' manoeuvre or no Gowers', and then remaining static for several years. There was then a rapid increase in Gowers' time followed by increasing difficulty with, and finally loss of, ambulation. He did not have any data on whether these children lost ambulation any later than they might have without intervention. At that stage he did not recommend orthoses but provided a wheelchair and advised surgical fixation of the spine prior to the onset of scoliosis.

In a subsequent randomized, controlled trial of surgical intervention along these lines versus conservative treatment, we found no difference between the two groups of Duchenne boys in the rate of decline of their muscle force and function, and apart from the improved posture of their feet there seemed to be no advantage in this fairly extensive surgical intervention (Manzur *et al.*, 1992). The same conclusions have recently been drawn by Granata *et al.* (1994) in an open study of surgical intervention in seven Duchenne boys.

Scoliosis and other deformities

Once the child becomes chairbound he is very prone to develop various deformities which can be rapidly progressive (see Figure 2-10). These deformities can be partly prevented by adequate attention to the posture of the spine and limbs (Figure 2-26). The back should be maintained in a vertical position with a slightly backward incline in the wheelchair, to avoid rotation and lateral flexion to one or the other side. The backrest of the wheelchair should be of a soft material and sufficiently flexible to give support to the spine. In addition, moulded jackets can be applied direct to the trunk to help to maintain it in a straight position. It is useful to take an X-ray of the whole dorsolumbar spine in a sitting position when the child goes off his feet to detect any early sign of scoliosis, and to monitor it by serial X-ray at regular intervals.

Recent advances in the instrumentation for surgical immobilization of the spine, and the use of

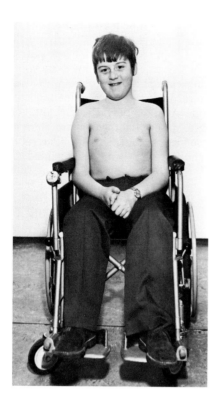
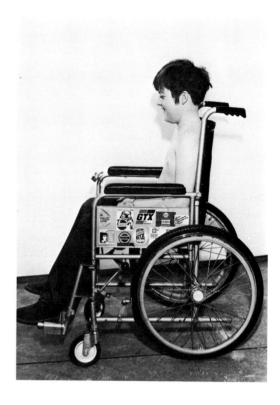

Figure 2-26   Child with Duchenne dystrophy in wheelchair after loss of ambulation. Note good vertical posture of spine. Wheelchair has soft curved backrest and slight backward incline to support the child's back. Seat is firm to prevent tilting of pelvis. Feet are in good resting posture at approximately 90° angle.

techniques such as the Luque procedure for anchoring of individual vertebrae to the metal rods, has greatly expedited the postoperative rehabilitation and allowed early sitting without the need for any prolonged immobilization or use of a spinal brace (Boachie Adjei *et al.*, 1989; Miller *et al.*, 1991; Galasko *et al.*, 1992; Miller *et al.*, 1992a; Shapiro *et al.*, 1992; Bellen *et al.*, 1993). This has made surgical intervention for scoliosis more feasible in Duchenne dystrophy and with increasing experience with this approach it would seem logical to intervene at an earlier stage of incipient progressive scoliosis, when the Cobb angle is around 30° and the respiratory function still good, rather than deferring it to a stage when the scoliosis is much more advanced, the operation technically more difficult and the respiratory reserve further compromised. Once scoliosis develops it is much more difficult to treat and arrest and tends to be steadily progressive.

Equinovarus deformity of feet. The feet should be kept as close as possible to a right angle. The fitting of supportive boots is helpful and attention should be given to the proper position of the footrests of the wheelchair to maintain the ankles at 90°.

Deformities can be a source of marked discomfort to the child in the late stages of Duchenne dystrophy and it is worth making an effort to prevent them.

Drug therapy

Ever since the time of Duchenne himself, there have been claims for the successful treatment of muscular dystrophy, with a wide variety of drugs and an equally variable degree of logic or rationale for their use. The trials were almost invariably inadequate and uncontrolled and it often took a subsequent well-controlled and more objective study to negate the initial results.

Following an invitation to contribute a review on therapy of Duchenne dystrophy to a special issue of the *British Medical Bulletin*, we reviewed all the available reports in the literature from 1940 to 1980 (Dubowitz and Heckmatt, 1980). In order to assess the value of the individual studies, we devised a 5-point 'quality control score', with a point for each of the following criteria: careful selection and definition of cases; adequate controls; objective ('blind') study; objective measurement of changes in muscle function; adequate duration of the trial (at least 2 years). Of 34 drug trials reviewed, 17 scored 0, seven scored 1, three scored 2, three scored 3, four scored 4, and none scored 5. It is of interest that the drug was considered to be of value in 15 of the 17 trials which had a quality score of 0, four of the seven with a score of 1, two of the three with a score of 2, but none of the three somewhat better constructed trials with a score of 3, or of the four with a score of 4 (see Table 2-3).

We suggested at the time that much time, energy and expense could be spared if editors of journals refused to publish any therapeutic claims which scored under 3. In a further review some 10 years later, we undertook a similar appraisal of publications during the 10 years since our first review (Heckmatt *et al.*, 1989). We added an additional scoring point for prospective trials which were shown statistically to have an 80% chance of detecting a 75% slowing of the disease process. We were impressed with the overall improvement in the quality of the trials, but there were still some publications with poor standards of control. Of ten reports reviewed, none scored 0, one scored 1, one scored 2, one scored 3, three each 4 and 5, and one scored 6. It is of interest that in none of the trials scoring 3 or more was the drug thought to be of benefit, in contrast to both trials scoring 1 or 2 (see Table 2-4).

A major contribution in the standardization of therapeutic trials in muscular dystrophy came from the multicentric trials introduced by Brooke and his colleagues (Brooke *et al*, 1981a,b; 1983). Methods were devised for working out the statistical power of a trial and the number of patients required to achieve a particular percentage improvement in a particular function over a set time period. In order to recruit the required number of subjects, a wide range of age and severity were included, ranging from early ambulant cases to late chairbound ones. This added to the complexity of standardizing the criteria for assessment.

In a double-blind therapeutic trial of isaxonine, a drug claimed to stimulate nerve growth and to have some beneficial effect both clinically and pathologically in dystrophic chicks, we were able to achieve a statistical power comparable with the large multicentric trials, with a small well-controlled unicentric trial, by careful selection of subjects within a narrow range of age and severity (Heckmatt *et al.*, 1988), and to demonstrate that the drug had no therapeutic benefit.

The same rigid criteria apply to all therapeutic trials, whether they be drugs, physical interventions, or novel experimental procedures, such as myoblast transfer (see below).

Table 2-3 Drug trials (1940–1979) (n = 34)

Quality control score	No.	Considered of value by authors
0	17	15
1	7	4
2	3	2
3	3	0
4	4	0
5	0	0

Table 2-4 Drug trials (1980–1989) (n = 10)

Quality control score	No.	Considered of value by authors
0	0	0
1	1	1
2	1	1
3	1	0
4	3	0
5	3	0
6	1	0

The current situation. Of all the drugs that have fallen by the wayside over the years the only one that still seems to be holding its own is prednisone.

Some 20 years ago, in an uncontrolled study of 14 Duchenne patients, Drachman and his colleagues (1974) concluded that steroids might have some palliative value and that further trials were indicated. It was 13 years before Brooke and his colleagues took up the challenge (Brooke *et al.*, 1987). In a multicentric study of 33 cases of Duchenne dystrophy, aged 5 to 15 years (12 of whom had already lost ambulation), they found a definite improvement in muscle function on prednisone, at a dose of 1.5 mg/kg/day for 6 months, in comparison with the natural history of 170 historical controls from their earlier studies.

Brooke and his colleagues (Mendell *et al.*, 1989) subsequently undertook a randomized, double blind, multicentric, controlled study of 103 Duchenne boys, aged 5 to 15 years, over a 6-month period, comparing two steroid dosage levels (0.75 and 1.5 mg/kg/day) with placebo. They found a definite increase in muscle strength in the two prednisone groups, compared with the control, at 1, 2 and 3 months, after which the strength levelled off.

The rate of loss of muscle strength in the control group was similar to the natural history of the disease. They concluded, however, that the relatively short-lived beneficial effect on the muscle strength was outweighed by the not-inconsiderable side-effects of prolonged steroid therapy, and did not at the time feel able to recommend steroids as a general long-term therapy for muscular dystrophy.

In a further multicentric study (Griggs *et al.*, 1991 a,b), a randomized controlled trial of daily prednisone was undertaken in 99 boys with Duchenne dystrophy, aged 5–15 years, in order to define the time course of improvement and the dose response to treatment. Prednisone at 0.75 mg/kg (n = 34), 0.3 mg/kg (n = 33) or placebo (n = 32), was given for 6 months. As early as 10 days after commencing treatment, there was a significantly higher average muscle strength score in the two groups on prednisone treatment, compared with the placebo. This improvement increased at 1 month and then reached a plateau that persisted for 6 months and contrasted with the placebo group that became steadily weaker. At 3 months the boys in the 0.75 mg/kg group showed a significantly better average muscle strength than those at 0.3 mg/kg, indicating a dose response. At 10 days and 1 month of treatment there were no side-effects of the prednisone, despite improvement in muscle strength and function. At 6 months there were significant side-effects in the group on 0.75 mg/kg, including weight gain, cushingoid appearance and excessive hair growth, whereas the 0.3 mg/kg group showed only weight gain.

An attempt was made to maintain 89 boys from these multicentric trials on continued therapy for a year or longer (Fenichel *et al.*, 1991). At the end of a year, 49 were taking at least 0.65 mg/kg/day and 40 a greater dose. The rate of decline in average muscle score (0.017 units/year) was significantly better in the first group than in the lower dosage group (0.164 units/year) (p = 0.0021) and both did better than natural history controls (0.4 units/year).

In a further controlled trial, Griggs *et al.* (1993) randomized 99 boys with Duchenne dystrophy, aged 5–15 years, into one of three groups: (1) placebo; (2) prednisone 0.3 mg/kg/day; (3) prednisone 0.75mg/kg/day. After 6 months, azathioprine was added in groups 1 and 2 and placebo in group 3. As in their earlier studies, the results showed an increase in muscle strength with prednisone within 10 days. It was significantly greater with 0.75 mg/kg/day and reached a maximum at 3 months and then plateaued. The beneficial effect was maintained over the 18 months of this prednisone therapy, but there were significant side-effects, particularly weight gain and growth retardation. Azathioprine had no effect on muscle strength. The authors now concluded that

prednisone was of sufficient benefit to be recommended for ambulatory patients over age 5 years, and continued if side-effects were not severe.

It is difficult from a clinical point of view to translate into actual functional benefit for the patient the statistically significant rise from 5.7 to 6.0 in the average muscle strength score, based on the assessment of 34 muscle groups on a 10-point MRC grading. On the other hand, it is extremely impressive that the score remained static over the 18 month period of treatment, compared with a decline of about 0.4 points in the placebo group, and might presumably continue to remain stable on continued treatment.

In addition to the gain in muscle strength, parallel studies in these various trials also showed an increase in muscle mass, based on creatine excretion, and a fall in the rate of muscle breakdown, based on a decreased excretion of 3-methyl histidine. There was no increase in the expression of dystrophin in the muscle or reduction in the number of necrotic fibres, but there was a significant reduction in the total number of T-cells (CD2 +), and selectively of the subsets of CD8 + cytotoxic suppressor T-cells (Kissel *et al.*, 1991). This suggested that the beneficial effect of prednisone might be through suppression of the immune attack on necrotic fibres. Somewhat surprisingly, Kissel *et al.* (1993) subsequently found no differences between the three groups of patients receiving prednisone or azathioprine with respect to the total T-cells, T-cell subsets, B-cells, natural killer cells, total mononuclear cells, necrotic muscle fibres, or fibres focally invaded by mononuclear cells. Since the azathioprine-treated patients did not show any associated clinical improvement, this was considered to imply that the therapeutic effect of the prednisone was not primarily through the effect on the cellular infiltrates.

Although muscular dystrophy is not normally considered as an immunological disorder, there is considerable evidence that both humoral and cellular immune responses contribute to the pathological process. Whilst it has been recognized for years that necrotic fibres in muscular dystrophy were invaded by macrophages, Arahata and Engel (1984) showed with selective monoclonal antibodies that many of these mononuclear cells were in fact cytotoxic T-cells. In addition, complement activation with deposition of membrane attack complex was observed on necrotic fibres (Engel and Biesecker, 1982). Furthermore, it has been found that HLA class I antigens (MHCI) are expressed in Duchenne dystrophy fibres, as in polymyositis, but not in normal muscle (Appleyard *et al.*, 1985; Emslie–Smith *et al.*, 1989). This would render the dystrophic muscle susceptible to T-cell-mediated attack.

If prednisone proves to be beneficial in arresting the disease process on a long-term basis, it might be worth devising alternative therapeutic regimes aimed at achieving the benefits but avoiding the side-effects, such as an intermittent schedule of prednisone at 0.75 mg/kg/day for, say, 10 days each month (Dubowitz, 1991). In an open, pilot study of this low dosage intermittent schedule in 32 cases of Duchenne dystrophy, all of whom were still ambulant, either independently or in orthoses, Sansome *et al.* (1993) showed some initial improvement in the average scores over the first 6 months, followed by a steady decline. There was a substantial reduction in amount of weight gain and other side-effects, compared with the daily dosage regimes. Adequately controlled studies will be necessary to assess the relative benefit of this regime against other schedules.

Similar beneficial results to those with prednisone have been obtained in two small randomized trials with deflazocort, an oxazoline derivative of prednisolone claimed to have fewer side-effects (Angelini *et al.*, 1991; Mesa *et al.*, 1991).

Of additional interest in this therapeutic context is a recent report by Sharma *et al.* (1993) of a comparable response in Duchenne dystrophy to another immunosuppressive drug, cyclosporine, which, like prednisone, also reduces the number of cytotoxic lymphocytes and may also interfere with the production of interleukin, various cytokines, and gamma-interferon by T-lymphocytes, possibly preventing muscle fibre degeneration or allowing damaged fibres to regenerate. In a study of 15 Duchenne boys they showed an increase in the maximum voluntary contraction, the tetanic tension, the twitch tension and the maximum compound muscle action potential of the anterior tibial muscles bilaterally, during a 2-month period on cyclosporine (5mg/kg/day), compared with a steady decline during a prior 4-month natural history phase and a subsequent 4-month drug washout phase.

If this approach with immunosuppressive drugs is able to arrest the disease, this could provide a very valuable moratorium for patients while the potential benefits of cell or gene therapy are currently still being explored (see below).

CARRIER DETECTION ————————

The female carrier of the X-linked Duchenne gene usually shows no clinical signs of the disease, but may on occasion manifest minor features such as muscle enlargement, especially of one calf, or even minor or more severe degrees of weakness.

Prior to the advent of recombinant DNA technology, the most reliable method of carrier detection was the elevated CK (Ebashi *et al.*, 1959; Dreyfus *et al.*, 1960). About 70% of genetically obligate carriers show a raised CK. The degree of elevation may be only slight to moderate, so reliable technique is essential. Whilst an elevated CK in a potential carrier would thus suggest a presumptive carrier, a normal CK could not exclude a carrier status.

Muscle biopsy also had a place in carrier detection (Dubowitz, 1963a,b; Emery, 1963; Pearson *et al.*, 1963) and, as in the case of CK, abnormality could be detected in some definite carriers and not in others, and comparative studies showed that the biopsy might show unequivocal abnormality even when the serum enzyme levels were normal (Dubowitz, 1963b; Dubowitz and Roy, 1970; Maunder–Sewry and Dubowitz, 1981). The changes were usually of a relatively mild and focal nature and it was often difficult to decide whether such changes were within the normal range. This was helped by objective quantitation of some of the aberrant features (Maunder–Sewry and Dubowitz, 1981).

All this has now been overtaken and largely superseded by the application of the new molecular genetic techniques to the study of muscular dystrophy. However, the routine estimate of the serum CK in potential carriers still remains useful in separating those with elevated levels, who are presumptive carriers, from those with normal levels, who may still be carriers. As will be seen below, not all cases can be clearly resolved by the DNA studies in themselves either.

Monozygotic twin carriers

There have been several reports of monozygotic twins carrying a mutation in the Duchenne gene, but with discordant clinical phenotype (Gomez *et al.*, 1977; Burn *et al.*, 1986; Chutkow *et al.*, 1987; Pena *et al.*, 1987; Ionasescu *et al.*, 1989; Bonilla *et al.*, 1990; Richards *et al.*, 1990; Lupski *et al.*, 1991; Zneimer *et al.*, 1993). This has been ascribed to unequal lyonization in the twins, with the paternal X-chromosome being preferentially inactivated in the manifesting carrier, and the maternal X-chromosome, carrying the mutation, in the normal one. The manifesting twin has often shown a full-blown pattern of severity comparable with a Duchenne phenotype in affected boys. Tremblay *et al.* (1993) recently attempted a therapeutic myoblast transfer with cultured muscle from the unaffected twin into the extensor carpi radialis muscle of the affected twin, a control injection being given into the other side. There was only a very slight difference in the proportion of dystrophin-positive fibres in the experimentally injected versus the control extensor carpi radialis, but they apparently found a significant gain in force of the wrist extensors on that side.

THE MOLECULAR GENETIC EXPLOSION

Locating the gene

The discovery of the gene locus for Duchenne dystrophy at Xp21 came, almost simultaneously, from three sources. Through the application of the new techniques of molecular genetics, it became possible to isolate DNA sequences from cloned fragments derived from the human X chromosome and to determine their exact location. Duchenne dystrophy was the first disease to be localized in this way by linkage with these restriction fragment length polymorphisms (RFLPs) (Murray *et al.*, 1982). Secondly, a number of documented females with Duchenne dystrophy, associated with an X:autosomal translocation, all had the breakpoint on the X chromosome at this locus (Figure 2-27). (For review see Dubowitz, 1986.) Thirdly, a number of cases of Duchenne dystrophy with associated X-linked disorders, such as chronic granulomatous disease, retinitis pigmentosa and McLeod's syndrome, were found to have a cytogenetically visible deletion at the same site (Francke *et al.*, 1985). Linkage studies in cases of Becker dystrophy pointed to the same locus, confirming that the two conditions are allelic and due to abnormalities in the same gene. This fits in with the clinical observation that Becker dystrophy has a similar clinical pattern to Duchenne apart from its later onset and milder course and that there is an overlap of cases between the two (Dubowitz, 1978).

Isolating, cloning and characterizing the gene

Two different strategies were used to try and isolate the Duchenne gene. Worton and his co-workers isolated the junctional region from a Duchenne female with an X:21 translocation, documented by Verellen–Dumoulin *et al.* (1984). They cloned the region spanning the translocation breakpoint, which at least contained part of the Duchenne locus. A sequence derived from this clone (XJ1.1) detected an RFLP closely linked to Duchenne dystrophy and also failed to hybridize with DNA from some patients with Duchenne dystrophy, indicating the presence of a deletion of the region complementary to the probe (Worton *et al.*, 1984; Ray *et al.*, 1985).

The isolation of the gene was achieved by Kunkel and his colleagues by an ingenious approach of preparing a library of cloned sequences (the pERT probes, 'phenol enhanced recombination technique') from the region of the normal X chromosome corresponding to the DNA deleted in a patient with Duchenne dystrophy, chronic granulomatous disease, retinitis pigmentosa and McLeod's syndrome and a visible deletion in the Xp21 region

(Kunkel *et al.*, 1985). This was followed within a comparatively short period of time by the complete cloning of the gene (Koenig *et al.*, 1987), and the discovery of the protein product of the gene, which they named dystrophin (Hoffman *et al.*, 1987a). The gene is a gigantic size, encompassing over 2000 kilobases (2 million base pairs), with around 80 exons spanning the gene. Dystrophin is a correspondingly large, 3685 amino acid, protein of 427 kilodaltons in size, but with very low abundance, comprising only about 0.002% of total striated muscle protein, but with obvious importance in relation to the muscle membrane. It is structurally related to the cytoskeletal proteins β-spectrin and α-actinin.

This major breakthrough generated a considerable amount of interest and further research, gradually unravelling the complexities of the gene, of dystrophin and also of its associated proteins, which have recently proved important in relation to some of the other forms of dystrophy, such as limb girdle dystrophy and congenital muscular dystrophy (see below). We now know that there are at least five different forms of dystrophin, which are specific in their cellular localizations and also have separate promoters. Three of these dystrophins are full-length, the muscle (M), cortical (C) and purkinje cell (P), and have their own first exons in addition to their distinct promoters. The other two promoters, Schwann cell (S) and general or glial (G) encode smaller proteins near the C-terminal end, which are not expressed in muscle. Ahn and Kunkel (1993) have provided an exhaustive review of all these advances, together with a series of colour-coded illustrations which I found extremely illuminating and helpful in understanding and visualizing this complex subject (Colour plate 1A, B, C, facing p. 64).

Clinical application

These advances found immediate application to clinical practice. With the flanking markers it became possible to detect carriers within affected families with a far greater precision than had previously been possible on the basis of CK estimation. This was further refined by the development of intragenic probes (Hodgson and Bobrow, 1989). Once the gene was isolated and sequenced, Kunkel made available to laboratories around the world a series of cDNA probes which made possible the screening in index cases for deletion of individual exons within the gene. Some 65–70% of cases of Duchenne or Becker cases had deletions in the gene, and a further small proportion had duplications. The remainder presumably had point mutations not detectable by existing techniques.

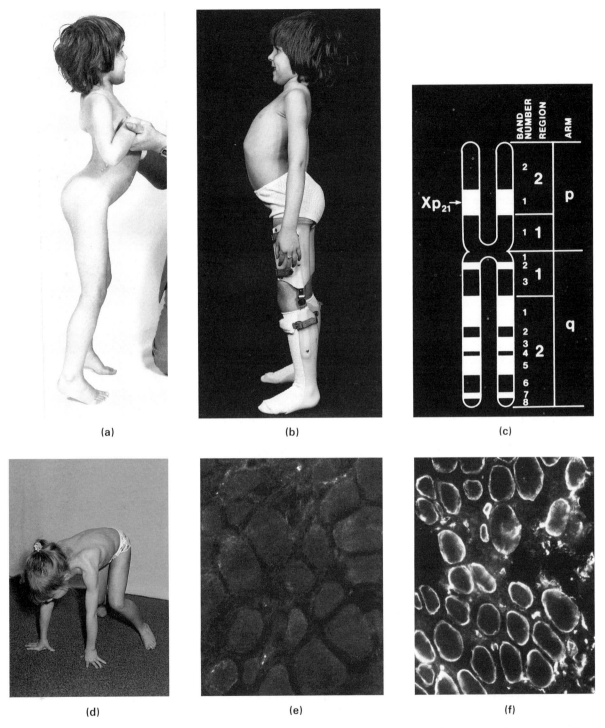

Figure 2-27a-f Female with classical Duchenne dystrophy associated with a translocation between chromosomes X and 1. Loss of ambulation at 7 years and rehabilitation in callipers (a,b). Muscle biopsy showed typical features of Duchenne type dystrophy with marked variation in fibre size, proliferation of connective tissue and some associated adipose tissue. In females with Duchenne dystrophy and X-autosome translocation, the break on the X chromosome is always in the region of Xp21, the locus of the Duchenne gene (c). (d-f) Another girl, aged 7 years, with a Duchenne-type muscular dystrophy, getting up with a Gowers' manoeuvre (d). She has an X-9 translocation with breakpoint at Xp21, and her muscle biopsy showed a dystrophic picture and was completely negative for dystrophin (e, Dys 1 antibody) but had a normal sarcolemmal stain with spectrin antibodies (f).

Contrary to early speculations, neither the size of the deletion nor its location bears any consistent relation to the severity of the clinical condition. In a review of 218 of our patients with Duchenne, Becker or intermediate phenotypes, 124 had deletions with the cDNA probes (Hodgson *et al.*, 1989). Seventy-four separate deletions were found, with 55 being unique to one patient and the remaining 19 occurring in at least two unrelated patients. Some deletions such as of exons 33–34 and 33–35 occurred only with Becker patients, and of exons 3–7 in four patients with intermediate severity and one Becker. We also found no correlation of associated mental retardation with any selective deletions.

In order to explain the varying clinical severity, Monaco *et al.* (1988) postulated that in Duchenne dystrophy the deletion, irrespective of size, leads to a frame shift of the triplet codons for amino acids, resulting in a severely truncated non-functional protein, whereas in Becker dystrophy the nucleotides remain in frame, and can produce a functional protein, although reduced in size (see p. 79). Over 90% of cases with deletions conform to this hypothesis. There have, however, been some exceptions. Thus deletion of exons 3–7, which is out of frame, usually seems to be associated with a milder phenotype, mostly of intermediate severity but at times even well within the Becker range (Malhotra *et al.*, 1988; Gangopadhyay *et al.*, 1992) (Figures 2-28 to 2-30).

Technological advances

It was of particular interest that these deletions tended to cluster around two particular 'hot-spot' regions of the gene, one encompassing exons 3–30 and the other exons 44–55. This meant that the majority of deletions could be detected by focusing on a relatively small number of exons within the gene. A method was developed by Chamberlain *et al.* (1988) for rapid screening for these deletions by the application of the polymerase chain reaction for amplifying the DNA in these regions, simultaneously using a number of appropriate primers which flank these hot spot regions, the so-called multiplex PCR technique. The method can be completed within 24 hours and, with the addition of further groups of primers, is now capable of detecting over 98% of the existing deletions (Chamberlain *et al.*, 1991; Beggs and Kunkel, 1990; Abbs *et al.*, 1991).

Presumably the remaining third or so of patients without a detectable deletion have point mutations. Roberts *et al.* (1991) have recently devised a method for detecting these point mutations by a complex method using RNA from lymphocytes.

Colour plate 1

A: Schematic diagram of dystrophins and their relatives. The actin-binding domain (red) is shared among a large number of actin-binding cytoskeletal proteins. The long internal region (green) consists of 24 homologous repeats of 109 amino acids, hypothesized to form a long flexible rod-like domain. The cysteine-rich region (purple) is homologous to the Ca^{2+}-binding EF-hand region of α-actinin. The C-terminus (yellow) is homologous only to dystrophin-related protein (DRP) and may participate in dystrophin association with the membrane.

B: The dystrophin gene. *Top line*: at least five distinct promoters drive independent cell-type specific expression of dystrophin. The C (cortical)-, M (muscle)- and P (Purkinje cell)-dystrophins, the 'full-length' forms, each use their own first exon. The S(Schwann cell)- and G (general or glial)-dystrophin promoters encode C-terminal proteins Dp116 and Dp71 respectively. *Middle line*: a map of the 79 (plus 4 additional first) exons of dystrophin, spanning 2.4 million bases. Bars represent approximate relative exon positions, and their colours represent the encoded domain. *Bottom line*: schematic domain map of the dystrophin polypeptide (see A).

C: Interactions of dystrophin. Schematic diagram of some of the proposed intermolecular interactions of dystrophin. Dystrophin is proposed to aggregate as a homo-tetramer and associate with actin at its N-terminus and the dystrophin-associated glycoprotein (DAGC) complex near the C-terminus. In skeletal muscle, dystrophin localizes at the costameres, which contain α-actin and vinculin and their associated proteins.

From Ahn and Kunkel 1993, courtesy of the authors and by permission of *Nature Genetics*.

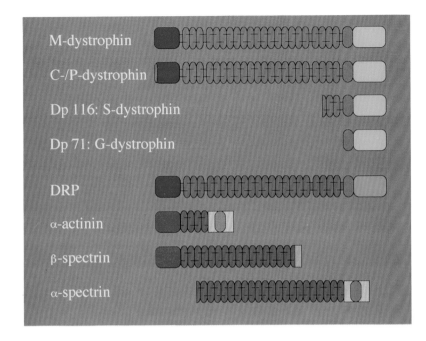

A

B

C

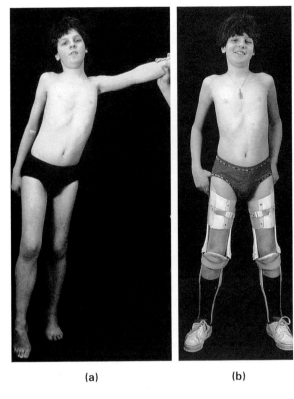

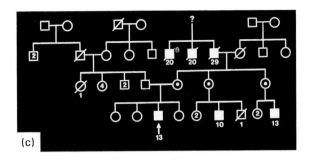

(c)

(a)　　　　　　　　　**(b)**

Figure 2-28a-c Intermediate severity Duchenne/Becker muscular dystrophy. This patient referred at 14 years of age for rehabilitation was still able to stand and walk short distances on the level but mobility was severely limited (a). Rehabilitation with percutaneous tenotomy of tendo Achilles and provision of callipers (b). He had an interesting family history (c). His maternal grandfather was affected by muscular dystrophy and died at 29 years of age. His mother was very young when her father died and cannot recall any detail about his disability. Her father also had two brothers who were affected. His other two daughters who would be obligate carriers, each has an affected son (aged 10 and 13 years at the time). The 13-year-old cousin remained ambulant until 16 years. A deletion of exons 3–7 was found.

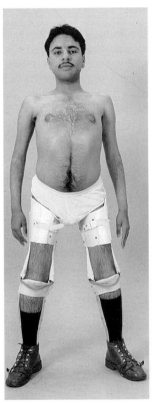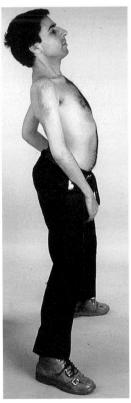

(a)　　　　　　　　　**(b)**

Figure 2-29a,b Intermediate muscular dystrophy. In this patient biopsy at 5 years of age showed marked dystrophic change with adipose and connective tissue proliferation. He subsequently was losing the ability to walk at 12 years of age and was remobilized in callipers. He continued to be ambulant until 20 years of age with five intervening replacements of callipers to allow for growth (a,b). At 20 years he was still able to stand but no longer able to walk. At 26 years he is currently still able to stand in callipers and sway his back from side to side. He has no scoliosis. He has a 3–7 exon deletion (see Figure 2-30).

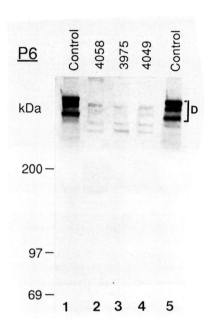

Figure 2-30 Western blot showing normal dystrophin band (D) (437 kD), lane 1 and 5. Note three bands normally present with polyclonal antibody P6 to rod domain. Lanes 3, 4 and 5 show three cases with 3–7 exon deletion. Note reduction in size of the dystrophin to about 380 kD and marked reduction in amount (about 10–15% of normal). Column 2 (4058) is from the patient in Figure 2.29 and column 3 (3975) from the asymptomatic 6-year-old boy with fatal post-anaesthetic rhabdomyolysis, documented by Bush and Dubowitz (1991).

Carrier detection

The advent of linked markers with the Duchenne gene already made a tremendous impact on the accuracy with which one could either confirm or exclude the possibility of carrier status in an at risk female within a family. This applied particularly in those cases where the CK was normal, which in itself could not exclude a carrier status as there was still a 30% risk of being a carrier with a normal level. In most of these cases one could convert a residual risk of around 10–15% based on CK and Bayesian calculations to a more than 95% confidence either for or against carrier status (Hodgson and Bobrow, 1989).

The isolation and characterization of the gene and possibility for identifying mutations in individual cases further extended the sensitivity of carrier detection. Once a deletion is detected in an index case this of course provides a direct marker for antenatal diagnosis or carrier detection. Current progress in detecting point mutations in index cases without deletions is opening the way for carrier detection in such families as well. The technology is rapidly moving from the research plane to clinical application.

Dystrophin in muscle biopsies

The recognition of the protein gene product of the Duchenne gene provided another means for the diagnosis of Xp21 myopathies by direct examination of the muscle. This was initially done with *Western blot* analysis, the proteins in the muscle being separated by electrophoresis and then probed with antibodies raised to fusion proteins corresponding to part of the dystrophin molecule. In their initial studies of dystrophin in relation to Duchenne and Becker muscular dystrophies and other neuromuscular disorders, using a single polyclonal antibody to a fusion protein derived from dystrophin, Hoffman and his colleagues (1988) concluded that dystrophin was absent in severe Duchenne dystrophy, was present but of abnormal molecular size in mild Becker muscular dystrophy, and was present in normal amounts in other forms of muscular dystrophy. It was thus a valuable tool not only for the confirmation of Duchenne or Becker dystrophy, but also for the exclusion of other forms of dystrophy, such as limb girdle dystrophy, that might have a similar clinical presentation but normal dystrophin. Hoffman also claimed that one might be able to prognosticate in Duchenne and Becker dystrophy on the basis of the dystrophin in the muscle. It almost looked as if the clinician had become redundant and all that was needed was a competent operator to take the muscle biopsy and a well-informed biochemist, working in the splendid isolation of his laboratory, to do the rest. However, not all their cases fitted into this neat compartmentalization. Thus one case of Becker dystrophy had absent dystrophin, which they ascribed to a deletion corresponding to the same DNA region as the fusion proteins used in preparing the original antibodies. By extrapolation this would imply that one would need to know the deletion status of the gene, based on the DNA studies of the patient's blood, before one could draw any conclusions in relation to prognosis from the absence of dystrophin, particularly in a clinically milder case. Conversely, although there was little or no significant dystrophin present in 35 of their 38 cases of Duchenne dystrophy, there were three samples which had detectable levels above 3% of normal. Similarly, in Becker muscular dystrophy the suggestion of altered size or molecular weight of dystrophin did not allow for the possibility of a normal sized protein of reduced amount.

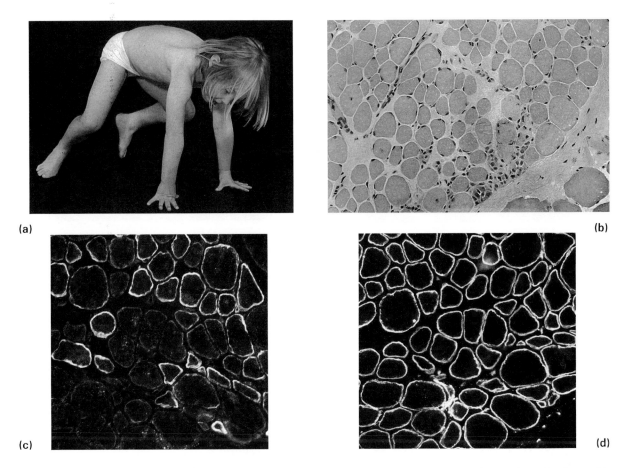

Figure 2-31a-d This 5-year-old girl presented with a Duchenne-like muscular dystrophy, getting up from the floor with a Gowers' manoeuvre (a). The CK was grossly elevated (6800 iu/litre) and muscle biopsy showed a dystrophic pattern on routine stains, with variation in fibre size, focal necrosis and regeneration, and proliferation of connective tissue, (b, H & E). Immunofluorescent staining with dystrophin antibodies showed a mosaic pattern of positive and negative fibres (c), confirming she was a manifesting Duchenne carrier. Spectrin antibodies showed a normal sarcolemmal staining in all fibres (d), confirming the integrity of the sarcolemmal membrane.

The application of *immunocytochemical techniques* to the study of dystrophin in muscle sections added a new dimension to the interpretation. In contrast to the early suggestion based on the biochemical fractionation studies that dystrophin might be localized to the triads, the cytochemical studies showed a clearcut localization to the sarcolemmal membrane (Zubrzycka–Gaarn *et al.*, 1988; Arahata *et al.*, 1988).

While confirming the general absence of any staining for dystrophin in Duchenne biopsies, it has also consistently revealed small numbers, usually less than 1%, of positive staining fibres in some Duchenne biopsies (see Figure 2-22). It has been suggested that these so-called revertant fibres may represent a somatic mutation, with reversion to normal, in individual fibres. Recent studies suggest that the deletion is put back in frame again by a

process of exon skipping (Sherratt *et al.*, 1993). In Becker biopsies there may be a variation in the intensity of stain in the positive fibres and also the presence of patchy, rather than continuous, staining of the membrane in individual fibres (Figure 2-22).

In *female carriers* the results are also interesting, but somewhat complex. Although manifesting carriers may show a mosaic pattern of positive and negative fibres (Figure 2-31) (Bonilla *et al.*, 1988; Arahata *et al.*, 1989; Nicholson *et al.*, 1990; Hoffman *et al.*, 1992; Sewry *et al.*, 1993), the majority of non-manifesting carriers that we have reviewed have shown an essentially normal dystrophin pattern with practically all fibres showing a normal staining pattern (Clerk *et al.*, 1991). Some carriers may show a varying degree of change with either patchy staining of the sarcolemma or a reduction in the intensity of staining (Figure 2-32).

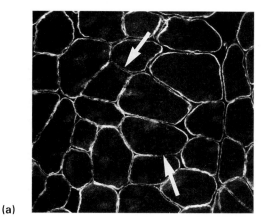
(a)

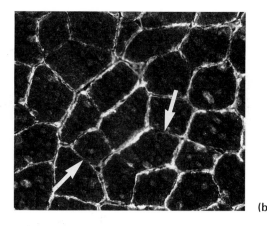
(b)

Figure 2-32a,b Biopsies from a possible carrier (a) and an obligate carrier (b) immunolabelled with dystrophin antibodies, showing weak and uneven labelling of the sarcolemmal membrane on some fibres in both cases (arrows).

In addition to the original Hoffman antibodies, a number of laboratories have produced antibodies to different parts of the dystrophin molecule, which has allowed a more comprehensive appraisal of the changes in dystrophin in the muscle in parallel with the deletion studies in the gene. Nicholson *et al.* (1990) recently reported their experience in a comparative study of immunoblotting and immunocytochemistry in a large series of 226 muscle biopsies, including 85 Duchenne and 55 Becker muscular dystrophies, using a monoclonal antibody to the rod domain of dystrophin, which was specific for dystrophin and did not cross-react with spectrin or α-actinin. They found isolated positive fibres in 40% of the Duchenne biopsies and a further 20% had weak labelling of a large number of fibres. Of the 54 Duchenne and 52 Becker biopsies showing a positive band on immunolabelling, 85% had a protein of abnormal size, whereas the remaining 15% had a protein of normal size but reduced abundance. They found that overall there was a good correlation between the abundance of dystrophin and clinical severity. Three of Nicholson's antibodies (Dys 1 to the rod region of the molecule, Dys 2 to the C terminal region, and Dys 3 to the N terminal region) are commercially available and have found wide usage.

Much more cumulative experience is still required comparing the severity of the clinical disease with the deletion data in relation to the gene and the changes in the dystrophin in the muscle. Meanwhile it would be prudent (for biochemists as well as physicians) not to lose sight of the importance of careful clinical assessment of the patient in relation both to the extent of weakness and the rate of progression of the disease, rather than trying to predict these from the laboratory data in isolation.

ANIMAL MODELS OF X-LINKED (Xp21) DYSTROPHIES

A number of animal models of the Xp21 dystrophy have been identified in recent years and have already attracted much research interest, both from the investigative and from the therapeutic point of view (Figure 2-33).

The mdx mouse

An X-linked dystrophy in the mouse was picked up purely by chance during a mutagenesis screen of serum enzymes (Bulfield *et al.*, 1984). Following a period of necrosis of the muscle at about 2–3 weeks of age there is active regeneration and recovery and the mice then remain essentially normal and have a normal lifespan (Dangain and Vrbova, 1984). The gene for the mouse dystrophy is homologous to the human dystrophin gene (Hoffman *et al.*, 1987b), and dystrophin is also absent in the *mdx* mouse muscle (Hoffman *et al.*, 1987a). It has recently been shown that the genetic abnormality is a point mutation at nucleotide position 3185, with the replacement of the nucleotide cytosine by a thymine, resulting in a stop codon (TAA) in place of a glutamine codon (CAA) (Sicinski *et al.*, 1989). This results in premature termination of translation at 27% of the length of the dystrophin polypeptide and the production of a truncated protein. Presumably this residual protein is sufficiently stable and functional to sustain regeneration and fibre integrity in the mouse dystrophy.

The XMD dog

An X-linked muscular dystrophy has been dis-

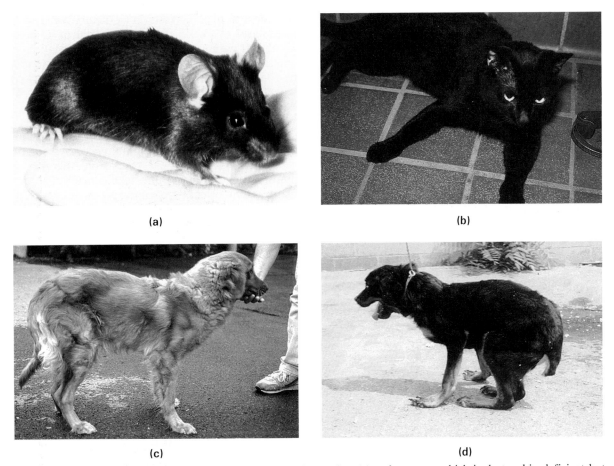

(a)   (b)

(c)   (d)

Figure 2-33a-d Animal models of Duchenne muscular dystrophy. (a) *mdx* mouse, which is dystrophin-deficient but clinically normal; (b) XMD cat, which is dystrophin-deficient but clinically normal and has remarkable muscle hypertrophy; (c) XMD dog. Golden Retriever with Duchenne-like muscular dystrophy, with marked clinical weakness and dystrophin deficiency; (d) XMD dog. Rottweiler with very severe Duchenne-like dystrophy with loss of ambulation by 6 months. (I am grateful to Dr Terry Partridge for the *mdx* mouse and to Dr Barry Cooper for the opportunity of personally examining the dystrophic cat, retriever and Rottweiler during visits to Ithaca.)

covered in a Golden Retriever strain of dogs which is also genetically homologous to the human disease and lacks dystrophin in the muscle (Valentine *et al.*, 1986; Cooper *et al.*, 1988). Clinically the dog manifests a severe weakness with an early onset and steady progression, comparable to the Duchenne type. From an early stage there is also marked wasting of the muscles, but none of the prominence and apparent enlargement of the muscles one sees in the human disease. The histological picture is identical to that in Duchenne dystrophy, including the early proliferation of endomysial connective tissue. Selective involvement of some muscles at an earlier stage than others has been demonstrated in the neonatal period (Valentine and Cooper, 1991), comparable with the selective involvement from an early stage in Duchenne dystrophy.

Sharp *et al.* (1992) have recently demonstrated an RNA processing error that results from a single base change in the 3′ consensus splice site of intron 6. The 7th exon is then skipped, which predicts a termination of the dystrophin reading frame with its N-terminal domain in exon 8. This is the first example of dystrophin deficiency caused by a splice site mutation.

A more severe, Duchenne-like, dystrophin-deficient muscular dystrophy, with loss of ambulation by 6 months and death within the first year, has recently been studied by Cooper's group in a family of Rottweiler dogs (Winand *et al.*, 1994a). A point mutation was identified in exon 58, resulting in conversion of glutamate to a stop codon.

The XMD cat

A dystrophin-deficient muscular dystrophy has been discovered in a single neutered male cat, which was not clinically weak and had marked prominence of the muscles (Carpenter *et al.*, 1989). A further two similar cats were subsequently documented by Gaschen *et al.* (1992) which also had generalized muscle hypertrophy and developed feeding problems as a result of obstruction of the oesophagus by the hypertrophied diaphragm. A similarly affected cat with striking muscle hypertrophy and associated stiffness, but no apparent clinical weakness, has also been studied by Cooper (personal communication). Muscle biopsy showed low levels of full-length dystrophin on Western blot and a mosaic pattern on immunocytochemistry. Further studies revealed a deletion of the muscle dystrophin promoter and exon 1, with the cortical neuronal promoter being intact (Winand *et al.*, 1994b). They concluded that the full-length dystrophin detected in the muscle by Western blot is probably the cortical neuronal isoform. This is reminiscent of a 10-year-old patient reported by Boyce *et al.* (1991) with a mild Becker phenotype and normal intellect, who had a deletion of the muscle promoter and exon 1, while retaining the brain promoter and exon 2, and showed a reduced level of normal sized dystrophin in the muscle biopsy.

This feline model of muscular dystrophy is of special interest, in parallel with the mouse dystrophy, for its absence of clinical weakness and its marked muscle hypertrophy, which probably also occurs in the *mdx* mouse, and is, of course, also a feature of selected muscles in the human disease, the so-called pseudohypertrophy already noted by Duchenne, who coined the term.

GENE THERAPY

In his inaugural lecture as Galton Professor of Eugenics at University College, London, Penrose (1946) considered the eugenic approach to disease pioneered by his eminent predecessors as wrong, not because of their statistical and genetic errors, not because of their inherent racial bias, not because of the apocalyptic consequences of the eugenic vision; rather he realized that the genetically determined phenotype of a metabolic disease such as phenylketonuria could be amenable to conventional allopathic medical therapy (Ledley, 1987). He wrote, 'There may be methods of alleviating the condition, even though it is inborn, in a manner analogous to the way in which a child with clubfoot may be helped to walk or a child with cataract may be helped to see' (Penrose, 1946). Within a few years the palliative

treatment of phenylketonuria by dietary means was introduced by Bickel, based on a trial in a single patient. If we adopt the same analogy in relation to muscular dystrophy, it is possible that a crutch may be found in order to keep our patients ambulant, independent of the direct genetic approach to curing the disease.

Recombinant DNA and molecular cloning technologies have introduced the exciting new possibility of selectively replacing abnormal genes by somatic gene therapy. This could be a truly therapeutic option in which the fundamental biochemical abnormality would be corrected in the patient's own cells.

Methods for gene transfer

It is a fundamental principle of molecular biology that if a gene is isolated and introduced into a suitable environment, it will continue to express its gene product. The transfer of genes among organisms is common in nature and is best exemplified by viruses, whose life cycle involves the transfer of viral genes into the infected cells and the consequent transformation of the infected cell to produce a new generation of viruses. The principle of somatic gene therapy is similar to viral infection.

There are several ways to transfer a gene into a cell. Purified DNA may be introduced into cells by direct microinjection (Capecchi, 1980), electroporation, in which a powerful electric current pulse disrupts the membrane and pushes DNA into a cell (Chu *et al.*, 1987), or transfection, in which particles containing DNA precipitates are taken up by a cell. These methods are referred to as DNA-mediated gene transfer. Viruses have evolved efficient means of introducing genes into a cell and integrating their genes into the host genome. Research on somatic cell therapy has concentrated on adapting viruses as vectors for gene transfer (viral-mediated gene transfer).

However, introducing a gene into a cell is only the first step in the somatic gene replacement therapy. It is essential that this gene be expressed and that the gene product be biologically active. The expression of a recombinant gene requires a promoter to direct transcription of the integrated DNA into mRNA and the signals for translation of the mRNA into protein.

Somatic cells versus germ cells

In gene therapy it is important to distinguish between introduction of genes into the germ cells where the recombinant cells may become part of the host genome and be passed onto future generations, and introduction of genes into somatic cells where the recombinant gene will only alter the phenotype of the individual. For technical and ethical reasons the consideration of gene therapy in the human context is restricted to somatic cells, although recent experiments have involved germ cell transfection in the *mdx* mouse (Wells *et al.*, 1992).

Clinical application of gene and cell therapy: myoblast transfer

Following the spectacular molecular genetic advances, there was understandably a wave of enthusiasm and optimism, both among patients and among scientists, that this would open the way for potential treatment, perhaps underestimating the major technical hurdles to be overcome.

Somatic cell therapy seemed to offer a possible shortcut for delivering the normal gene or its product direct to the muscle. It entailed transplanting normal muscle cells directly into the diseased muscle, with a view to obtaining fusion of the donor myoblasts with the host myoblasts, the so-called satellite cells, which are normally quiescent in muscle until activated to proliferate, divide and fuse. This should then produce a mixture of dystrophin-positive and dystrophin-negative fibres comparable with the heterozygote female carrier of the Duchenne gene.

The discovery of several animal models of Duchenne dystrophy provided an extra boost for this research.

In a key experiment, Partridge and his colleagues (Partridge *et al.*, 1989) were able to demonstrate that the direct injection into the muscle of the *mdx* mouse of myoblasts from dissociated normal neonatal muscle produced dystrophin-positive fibres and also hybrid fibres, identified by isoenzyme markers, indicating a fusion between donor and host myoblasts and not merely between the donor myoblasts themselves. Partridge's experimental mouse model was somewhat special and remote from the reality of the human disease. It combined the *mdx* with a nude mouse strain, thus eliminating the possibility of immunological rejection of the donor muscle. In addition, the small size of the mouse muscle made such an experiment more feasible in relation to the number of myoblasts introduced relative to the host muscle. A particular disadvantage of the mouse model was the absence of weakness, so that it would not be possible to assess the potential benefit of any treatment at a clinical level.

The canine model, on the other hand, provided a good model in which to assess any potential therapeutic benefit, given its similarities to the human disease, and it could help to resolve such fundamental questions as the potential viability of the technique in dystrophic muscle, the number of donor myoblasts required in relation to the size of the host muscle, the need for immunosuppression, and the possible importance from a therapeutic point of view of the stage of the disease and the age of the donor muscle.

Fired by the apparent success in the limited *mdx* mouse experiments, a number of North American centres opted to pursue further therapeutic experiments directly in the human disease, despite the notes of caution voiced by a number of scientists at a workshop on gene therapy at the time (Griggs and Karpati, 1990). In the most comprehensive study to date, Karpati and his colleagues in Montreal recruited into a double-blind study eight young boys with Duchenne dystrophy, all of whom had a deletion in the gene and absence of dystrophin in the muscle. Ten million cultured myoblasts from the father's muscle, of proven purity by cell sorting, were injected into each of 55 sites in one biceps, whereas a comparable injection, but without the myoblasts, was made into the other biceps as control. Neither patients nor parents nor personnel were aware which side was which. Immunosuppression was provided with cyclophosphamide (for reasons of local preference) for 6–12 months. The power of the muscle was assessed by sequential myometry and the dystrophin status of the muscle on repeat biopsy at 3 and 12 months by Western blot and immunocytochemistry. At the end of a 1-year follow-up, there were no significant differences between the two sides in the individual cases at either a clinical level or in the dystrophin status, and there was no significant increase in donor-derived DNA and dystrophin messenger RNA in the injected muscle (Karpati *et al.*, 1993).

In an uncontrolled study, Tremblay's group performed myoblast transfer with repeated injections into several different muscles in four advanced, non-ambulant, cases of Duchenne dystrophy (Huard *et al.*, 1992). Meticulous attention was paid to histocompatibility of the donor and recipient for HLA classes I and II-DR and no immunosuppression was used. In one case the donor was a brother, in the other three sisters, including one Duchenne carrier. Three of the four patients were shown to form antibodies against the donor's myotubes. Muscle biopsies of the injected tibialis anterior showed some degree of dystrophin immunostaining in 80%, 75%, 25% and 0% respectively of the muscle fibres, and in the contralateral uninjected muscle in 16% of the first case and none in the other three.

Law and his colleagues injected into eight foci in the extensor digitorum brevis muscle of three boys with Duchenne dystrophy 8 million cultured myoblasts obtained from a 1g biopsy from the father or brother (Law *et al.*, 1991). In the first patient the donor was the non-biological adoptive father. A comparable volume of carrier fluid without myoblasts was sham-injected into the other side. In the second and third patients this was double-blinded. After 3 months there was claimed to be an increase in twitch tension in the myoblast-injected side compared with a reduction on the sham-injected side, and bilateral open biopsy showed the presence of dystrophin by immunoblot and immuno-cytochemistry on the myoblast injected side only. Eight further patients were also included in this study but were not analysed. Fired by the success of this limited series of experiments, Law established a Cell Therapy Research Foundation and proceeded to his phase 2 therapeutic trials of myoblast transfer into several major muscles in Duchenne dystrophy. They subsequently reported the results of a 3-month follow-up on 18 of their 21 cases (Law *et al.*, 1992). Five billion cultured, normal myoblasts were transferred via 48 intramuscular injections into 22 major muscles of both lower limbs. Immuno-supression was provided by cyclosporin. Dyna-mometer measurements of the isometric tension in the knee flexors, knee extensors and plantar flexors, before and 3 months after myoblast transfer in 18 subjects, showed a mean increase of 41.3% in 43% of the 69 muscle groups measured, no change in 38% and a reduction of 23.4% in 19%. When he presented his data at the first meeting of the Society for Cell Transplantation, Law came under considerable fire from his scientific colleagues about the validity of his data in this uncontrolled study (Thompson, 1992).

Blau and her colleagues studied the tibialis anterior muscle from eight cases of Duchenne dys-trophy, with a documented deletion in the dystro-phin gene, 1 month after the injection of 100 million cultured myoblasts into 80–100 injection sites (Gussoni *et al.*, 1992). In three of the eight they were able to show by polymerase chain reaction the expression of dystrophin messenger RNA derived from the donor myoblast DNA. Given the extreme sensitivity of this technique, this result presumably reflects the persistence of donor DNA from a few of the implanted myoblasts. Immunocytochemically the number of dystrophin-positive fibres was only about 10 per 1000 fibres counted, which was no greater than the frequency of spontaneously occur-ring dystrophin-positive 'revertant' fibres in some of the control side muscles.

So where do we currently stand in relation to myoblast therapy in Duchenne dystrophy? Could the essentially negative results merely reflect the birth pangs reminiscent of earlier transplantation procedures such as kidney, bone marrow and heart? There may be simple technical reasons for the failure in relation to the culture of the donor cells, or the state of proliferative activity of the recipient satellite cells, which further systematic studies with the canine model could help to resolve.

On the other hand, cell therapy may turn out to be a non-starter in the treatment of muscular dystrophy and alternative approaches, such as the introduction of gene constructs either directly into the muscle or via appropriate viral vectors, may need to be pursued (Dubowitz, 1992).

Animal experiments on gene therapy

In an interesting experiment, Wolff *et al.* (1990) demonstrated that injection of plasmid DNA directly into rodent skeletal muscle expressed reporter genes such as β-galactosidase or luciferase, suggesting one might be able to circumvent the need for viral or other vectors for the DNA. In a similar study, Wolff's group have subsequently shown that non-human, primate muscle is also able to take up and express intramuscularly injected plasmid DNA, but the level of expression of luciferase was considerably lower than in rodent muscle. This does not augur well for this approach in human muscle.

Meanwhile, a number of laboratories have succeeded in producing constructs of the 12 kb full-length human dystrophin complementary DNA gene, containing all the 80-odd exons necessary for protein production. This provided the possibility for attempting to introduce the dystrophin gene into the muscle cell.

Lee *et al.* (1991) were able to introduce DNA constructs of mouse dystrophin into cultured COS cells (a kidney cell line) which then expressed dystrophin, thought to be membrane-bound, in about 3–5% of cultured cells. Acsadi *et al.* (1991) were subsequently able to show that either a 12 kb full-length human dystrophin complementary DNA gene or a 6.3 kb minigene, derived from a mildly affected Becker patient with a large deletion of the gene, could be expressed in cultured cells *in vitro*. When human dystrophin expression plasmids were injected intramuscularly into dystrophin-deficient *mdx* mice, the human dystrophin was present in about 1% of myofibres. From a purely technical point of view this was a further important step in demonstrating that dystrophin could be expressed either *in vivo* or by transfection of cultured myo-blasts *in vitro*. However, in spite of the wide ex-posure of this 'break-through' in both the scientific and lay press, this was still a far cry from producing any clinical benefit.

It is rather frustrating that none of these sophisti-cated studies have surpassed nature's spontaneous correction of the defect in individual muscle fibres in Duchenne dystrophy. Moreover, the *mdx* mouse, with its normal clinical phenotype, cannot tell us whether the dystrophin expressed is functional and therapeutically viable, and comparable experiments will have to be done in the dystrophic dog or the dystrophic human, once a greater yield of dystrophin-positive fibres can be achieved.

In a recent study along similar lines with the use of a DNA adenoviral vector, Ragot *et al.* (1993) were able to achieve up to 50% of conversion to dystrophin-positive fibres in the neonatal *mdx* mouse, using the same Becker minigene as Acsadi *et al.* (1991). The adenoviral vector has the advantage that it can enter non-dividing cells, in contrast to retroviral vectors which are only effective in dividing cells. If these early studies in the *mdx* mouse prove to be consistent it would be important to repeat them in the dystrophic dog with a view to possible human application.

One of the major problems with somatic cell therapy in muscle diseases is to target the donor cells to the muscles by some more practical means than direct injection into individual muscles.

Earlier pilot studies of injection of myoblasts into the circulation were unsucccessful, but in a recent study in the rat of intra-arterial injection via the abdominal aorta of myoblasts labelled with *lac Z* via a retroviral vector, Neumeyer *et al.* (1992) were able to demonstrate the presence of a few galactosidase-positive fibres in the tibialis anterior muscle both on the pre-injured (buvicaine injection) side and on the control (saline injection) side. This suggests that transformed myoblasts may be able to migrate from the arterial circulation to muscle and fuse there to form differentiated muscle cells.

Much more basic experimental work needs to be done to establish whether or not these exciting new techniques may have a practical role in the treatment of Duchenne dystrophy.

BECKER MUSCULAR DYSTROPHY

Becker muscular dystrophy is a photocopy of Duchenne dystrophy, with a similar clinical appearance and distribution of weakness but milder in severity. It is also inherited through an X-linked mechanism and recent studies with recombinant DNA techniques initially showed that it has the same location as the Duchenne gene and is thus allelic. Subsequent studies have confirmed that both Duchenne and Becker dystrophy are due to deletions or other mutations in the same gene.

The benign phenotype was first described by Becker and Kiener (1955) in several members of Kiener's own family, and further families were later documented by Becker (1962). There have been many subsequent reports in the literature. Emery and Skinner (1976) documented 29 cases from 10 families; Ringel *et al.* (1977) 19 from 12 families; and Bradley *et al.* (1978) 17 from 8 families.

In the series of Emery and Skinner (1976) the mean age of onset of symptoms was 11 years, ranging from as early as 2½ years to 21 years. Early onset is thus not necessarily indicative of severe disease. As in the case of Duchenne dystrophy, it is also possible to identify preclinical cases in affected families by grossly elevated CK. They also noted variation in severity within some families. Fourteen of 38 affected relatives became chairbound at ages ranging from 12 to 30 years (mean 27) and 10 died, usually of respiratory or cardiac failure, at ages ranging from 23 to 63 years (mean 42 years).

CLINICAL FEATURES ————————————————

The onset of symptoms is usually later than in Duchenne dystrophy but some cases may be already manifest in early childhood. The course is a much more benign one and compatible with the continuation of ambulation into adolescence and adult life. The distinction from Duchenne dystrophy is usually suspected on clinical grounds because of the milder weakness compared with a Duchenne case of similar age. If there are affected maternal uncles who are still ambulant the diagnosis is easy (Figures 2-34 to 2-37).

The most useful clinical criterion is the ability of the patient to walk. Whereas all children with Duchenne dystrophy are off their feet by the age of 13 years, those with Becker type will remain ambulant beyond 16 years. However, there is considerable variability within the range of Becker dystrophy (Figures 2-38, 2-39). Some patients may become chairbound in their late teens or 20s, whereas others may continue walking into their 40s or 50s or later. It is also noteworthy that some sufferers of Becker dystrophy, despite the later age of onset, may follow a pretty rapid course and lose the ability to walk within 10 to 12 years of onset of clinical weakness, which is not all that different from the progression of Duchenne dystrophy.

If one arbitrarily defines the Duchenne phenotype as losing ambulation before the 13th birthday and the Becker as being ambulant beyond the 16th, there will inevitably also be some intermediate subjects who stop walking between 13 and 16 years (see Figures 2-28, 2-29).

As all these cases are due to abnormalities within the same gene, one could call them all Xp21 dystrophies. It is still useful, however, to try and recognize the severe and benign phenotypes in order to give an appropriate prognosis and institute appropriate management. It is also important in any therapeutic trials to select a clearly defined population of cases.

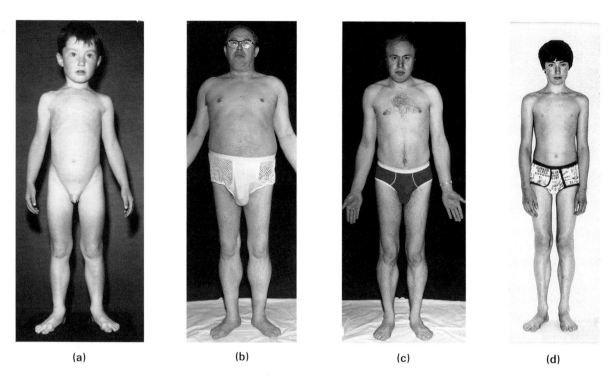

(a) (b) (c) (d)

Figure 2-34a-d Becker muscular dystrophy in (a) a 5-year-old boy presenting with mild muscle weakness, and (b and c) his two ambulant, affected uncles aged 39 and 24 years. The index case showed very little progression at follow-up over the ensuing years and was still very active and mobile at 14 years (d). He was recently reviewed again at 25 years and is still ambulant, although he has had increasing difficulties. The older uncle is now 58 years and has recently become wheelchair-bound. The younger uncle at 43 years is still ambulant.

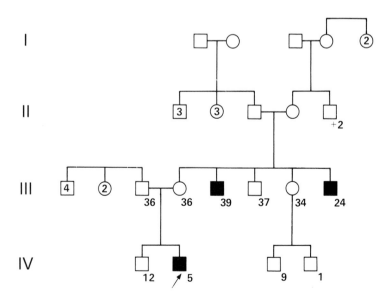

Figure 2-35 Pedigree chart of family in Figure 2-34.

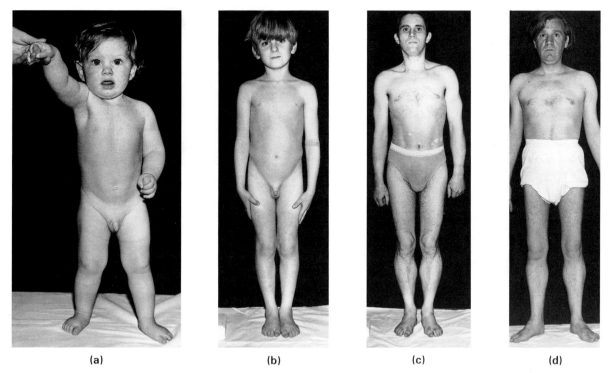

Figure 2-36a-d   Preclinical Becker dystrophy in (a) a 10-month-old symptom-free child with CK of 2400 iu/litre and (b) his 8-year-old brother with muscle cramps in the calves on exercise, with no associated weakness, and a CK of 1600 iu/litre. The mother's brother (c), aged 32, and half-brother (d), aged 42, had a slowly progressive muscular dystrophy. Note the prominence of the calves.

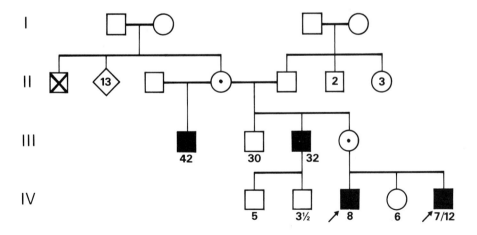

Figure 2-37   Pedigree chart of family in Figure 2-36.

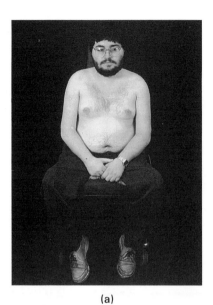

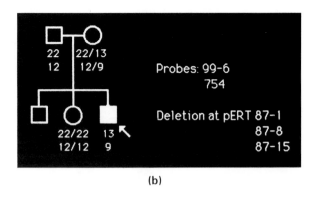

(b)

(a)

Figure 2-38a,b Becker dystrophy; severe end of spectrum. This patient, an isolated case of muscular dystrophy, was late walking (21 months), had a clumsy gait and was never able to run. He walked on his toes from 8 years and had marked prominence of the calves. He had increasing difficulty and lost ambulation at 16 years 2 months. He has subsequently remained fairly stable (a) and currently at 30 years of age is still mobile in his wheelchair, has a straight spine and has been free of respiratory and cardiac complications. He was of some historical interest in being the first Becker patient to show an intragenic deletion in the Duchenne gene with the pERT probes (b) (Hodgson *et al.*, 1986a), and subsequently found to have a deletion of almost half the gene.

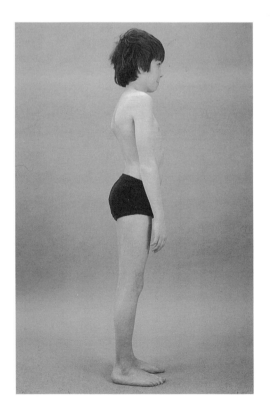

Figure 2-39 Becker dystrophy; mild end of the spectrum. This 11-year-old boy presented with a 1-year history of cramps and tiredness after strenuous exercise, associated with myoglobinuria. He had no overt weakness or limitation of physical activity but subsequently stopped cycling because of discomfort. He had a minimal Gowers' sign getting up from the floor. His CK was grossly elevated (14 300 iu/litre). Muscle biopsy showed an overtly dystrophic picture with variation in fibre size and evidence of necrosis as well as regeneration. Phosphorylase and phosphofructokinase reactions were normal. On follow-up over the next 4 years, he remained stable and symptom-free apart from cramps on strenuous exercise. When reviewed recently at 23 years he still had no weakness and was able to avoid cramps by limiting his physical activity.

As in Duchenne dystrophy, contractures of multiple joints are not a feature of the ambulant patient with Becker dystrophy but occur in those who become chairbound. Tightness of the heel-chords with a tendency to toe-walking and some tightness of the hips is fairly common, but more marked contractures, and particularly of the elbow flexors and spinal muscles, should raise the possibility of Emery–Dreifuss dystrophy (see below).

Cardiac involvement, if it occurs, is usually, but not invariably, a late manifestation (Kuhn *et al.*, 1979; Lazzeroni *et al.*, 1989).

It has been assumed in the past that with the milder nature of Becker dystrophy, the degree of cardiac involvement is also less than in Duchenne dystrophy. It is likely that the risk of cardiomyopathy has been underestimated. Steare *et al.* (1992) studied 19 patients, two of whom had dyspnoea on effort, the remainder being asymptomatic. The ECG was abnormal in 74%, with intraventricular conduction delay or right bundle branch block in 42%. Echocardiography demonstrated left ventricular dilatation in 37%, while 63% had subnormal systolic function due to global hypokinesia.

Melacini *et al.* (1993) recently reported their results of a comprehensive study of cardiac function by electrocardiographic and echocardiographic assessment and 24-hour Holter monitoring in 31 patients with Becker muscular dystrophy, who had undergone detailed clinical assessment, DNA analysis for deletions and dystrophin assay in their muscle biopsies. Deletions were found in 19 patients, no detectable deletion in 10, and duplication in two. Only one patient, aged 36 years, was symptomatic, with syncope and exertional dyspnoea, and died suddenly 6 months later. He had a deletion of exons 45–48 and mild muscle weakness. No correlation was found between the skeletal muscle disease, the cardiac involvement and the dystrophin abnormalities. There was abnormality of the electrocardiogram in 68% and of the echocardiogram in 62%. Right ventricular involvement was detected in 32%, left ventricular in 10% in isolation and in 29% in association with right ventricular dysfunction. The right ventricular involvement was manifested in teenagers, the left ventricular impairment in older patients. Four patients had life-threatening ventricular arrhythmias. Of the patients with a deletion, all five patients deleted for exon 49 had cardiac involvement, and all but two of the 12 deleted for exon 48.

Some patients who are still active and mobile may develop a severe dilated cardiomyopathy in their late teens or early adult life and this may lead to cardiac failure and be very difficult to control (Figure 2-40). Not only may cardiomyopathy be a prominent feature in cases with mild dystrophy, but some cases presenting with isolated cardiomyopathy have been found to have an underlying Becker dystrophy, with elevated serum creatine kinase and confirmatory evidence of Becker dystrophy on DNA and dystrophin analysis (Muntoni *et al.*, 1993).

The place for heart transplant has recently been reviewed in cases of Becker dystrophy with end-stage cardiac failure, whose prognosis would otherwise be hopeless (Quinlivan and Dubowitz, 1992). Five successful transplants in Becker dystrophy have been recorded in the literature to date (Casazza *et al.*, 1988; Donofrio *et al.*, 1989; Sakata *et al*, 1990).

Intellectual function: A proportion, as yet not precisely determined, have some impairment of intellect (Bushby and Gardner–Medwin, 1993).

SPECIAL INVESTIGATIONS ——————

The *serum CK* level is substantially raised, especially in the early stages, and gradually falls as the disease progresses. In the preclinical stage of the disease, which may last 10 years or more, when the only abnormality is calf enlargement and there is no apparent muscle weakness, the serum level is grossly elevated to levels comparable with those found in boys with Duchenne muscular dystrophy of the same age but who are clinically affected. Why in Becker muscular dystrophy there should be this lag period before the onset of muscle weakness remains unexplained. Female carriers of Becker dystrophy also show elevated CK levels.

The *muscle biopsy* in Becker dystrophy does show some differences in pattern from those of Duchenne (Dubowitz and Brooke, 1973), with less severe involvement and more evidence of regeneration for the comparable age and differences in distribution of the fibre types, but this can be difficult to distinguish in borderline cases and the clinical distinction is a more dependable one. In addition to the overall dystrophic pattern of change, there may be clusters of atrophic fibres, which have confused some earlier authors into diagnosing a denervation process.

MOLECULAR GENETICS ——————

In the isolated male case the clinical distinction between the X-linked Becker dystrophy and the autosomal limb girdle dystrophy is difficult, if not impossible. Both have a similar distribution and severity of weakness, and the prominence of the calves or the gross elevation of CK, which are more marked in the Becker, are not absolute. The demonstration of a deletion in the Xp21 gene with the cDNA probes is one way of confirming a Becker dystrophy, but about 30% of cases of known Becker dystrophy do not have a demonstrable deletion.

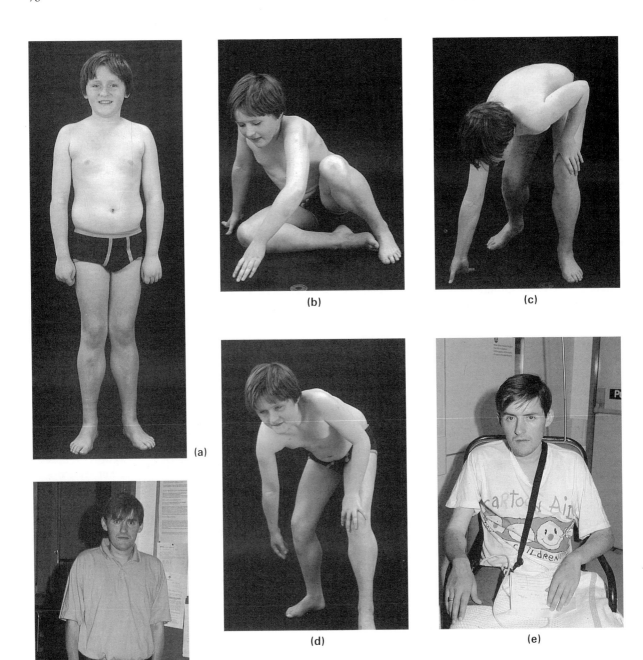

Figure 2-40a-f Becker dystrophy; Cardiomyopathy. This boy presented at 14 years with mild disability and got up fairly rapidly from the floor with a Gowers' manoeuvre (a-d). His CK was grossly elevated and his muscle biopsy dystrophic. The family history was positive; a maternal uncle had been similarly affected and died suddenly at 31 years. He subsequently remained well and active until he suddenly went into cardiac failure with a dilated cardiomyopathy at age 24 (e). He responded well to medical treatment and regained his mobility (f) but subsequently went into acute failure again a year later. He was put on the waiting list for a heart transplant but once again has gradually responded to medication and is currently well and mobile, some 6 months on, and has opted to bide his time before surgery. He has no detectable deletion in his DNA and the dystrophin analysis has been somewhat complex, with an absence of dystrophin on Western blot and also immunocytochemically with Dys 1 antibody, but presence of a reasonable amount of dystrophin, with slightly reduced molecular mass, with the antibodies to other parts of the dystrophin molecule.

Alteration in dystrophin in the muscle will also help to identify a Becker type dystrophy and to exclude limb girdle dystrophy, in which dystrophin is normal. Screening the mother or female siblings for carrier status by serum CK elevation is a simple and still useful technique.

In 1988, Monaco and colleagues proposed that the milder Becker muscular dystrophy resulted from mutations at Xp21 which maintained the translational reading frame (in-frame mutations), resulting in an abnormal, but partially functional dystrophin, whereas in Duchenne muscular dystrophy the mutations shifted the reading frame (frame-shift mutations) so that virtually no dystrophin was produced (Monaco *et al.*, 1988). This 'reading frame' hypothesis holds up in 90% of cases and is of diagnostic and prognostic significance (Gillard *et al.*, 1989; Koenig *et al.*, 1989).

The following analogy shows the effects of an 'in frame' and 'out of frame' deletion respectively:

THIS LINE CAN BE READ WELL

THIS LINE BE READ WELL

THIS LNEC ANB ER EADW ELL

These molecular approaches to diagnosis and prognosis will become increasingly refined with time. Meanwhile an approach involving muscle immunohistochemistry can also provide valuable information. We have seen already that with this technique, as well as Western blotting, in Duchenne muscular dystrophy there is a virtual absence of dystrophin whereas in Becker muscular dystrophy dystrophin is present but of abnormal size and/or abundance.

A further refinement is the use of antibodies *specific* to the C-(carboxy-) terminal region of dystrophin. Using such antibodies, immunohistochemistry reveals that the C-terminal region is almost always absent in Duchenne but invariably present in Becker muscular dystrophy (Arahata *et al.*, 1991). Thus when this region of the molecule is missing, a more severe phenotype is likely. Such truncated dystrophins have also been found in male fetuses with Duchenne muscular dystrophy (Ginjaar *et al.*, 1991). In these studies, however, it is essential that the antibodies used are carefully characterized and are specific for the C-terminal region of dystrophin (Ellis *et al.*, 1990).

ATYPICAL CLINICAL PRESENTATIONS —————————————

Cramps on exercise

The presentation of cases of Becker dystrophy, usually the mildly affected energetic ones, with cramps on exercise is well recognized (Dubowitz, 1978) and has recently been rediscovered in America

(Gospe *et al.*, 1989). The diagnosis is suspected if one finds an associated muscle weakness and is further supported by a very high serum CK and a dystrophic muscle biopsy. The diagnosis can now be consolidated by the demonstration of a deletion in the Xp21 gene or abnormality in the expression of dystrophin in the muscle.

Focal myopathy

There have been intermittent reports over the years of focal myopathies, such as quadriceps myopathy. Recent studies with the new molecular tools have established that many of these are in fact variants of Becker dystrophy. Carriers of Duchenne or Becker dystrophy can also present with a focal weakness in addition to asymmetrical calf hypertrophy.

Cardiomyopathy

In addition to the incidental cardiomyopathy which is an integral component of Becker dystrophy, some cases may present with an isolated cardiomyopathy with no clinical manifestation of skeletal muscle involvement. The diagnosis can be established by demonstration of a deletion in the Xp21 gene. This opens the door for routine screening of isolated cases of cardiomyopathy for possible Becker dystrophy by an initial serum CK estimation and subsequent search for a deletion in the Xp21 gene.

LIMB GIRDLE MUSCULAR DYSTROPHY

The term limb girdle dystrophy was originally used to include those patients with muscle weakness of girdle distribution mainly affecting the proximal muscles of the limbs. It embraced the pelvifemoral type with weakness predominantly in the pelvic girdle, and the scapulohumeral with weakness predominantly in the shoulder girdle (Walton and Nattrass, 1954).

There is no doubt that before the days of adequate investigation of muscle disorders this diagnosis included many cases of the benign spinal muscular atrophy (Kugelberg–Welander form) and of various congenital myopathies. Some recent authors have even gone so far as to doubt the existence of a true limb girdle dystrophy at all.

There are, however, cases of autosomal muscular dystrophy, with elevated CK, unequivocal myopathic changes on EMG and dystrophic changes on muscle biopsy, which comprise a separate group. Recent advances in molecular genetics have now helped to firmly establish a number of different syndromes with autosomal inheritance and different gene loci (Table 2-1).

Isolated male cases of limb girdle dystrophy may be difficult to distinguish clinically from Duchenne or Becker dystrophy, and appropriate DNA or dystrophin studies may now help to diagnose or exclude these. Similarly, in isolated cases females presenting as having a limb girdle dystrophy may turn out to be manifesting carriers of the Duchenne gene (see Figure 2-31).

CLINICAL FEATURES

The range of severity in limb girdle dystrophy is wide. Some cases have an early onset and rapid progression and conform clinically in pattern to the Duchenne type. This probably accounts for cases of Duchenne type dystrophy seen from time to time in females (Dubowitz, 1960b) (Figure 2-41) and is well documented in the literature (Penn *et al.*, 1970).

Other patients with a childhood onset can be very slowly progressive and remain ambulant into adult life, whereas some with relatively late onset may have a very rapid progression. As in other forms of dystrophy, prominence of various muscles can also be a feature of limb girdle dystrophy. Some subjects may present with a marked toe-gait and progressive tightness of the tendo Achillis, in association with relatively mild weakness. In some of the very mild cases, patients who have very little apparent deficit

in muscle power and are able to participate in active sports may present with severe cramps on exercise, comparable with the presentation in some cases of Becker dystrophy, and resembling McArdle's disease (see Chapter 4). The CK is usually grossly elevated, the EMG myopathic and the muscle biopsy similar to other cases of limb girdle dystrophy.

It is likely that many of the isolated male cases which have been labelled in the past as limb girdle dystrophy are probably Becker dystrophy, which is more common, and it is important to check for mutations in the Duchenne gene and also the dystrophin status in the muscle biopsy. In a recent application of dystrophin immunohistochemistry and immunoblotting in 41 cases of presumed limb girdle dystrophy, Arikawa *et al.* (1991) found that five men had Becker muscular dystrophy and two women were probably manifesting carriers of Duchenne muscular dystrophy. Misclassification had occurred in four out of 13 isolated men (31%) and two out of 15 women (13%). Similarly Norman *et al.* (1989) reviewed 33 male patients (30 isolated and three with affected brothers), previously diagnosed as Becker or limb girdle dystrophy. Molecular deletions were found in 13 of the 18 patients with a diagnosis of Becker muscular dystrophy (72%) and in four of the 15 (27%) thought to have limb girdle dystrophy. The results of such studies have important implications for genetic counselling.

(a) (b) (c)

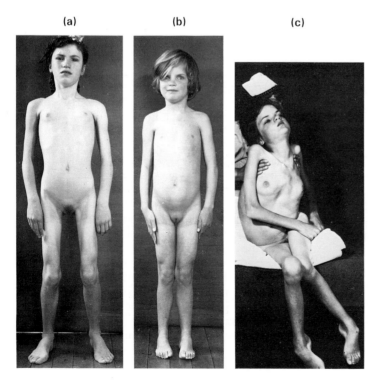

Figure 2-41a-c Limb girdle dystrophy resembling Duchenne type in (a) an 11-year-old girl with onset of symptoms at 5 years and subsequent loss of ambulation before her 12th birthday; and (b) her 8-year-old sister with onset of weakness at 6 years and subsequent loss of ambulaton at 11 years and rapid deterioration (c). Parents are first cousins.

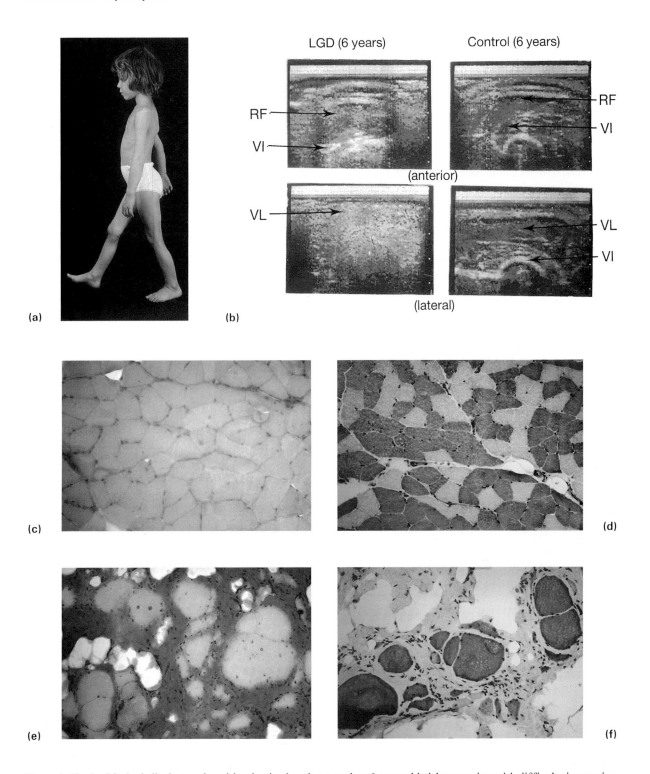

Figure 2-42a-f Limb girdle dystrophy with selective involvement in a 6-year-old girl presenting with difficulty in running and going up stairs and minimal proximal lower limb weakness (a). Ultrasound imaging showed sparing of rectus femoris but markedly increased echogenicity in vastus intermedius and vastus lateralis (b). Concurrent needle biopsy of the rectus femoris and vastus lateralis showed a practically normal histological and histochemical picture in the rectus femoris (c, Verhoeff-van Gieson stain; d, ATPase) apart from some variability in fibre size and occasional atrophic fibres ('minimal change myopathy'), and a strikingly dystrophic picture in the vastus lateralis (e, f) with marked proliferation of connective and adipose tissue and loss of muscle fibres.

Passos-Bueno *et al.* (1991a) reported a comprehensive study of autosomal recessive limb girdle dystrophy in 22 Brazilian families, with 62 patients diagnosed as limb girdle dystrophy. In 19 families the clinical course was mild, in the remaining three, progression was comparable with X-linked Duchenne muscular dystrophy. The parental consanguinity rate was high (77%). No major clinical differences were observed in this series of autosomal recessive dystrophy compared with X-linked dystrophies and several patients had calf hypertrophy and/or serum creatine kinase activity as high as that observed in Becker muscular dystrophy. However, muscle dystrophin was found to be qualitatively and quantitatively normal in the autosomal forms but absent or abnormal in the X-linked ones.

While female patients with limb girdle dystrophy with normal chromosomes might be presumed to have an autosomal recessive disorder, some may in fact be manifesting carriers of Duchenne/Becker dystrophy and studies of the status of dystrophin in the muscle is essential to distinguish them.

SEVERE AUTOSOMAL RECESSIVE MUSCULAR DYSTROPHY OF CHILDHOOD ('SCARMD')

A rapidly progressive autosomal recessive dystrophy seems to be particularly prevalent in North Africa and extensive families were reported from the Sudan (Salih *et al.*, 1983) and Tunisia (Ben Hamida *et al.*, 1983). The latter documented 93 cases, aged between 6 and 30 years, from 28 families. The age of onset of symptoms ranged from 3 to 12 years. The clinical severity varied and they were able to define roughly three groups – one with onset between 3 and 8 years and loss of ambulation between 10 and 15 years, approximating to Duchenne dystrophy in severity and accounting for about 20% of the cases; a second less severe group with onset between 4 and 9 years and loss of ambulation between 15 and 20 years and accounting for about 55% of the cases; and a milder group with onset between 4 and 12 years and loss of ambulation between 20 and 30 years, comprising the remaining quarter.

INVESTIGATIONS

Detailed investigation is essential in all cases of possible limb girdle dystrophy to exclude the specific congenital myopathies, metabolic myopathies or spinal muscular atrophy which can all present as a limb girdle weakness.

The *EMG* will usually show a myopathic pattern with low amplitude, polyphasic potentials. Usually *CK* is elevated but the range may vary from practically normal to a gross elevation.

Ultrasound imaging shows increased echogenicity in the muscle and there may also on occasion be selective involvement of some muscles and sparing of others, which is helpful in choosing an appropriate muscle for biopsy (Figure 2-42).

Muscle biopsy shows characteristic features of a dystrophic pattern of change with variation in fibre size, splitting of fibres, internal nuclei and evidence of degeneration and regeneration of fibres. In addition one frequently sees structural changes in the fibres with the histochemical preparations for oxidative enzymes, such as 'moth-eaten' fibres, whorled fibres and lobulated fibres. Striking hypertrophy of fibres is also a common feature in some cases. It is not possible to draw any correlation between the extent of the pathological changes in the muscles and the degree of clinical weakness. Indeed, some almost subclinical cases may have very marked pathological changes and some very weak patients may show very little change.

MOLECULAR GENETIC STUDIES

Application of the new techniques of molecular genetics in the past few years has helped to delineate a number of specific limb girdle syndromes, either on the basis of gene location or specific changes in the muscle itself (see Table 2-1).

In a study of four North African cases of severe autosomal recessive muscular dystrophy of childhood with antibodies to dystrophin and also to the various dystrophin-associated glycoproteins (Figure 2-43), Campbell's group (Matsumura *et al.*, 1992) found normal expression of dystrophin but selective loss of the 50kD dystrophin-associated glycoprotein (50 DAG).

Whilst originally thought to be a specific North African disease, and even given a title 'Mahgrebian muscular dystrophy' to reflect the ethnic origin, it is now obvious that it is probably a universal disorder and cases have been identified amongst Europeans in France (Fardeau *et al.*, 1993) (who suggested calling the 50 kD glycoprotein 'adhalin' from the Arabic word *adhal* = muscle) and in England in a family of Asian origin (Sewry *et al.*, 1994a) (Figure 2-44) and in an isolated English girl (Figure 2-45). Once Campbell's antibody to the 50 DAG is made more generally available for screening of other potential cases, SCARMD will almost certainly be found to be a disorder of much wider geographic distribution, although perhaps less prevalent than in some of the inbred communities of North Africa.

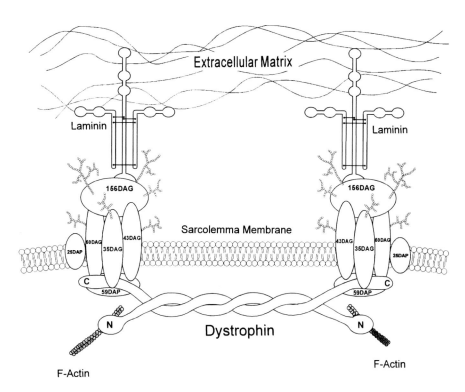

Figure 2-43 Schematic model of the dystrophin–glycoprotein complex as a trans-sarcolemmal link between the subsarcolemmal actin cytoskeleton and the extracellular matrix component laminin, showing the various dystrophin-associated glycoproteins (DAG), and dystrophin-associated proteins (DAP), of different molecular size, which straddle the membrane (the numbers reflect the molecular size in kD). (Reproduced from Matsumura and Campbell, 1994, with the courtesy of the authors and by permission of *Neuromuscular Disorders* and *Muscle and Nerve*.)

In a recent study of the severe autosomal recessive, Duchenne-like muscular dystrophy in three large, highly inbred, Tunisian families, Ben Othmane *et al.* (1992) found, by homozygosity screening, a linkage to the pericentromeric region of chromosome 13q (13q12) and this has since been confirmed in other North African families (Azibi *et al.*, 1993; El Kerch *et al.*, 1994). There was no linkage with chromosome 6q, the locus of the dystrophin related protein (DRP; utrophin), with chromosome 15q, associated with the milder autosomal recessive limb girdle dystrophy, or with the chromosome 5q locus of the dominant limb girdle dystrophy.

Recent linkage studies on the 50 DAG have shown that it is not located on chromosome 13q, so that it is not the gene product of the SCARMD gene, and presumably the loss of the 50 DAG is a secondary phenomenon. It is now also emerging that not all SCARMD families with 50 DAG deficiency localize to 13q (Passos-Bueno *et al.*, 1993), so there may be additional genes also causing deficiency of the 50 DAG (Romero *et al.*, 1994). In addition, there are still families with a similar clinical phenotype who do not have any abnormality of the 50 DAG or of dystrophin (Figures 2-46, 2-47).

One large French family with four affected siblings with SCARMD did not show linkage to chromosome 13q (Romero *et al.*, 1994) and has now been found to be linked to the locus for adhalin (the 50 DAG) on chromosome 17q12-q21.33 and to have a missense mutation in the adhalin gene (Roberds *et al.*, 1994).

It is of interest that all the DAGs are reduced in Duchenne dystrophy (see Figure 2-44) (Matsumura and Campbell, 1993, 1994; Mizuno *et al.*, 1994) and also in the dystrophin-negative fibres in symptomatic Duchenne carriers (Matsumura and Campbell, 1994; Sewry *et al.*, 1994b).

It is also of interest in this context that all the DAGs are reduced in Duchenne dystrophy, considered to be secondary to the absence of dystrophin.

Matsumura *et al.* (1993) have recently reviewed the potential role of the dystrophin–glycoprotein complex in the pathogenesis of various muscular dystrophies. The 156 kD and 43 kD dystrophin-associated glycoproteins are encoded by a single gene and the term dystroglycan has been suggested for them. In a recent study of the direct interaction between the C-terminal portion of dystrophin and the dystrophin-associated proteins, Suzuki *et al.*

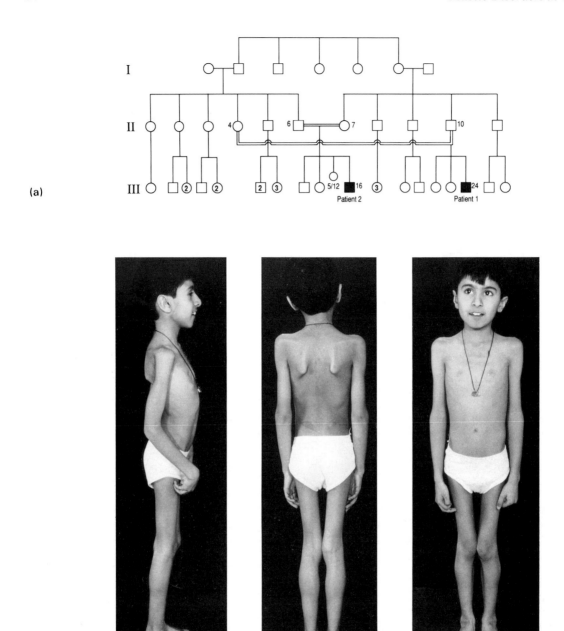

(a)

(b)

Figure 2-44a,b Limb girdle dystrophy; SCARMD; 50 DAG ('adhalin') deficiency. (a) Pedigree chart showing the two affected cousins, Patient 1 III, 24 and Patient 2 III, 16, and the consanguinity of their parents, the father and mother of Patient 1 being siblings respectively of the mother and father of Patient 2 (b). Patient 1 was delayed in walking (18 months) and noted at 2½ years to walk on his toes with a waddling gait. During childhood he was generally weak and fell frequently. His intellect was normal. When referred at 9 years he had a waddling gait, could not jump (both legs) or hop (one leg) and got up from the floor with a Gowers' manoeuvre in 5 seconds. His motor ability score was 30 out of 40. There was no calf hypertrophy and no cardiac abnormality; CK was 9925 (N <170) iu/litre. When recently assessed at 12 years his weakness was fairly stable, but his Gowers' manoeuvre took 20 seconds and his motor ability score was down to 27. His cousin (III,16) was referred at 10 years. His motor milestones had been normal and first symptoms were at 8 years with difficulty running. He had a waddling gait, difficulty going up stairs, a Gowers' manoeuvre of 4 seconds and a motor ability score of 38, with ability to jump and to hop on one leg, with difficulty. He had no calf hypertrophy or cardiac involvement; CK was 7360 iu/litre. He was noticeably less severely affected than his cousin.

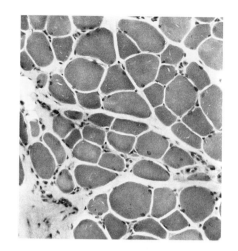

(c)

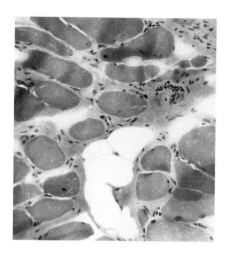

(d)

	Dystrophin	156DAG	59DAP	50DAG	43DAG	35DAG
Normal						
DMD						
Patient 1						
Patient 2						

(e)

Figure 2-44c-e Needle biopsy of the quadriceps at 9 and 10 years respectively showed a dystrophic picture (c,d; H & E) and complete absence of the 50 DAG (e). (e) The various dystrophin-associated glycoproteins (DAG) and the dystrophin-associated protein (DAP) and also dystrophin are shown in the two patients (horizontal columns 3 and 4 across), in comparison with a control biopsy (column 1 across) and a patient with Duchenne dystrophy (column 2 across). Note the absence of dystrophin in Duchenne dystrophy and the reduction in all the glycoproteins, and in the two cousins the total absence of the 50 kD glycoprotein (50 DAG), and the slight reduction also in the 43 DAG and the 35 DAG. (Illustration courtesy of Dr K. Matsumura.)

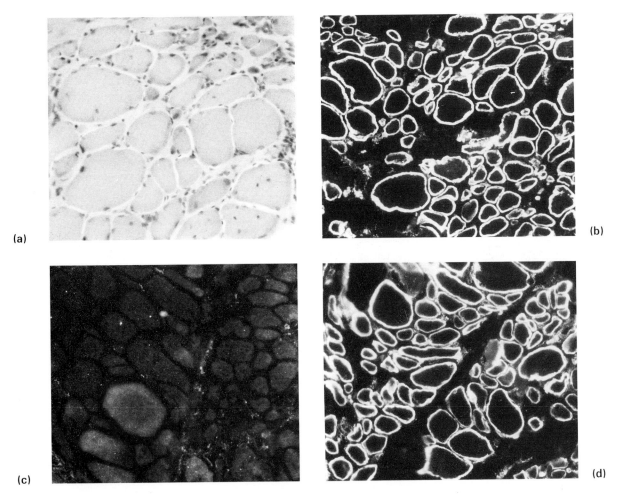

(a)

(b)

(c)

(d)

Figure 2-45a-d   Limb girdle dystrophy; SCARMD; 50 DAG deficiency. Needle biopsy from a 4-year-old English girl presenting with a Duchenne-like dystrophy, showing the dystrophic picture on routine staining (a, H & E), normal dystrophin pattern (b), complete absence of the 50 kD dystrophin-associated glycoprotein (c), and normal staining for the 43 DAG (d). (Courtesy Drs S. Robb and N. Fagg.)

facing page

Figure 2-46a-e   Limb girdle dystrophy; normal dystrophin; normal 50 DAG. Four affected children (a,b,c,d; aged 10½, 9½, 9½ and 6½ years) with variable severity in the same sibship (e). Note the varying degree of lordosis with normal posture in the third child. The parents and rest of the family were normal, with no previous history of any neuromuscular disorder.

Figure 2-46f-i   The eldest boy (III, 4) had a course similar to Duchenne dystrophy and lost the ability to walk at 12 years; after being remobilized in callipers, he subsequently became chairbound (f). Another brother (g: III, 5) also had a similar course but somewhat milder, and remained ambulant until 14 years and was kept mobile subsequent to that for about a year in callipers, after which he became chairbound. He later developed a progressive scoliosis and underwent a Luque operation. His twin brother (h: III, 6) had practically no disability but was found to have a mild scoliosis and his CK was also elevated (2300 iu/litre) at 11 years of age. He subsequently showed a relatively mildly progressive course but was still ambulant at 17 years with very little progression of the scoliosis. His muscle biopsy at 12 years showed an overtly dystrophic picture. The sister (i: III, 7) followed a somewhat similar course and lost the ability to walk at 11½ years. She developed a scoliosis which stabilized without requiring surgery. Her chromosomes were normal and CK was 1500 at 8 years of age. The three severely affected siblings subsequently developed nocturnal hypoventilation. There was no cardiac abnormality. The muscle biopsies showed normal dystrophin as well as normal 50kD dystrophin-associated glycoprotein.

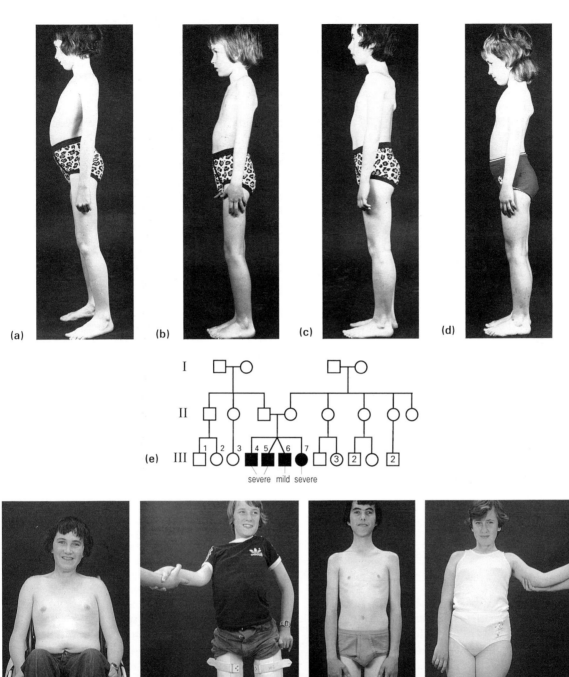

(a)   (b)   (c)   (d)

(e)

(f)   (g)   (h)   (i)

(1994) found that the 43 kD dystrophin-associated glycoprotein binds directly to dystrophin, as do two other proteins, and they have proposed a model for the molecular architecture at the binding site for the complex on dystrophin.

It seems likely that in the future some of these autosomal muscular dystrophies, not due to the X-linked dystrophin gene and not having an abnormality in the 50 DAG, may be found to have an abnormality in the other glycoproteins associated with dystrophin or in the laminin/merosin complex attached to the glycoproteins on the outside of the muscle membrane (see Figure 2-43).

PROGNOSIS

It is difficult to prognosticate in such a variable condition as limb girdle dystrophy, and prognosis in general should be based on the degree of clinical weakness and the rate of progression in the individual case. Even within the genetically distinct entities such as the 13q severe autosomal recessive form in childhood there is considerable variability in clinical severity between families and even within the same sibship. As in other neuromuscular syndromes, respiratory deficit and scoliosis will influence the prognosis. Cardiac involvement is not a usual feature of limb girdle dystrophy but abnormal ECG patterns are found in occasional cases. It is of interest in this context that a deficiency of the 50 DAG has recently been found in the dystrophic hamster (BIO 14.6), in which cardiomyopathy is a predominant feature (Roberds *et al.*, 1993; Yamanouchi *et al.*, 1994). This should provide a valuable animal model for the further molecular genetic study of SCARMD.

MANAGEMENT

As in Duchenne dystrophy, it is important to encourage these patients to remain ambulant, as periods of immobility may lead to deterioration. It is also important to give them encouragement and psychological back-up support, particularly in the milder cases with very little functional deficit. When patients hear the term dystrophy they often become very anxious about the diagnosis and prognosis and may fear complete loss of motor ability. In some of the very mild cases, presenting with muscle cramps and very little weakness, it may be preferable to avoid the term dystrophy and rather refer to the condition as a myopathy and give a good general outlook and prognosis, or if one is going to use the term dystrophy to at least assure the patient and family that this is a much more benign form.

Patients with fixed equinus of the feet from shortening of the tendo Achillis, associated with relatively mild weakness, often benefit from tenotomy, but careful assessment is necessary to ensure that the deformity of the feet and not the degree of weakness is the major factor in the difficulty with walking.

GENETIC COUNSELLING

As the condition is usually inherited through an autosomal recessive mechanism, both parents are heterozygote carriers and there is a 25% risk of any further child being similarly affected. On the other hand, the affected patient will not pass the disease on to his/her own children unless he happens fortuitously to marry a carrier of the same gene. He can thus be reassured that from a genetic point of view it is comparatively safe to go ahead and have a family and that the children are unlikely to be affected. It is also advisable not to marry a blood relation, who would have a high risk of being a heterozygote carrier of the gene, and in such cases counselling needs to be more cautious and carrier detection may be helpful.

In all cases of limb girdle dystrophy it is essential to ensure that both parents of the affected child are unaffected, both on clinical and possible serum enzyme and EMG assessment, since rare cases of a limb girdle type of dystrophy may have a dominant inheritance. The recent advances in molecular genetics in defining some specific disorders within this group have certainly opened the way for more accurate diagnosis and counselling, and more gene loci will undoubtedly be found in the future.

facing page

Figure 2-47a-i Limb girdle dystrophy; normal dystrophin; normal 50 DAG. These three siblings were the only children of consanguinous Arabic parents and were referred because of delay in motor milestones and motor difficulties. The oldest child (a,b,c), aged 4 years, had not walked independently till 2 years. She had a lordotic posture, a waddling gait and got up from the floor with a Gowers' manoeuvre. The second child (d,e,f) aged 2 years 7 months, had walked at 2 years 4 months and was unable to run or climb steps. She also had a waddling gait and got up with a Gowers' manoeuvre. The youngest child (g,h) at 13 months, was just able to stand with support. All three had grossly elevated CK (4460, 7650 and 2270 iu/litre respectively; N <200). Ultrasound imaging showed increased muscle echogenicity in all three and their needle biopsies showed a dystrophic picture with a normal staining for dystrophin (i) and for the dystrophin-associated glycoproteins.

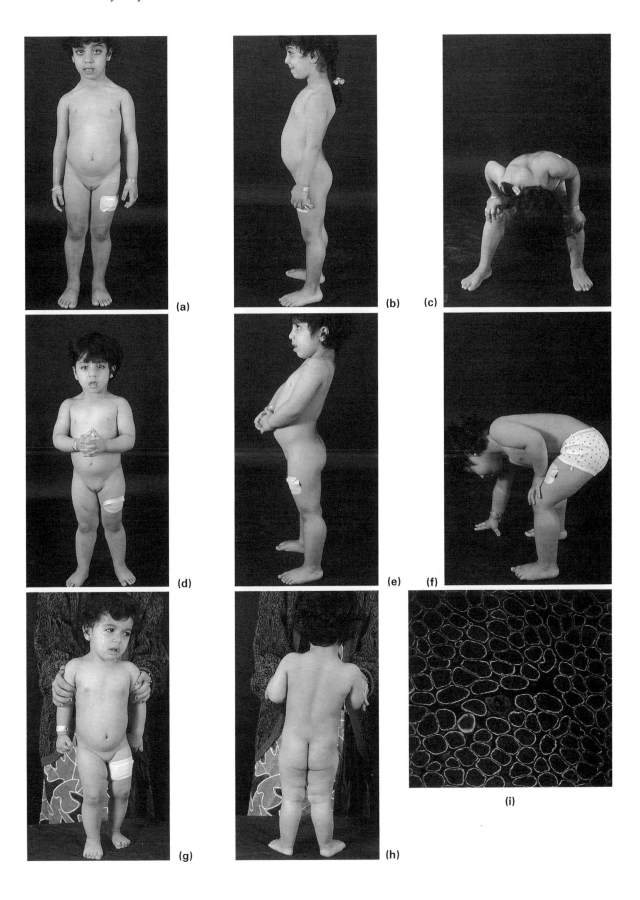

(a)

(b)

(c)

(d)

(e)

(f)

(g)

(h)

(i)

MILD AUTOSOMAL RECESSIVE MUSCULAR DYSTROPHY

A genetically homogeneous group of inbred families from Reunion Island, comprising individuals at high risk of a mild form of autosomal recessive limb girdle dystrophy, was systematically analysed using a panel of 85 polymorphic markers spanning approximately 30% of the human genome (Beckmann *et al.*, 1991). Linkage was established on chromosome 15. Young *et al.* (1992) subsequently confirmed this linkage in an isolated Old Order Amish community in Indiana. They obtained genotype data on 12 nuclear families, totalling 116 individuals from a highly inbred kindred, which could be traced through nine generations. The phenotype of this limb girdle dystrophy in this community has previously been well documented (Jackson and Strehler, 1968). The clinical course in both the Reunion and the Amish populations was characterized by onset in late childhood and a moderate progression. It is currently unknown how many families from different communities may also map to this locus. Exclusion of linkage to chromosome 15 has been clearly shown in some families, though preliminary results suggest that some families from Brazil may also show linkage (Bushby, 1992).

An additional gene locus for the mild autosomal recessive limb girdle dystrophy has recently been identified by Bashir *et al.* (1994) on chromosome 2p in two large inbred families of different ethnic origin.

DOMINANT LIMB GIRDLE DYSTROPHY

There have been occasional reports of a dominantly inherited limb girdle muscular dystrophy, usually of late onset and mild course. Chutkow *et al.* (1986) reported a kindred with an insidious onset any time from the late second to the sixth decade and followed by slow progression. Pelvifemoral weakness preceded scapulohumeral and there was marked variation in expressivity, including an asymptomatic myopathy (pre- or sub-clinical) and a non-manifesting carrier state extending into the eighth decade. The muscle biopsy was characterized by the presence of rimmed vacuoles. Marconi *et al.* (1991) described a similar clinical pattern running through four generations of a family and also associated with vacuoles in the biopsy. Gilchrist *et al.* (1988) reported a large family with autosomal dominant inheritance, affecting 16 members with a proximal girdle weakness affecting the legs more than the arms, with onset in the third decade. They were unable to establish a conclusive linkage.

Further families have been recorded by Somer *et al.* (1989). Miller *et al.* (1992b) have recently documented an affected father and son with a Becker-like clinical picture, with normal results on DNA studies of the dystrophin gene and normal expression of dystrophin in the muscle. The father lost ambulation at 30 years. In both, CK was grossly elevated and the muscle biopsy overtly dystrophic. On the face of it this looked like a dominantly inherited, childhood onset, dystrophy.

MOLECULAR GENETICS

A gene locus on chromosome 5q22.3-31.3 has recently been recorded by Speer *et al.* (1992) in a large dominant pedigree with a very mild dystrophy, onset after the age of 20 and CK normal or only moderately elevated, using a series of CA(n) microsatellite repeat markers. They also excluded linkage to the 15q locus. The gene has recently been further refined (Yamaoka *et al.*, 1994).

MOLECULAR STUDIES: DYSTROPHIN-RELATED PROTEIN (DRP); UTROPHIN

In view of the clinical similarities between the limb girdle and the X-linked dystrophies and the unique homology between the autosomally inherited gene on chromosome 6 and the 1.8 kb sequences at the carboxyterminal domain of the dystrophin gene (Love *et al.*, 1989; Tinsley *et al.*, 1992), it seemed likely that this 6q sequence might be a strong candidate for an autosomal recessive dystrophy. However, in a linkage study of 226 individuals (57 patients/169 unaffected) from 19 large, unrelated Brazilian families, Passos–Bueno *et al.* (1991b) were able to exclude linkage of limb girdle muscular dystrophy with the gene for the autosomal homologue of dystrophin (dystrophin related protein, DRP) in the chromosome 6q 23-q27 region.

At present utrophin is still a protein in search of a disease and has not been found to be associated with any of the neuromuscular disorders. This is perhaps not surprising given that it is not expressed in the sarcolemma of skeletal muscle but only at the neuromuscular junctions and myotendinous junctions (Khurana *et al.*, 1991). Utrophin is expressed in the sarcolemma of dystrophin-deficient fibres in Duchenne dystrophy (Tanaka *et al.*, 1991; Mizuno *et al.*, 1993). If this is nature's effort to compensate for the deficiency of dystrophin, it has not been very effective at a clinical level.

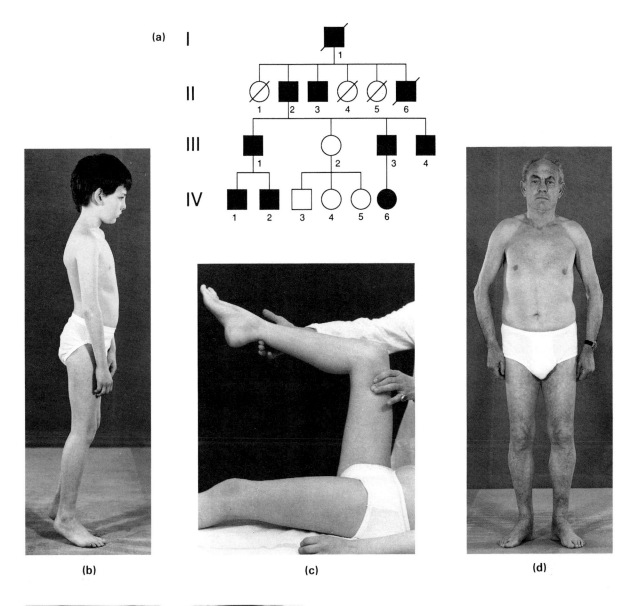

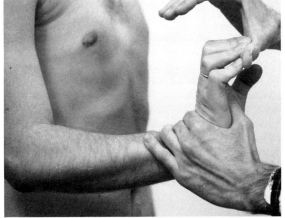

(b)　　　　　　　　　(c)　　　　　　　　　(d)

(e)

Figure 2-48a-e Bethlem myopathy. (a) Family tree showing dominant inheritance. The index case (IV,1) presented at 9 years with toe-walking and tightness of the heel cords (b) and minimal disability. Note the flexed posture of the fingers at rest. There were associated contractures of the hamstrings (c) with limited passive extension of the knees. There was a slightly limited extension to his fingers when the wrist was held fully extended to 90°, and mild weakness of the biceps and extensor digitorum muscles. His 59-year-old great uncle (II, 3) (d) had fixed flexion contractures of the elbows and fingers (e) but was fully active with minimal disability, as were various other adult affected members in the family, confirming the mild nature of the disorder, which is readily missed if family members are not carefully assessed. (Courtesy of Professor Luciano Merlini and by permission of *Neuromuscular Disorders*.)

EARLY-ONSET, BENIGN AUTOSOMAL DOMINANT LIMB-GIRDLE MYOPATHY WITH CONTRACTURES (BETHLEM MYOPATHY)

In 1976 Bethlem and van Wijngaarden described three Dutch families in which 28 individuals suffered from a very benign myopathy with autosomal dominant inheritance. The onset was in early childhood (around the fifth year of life) with difficulty in running, getting up from the floor, and climbing stairs. Progression was slow but without significant disability and with many patients living into old age. There was mild weakness and atrophy of the muscles of the trunk and extremities, with the proximal muscles more involved than the distal muscles, the extensors more than the flexors. Most of the patients showed early flexion contractures of elbows and ankles, and of the interphalangeal joints of the fingers, the latter being the most constant and associated with a marked paresis of the extensor digitorum muscles. Four of 28 had a congenital torticollis. Usually CK was not elevated. Muscle biopsy findings were nonspecific but remarkably uniform, with marked variation in fibre size and a very marked increase of fatty tissue.

Bethlem and his colleagues subsequently reported a family of Polish descent in which six members over four generations showed a similar benign myopathy with onset in early infancy but no hypotonia at birth (Arts *et al.*, 1978). Serum CK was slightly increased (from two up to seven times the upper value of normal). One of the six had congenital torticollis. They considered this myopathy a specific new disease entity.

Mohire *et al.* (1988) documented a large French-Canadian kindred with 33 affected members in six generations showing early-onset, autosomal dominant, limb girdle myopathy and contractures. The course was very benign with many members only minimally impaired, even in old age. Contractures of ankle and elbow were present in all while in some they were more widespread. Serum CK was normal or only slightly raised and the muscle biopsy showed non-specific myopathic changes without fibre necrosis or regeneration. Cardiac involvement was absent clinically in all patients and at autopsy in two affected individuals. In view of the striking similarity between the four previously reported families and their own they considered this myopathy to be a distinct clinicogenetic entity and proposed the eponymous name 'Bethlem myopathy'.

A sixth family was reported from Japan by Tachi *et al.* (1989). A mother and her son had an early-onset, benign, limb girdle myopathy with contractures, increasing with age, and absence of cardiac involvement. Computed tomography of muscles revealed a mild diffuse involvement. Muscle histology revealed non-specific myopathic changes, without dystrophic features.

A further two families have recently been documented by Merlini *et al.* (1994) (Figure 2-48). Early contractures of the fingers in childhood are readily missed and can be detected by passively extending the wrist and then the fingers after placing the forearm in a flexed and pronated position.

DISTAL MUSCULAR DYSTROPHY (AUTOSOMAL DOMINANT) (Welander)

Although the distal type of muscular dystrophy was first described by Gowers (1902), it is usually associated with the name of Welander (1951) in Sweden, who documented 249 cases from 72 families. It is a disease of adult life with onset usually after the age of 40 and a relatively mild disorder with a slow progression and usually affecting the arms before the legs. The CK is usually normal or slightly elevated and the biopsy shows myopathic changes (Edström, 1975). This condition appeared to be very rare outside Sweden but cases have been recorded (Sumner *et al.*, 1971; Markesbury *et al.*, 1974). Some of these cases had the onset of weakness in the legs before the arms and it has been suggested that these may represent a different type to the Welander form (Barohn *et al.*, 1991). This should be resolved once the gene is identified.

There have also been a number of reports of familial cases of distal myopathy with onset in infancy (Magee and DeJong, 1965; van der Does de Willebois *et al.*, 1968; Lapresle *et al.*, 1972; Bautista *et al.*, 1978).

DISTAL MUSCULAR DYSTROPHY (AUTOSOMAL RECESSIVE) (Miyoshi Myopathy)

In recent years a distal form of muscular dystrophy has been well documented, which seems to be particularly prevalent in Japan (Miyoshi *et al.*, 1974, 1986; Nonaka *et al.*, 1985). Miyoshi *et al.* (1986) reviewed 17 cases from eight families. It has an autosomal recessive pattern of inheritance, and is characterized by an onset in the teens or early adult life, with early selective involvement of the gastrocnemius muscles and subsequent spread to the thighs and glutei and also the forearm muscles. An initial characteristic feature is the inability to stand on the toes, with retention of the ability to stand on the heels. This is followed by a progressive course, with increasing difficulty climbing stairs, getting up from the floor and running. Most cases retain the ability to walk independently. There is striking atrophy of the lower legs and there may also be mild atrophy of the forearms and some loss of grip strength. An interesting feature is the selective involvement of the flexors of the distal interphalangeal joints so that they are unable to make a clenched fist and the fingers remain extended.

The creatine kinase is grossly elevated and usually between 10 and 100 times normal (comparable with Duchenne dystrophy). It also shows marked elevation in the preclinical stages of the disease as well as a mild elevation in some heterozygotes, who do not show any weakness or atrophy.

Muscle biopsy shows an overtly dystrophic picture with fibre necrosis, loss of muscle fibres, marked variation in fibre size, presence of opaque fibres and proliferation of adipose and connective tissue. The changes are most marked in the gastrocnemius and less striking in the quadriceps or other muscles. In an autopsy on one of their patients who died of pneumonia at the age of 68 years, Miyoshi *et al.* (1986) found no abnormality in the central or peripheral nervous system or in the heart.

A number of reports in the past few years have documented cases in Europe and America. Kuhn and Schröder (1981) described two affected brothers, Scopetta *et al.* (1988) two affected sisters, Galassi *et al.* (1987) three cases picked up on their high serum CK, and Barohn *et al.* (1991) four sporadic and one familial case, whose sibling was reported by Galassi *et al.* The clinical and laboratory features were identical to the Japanese cases. One of Barohn's cases had three muscle biopsies; the vastus lateralis showed only mild myopathic changes, the gastrocnemius a strikingly advanced dystrophic picture with marked connective tissue proliferation and only a few islets of residual fibres, and the biceps changes intermediate between the two. Although not reported in the literature, ultrasound imaging of the muscle would probably be very helpful in showing the relative extent of pathological change in different muscles by the increasing echogenicity. Barohn *et al.* (1991) suggested a classification of four separate distal myopathies, two with dominant and two with recessive inheritance.

It will be of interest in the future to see if any of these distal forms of muscular dystrophy are associated with an abnormality in the dystrophin-associated glycoproteins, in view of the striking pathological resemblance of the Miyoshi type to Duchenne dystrophy. In view of the gross elevation in serum CK it is also important that preclinical and early symptomatic cases are not mistaken for Duchenne or Becker dystrophy if picked up on screening programmes.

DISTAL MUSCULAR DYSTROPHY (AUTOSOMAL RECESSIVE)

Nonaka *et al.* (1981) reported a distal form of myopathy with autosomal recessive inheritance and a very similar clinical picture to the distal muscular dystrophy, but with the anterior tibial and peroneal muscles more affected than the calves, and with only a slight elevation of the serum CK and a muscle biopsy characterized by fibre atrophy and rimmed vacuoles and no striking necrosis and degeneration. They looked upon this as a separate disorder and subsequently documented the differences in the pathological features in four cases of each condition (Nonaka *et al.*, 1985). It needs to be distinguished from inclusion body myopathy, which also presents as a chronic myopathy, selectively involving distal muscles and characterized histologically by rimmed vacuoles containing inclusions (Carpenter *et al.*, 1978). It will be of interest to know whether this vacuolar myopathy has anything in common with oculopharyngeal myopathy which is also characterized by rimmed vacuoles.

TIBIAL MUSCULAR DYSTROPHY

A dominantly inherited distal myopathy of late adult onset, mainly affecting the anterior tibial compartment muscles, has been documented in recent years in Finland, particularly by Udd and his colleagues (Udd *et al.*, 1991). Moreover, the occurrence of a severe proximal limb girdle syndrome within the same large pedigree appeared to have an autosomal recessive inheritance but was compatible with the monozygous state of the dominant gene in affected individuals (Udd, 1992).

CONGENITAL MUSCULAR DYSTROPHY

The term congenital muscular dystrophy has been widely used for a group of infants presenting with muscle weakness at birth or within the first few months of life in association with a dystrophic pattern on muscle biopsy (Figures 2-49 to 2-53). There is often an associated hypotonia on clinical presentation but other patients may present with arthrogryposis and associated contractures of various joints. The condition tends to remain relatively static, but some subjects may show slow progression whereas others may have actual functional improvement and pass various motor milestones and achieve the ability to walk. There may be variable respiratory and swallowing

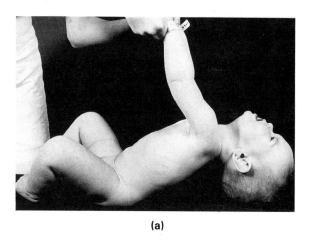

(a)

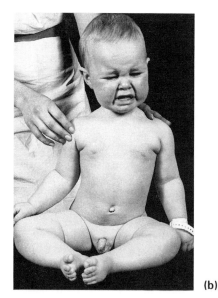

(b)

(c)

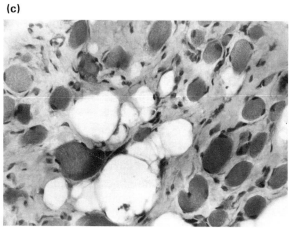

Figure 2-49a-g Congenital muscular dystrophy in a 9-month-old boy with hypotonia and weakness from birth. No contractures. No deterioration. Still has marked head lag (a), but can sit with support (b). Biopsy of rectus femoris (c, van Gieson) showed extensive replacement of muscle by connective tissue (grey areas) and fat (clear areas) and complete disruption of bundle pattern of fibres. He showed steady physical improvement and by 2 years was able to sit unsupported (d) and to stand with support (e). He subsequently walked unaided, by 4 years, and developed flexion contractures of the hips (f,g). We kept him at a safe distance from orthopaedic surgeons and the contractures improved with passive stretching and did not limit his mobility.

(d)

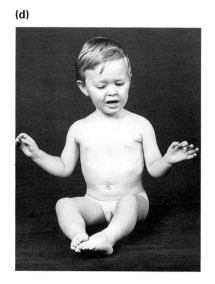

(e)

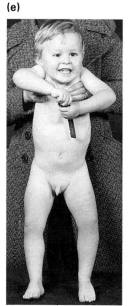

(f)

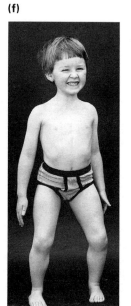

(g)

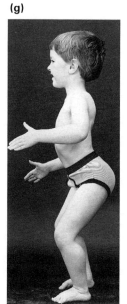

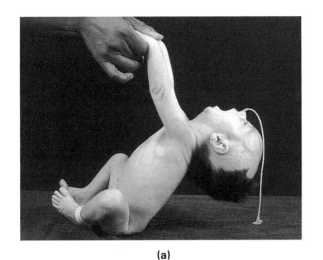

(a)

Figure 2-50a-g Congenital muscular dystrophy. This boy was floppy from birth with associated facial weakness and swallowing difficulties, but had reasonable mobility of the limbs (a). Needle biopsy of quadriceps at 3 weeks showed extensive atrophy and degeneration of muscle fibres (b) with associated cellularity and connective tissue proliferation. A short course of steroids, on grounds of infantile myositis, produced no benefit. When reviewed at 9 months he showed remarkable improvement, with ability to sit unaided, to raise legs against gravity and to take weight on his legs, but was still hypotonic (d, e). Ultrasound showed persistent abnormality of the quadriceps and a repeat needle biopsy (c) was still grossly abnormal with a remarkable dystrophic picture. He walked unaided at 2 years of age (f) and continued to improve. There were persistent flexion contractures of the hips but operative release was not recommended. He has continued to improve and currently at 5 years of age has practically no disability (g).

(b)

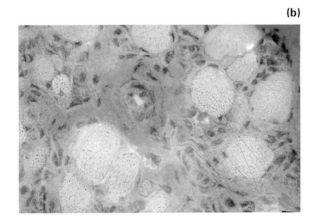

(c)

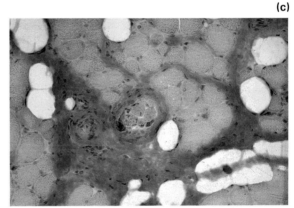

(d)   **(e)**   **(f)**   **(g)**

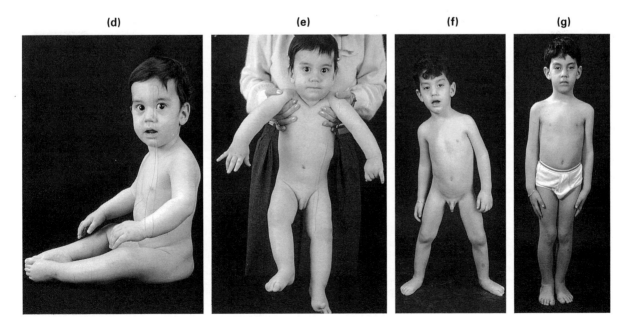

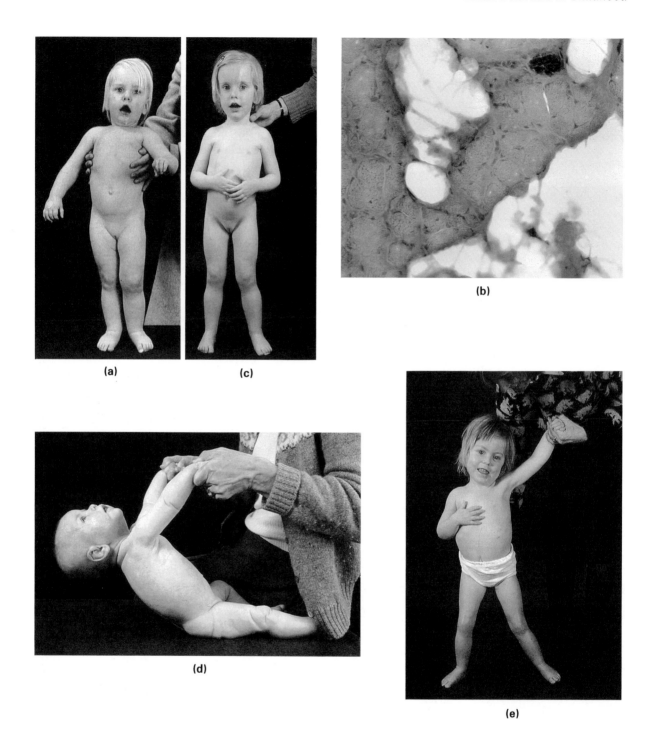

(a)   (c)

(b)

(d)

(e)

Figure 2-51a-e Congenital muscular dystrophy. This 13-month-old child had marked hypotonia from birth and delayed motor milestones (a). Needle biopsy of quadriceps showed severely dystrophic muscle with marked adipose tissue and connective tissue proliferation (b). She showed subsequently improvement in motor function with ability to stand unaided by 2½ years of age, and was able to walk well by 4 years of age (c). Her 4½-month-old sister presented with a similar problem. Note the hyptonic posture and poor head control (d). She subsequently sat unsupported at 12 months and was taking good weight on her legs, and standing with support at 2 years (e).

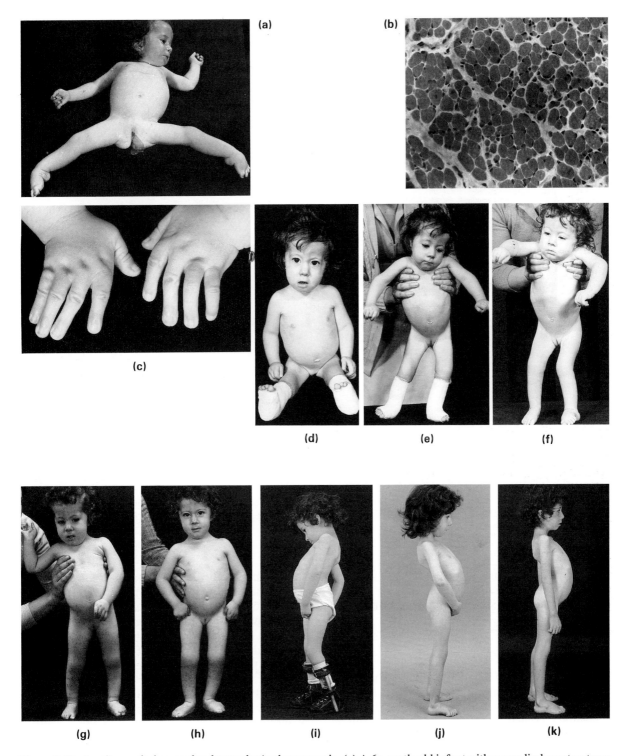

Figure 2-52a-k   Congenital muscular dystrophy/arthrogryposis. (a) A 6-month-old infant with severe limb contractures and deformities from birth. Note fixed flexion of hands and equinus of feet. The knees were still extended with limited flexion, reflecting the *in utero* posture (breech presentation with extended legs). Muscle power was good and she was able to sit unaided. Muscle biopsy showed mild myopathic change with variation in fibre size and some connective tissue proliferation (b). Marked improvement of flexion deformity of fingers following regular daily passive extension by parents (c). Some improvement in fixed equinus deformity of feet but needed operative correction (d, e, 9 months). Gradual improvement in posture and function of legs (f, 12 months; g, 18 months; h, 2 years; i, 3½ years; j, 4 years; k, 8 years).

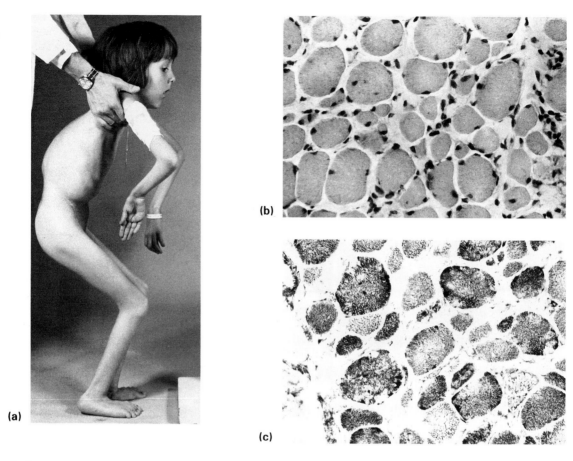

Figure 2-53a-c Congenital muscular dystrophy. (a) A 7-year-old boy with hypotonia from birth and progressive contractures. He was never able to stand unaided. EMG: myopathic; CK 24 iu/litre. (b) Biopsy of deltoid showed a dystrophic pattern, with marked variation in fibre size, internal nuclei and extensive proliferation of connective tissue (lighter areas) and to a lesser extent, fat (H & E). (c) Oxidative enzyme preparation shows marked disruption of fibre pattern ('moth-eaten' fibres) (NADH-TR).

problems at the time of presentation and the associated diaphragmatic involvement may lead to respiratory failure in later childhood or adolescence.

HISTORICAL REVIEW

Although Batten (1903) had already introduced the concept of a congenital form of myopathy, Howard (1908) was probably the first to use the term congenital muscular dystrophy for his case of muscle weakness with associated talipes equinovarus.

It is difficult in this context to assess some of the early reports in the literature, such as the two cases of 'atonic-sclerotic muscular dystrophy' described by Ullrich (1930) or the three infants from the same family who had congenital muscular dystrophy and died by 6, 8 and 10 weeks of age, described by de Lange (1937), since modern histochemical and

electron microscopic studies may well have revealed one of the recognizable congenital myopathies and more intensive neonatal care may have tided these infants over their early problems and improved the longterm prognosis. Some of these severely affected cases might well be examples of congenital myotonic dystrophy rather than congenital muscular dystrophy.

Several reviews of large series of cases in recent times have helped to define more clearly the pattern of disease and have also highlighted some striking differences.

Vassella *et al.* (1967) described in detail eight cases and reviewed 27 from the literature. They defined congenital muscular dystrophy as a primary myopathy already present at birth, with the same features as seen in progressive muscular dystrophy. They drew attention to the variability in the clinical severity and also to the high incidence of affected siblings, suggesting an autosomal recessive pattern of inheritance. Zellweger *et al.* (1967a, b) reported separately three cases of benign congenital muscular dystrophy and three with a severe form of disease. The exact criteria for the subdivision into benign and severe are not clear since one of the severe cases did achieve the ability to walk. Rotthauwe *et al.* (1969) reviewed eight personal cases, using the same diagnostic criteria as Vassella *et al.* They categorized seven as severe and one as benign. All subjects had weakness and hypotonia at birth, and sucking and swallowing difficulty was also common.

Donner *et al.* (1975) reviewed 15 cases of congenital muscular dystrophy from Finland followed for up to 15 years. These constituted 9% of 160 cases of neuromuscular disorders seen at the same hospital over a 10-year period. Muscle weakness was generalized and included the face and respiratory muscles. Contractures were present at birth in nine and were amenable to treatment. There was a tendency for new contractures to develop in the second and third years. The CK tended to be high in the early stages (1–2 years) and normal or near normal later. Histopathological changes varied from slight to a very extensive, apparently inactive or burnt-out picture. Seven of their patients achieved the ability to walk unaided. Two died. In three ECG abnormalities were noted. The IQs ranged from 78 to 130. They concluded that the active phase of the disease process was at its height during intrauterine or early postnatal life and then tended to wane, leaving a burnt-out state in which new contractures might develop and cause possible deterioration with time. Two families contained more than one affected child and in a third family the parents were first cousins, supporting an autosomal recessive inheritance.

INVESTIGATIONS

Ultrasound imaging of the muscle usually shows a very striking and diffuse increase in echo throughout the muscle, much more marked than that in Duchenne dystrophy (Figure 2-54). This probably reflects the common proliferation of adipose tissue in the muscle. In some cases, ultrasound imaging may show striking differential involvement of the quadriceps muscle, with sparing of the rectus femoris and marked increase in echo in the vasti. Selective multiple needle biopsies through the same small incision have shown striking histological abnormality in the vasti and sparing of the rectus (Figure 2-55) (Heckmatt and Dubowitz, 1987).

Electromyography reveals a myopathic pattern.

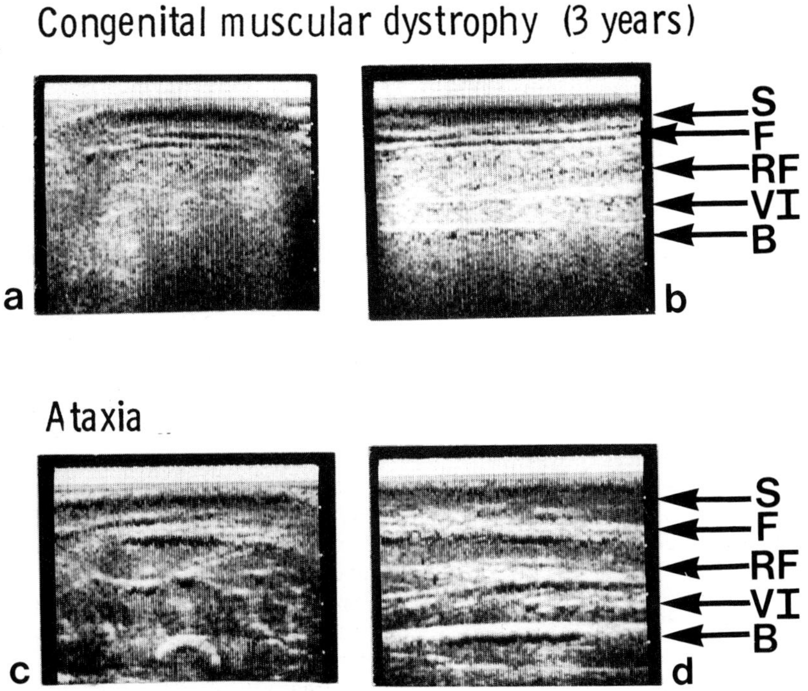

Figure 2-54 (a, b) Congenital muscular dystrophy (3 years). (c, d) Ataxia. (S: skin; F: facia; RF: rectus femoris; VI: vastus internis; B: bone)

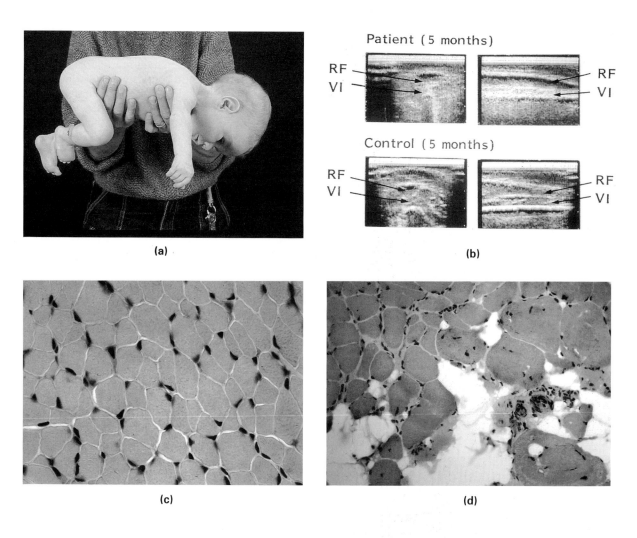

(a)

(b)

(c)

(d)

(e)

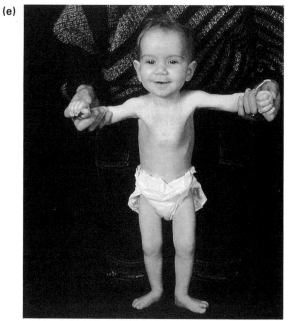

Figure 2-55a-e Congenital muscular dystrophy (differential involvement). This 5-month-old floppy infant presented with delay in motor milestones (a). Ultrasonography of the quadriceps showed a striking differential involvement with sparing of rectus (c) and involvement of vasti (b). Selective needle biopsy of both components through the same incision confirmed this, with an essentially normal picture in the rectus, and a striking dystrophic picture in the vastus lateralis (d). The pathology would have been completely missed by a standard open biopsy of the rectus or interpreted as a 'minimal change myopathy'. At subsequent follow-up she showed marked improvement in muscle function and was able to stand well with support by 8 months (e). She walked at 18 months and currently, 4 years later, continues to be ambulant.

The *CK* may be moderately elevated, especially in the early phase, but can be within normal limits or only slightly elevated and does not attain the levels seen in Duchenne dystrophy. In cases with an unduly high CK it is important to exclude a Duchenne dystrophy by DNA deletion studies, or dystrophin in the muscle, which should be normal.

Muscle biopsy usually shows marked pathological changes consistent with a dystrophic process. A striking feature of many biopsies is the remarkable replacement of muscle by adipose tissue, and connective tissue proliferation is also usual. Some, however, show mainly connective tissue proliferation and little adipose tissue. The muscle biopsy often looks much worse than the clinical picture and one may be surprised that a patient with such extensive pathological change in a limb muscle may actually be ambulant. Under no circumstances, therefore, should the biopsy picture be used as an index of severity of the disease or as a means of prognosis.

MANAGEMENT —————————————————

In view of the relatively static or non-progressive course the disease is likely to follow, it is important to try to correct existing contractures by passive stretching, night splints and serial plaster casts and to prevent progression of contractures by active and passive exercises. In some cases patients may need tenotomies in order to achieve an upright posture and consequent ambulation. Early surgical intervention should be avoided, as the deformities are likely to recur, and it is better to defer surgical correction, particularly of equinovarus deformity of the feet, until the child has achieved the ability to take some weight on the legs. If one corrects the deformities at that stage the child is likely to maintain the corrected posture.

The patient should be encouraged from an early stage to be mobile and active since immobility is always conducive to progression of contractures. In late cases which have had no active treatment, one frequently finds that the fixed deformities of the limbs are more of a handicap than the degree of muscle weakness present.

Some patients whose power is too weak to sustain their body weight may achieve ambulation with callipers, and the same principles apply as in the management of cases of spinal muscular atrophy of intermediate severity (see Chapter 8).

One difficult problem to deal with is the commonly associated dislocation of the hips. Over-enthusiastic orthopaedic intervention with immobilization of the hips in a plaster spica may result in a fixed flexion deformity and negate any hope of ever becoming ambulant. I have generally preferred to concentrate on trying to promote mobility and ambulation as a first priority in these children and to defer any intervention on the hips until locomotion is achieved. If ambulation is not achieved, the need for doing anything operative on the hips is doubtful anyway.

SYNDROMES OF CONGENITAL MUSCULAR DYSTROPHY WITH CENTRAL NERVOUS SYSTEM ABNORMALITY

In recent years a number of syndromes have been reported of congenital muscular dystrophy in association with central nervous system involvement.

FUKUYAMA TYPE CONGENITAL MUSCULAR DYSTROPHY —————————

A series of publications from Japan reviewed over 100 cases of congenital muscular dystrophy, suggesting that the condition may be more prevalent there (Fukuyama *et al.*, 1960; Matsumoto *et al.*, 1970; Segawa, 1970; Segawa *et al.*, 1970; Nonaka *et al.*, 1972). The type originally described in 15 cases by Fukuyama *et al.* (1960) is distinctive in its associated severe mental retardation and frequently associated febrile or afebrile convulsions. The muscular dystrophy itself affects the facial as well as the limb muscles and has the usual associated joint contractures.

In addition to the Fukuyama type congenital muscular dystrophy, a number of syndromes associated with congenital muscular dystrophy have been documented that have consistent structural abnormalities of the brain and may represent separate genetic disorders.

MUSCLE-EYE-BRAIN DISEASE —————————

Santavuori *et al.* (1977) described a syndrome comprising congenital muscular dystrophy, mental retardation and ocular abnormality in nine children, including two affected brothers, and suggested it may be genetically determined through an autosomal recessive mechanism.

Santavuori *et al.* (1989) further reviewed the syndrome of muscle-eye-brain disease in 19 patients, who presented with congenital hypotonia and muscle weakness. The CK was elevated, EMG myopathic and biopsy showed slight or moderate changes of muscular dystrophy. Ophthalmological findings included severe visual failure and uncontrolled eye movements associated with severe myopia. Flash visual evoked potentials were exceptionally high. Psychomotor development was slow during the first year of life and there was severe mental retardation. Most patients began to deteriorate around 5 years of age, including contractures and spasticity. In several patients CT scans showed ventricular dilatation and low density of the white matter. The authors considered that the spasticity and the ocular features differentiated muscle–eye–brain disease from the Fukuyama type of congenital muscular dystrophy.

WALKER–WARBURG SYNDROME —————

This is an autosomal disorder with characteristic brain and eye abnormalities. Dobyns *et al.* (1989) reviewed the data on 21 personal cases and an additional 42 from the literature, extended the phenotype to include congenital muscular dystrophy, and cleft lip and/or palate, and further revised the diagnostic criteria. Four anomalies were consistently present in all the cases assessed: type II lissencephaly (21/21), cerebellar malformation (20/20), retinal malformation (18/18) and congenital muscular dystrophy (14/14). Two other frequently observed abnormalities were ventricular dilatation (with or without hydrocephalus) (20/21) and anterior chamber malformation (16/21). All other malformations occurred less frequently. Congenital macrocephaly with hydrocephalus (11/19) was more common than microcephaly (3/19). Dandy–Walker malformation (10/19) was sometimes associated with posterior encephalocoeles. Additional abnormalities included microphthalmia (8/21), ocular colobomas (3/15), congenital cataracts (7/20), genital anomalies in males (5/8) and cleft lip or palate (4/21). Median survival in their series was 9 months. They considered Fukuyama congenital muscular dystrophy to be distinct from Walker–Warburg because of less frequent and severe cerebellar and retinal abnormality, but that Walker–Warburg is identical to muscle–eye–brain disease. In a response to this latter suggestion, Santavuori *et al.* (1990), while agreeing that there were certain similarities between the two syndromes, drew attention to some of the significant differences.

CENTRAL NERVOUS SYSTEM INVOLVEMENT IN 'PURE' CONGENITAL MUSCULAR DYSTROPHY ——————

The form of congenital muscular dystrophy seen in the West is usually associated with normal intellectual development and no evidence of neurological dysfunction.

However, some cases of congenital muscular dystrophy do have some degree of intellectual retardation, usually mild. In addition, a number of brain imaging studies in recent years have shown a fairly consistent change in the white matter, with either CT or magnetic resonance imaging, in a proportion of cases of pure congenital muscular dystrophy with normal intellect. Yoshioka *et al.* (1980) found low density areas in the white matter on CT scanning in 14 out of 25 cases of congenital muscular dystrophy. Echenne *et al.* (1986) reported a brain CT scan of 10 cases of congenital muscular dystrophy, seven of whom showed hypodensity in the white matter. Two of the patients corresponded to muscle–eye–brain syndrome, one to Fukuyama type, and some of the remainder had associated mental retardation. This series seems to have been selected for central nervous system involvement. Oliviera *et al.* (1990) found diffuse bilateral hypodensity of the white matter, particularly in the frontal lobes, in 10 out of 12 cases of congenital muscular dystrophy in Brazil.

A recent workshop on congenital muscular dystrophy brought together a number of experts in the field in order to try and achieve some consensus in relation to defining the various syndromes (Dubowitz, 1994). The following clinical phenotypes could currently be defined. Whether they will prove to be completely independent entities or possibly allelic variations from a single gene will have to wait resolution by linkage studies of the individual disorders, which is currently in progress.

I. 'Pure' congenital muscular dystrophy

The main features are:

i. Muscle weakness with hypotonia or arthrogryposis.
ii. Histological changes of a dystrophic nature, often with extensive connective tissue or adipose proliferation but no substantial evidence of necrosis or regeneration.
iii. The CK may be normal or moderately elevated.
iv. The intellect is usually normal.
v. Brain imaging may show a normal picture or evidence of changes in the white matter on CT or magnetic resonance imaging.

The association of intellectual retardation in some cases, or of associated epilepsy, does not seem to correlate with the presence or absence of imaging changes in the central nervous system.

II.   *Fukuyama type congenital muscular dystrophy*

In addition to muscle weakness and a dystrophic muscle biopsy, this form of congenital muscular dystrophy is characterized by:

i.   The consistent association of mental retardation which is often severe in degree.
ii. The CK is consistently elevated.
iii. There are consistent structural changes in the brain at autopsy or on imaging.
iv. There is no significant ocular involvement.
v.   Seizures are frequently associated with the condition (about 40%).
vi. Most cases survive beyond infancy and childhood and into adolescence.

III.   *Muscle–Eye–Brain disease (Santavuori)*

In addition to the muscle weakness and associated dystrophic changes in the muscle, there is consistent ocular and central nervous system involvement.

The most consistent ocular abnormality is severe myopia but others include strabismus, glaucoma, lens opacity, retinal atrophy and optic atrophy.

There is associated mental retardation which is often severe. Epilepsy is also commonly associated and the EEG is always abnormal after the age of 1 year. Hydrocephalus is present in the majority of cases. The CK may be normal within the first year but is always elevated after that.

IV.   *Walker–Warburg syndrome*

This is characterized by structural changes and associated mental retardation in addition to the muscle weakness and dystrophic changes.

The consistent central nervous system abnormalities on imaging are a type II lissencephaly, comprising variable gyral malformations together with an abnormally thick cortex and decreased interdigitations between white matter and cortex. There may also be other structural changes within the nervous system. Ocular malformations are also common but are thought to be less severe and less consistent than in the muscle–eye–brain disease.

There is divergence of opinion as to whether the Walker–Warburg syndrome and the muscle–eye–brain disease are one entity with variable severity, or whether they represent two separate entities in view of the more striking ocular involvement in the muscle–eye–brain disease. There is certainly some degree of overlap in the structural changes within the central nervous system.

MOLECULAR GENETICS ——————————

Dystrophin and associated proteins

Dystrophin in the muscle is usually normal, both on Western blot and on immunocytochemical assessment of sections. Matsumura *et al.* (1993) recently

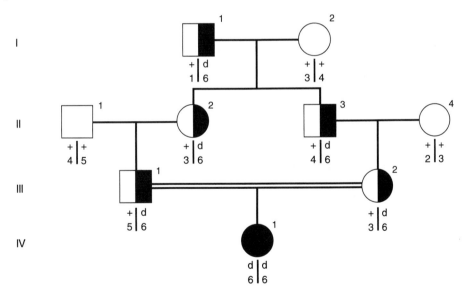

Figure 2-56 Homozygosity by descent. Hypothetical inbred pedigree demonstrating cosegregation of a disease (with two alleles d and +) with an informative DNA-marker (with six alleles, 1-6). The 'affected' daughter (IV-1) is homozygous-by-descent for both loci (dd, 66); she has inherited two copies of an identical chromosomal fragment from her great grandfather (I-1). (From Farrall *et al.*, 1993 with the courtesy of the author and by permission of *Nature Genetics*.)

reported a reduction in all the dystrophin-associated glycoproteins together with a selective marked reduction of the 43kD glycoprotein, with normal dystrophin, in four cases of Fukuyama congenital muscular dystrophy (FCMD), but not in cases of non-Fukuyama muscular dystrophy. However, Arahata *et al.* (1993a) were unable to confirm these results in a study of 10 cases of FCMD, finding a reduction in 43 kD glycoprotein (43 DAG) only in the occasional fibres with reduction in dystrophin. In addition they noted a more consistent reduction in laminin M (merosin), a protein attached to the dystrophin associated glycoproteins on the outside of the muscle membrane, which they considered might have an early or primary role in the pathogenesis of FCMD.

Gene location for FCMD

In a recent study of gene linkage in Fukuyama type muscular dystrophy, Toda *et al.* (1993) identified the gene locus for FCMD on chromosome 9q31-33 by a remarkable bit of serendipidity. In a systematic study of 21 families they noted that in one particular consanguinous family there was a coincidental involvement of FCMD and xeroderma pigmentosum in the same isolated index case; no other member of the family showed either FCMD or xeroderma pigmentosum by itself. They reasoned that the genes for the two diseases might be closely linked and that, as a result of consanguinity within the family, the affected case had inherited both genes from a single ancestor carrying both genes – an example of homozygosity by descent (see Figure 2-56). As the gene location of xeroderma pigmentosum was already known (9q34) and there were some DNA probes available in this region, they went directly for linkage of FCMD at this site – and struck oil. They were also able to exclude the site for the 43 DAG gene on chromosome 3p21 as a possible location, so that 43 DAG is not a candidate protein for FCMD, and any reported changes must be secondary. Work is currently in progress to see whether any of the other forms of congenital muscular dystrophy, and especially those with central nervous system involvement, also locate to 9q, and this should at least help to resolve whether these individual disorders are allelic or not.

MEROSIN AND CONGENITAL MUSCULAR DYSTROPHY ——————————

Following the observation above of Arahata *et al.* (1993a) of a reduction in laminin M (merosin) in some of their cases of Fukuyama muscular dystrophy, Tomé *et al.* (1994) screened a series of biopsies from classical congenital muscular dystrophy and found a complete absence in 13 of 20 cases. In a similar study of our own cases we found absent merosin in 10 of 22 cases (C.A. Sewry unpublished data). These results and the current gene linkage studies were presented at the recent Second Workshop of the International Consortium on Congenital Muscular Dystrophy (Dubowitz and Fardeau, 1995). A possible linkage to chromosome 6, the locus for the merosin gene, was pursued using homozygosity mapping in consanguinous families with multiple affected children (Hillaire *et al.*, 1994) and the data suggests that the merosin-negative cases link to this locus. Merosin-positive families do not link to either 6q or 9q.

In a study of MRI brain imaging changes in four sibling pairs we found concordance in either negative or positive white matter changes in each of the pairs and similar observations were found by Topaloglu in these three sibling pairs (Philpot *et al.*, 1995a). In a correlative study of our patients to date who have had both merosin studies as well as MRI imaging, all 11 cases with merosin-positive muscle biopsies had normal brain imaging, whereas all seven merosin-negative cases who have had brain imaging showed abnormality (Philpot *et al.*, 1995b). It thus looks as though the merosin-negative cases are those with associated MRI changes in the cerebral white matter, which correlates well with the tissue specific localization of merosin in muscle and Schwann cells.

THE dy/dy MOUSE – AN ANIMAL MODEL FOR CONGENITAL MUSCULAR DYSTROPHY ——————————

The *dy/dy* dystrophic mouse (dystrophia muscularis), with autosomal recessive inheritance, was extensively studied in the 1960s and 1970s as a model for the human Duchenne dystrophy, but was shunted into the wings after a study by Bradley and his colleagues (Bradley and Jenkison 1973; Madrid *et al.*, 1975) found evidence for focal demyelination in the ventral roots of the spinal cord and suggested the disease was a neuropathy rather than a myopathy. A recent study by Arahata *et al.* (1993b) found a complete deficiency of merosin in the muscle of the homozygous *dy/dy* mouse and demonstrated a comparable absence in the ventral roots of the spinal cord. No studies were made of merosin in the central nervous system. In a parallel study, Campbell and his colleagues (Sunada *et al.*, 1994) found a similar deficit in merosin in the *dy/dy* mouse. Merosin was completely absent in the nerves but seemed to be present in trace amounts in muscle.

As the gene locus for the *dy/dy* mouse was already known to be on chromosome 10, and this was also the locus for the merosin gene, it seemed extremely likely that the two would concur, and this was demonstrated by Sunada *et al.* (1994). It is also of interest that human chromosome 6 corresponds to mouse chromosome 10.

The *dy/dy* mouse should be a good model for congenital muscular dystrophy for any further studies on the pathogenesis of the disease or possible therapeutic efforts. After a period of reasonable motor function in the newborn period, it develops a severe muscle weakness at a few weeks of age, affecting the lower limbs more than the upper. It is rapidly progressive and leads to difficulty with ambulation and dragging of the hind limbs and shortens the lifespan, usually to less than a year.

EMERY–DREIFUSS MUSCULAR DYSTROPHY

This X-linked muscular dystrophy is clinically distinct from the Duchenne/Becker type and is characterized by a relatively mild skeletal muscle weakness, with a distinct distribution, in association with contractures of various muscles and cardiomyopathy.

In 1961, Dreifuss and Hogan described a large family in Virginia in the USA with an X-linked form of muscular dystrophy which they considered at the time to be a benign type of Duchenne muscular dystrophy. However, on reinvestigating the family a few years later, Emery and Dreifuss (1966) considered it to be a very different disease from either Duchenne or Becker muscular dystrophy. Emery (1989a,b) has reviewed it again in recent years.

CLINICAL FEATURES —————————————————

Although the condition usually presents in adolescence or early adult life it may already present in early childhood and also be detectable in families with previously affected members (Figure 2-57).

The initial presenting feature is usually the tightness of various muscle groups as a result of the contractures, and this may cause tightness of the tendo Achilles with consequent toe walking, tightness of the spinal extensor muscles with consequent limitation of full flexion, with inability to approximate the chin to the sternum and to touch the toes. There are also early contractures of the elbow flexors with limitation of full extension.

The associated weakness may be relatively mild and has a selective scapulohumeroperoneal distribution. There is often very striking wasting of the upper arms, accentuated by the sparing of the deltoids and the forearm muscles. There may also be focal wasting of the calf muscles (Figure 2-58).

Cardiac involvement

The asssociated cardiomyopathy usually presents with arrhythmia and may lead to sudden death in early adult life. One of the special features is an atrial paralysis. Prior to the age of 20 the electrocardiogram is usually normal, but evidence of arrhythmia, sometimes only at night, may be detected on 24-hour Holter monitoring. It is important to detect the arrhythmia, which is sometimes the presenting feature, as the provision of a cardiac pacemaker may be life-saving and considerably improve the prognosis.

In patients with no cardiac symptoms, the earliest ECG change consists of low-amplitude P waves and first degree heart block, while the most advanced state consists of 4-chamber dilated cardiomyopathy with complete heart block and ventricular arrhythmias (Emery and Dreifuss, 1966; Rotthauwe *et al.*, 1972; Thomas *et al.*, 1972; Waters *et al.*, 1975; Oswald *et al.*, 1987; Yoshioka *et al.*, 1989). Initial depolarization (tall R waves in lead V1 and Q waves in inferolateral leads), so characteristic of Duchenne dystrophy, is not a feature of Emery–Dreifuss dystrophy (Hassan *et al.*, 1979).

Atrial arrhythmia usually appears prior to complete heart block. Reported features include first degree heart block, followed by Wenckebach phenomenon and then, complete atrioventricular dissociation (Hassan *et al.*, 1979) and atrial fibrillation or flutter with progressive slowing of the rate (Emery and Dreifuss 1966; Waters *et al.*, 1975; Voit *et al.*, 1988). Syncope or near-syncope commonly occurs late in the second decade or early in the third (Waters *et al.*, 1975). Subsequently, with more prolonged survival, a generalized cardiomyopathy appears (Thomas *et al.*, 1972; Voit *et al.*, 1988). Some patients develop generalized left ventricular hypokinesis, perfusion defects in the cardiac muscle, and tricuspid and mitral valve regurgitation (Yoshioka *et al.*, 1989).

Respiratory involvement

Some cases may show evidence of nocturnal hypoventilation, presumably as a result partly of the restricted expansion of the chest in association with the rigid spine, and partly due to involvement of the diaphragm. In one of our patients a marked bradycardia at night, dropping as low as 15 beats per minute, was detected on a 24-hour Holter monitor and a cardiac pacemaker was initially recommended, which the patient refused. He was also found to have associated hypoxia at night on percutaneous

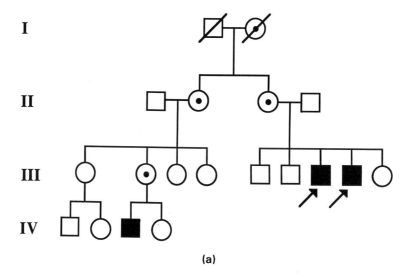

(a)

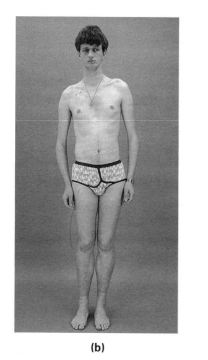

(b)

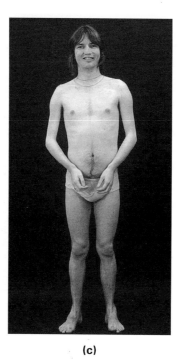

(c)

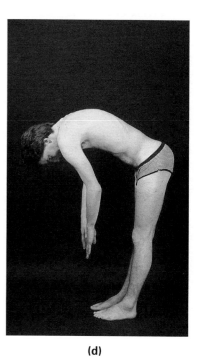

(d)

Figure 2-57a-d Emery–Dreifuss dystrophy. Two brothers (a: III, 7 and 8), aged 21 and 20 years, were referred for investigation of mild muscle weakness, affecting particularly the distal parts of the legs and associated with limitation of elbow extension (b,c) and limited neck and trunk flexion (d). Both brothers had previously had pacemakers inserted following discovery of arrhythmia during an insurance medical examination. Their physical disability was minimal and one was able to cope with a heavy labouring dockworker's job without difficulty. CK was 625 iu/litre and 620 iu/litre respectively. Muscle biopsy showed an overtly pathological picture, with variation in fibre size and focal areas of atrophic fibres with associated internal nuclei, and also some splitting and whorling of fibres (e).

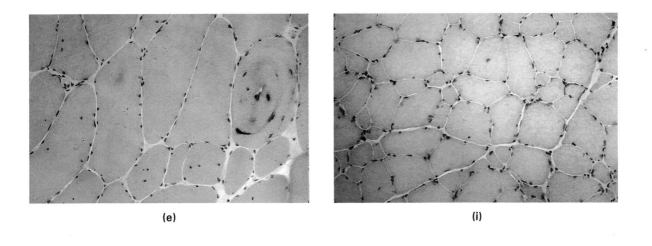

(e)

(i)

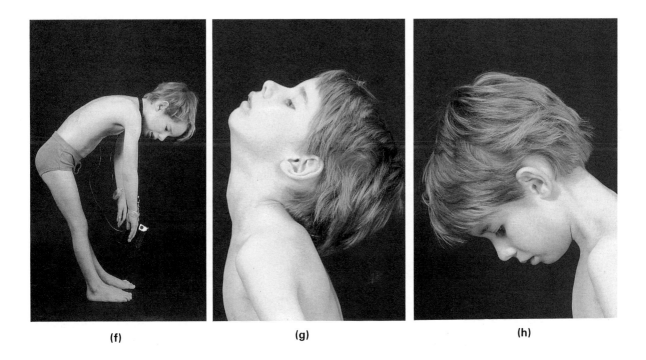

(f)

(g)

(h)

Figure 2-57e-h A 6-year-old cousin on the maternal side was subsequently found to be affected (IV, 3). His early milestones were normal, but he had experienced mild weakness of the legs since 2 years of age, and began to fall and have breath-holding attacks after falling. From 5 years of age he developed a waddling gait and had difficulty climbing stairs. On examination there was a slight limitation of elbow extension and also trunk and neck flexion (f-h). CK was 1640 iu/litre. Muscle biopsy showed overt mild pathological changes (i). 24-hour Holter monitoring did not reveal any cardiac arrhythmia. Holter monitoring of the two mothers (II,3 and II,2) did not reveal any arrhythmia either.

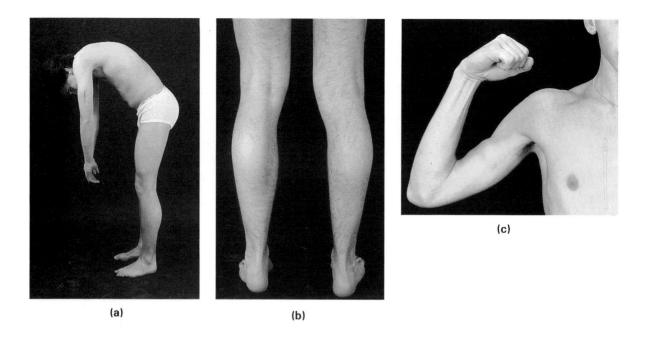

(a)   (b)   (c)

Figure 2-58a-c Emery–Dreifuss dystrophy. This young man, aged 18 years, presented with mild weakness of the legs, particularly affecting the lower parts. On examination he was found to have limitation of flexion of the spine (a), marked wasting of the medial aspects of both gastrocnemii (b), and focal wasting of the upper arms, affecting particularly the biceps with sparing of the deltoids (c). His older brother, aged 20 years, had a similar problem. Muscle biopsy in both brothers showed unequivocal dystrophic change but fairly mild and focal. Occasional fibres showed necrosis and phagocytosis and there was also some regenerative activity.

oximetry, which completely resolved on nocturnal mask ventilation, as did the bradycardia, and he has continued well for several years since, even managing an African safari with his portable ventilator (Figure 2-59).

CARRIERS

Carriers of Emery–Dreifuss muscular dystrophy are usually free of muscle or spinal manifestations, but they may have arrhythmias and a pacemaker may be needed (Mawatari and Katayama, 1973; Dickey *et al.*, 1984; Emery, 1987; Pinelli *et al.*, 1987; Bialer *et al.*, 1991). In the original Virginia family, six of 34 carrier females (18%) had arrhythmia, two had pacemakers, and the frequency of heart disease increased with age. All five carriers over age 60 had an abnormal ECG (Bialer *et al.*, 1991). Merchut *et al.* (1990) recently reported a cardiac transplantation in a female with Emery–Dreifuss dystrophy.

SPECIAL INVESTIGATIONS

The *creatine kinase* may be moderately elevated, usually within the range of between twice and five times the upper limit of normal, and certainly not

reaching the very grossly elevated levels seen in Duchenne or Becker dystrophies. Ultrasonography of the muscles may show selective involvement with, for example, increased echogenicity of the vasti and sparing of the rectus femoris. This may also be demonstrated on other imaging methods such as CT scanning.

Electromyography

Electromyography usually shows a myopathic pattern.

Muscle biopsy

Muscle biopsy shows a myopathic process with variation in fibre size, including clusters of atrophic fibres, which should not be mistaken for denervation, mild proliferation of connective tissue and possibly some focal necrosis of fibres (Figures 2-57 to 2-59). The picture is not as overtly dystrophic as in Duchenne or Becker dystrophy but has enough changes to be classified for the present with the dystrophies. This may well need to be revised once the gene and its product are identified. Furthermore, autopsy studies indicate that the spinal cord is normal (Hara *et al.*, 1987).

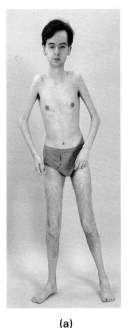
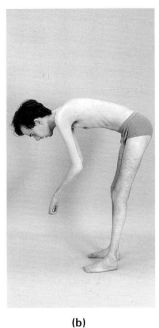

(a)   (b)

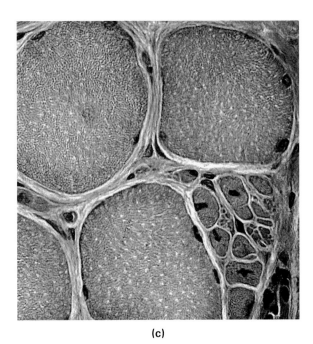

(c)

Figure 2-59a-c Emery–Dreifuss dystrophy: an isolated case. This 24-year-old young man with limitation of spinal flexion and elbow extension (a,b) was originally referred with mild limb weakness at 14 years of age. Muscle biopsy showed a dystrophic picture with focal atrophic (? split-up) fibres (c). He subsequently was found to have marked bradycardia (15/min) at night on his Holter monitoring, and also nocturnal hypoventilation, which was a more marked problem from his functional point of view. Following the provision of a cuirass ventilator at night, he improved considerably as did the bradycardia. He was able with his portable ventilator to go on safari in Africa across the Sahara.

MOLECULAR GENETICS ————————

The condition was shown early on to be unlinked to any of the probes of the Xp21 Duchenne and Becker dystrophies, and dystrophin is normal in the muscle. The gene was subsequently found to be located in the Xq28 region, very close to the factor VIII gene (Hodgson *et al.*, 1986b; Thomas *et al.*, 1986; Yates *et al.*, 1986; Müller *et al.*, 1991; Wehnert *et al.*, 1991; Cole *et al.*, 1992). Several laboratories are currently working on the further refinement of the location of the gene and its isolation and characterization and an international consortium has been established to monitor progress and pool resources (Yates, 1991).

A dominantly inherited disorder with a similar phenotype has been well documented (Witt *et al.*, 1988), with evidence of male to male transmission, thus excluding an X-linked inheritance with manifesting carriers, as may occur in some families. It is also likely that many of the reported cases of Rigid Spine syndrome (Dubowitz, 1973) may be isolated cases of Emery–Dreifuss syndrome in view of the marked predominance of males and the similar phenotype with associated contractures at the elbows and ankles. An associated scoliosis is also a common feature of both conditions.

SCAPULOHUMERAL MUSCULAR DYSTROPHY ————————

The scapulohumeral form of dystrophy is very uncommon. It overlaps in presentation with the more common facioscapulohumeral variety.

Many cases included in the earlier literature are probably not true cases of dystrophy but other neuromuscular disorders, which may present with scapulohumeral weakness. All cases thus need to be fully investigated to exclude one of the congenital myopathies or a neurogenic syndrome.

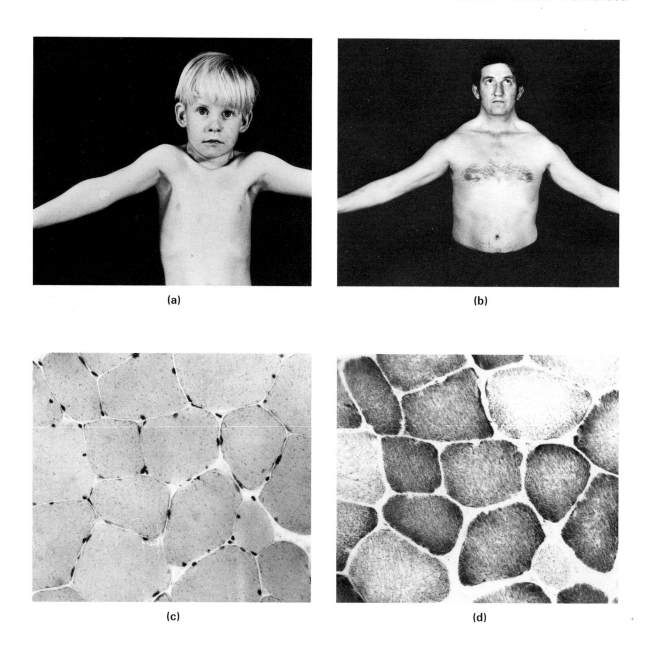

(a)

(b)

(c)

(d)

Figure 2-60a-d Scapulohumeral weakness without facial involvement in 5-year-old boy (a) and his 33-year-old father (b). CK and EMG normal. Compare Figure 2-61. Muscle biopsy from father shows mild myopathic change with variation in fibre size and normal histochemical pattern (c, d). Deltoid. (c, H & E × 240; d, NADH-TR × 240.)

As in the case of facioscapulohumeral 'dystrophy' (see next section), the changes in the muscle biopsy may be very slight, and not at all comparable with those seen in limb girdle dystrophy (Figure 2-60).

FACIOSCAPULOHUMERAL MUSCULAR DYSTROPHY

This form of muscular dystrophy predominantly affects the shoulder girdle and the facial muscles (Figures 2-61 to 2-70). The facial weakness may precede the scapulohumeral, as already noted by Duchenne (1872) who gave a detailed description of the disease some years ahead of Landouzy and Dejerine (1884), whose names are usually associated with it. In some cases the weakness may be more widespread and affect the lower limbs as well.

The inheritance is autosomal dominant. As in so many other dominant conditions, variation in clinical severity within a pedigree is common and subclinical cases may be identified on careful assessment (Figures 2-62 to 2-65).

CLINICAL FEATURES

As the condition is frequently a relatively mild one, with a very slow progression, presentation is commonly in adolescence or adult life. Childhood cases do occur, however, and are also readily identified in affected families.

The early symptoms may relate to the weakness of the facial or of the scapulohumeral muscles. In some the weakness may be very slight and focal. On clinical examination the diagnosis can usually be made quite readily by identifying the facial weakness, even if mild, with inability to screw the eyes closed and bury the eyelashes, or to purse the lips, puff out the cheeks, blow or whistle. A fairly typical double dimple at the angle of the mouth also often appears when the patient tries to smile.

With abduction of the shoulders there is difficulty in raising the arms and also a striking upward riding of the scapulae, giving a characteristic stepwise or terraced appearance to the shoulders (see Figure 2-61). Some subjects may have a more severe weakness, with more extensive involvement of the trunk and pelvic girdle muscles, often with a markedly lordotic posture, and may progress to loss of ambulation in early adult life or later.

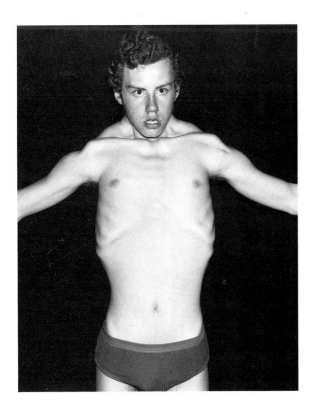
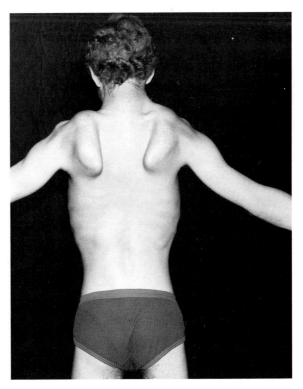

Figure 2-61   Facioscapulohumeral dystrophy in a 15-year-old male, showing facial weakness and upward riding of the scapulae on abduction of the arms.

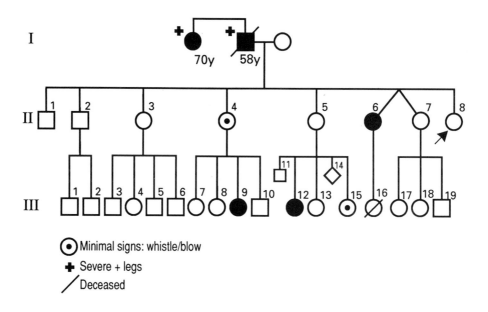

Figure 2-62 Facioscapulohumeral muscular dystrophy. Pedigree chart showing dominant inheritance and subclinical cases (II,5). Index patient (II,8) was clinically normal and requested genetic counselling. Figures 2-63 and 2-64 illustrate two branches of the family (II,4 and II,5).

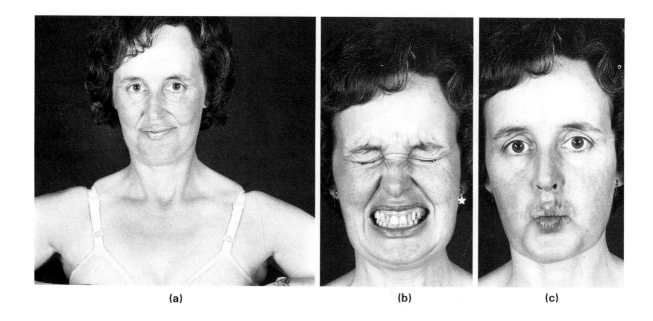

(a)   (b)   (c)

Figure 2-63a-c On examination II,4 showed normal shoulder girdle movements, and no apparent facial weakness (a). She had normal facial movements and complete closure of the eyelids, with burying the the eyelashes (b), but was unable to blow out the cheeks, to whistle or to purse the lips (c).

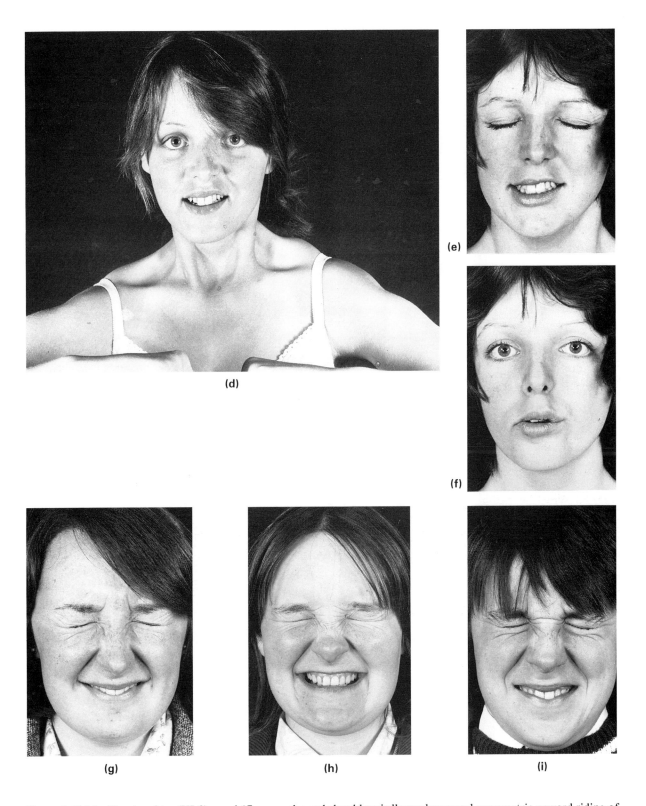

Figure 2-63d-i   Her daughter (III,9), aged 17 years, showed shoulder girdle weakness and asymmetric upward riding of the scapulae (d) and facial weakness, with inability to screw up the eyes and bury the eyelashes (e) or to whistle or blow out the cheeks (f). Her other two daughters, III,7 (g) and III,8 (h), aged 18 and 15 years, and her son, III,10 (i) aged 14 years, had no facial or shoulder weakness.

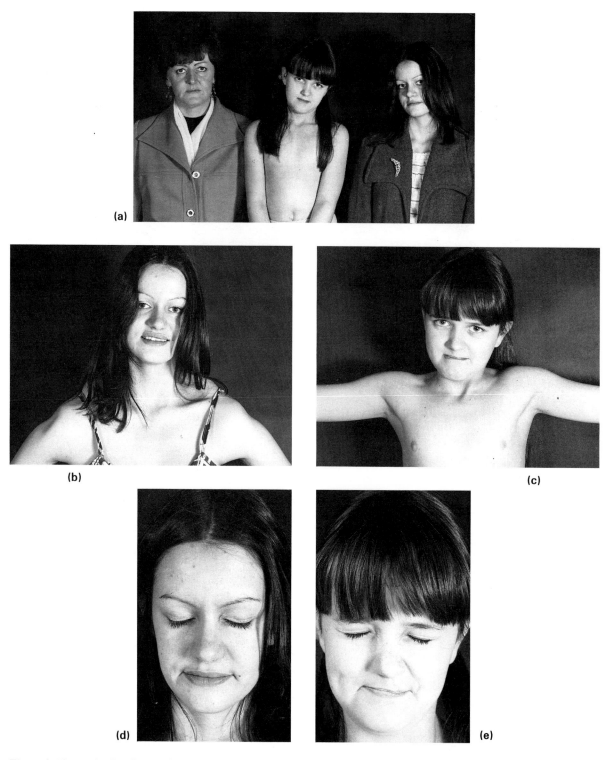

Figure 2-64a-e   (a) Family II,5 from pedigree chart in Figure 2-62, showing II,5 who has no detectable weakness of the face or shoulder girdle, and two of her daughters, III,15 and III,12. Her other daughter, III,13, was also examined and had no weakness. The older daughter, III,12, had shoulder girdle weakness and upward riding of the scapulae with abduction of the arms (b), whereas the younger daughter (III,15) had no shoulder girdle abnormality (c). Case III,12 showed overt facial weakness with limited facial movements and eye closure (d) and III,15 showed mild facial weakness with inability to screw the eyes up tightly and bury the eyelashes completely (e).

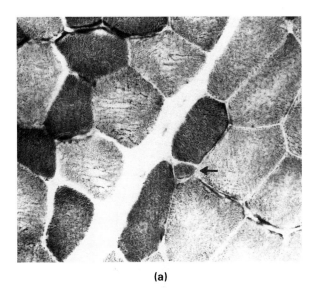

(a)

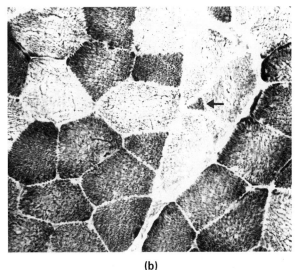

(b)

Figure 2-65a,b   Muscle biopsy of the deltoid from (a) II,5 (subclinical) and (b) III,12 (affected) showing a normal-looking muscle apart from focal very small fibres (arrows) (NADH-TR).

There is usually no associated cardiac or intellectual involvement in this myopathy. Some families may, however, have associated abnormality of the retina, with a vasculopathy producing capillary telangiectasia and microaneurysms, or a sensorineural hearing loss.

INVESTIGATIONS

As in other neuromuscular disorders, the facioscapulohumeral distribution of weakness is common to a number of underlying pathological conditions. Careful investigation with all the various techniques is essential. In a study of 17 cases of facioscapulohumeral syndrome, van Wijngaarden and Bethlem (1971) found that seven were due to muscular dystrophy, two to myasthenia, five to myotubular myopathy, one to nemaline myopathy, one to mitochondrial myopathy and one to central core disease.

Some cases have a denervation pattern and others may show a very striking inflammatory response suggestive of a 'myositis', but usually unresponsive to steroids. In most of the myopathic cases the changes on muscle biopsy are relatively slight, the most consistent being the presence of isolated small atrophic fibres (see Figure 2-65). In association with this focal fibre atrophy other fibres may be hypertrophied. One is frequently surprised by the relatively minimal pathological change in the muscle in contrast to the striking clinical weakness of the same muscles.

Much confusion has been caused in recent years by attempts to define a facioscapulohumeral spinal muscular atrophy on the basis of the muscle biopsy suggesting a denervation process, often on rather insecure grounds such as grouping of small fibres (which is also common in Becker dystrophy and does not in itself constitute a neurogenic atrophy), or fibre type predominance or fibre type grouping. In a detailed immunocytochemical study of biopsies from facioscapulohumeral dystrophy, we have shown that the isolated very small fibres are in fact regenerating rather than atrophic or denervating (Sewry and Dubowitz, unpublished data). One may question whether the term dystrophy is indeed justified for these cases, since the muscle does not show the usual changes associated with dystrophy. Until more insight and understanding are available for the interpretation of these pathological changes, the common usage of the term facioscapulohumeral dystrophy for these cases is probably convenient and worth retaining. With the recent advances at the molecular genetic level and location of the gene, further understanding should come once the gene is isolated and its product identified.

It is particularly noteworthy that, following the recent discovery of the gene location on chromosome 4q, all the dominantly inherited families studied conformed to this single locus, despite the varying pathological features of the muscle biopsies (Padberg *et al.*, 1991). This consortium also defined clinical criteria for the diagnosis of facioscapulohumeral dystrophy.

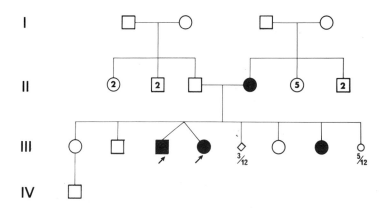

Figure 2-66. Pedigree chart of family with dominantly inherited facioscapulohumeral dystrophy and marked variation in clinical severity as illustrated in Figures 2-67a-e.

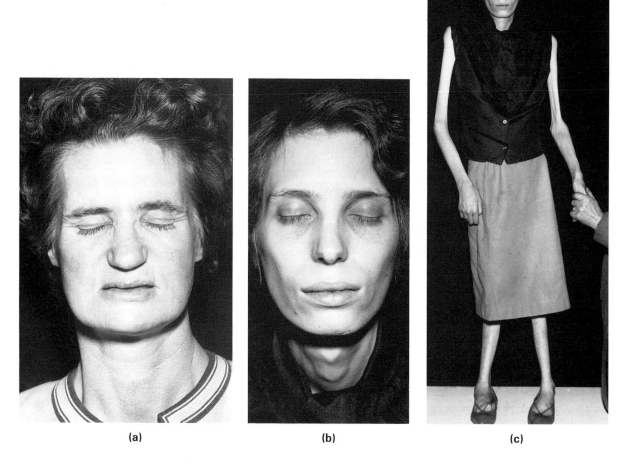

(a)   (b)   (c)

Figure 2-67a-c   The mother, II,4 in pedigree chart in Figure 2-66, had no clinical disability and showed minimal facial weakness with inability to close the eyes tightly and bury the eyelashes (a). Her daughter, III,4 (b, c), was severely affected, with marked generalized wasting and weakness and a myopathic facies with inability to close her eyes tightly. Her twin brother (III,3) was only mildly affected. The younger daughter (III,7) (see Figure 2-67d,e) had no clinical disability but on examination had a mild degree of shoulder and facial muscle involvement (d,e).

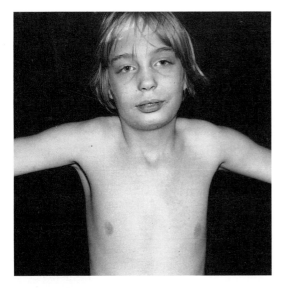
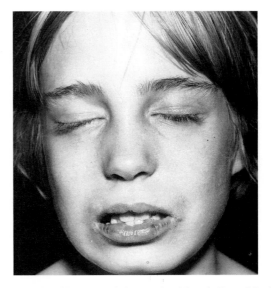

Figure 2-67d,e   Case III, 7 in Figure 2-66. The patient has no clinical disability and minimum shoulder girdle and facial weakness on examination.

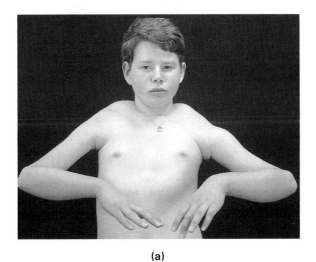

(a)

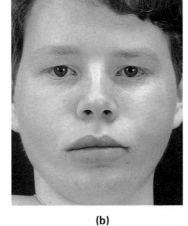

(b)

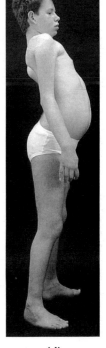

(d)

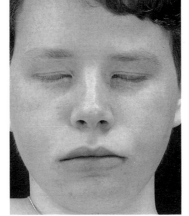

(c)

Figure 2-68a-d   Facioscapulohumeral dystrophy with typical shoulder girdle abnormality with upward riding of the scapulae on abduction of the arms (a), as well as facial weakness with limited smile and eye closure and pouting of the lips (b,c). The patient also has marked trunk weakness and associated lumbar lordosis (d). He subsequently had increasing difficulty with ambulation and became wheelchair bound.

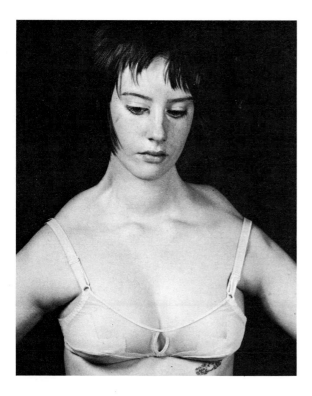

Figure 2-69 Facioscapulohumeral muscular dystrophy in a 16-year-old girl with 2-year history of shoulder weakness and associated thyrotoxicosis. The shoulder girdle weakness improved both subjectively and on quantitative myometry after treatment of the thyrotoxicosis but no change occurred in her facial weakness and residual shoulder girdle signs.

A survey by Lunt and Harper (1991) of 41 families with facioscapulohumeral muscular dystrophy, containing 168 affected subjects, provided useful data for genetic counselling. Penetrance was 95% by the age of 25 years; very occasionally obligate carriers are clinically normal in middle age. One-third of heterozygotes were mildly affected over the age of 40 years, but about one-fifth in this age group needed wheelchairs. It was shown that estimation of serum creatine kinase activity is limited as a pre-symptomatic test for facioscapulohumeral dystrophy as this was normal in a substantial proportion of patients.

MOLECULAR GENETICS

The locus for autosomal dominant facioscapulo-humeral dystrophy has been mapped to the distal long arm of chromosome 4 in the region of 4q35-ter (Wijmenga *et al.*, 1990, 1991). A number of closely linked markers have subsequently been identified which have provided a means of accurate diagnosis or exclusion of subclinical and equivocal cases in affected families, and also of sporadic cases, and have opened the way for prenatal diagnosis.

Upadhyaya *et al.* (1990) reported presymptomatic and prenatal diagnosis with 98% accuracy using a closely linked, highly polymorphic DNA marker, D4S139.

Gene mapping studies have not, to date, provided any evidence for genetic heterogeneity in facio-scapulohumeral dystrophy, and families thought to have 'facioscapulohumeral SMA' appear to show linkage to the same region.

A recent workshop of the International Consortium on Facioscapulohumeral Muscular Dystrophy (Lunt, 1994) reported the cumulative experience of the various participating centres with the various probes in relation to family studies and also the recognition of *de novo* fragments in isolated cases.

Although the gene has not yet been isolated or characterized, Wijmenga *et al.* (1992) have recently identified rearrangements at the gene locus.

MANAGEMENT

Many of these patients are relatively mildly affected, with little disability, and cope well with everyday routines. One can usually give them a reassurance that this is one of the mildest forms of dystrophy that tends to have a very long course, a good prognosis and very little tendency to progression. Others, however, may have significant trunk and lower limb weakness with progressive difficulty in ambulation.

In cases where patients have marked difficulty in elevation of the shoulders and use of the arms, benefit may be derived from orthopaedic efforts to try to fixate the scapulae, since it is the mobility of the scapulae that often contributes most of the disability. This can be tested clinically by trying to immobilize the scapula by firm pressure with one's hands and seeing whether this improves the patient's ability to abduct the arm. If this is the case, one may get considerable functional benefit by surgical fixation of the scapula.

GENETIC COUNSELLING

As the condition has a dominant pattern of inheritance there is a 50% risk of any child being affected. Due to the marked variability in the clinical severity it can at times be difficult to be sure that a relative requesting genetic counselling is not subclinically affected (see Figure 2-62). In these cases EMG, CK and biopsy may also be normal. The advances in the molecular genetics have now opened the way for accurate ascertainment in such cases and also for providing prenatal diagnosis.

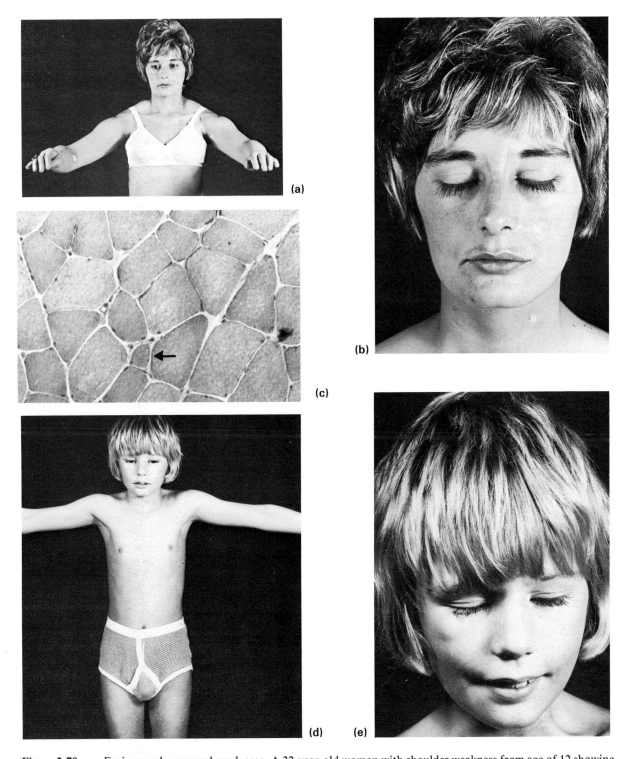

Figure 2-70a-e Facioscapuloperoneal syndrome. A 32-year-old woman with shoulder weakness from age of 12 showing (a) limited abduction of shoulders and overriding of scapulae, and (b) associated facial weakness with inability to close eyes fully or bury eyelashes. She also has a bilateral footdrop with marked weakness of ankle dorsiflexors. CK normal. EMG (deltoid) borderline myopathic. A muscle biopsy from her deltoid (c) looked normal apart from variation in fibre size and isolated small fibres (arrow). Her 9-year-old son (d,e) showed no shoulder girdle or lower limb weakness but overt weakness of the face with inability to close the eyes tightly or purse the lips or say 'oo'. Future molecular characterization of the FSH gene should help to identify cases such as these as variants of the FSH gene.

OCULAR SYNDROMES

A number of myopathies with involvement of the external ocular muscles have traditionally been classified with the muscular dystrophies. In some cases the weakness of the ocular muscles occurs in isolation; in others it is part of a more generalized neuromuscular problem or part of a more complex syndrome involving other systems as well.

In a patient presenting with progressive external ophthalmoplegia it can be very difficult to decide whether the lesion is in the nerve nucleus, the nerve, the neuromuscular junction or the muscle.

External ophthalmoplegia is not a feature of Duchenne, limb girdle or facioscapulohumeral dystrophy or of the spinal muscular atrophies. It is, however, a common component of myasthenia gravis and may at times be the only clinical manifestation, and is also an occasional feature of myotonic dystrophy. It is thus important to exclude these two conditions. Ocular muscle involvement also occurs in some of the congenital myopathies, particularly myotubular myopathy (see Chapter 3) and is a key component of some of the mitochondrial myopathies (see Chapter 5).

Patients are usually much more conscious of the ptosis than of external ophthalmoplegia and it is surprising at times to find almost complete limitation of the movement of the eyes in all directions without the patient being aware of either any deficit in mobility or of diplopia. The absence of diplopia may reflect the relatively symmetrical involvement of muscle on the two sides. The head is often held extended to compensate for the ptosis.

Attempts have been made in the past to delineate various ocular syndromes on the basis of the clinical picture (Rowland, 1975). In all cases it is essential to assess carefully the extent of the ocular involvement, the association of pupillary changes, which would imply a neural rather than myopathic basis, the association of retinitis pigmentosa or other retinal pigmentations which occur in a number of mitochondrial syndromes, involvement of other cranial nerves, involvement of other muscles, presence of cardiomyopathy and the association of abnormality in the nervous system or any other system.

CONGENITAL PTOSIS ————————

This is a common paediatric problem and may be sporadic or inherited as a dominant trait. It usually remains static but may be more marked during illness or fatigue. It is often asymmetrical (Figure 2-71).

External ophthalmoplegia, with or without ptosis, may also occur in isolation. It is usually symmetrical and tends to be slowly progressive. In recent years

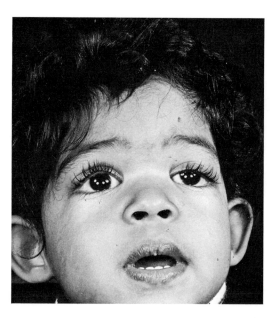

Figure 2-71 A 2-year-old child with isolated left ptosis. There was no other muscle weakness. The family history was negative.

many of these cases of progressive external ophthalmoplegia (PEO) have been shown to have a mutation in the mitochondrial genome and will be discussed in detail in that section (see Chapter 5).

CONGENITAL FAMILIAL EXTERNAL OPHTHALMOPLEGIA ————————

'Congenital fibrosis of the extraocular muscles' or 'congenital familial external ophthalmoplegia' is an autosomal dominant, congenital, non-progressive disorder of the extraocular muscles, characterized clinically by bilateral ptosis and external opthalmoplegia. Affected individuals often have associated facial weakness. In contrast to the classical pathological description, recent work suggests that the extraocular muscles are not fibrotic (EC Engle, personal communication). The disorder has recently been mapped to the centromeric region of chromosome 12 in a study of several large families (Engle *et al.*, 1994).

OCULOPHARYNGEAL MYOPATHY ——

Victor *et al.* (1962) suggested the name oculopharyngeal muscular dystrophy for the late-onset association of dysphagia with ocular myopathy which they considered a separate entity. Several families were subsequently documented and Barbeau (1966, 1968) was able to trace the condition through ten generations of a French–Canadian family. The large concentration observed by Barbeau in Canada was thought to be a 'founder effect' of a French couple who emigrated to Quebec in 1634. A similar population concentration of oculopharyngeal dystrophy has recently been documented by Blumen *et al.* (1993) in a cluster of Jews in Israel coming from Bukhara (Uzbekistan). Although essentially a disease of late adult onset, genetic anticipation was suggested in some of the latter families, with onset in childhood in children of affected parents.

Inheritance follows an autosomal dominant pattern. As so often happens in dominantly inherited conditions, the clinical severity and expression show marked variation and cases occur with either dys-phagia or ocular involvement by itself. In some of the latter there may be only ptosis without external ophthalmoplegia. Some cases also have associated skeletal muscle weakness.

Limb muscle biopsy shows a striking and apparently characteristic picture with vacuolation of fibres, rimmed by red stain with the Gomori trichrome stain, the so-called 'rimmed vacuoles', resembling but not identical to the 'ragged-red' fibres of the Kearns–Sayre syndrome (Dubowitz and Brooke, 1973). Tomé and Fardeau (1980) subsequently described a pathognomonic morpho-logical feature on electron microscopy of intranuclear tubulofilamentous inclusions of 8.5 nm outer diameter.

APPENDIX:
CLASSIFICATIONS OF FUNCTIONAL ACTIVITY IN DUCHENNE MUSCULAR DYSTROPHY

1. Modified Swinyard Classification (Swinyard *et al.*, 1957; Inkley *et al.*, 1974)

1. Walks and climbs stairs without assistance.
2. Walks and climbs stairs using hand rail.
3. Walks and climbs stairs with difficulty.
4. Walks. Gets out of chair but does not climb stairs.
5. Walks but does not get out of chair.
6. Walks with help - or independently with braces.
7. Walks in long leg callipers - not independently.
8. Stands in long leg braces.
9. Only sits in wheelchair.

2. Archibald and Vignos (1959)

1. Walks and climbs stairs without assistance.
2. Walks and climbs stairs with aid of railing.
3. Walks and climbs stairs slowly with aid of railing.
4. Walks but cannot climb stairs.
5. Walks unassisted but cannot climb stairs or get out of chair.
6. Walks only with assistance or with braces.
7. In wheelchair. Sits erect, can roll chair and perform bed and wheelchair activities of daily living.
8. In wheelchair. Sits erect. Unable to perform bed and chair activities without assistance.
9. In a wheelchair. Sits erect only with support. Able to do only minimal activities of daily living.
10. In bed. Cannot perform activities of daily living without assistance.

3. Brooke *et al.* (1989)

Arms and shoulders

1. Starting with arms at the sides, patient can abduct the arms in a full circle until they touch above the head.
2. Can raise arms above head only by flexing the elbow (i.e. shortening the circumference of the movement) or by using accessory muscles.
3. Cannot raise hands above head but can raise an 8 oz glass of water (using both hands if necessary).
4. Can raise hands to mouth but cannot raise an 8 oz glass of water to mouth.
5. Cannot raise hand to mouth but can use hands to hold pen or pick up pennies from table.
6. Cannot raise hands to mouth and has no useful function of hands.

Hips and legs.

1. Walks and climbs stairs with assistance.
2. Walks and climbs stairs with aid of railing (<12 seconds).
3. Climbs stairs slowly (>12 seconds).
4. Walks unassisted and rises from chair but cannot climb stairs.
5. Walks unassisted but cannot rise from chair or climb stairs.
6. Walks only with assistance or walks independently with long leg braces.
7. Walks in long leg braces but requires assistance for balance.
8. Stands in long leg braces but unable to walk even with assistance.
9. Is in wheelchair.
10. Is confined to bed.

REFERENCES

Abbs, S., Yau, S.C., Clark, S. *et al.* (1991) A convenient multiplex PCR system for the detection of dystrophin gene deletions: a comparative analysis with cDNA hybridisation shows mistypings by both methods. *Journal of Medical Genetics* **28**: 304–311.

Acsadi, G., Dickson, G., Love, D.R. *et al.* (1991) Human dystrophin expression in *mdx* mice after intramuscular injection of DNA constructs. *Nature* **353**: 815–818.

Adriaenssens, K. and Vermeiren, G. (1980) Simple electrophoretic technique for creatine kinase MM isozyme in neonatal Duchenne muscular disease screening using dried blood samples. *Clinica Chimica Acta* **105**: 99–103.

Ahmad, M., Sanderson, J.E., Hallidie-Smith, K.A. and Dubowitz, V. (1977) Echocardiographic assessment of left ventricular function in Duchenne's muscular dystrophy. *British Heart Journal* **40**: 734–740.

Ahn, A.H. and Kunkel, L.M. (1993) The structural and functional diversity of dystrophin. *Nature Genetics* **3**: 238–291.

Allen, J.E. and Rodgin, D.W. (1960) Mental retardation in association with progressive muscular dystrophy. *American Journal of Diseases of Children* **100**: 208–211.

Angelini, C., Pegoraro, E., Perini, F. *et al.* (1991) A trial with a new steroid in Duchenne muscular dystrophy. In: Angelini, C., Danieli, G.A. and Fontanari, D. eds, *Muscular Dystrophy Research: From Molecular Diagnosis Toward Therapy*. Amsterdam: Excerpta Medica, pp. 173–179.

Appleyard, S.T., Dunn, M.J., Dubowitz, V. *et al.* (1985) Increased expression of HLA ABC class I antigens by muscle fibres in Duchenne muscular dystrophy, inflammatory myopathy and other neuromuscular disorders. *Lancet* i: 361–363.

Arahata, K. and Engel, A.G. (1984) Monoclonal antibody analysis of mononuclear cells in myopathies. I. Quantitation of subsets according to diagnosis and sites of accumulation and demonstration and counts of muscle fibers invaded by T cells. *Annals of Neurology* **16**: 193–208.

Arahata, K., Ishiura, S., Ishiguro, T. *et al.* (1988) Immunostaining of skeletal and cardiac muscle surface membrane with antibody against Duchenne muscular dystrophy peptide. *Nature* **333**: 861–863.

Arahata, K., Ishihara, T., Kamakura, K. *et al.* (1989) Mosaic expression of dystrophin in symptomatic carriers of Duchenne's muscular dystrophy. *New England Journal of Medicine* **320**: 138–142

Arahata, K., Beggs, A.H., Honda, H. *et al.* (1991) Preservation of the C-terminus of dystrophin molecule in the skeletal muscle from Becker muscular dystrophy. *Journal of the Neurological Sciences* **101**: 1488–156.

Arahata, K., Hayashi, Y.K., Mizuno, Y. *et al.* (1993a) Dystrophin-associated glycoprotein and dystrophin co-localisation at sarcolemma in Fukuyama congenital muscular dystrophy. *Lancet* **342**: 623–624.

Arahata, K., Hayashi, Y.K., Koga R. *et al.* (1993b) Laminin in animal models for muscular dystrophy: defect of laminin M in skeletal and cardiac muscles and peripheral nerve of the homozygous dystrophic *dy/dy* mice. *Proc Japan Acad* **69** Ser. B: 259.

Archibald, K.C. and Vignos, P.J. (1959) A study of contractures in muscular dystrophy. *Archives of Physical Medicine and Rehabilitation* **40**: 150–157.

Arikawa, E., Hoffman, E.P., Kaido, M. *et al.* (1991) The frequency of patients with dystrophin abnormalities in a limb-girdle patient population. *Neurology (Tokyo)* **41**: 1491–1496

Arts, W.F., Bethlem, J. and Volkers, W.S. (1978) Further investigation on benign myopathy with autosomal dominant inheritance. *Journal of Neurology* **217**: 201–206.

Azibi, K., Bachner, L., Beckmann, J.S. *et al.* (1993) Severe childhood autosomal recessive muscular dystrophy with the deficiency of the 50 kDa dystrophin-associated glycoprotein maps to chromosome 13q12. *Human Molecular Genetics* **2**: 1423–1426.

Barbeau, A. (1966) The syndrome of hereditary late onset ptosis and dysphagia in French Canada. In: Kuhn, E. ed., *Symposium über progressive Muskeldystrophie*. Berlin: Springer-Verlag, pp. 102–109.

Barbeau, A. (1968) Oculopharyngeal muscular dystrophy in French Canada. In: Brunette, J.R. and Barbeau, A. eds, *Progress in Neuro-ophthalmology* Vol. 2. Amsterdam: Excerpta Medica, p. 3.

Barohn, R.J., Levine, E.J., Olson, J.O. *et al.* (1988) Gastric hypomotility in Duchenne's muscular dystrophy. *New England Journal of Medicine* **319**: 15–18.

Barohn, R.J., Miller, R.G. and Griggs, R.C. (1991) Autosomal recessive distal dystrophy. *Neurology* **41**: 1365–1370.

Bashir, R., Strachan, T., Keers, S. *et al.* (1994) A gene for autosomal recessive limb-girdle muscular dystrophy maps to chromosome 2p. *Human Molecular Genetics* **3**: 455–457.

Batten, F.E. (1903) Three cases of myopathy, infantile type. *Brain* **26**: 147.

Bautista, J., Rafel, E., Castilla, J.M. *et al.* (1978) Hereditary distal myopathy with onset in early infancy: observation of a family. *Journal of the Neurological Sciences* **37**: 149–158.

Becker, P.E. (1962) Two new families of benign sex-linked recessive muscular dystrophy. *Revue Canadienne de Biologie* **21**: 551.

Becker, P.E. and Kiener, F. (1955) Eine neue X-chromasomale Muskeldystrophie. *Archiv für Psychiatrie und Nervenkrankheiten*, **193**: 427.

Beckmann, J.S., Richard, I., Hillaire, D. *et al.* (1991) A gene for limb-girdle muscular dystrophy maps to chromosome 15 by linkage. *C R Acad Sci III*, **312**: 141–148.

Beggs, A.H. and Kunkel, L.M. (1990) Improved diagnosis of Duchenne/Becker muscular dystrophy. *Journal of Clinical Investigation* **85**: 613–619.

Bellen, P., Hody, J.L., Clairbois, J. *et al.* (1993) The surgical treatment of spinal deformities in Duchenne muscular dystrophy. *The Journal of Orthopaedic Surgery* 7: 48–57.

Ben Hamida, M., Fardeau, M. and Attia, N. (1983) Severe childhood muscular dystrophy affecting both sexes and frequent in Tunisia. *Muscle and Nerve* 6: 469–480.

Ben Othmane, K., Ben Hamida, M., Pericak-Vance, M. *et al.* (1992) Linkage of Tunisian autosomal recessive Duchenne-like muscular dystrophy to the peri-centromeric region of chromosome 13q. *Nature Genetics* 2: 315–317.

Bethlem, J. and van Wijngaarden, K.G. (1976) Benign myopathy, with autosomal dominant inheritance. *Brain* 99: 91–100.

Bialer, M.G., McDaniel, N.L. and Kelly, T.E. (1991) Progression of cardiac disease in Emery–Dreifuss muscular dystrophy. *Clinical Cardiology* 14: 411–416.

Blumen, S.C., Nisipeanu, P., Sadeh, M. *et al.* (1993) Clinical features of oculopharyngeal muscular dystrophy among Bukhara Jews. *Neuromuscular Disorders* 3: 575–577.

Boachie Adjei, O., Lonstein, J.E., Winter, R.B. *et al.* (1989) Management of neuromuscular spinal deformities with Luque segmental instrumentation. *Journal of Bone and Joint Surgery (Am)* 71: 548–562.

Bonilla, E., Samitt, C.E., Miranda, A.F. *et al.* (1988) Normal and dystrophin-deficient muscle fibers in carriers of the gene of Duchenne muscular dystrophy. *American Journal of Pathology* 133: 440–445.

Bonilla, E., Younger, D.S., Chang, H.W. *et al.* (1990) Partial dystrophin deficiency in monozygous twin carriers of the Duchenne gene discordant for clinical myopathy. *Neurology* 40: 1267–1270.

Boyce, F.M., Beggs, A.H., Feener, C. *et al.* (1991) Dystrophin is transcribed in brain from a distant upstream promoter. *Proceedings of the National Academy of Sciences USA* 88: 1276–1280.

Bradley, W.G. and Jenkison, M. (1973) Abnormalities of peripheral nerves in murine muscular dystrophy. *Journal of Neurological Sciences* 18: 227–247

Bradley, W.G., Jones, M.Z., Mussini, J.-M. *et al.* (1978) Becker-type muscular dystrophy. *Muscle and Nerve* 1: 111–132.

Brooke, M.H., Griggs, R.C., Mendell, J.R. *et al.* (1981a) The natural history of Duchenne muscular dystrophy (DMD): a caveat for therapeutic trials. *Transactions of the American Neurological Association* 106: 195–199.

Brooke, M.H., Griggs, R.C., Mendell, J.R. *et al.* (1981b) Clinical trials in Duchenne muscular dystrophy: 1. The design of the protocol. *Muscle and Nerve* 4: 186–197.

Brooke, M.H., Fenichel, G.M., Griggs, R.C. *et al.* (1983) Clinical investigation in Duchenne dystrophy: 2. Determination of the 'power' of therapeutic trials based on the natural history. *Muscle and Nerve* 6: 91–103.

Brooke, M.H., Fenichel, G.M., Griggs, R.C. *et al.* (1987) Clinical investigation of Duchenne muscular dystrophy: Interesting results in a trial of prednisone. *Archives of Neurology* 44: 812–817.

Brooke, M.H., Fenichel, G.M., Griggs, R.C. *et al.* (1989) Duchenne muscular dystrophy: patterns of clinical progression and effects of supportive therapy. *Neurology* 39: 475–481.

Bulfield, G., Siller, W.G., Wight, P.A.L. *et al.* (1984) X chromosome-linked muscular dystrophy (mdx) in the mouse. *Proceedings of the National Academy of Sciences* USA 81: 1189–1192.

Burn, J., Povey, S., Boyd, Y. *et al.* (1986) Duchenne muscular dystrophy in one of monozygotic twin girls. *Journal of Medical Genetics* 23: 494–500.

Bushby, K. (1992) Report on the 12th ENMC-sponsored international workshop on the 'limb-girdle' muscular dystrophies. *Neuromuscular Disorders* 2: 3–5.

Bushby, K.M.D. and Gardner-Medwin, D. (1993) The clinical, genetic and dystrophin characteristics of Becker muscular dystrophy. 1. Natural history. *Journal of Neurology* 240: 998–104.

Campbell, K.P. and Kahl, S.D. (1989) Association of dystrophin and an integral membrane glycoprotein. *Nature* 338: 259–262.

Capecchi, M.R. (1980) High efficiency transformation by direct microinjection of DNA into cultured mammalian cells. *Cell* 22: 479–488.

Carpenter, J.L., Hoffman, E.P., Romanul, F.C. *et al.* (1989) Feline muscular dystrophy with dystrophin deficiency. *American Journal of Pathology* 135: 909–919.

Carpenter, S., Karpati, G., Heller, I. *et al.* (1978) Inclusion body myositis: a distinct variety of idiopathic inflammatory myopathy. *Neurology* 28: 8.

Carroll, N., Bain, R.J., Smith, P.E. *et al.* (1991) Domiciliary investigation of sleep-related hypoxaemia in Duchenne muscular dystrophy. *European Respiratory Journal* 4: 434–440.

Casazza, F., Brambilla, G., Salvato, A. *et al.* (1988) Cardiac transplantation in Becker muscular dystrophy. *Journal of Neurology* 235: 496–498.

Chamberlain, J.S., Gibbs, R.A., Ranier, J.E. *et al.* (1988) Deletion screening of the Duchenne muscular dystrophy locus via multiplex DNA amplification. *Nucleic Acids Research* 16: 11141–11156.

Chamberlain, J.S., Gibbs, R.A., Ranier, J.E. *et al.* (1991) Detection of gene deletions using multiplex polymerase chain reactions. In: Mathew, C. ed., *Methods in Molecular Biology* Vol. 9, *Protocols in human molecular genetics*. Clifton, NJ: Humana Press, pp. 299–312.

Chu, G., G., Hayakawa, H. and Berg, P. (1987) Electroporation for the efficient transfection of mammalian cells with DNA. *Nucleic Acids Research* 15: 1311–1326.

Chutkow, J.G., Heffner, R.R.Jr, Kramer, A.A. *et al.* (1986) Adult-onset autosomal dominant limb-girdle muscular dystrophy. *Annals of Neurology* 20: 240–248.

Chutkow, J.G., Hyser, C.L., Edwards, J.A. *et al.* (1987) Monozygotic female twin carriers discordant for the clinical manifestations of Duchenne muscular dystrophy. *Neurology* 37: 1147–1151.

Clerk, A., Rodillo, E., Heckmatt, J.Z. *et al.* (1991) Characterization of dystrophin in carriers of Duchenne muscular dystrophy. *Journal of the Neurological Sciences* **102**: 197–205.

Cole, C.G., Abbs, S.J., Dubowitz, V. *et al.* (1992) Linkage of Emery-Dreifuss muscular dystrophy to the red/green cone pigment (RGCP) genes, proximal to factor VIII. *Neuromuscular Disorders* **2**: 51–57.

Conte, G. and Gioja, L. (1836) Scrofola del sistema muscolare. *Annali Clinici dell'Ospedale degl'Incurabili (Napoli)* **2**: 66–79.

Cooper, B.J., Winand, N.J., Stedman, H. *et al.* (1988) The homologue of the Duchenne locus is defective in X-linked muscular dystrophy of dogs. *Nature* **334**: 154-156.

Dangain, J. and Vrbova, G. (1984) Muscle development in mdx mutant mice. *Muscle and Nerve* **7**: 700–704.

de Lange, C. (1937) Studien über angeborenen Lähmungen bzw. angeborenen Hypotonie. II. Über die angeborenen oder frühinfantilen Form der Dystrophie musculorum progressive (Erb). *Acta Paediatrica (Stockholm)* **20** (Suppl 3): 33.

Dickey, R.P., Ziter, F.A. and Smith, R.A. (1984) Emery-Dreifuss muscular dystrophy. *Journal of Pediatrics* **104**: 555–559.

DiMarco, A.F., Kelling, J.S., DiMarco, M.S. *et al.* (1985) The effects of inspiratory resistive training on muscle function in patients with muscular dystrophy. *Muscle and Nerve* **8**: 284–290.

Dobyns, W.B., Pagon, R.A., Armstrong, D. *et al.* (1989) Diagnostic criteria for Walker–Warburg syndrome. *American Journal of Medical Genetics* **32**: 195–210.

Donner, M., Rapola, J. and Somer, H. (1975) Congenital muscular dystrophy: a clinico-pathological and follow-up study of 15 patients. *Neuropädiatrie* **6**: 239-258.

Donofrio, D., Challa, V., Hackshaw, B. *et al.* (1989) Cardiac transplantation in a patient with Becker muscular dystrophy and cardiomyopathy. *Archives of Neurology* **46**: 705–707.

Drachman, D.B., Toyka, K.V. and Myer, E. (1974) Prednisone in Duchenne muscular dystrophy. *Lancet* **ii**, 1409–1412.

Dreifuss, F.E. and Hogan, G.R. (1961) Survival in X-chromosomal muscular dystrophy. *Neurology (Minneapolis)* **11**: 734.

Dreyfus, J.C., Schapira, G. and Demos, J. (1960) Étude de la créatine-kinase sérique chez les myopathes et leur familles. *Revue Française d'Études Cliniques et Biologiques* **5**: 384.

Dubowitz, V. (1960a) Progressive Muscular Dystrophy in Childhood. MD Thesis, University of Cape Town.

Dubowitz, V. (1960b) Progressive muscular dystrophy of the Duchenne type in females and its mode of inheritance. *Brain* **83**: 432–439.

Dubowitz, V. (1963a) Myopathic changes in a muscular dystrophy carrier. *Journal of Neurology, Neurosurgery and Psychiatry* **26**: 322–325.

Dubowitz, V. (1963b) Myopathic changes in muscular dystrophy carriers. *Proceedings of the Royal Society of Medicine* **56**: 810–812.

Dubowitz, V. (1965) Intellectual impairment in muscular dystrophy. *Archives of Disease in Childhood* **40**: 296–301.

Dubowitz, V. (1973) Rigid spine syndrome: a muscle syndrome in search of a name. *Proceedings of the Royal Society of Medicine* **66**: 219–220.

Dubowitz, V. (1978) *Muscle Disorders in Childhood* 1st edn. London, Philadelphia and Toronto: W.B. Saunders

Dubowitz, V. (1986) X;autosome translocations in females with Duchenne or Becker muscular dystrophy. *Nature* **322**: 291–292.

Dubowitz, V. (1989) The Duchenne dystrophy story: from phenotype to gene and potential treatment. *Journal of Child Neurology* **4**: 240–250.

Dubowitz, V. (1991) Prednisone in Duchenne dystrophy. *Neuromuscular Disorders* **1**: 161–163.

Dubowitz, V. (1992) Myoblast transfer in muscular dystrophy: panacea or pie in the sky? *Neuromuscular Disorders* **2**: 305–310.

Dubowitz, V. (1994) Report on 22nd ENMC Sponsored Workshop on Congenital Muscular Dystrophy, held in Baarn, The Netherlands, 14–16 May, 1993. *Neuromuscular Disorders* **4**: 75–81.

Dubowitz, V. and Brooke, M.H. (1973) *Muscle Biopsy: A Modern Approach*. London and Philadelphia: W.B. Saunders.

Dubowitz, V. and Crome, L (1969) The central nervous system in Duchenne muscular dystrophy. *Brain* **92**: 805–808.

Dubowitz, V. and Fardeau M. (1995) Proceedings of the 27th ENMC Sponsored Workshop on Congenital Muscular Dystrophy, Holland, 22–24 April 1994. *Neuromuscular Disorders* **5**: in press

Dubowitz, V. and Heckmatt, J. (1980) Management of muscular dystrophy: pharmacological and physical aspects. *British Medical Bulletin* **36**: 139–144.

Dubowitz, V. and Roy, S. (1970) Central core disease of muscle: clinical, histochemical and electron microscopic studies of an affected mother and child. *Brain* **93**: 133–146.

Duchenne, G.-B. (1855) De l'électrisation localisée et son application à la pathologie et à la thérapeutique 1st edn.

Duchenne, G.-B. (1861) De l'électrisation localisée et son application à la pathologie et à la thérapeutique 2nd edn. Paris: Baillière et Fils.

Duchenne, G.-B. (1868) Recherches sur la paralysie musculaire pseudohypertrophique ou paralysie myosclerosique. *Archives Générales de Médecine* 6 ser., **11**: 5, 179, 305, 421, 552.

Duchenne, G.-B. (1872) De l'électrisation localisée et son application à la pathologie et à la thérapeutique 3rd edn. Paris: Baillière et Fils.

Ebashi, T., Toyokura, Y., Momoi, H. *et al.* (1959) High creatine phosphokinase activity of sera of progressive muscular dystrophy patients. *Journal of Biochemistry (Tokyo)* **46**: 103–104.

Echenne, B., Arthuis, M., Billard, C. *et al.* (1986) Congenital muscular dystrophy and cerebral CT scan anomalies: Results of a collaborative study of the Société de Neurologie Infantile. *Journal of the Neurological Sciences* **75**: 7–22.

Edström, L. (1975) Histochemical and histopathological changes in skeletal muscle in late-onset hereditary distal myopathy (Welander). *Journal of the Neurological Sciences* **26**: 147–157.

El Kerch, F., Sefiani, A., Azibi, K. *et al.* (1994) Linkage analysis of families with severe childhood autosomal recessive muscular dystrophy (SCARMD) in Morocco indicates genetic homogeneity of the disease in North Africa. *Journal of Medical Genetics* **31**: 342–343.

Ellis, J.M., Nhuyen thi Man, Morris, G.E. *et al.* (1990) Specificity of dystrophin analysis improved with monoclonal antibodies. *Lancet* **336**: 881–882.

Emery, A.E.H. (1963) Clinical manifestations in two carriers of Duchenne muscular dystrophy. *Lancet* **i**: 1126.

Emery, A.E.H. (1972) Abnormalities of the electrocardiogram in hereditary myopathies. *Journal of Medical Genetics* **9**: 8–12.

Emery, A.E.H. (1987) X-linked muscular dystrophy with early contractures and cardiomyopathy (Emery–Dreifuss type). *Clinical Genetics* **32**: 360–367.

Emery, A.E.H. (1989a) Emery–Dreifuss muscular dystrophy and other related disorders. *British Medical Bulletin* **45**: 772–787.

Emery, A.E.H. (1989b) Emery–Dreifuss syndrome. *Journal of Medical Genetics* **26**: 637–641.

Emery, A.E.H. (1991) Population frequencies of inherited neuromuscular diseases – a world survey. *Neuromuscular Disorders* **1**: 19–29.

Emery, A.E.H. (1993a) *Duchenne Muscular Dystrophy* 2nd edn. Oxford Monographs on Medical Genetics, No. 24. Oxford: Oxford University Press.

Emery, A.E.H. (1993b) Duchenne muscular dystrophy – Meryon's disease. *Neuromuscular Disorders* **3**: 263–266.

Emery, A.E.H. and Dreifuss, F.E. (1966) Unusual type of benign X-linked muscular dystrophy. *Journal of Neurology, Neurosurgery and Psychiatry* **29**: 338.

Emery, A.E.H. and Skinner, R. (1976) Clinical studies in benign (Becker type) X-linked muscular dystrophy. *Clinical Genetics* **10**: 189–201.

Emslie-Smith, A.M., Arahata, K. and Engel, A.G. (1989) Major histocompatibiity complex class I antigen expression, immunolocalization of interferon subtypes, and T cell-mediated cytotoxicity in myopathies. *Human Pathology* **20**: 224–231.

Engel, A.G. and Biesecker, G. (1982) Complement activation in muscle fiber necrosis: demonstration of the membrane attack complex of complement in necrotic fibers. *Annals of Neurology* **12**: 289–296.

Engle, E.C., Kunkel, L.M., Specht, L.A. and Beggs, A.H. (1994) Mapping of a gene for congenital fibrosis of the extraocular muscles to the centromeric region of chromosome 12. *Nature Genetics* **7**: 69–73.

Erb, W.H. (1884) Ueber die 'juvenile form' der progressiven Muskelatrophie; ihre Beziehungen zur sogenannten Pseudo-hypertrophic der Muskeln. *Deutsches Archiv für klinische Medizin* **34**: 467–519.

Erb, W.H. (1891) Dystrophia muscularis progressiva. Klinische und pathologischanatomische Studien.

Deutsch Zeitschrift für Nervenheilkunde **1**: 13–94, 173–261.

Estrup, C., Lyager, S., Noeraa, N. *et al.* (1986) Effect of respiratory muscle training in patients with neuromuscular diseases and in normals. *Respiration* **50**: 36–43.

Eulenburg, A. von and Cohnheim, R. (1866) Ergebnisse der anatomischen Untersuchung eines Falles von sogenannter Muskelhypertrophie. *Verhandlungen der Berliner medizinischen Gesellschaft* **1**: 191

Fardeau, M., Matsumura, K., Tomé, F.M.S. *et al.* (1993) Deficiency of the 50 kDa dystrophin associated glycoprotein (adhalin) in severe autosomal recessive muscular dystrophies in children native from European countries. *Comptes Rendus de l'Academie des Sciences, Sciences de la vie* **316**: 799–804.

Farrall, M. (1993) Homozygosity mapping: familiarity breeds debility. *Nature Genetics* **5**: 107–108.

Fenichel, G.M., Florence, J.M., Pestronk, A. *et al.* (1991) Long-term benefit from prednisone therapy in Duchenne muscular dystrophy. *Neurology* **41**: 1874–1877.

Florek, M. and Karolak, S. (1977) Intelligence level of patients with the Duchenne type of progressive muscular dystrophy (PMD-D). *European Journal of Pediatrics* **126**: 275–282.

Francke, U., Ochs, H.D., de Martinville, B. *et al.* (1985) Minor Xp21 chromosome deletion in a male associated with expression of Duchenne muscular dystrophy, chronic granulomatous disease, retinitis pigmentosa and McLeod syndrome. *American Journal of Human Genetics* **37**: 250–267.

Fukuyama, Y., Kawazura, M. and Haruna, H. (1960) A peculiar form of congenital progressive muscular dystrophy. Report of fifteen cases. *Pediatria Universitatis Tokyo* No. 4: 5–8.

Galasko, C.S., Delaney, C. and Morris, P. (1992) Spinal stabilisation in Duchenne muscular dystrophy. *Journal of Bone and Joint Surgery* **74B**: 210–214

Galassi, G., Rowland, L.P., Hays, A. *et al.* (1987) High serum levels of creatine kinase: asymptomatic prelude to distal myopathy. *Muscle and Nerve* **10**: 346–350.

Gangopadhyay, S.B., Sherratt, T.G., Heckmatt, J.Z. *et al.* (1992) Dystrophin in frame-shift deletion patients with Becker muscular dystrophy. *American Journal of Human Genetics* **51**: 562–570.

Gaschen, F.P., Hoffman, E.P., Gorospe, J.R. *et al.* (1992) Dystrophin deficiency causes lethal muscle hypertrophy in cats. *Journal of the Neurological Sciences* **110**: 149–159.

Gilchrist, J.M., Pericak-Vance, M., Silverman, L. *et al.* (1988) Clinical and genetic investigation in autosomal dominant limb girdle muscular dystrophy. *Neurology* **38**: 5–9.

Gillard, E.F., Chamberlain, J.S., Murphy, E.G. *et al.* (1989) Molecular and phenotypic analysis of patients with deletions within the deletion-rich region of the Duchenne muscular dystrophy (DMD) gene. *American Journal of Human Genetics* **45**: 507–520.

Ginjaar, I.B., Bakker, E., van Paassen, M.M.B. *et al.*

(1991) Immunohistochemical studies show truncated dystrophins in the myotubes of three fetuses at risk for Duchenne muscular dystrophy. *Journal of Medical Genetics* **28**: 505–510.

Golbus, M.S., Stephens, J.D., Mahoney, M.J. *et al.* (1979) Failure of fetal creatine phosphokinase as a diagnostic indicator of Duchenne muscular dystrophy. *New England Journal of Medicine* **300**: 860–861.

Goldberg, S.J., Stern, L.Z., Feldman, L. *et al.* (1982) Serial two-dimensional echocardiography in Duchenne muscular dystrophy. *Neurology* **32**: 1101–1105.

Gomez, M.R., Engel, A.G., Dewald, G. *et al.* (1977) Failure of inactivation of Duchenne dystrophy X-chromosome in one of female identical twins. *Neurology* **27**: 537–541.

Gospe, S.M. Jr., Lazaro, R.P., Lava, N.S. *et al.* (1989) Familial X-linked myalgia and cramps: a non-progressive myopathy associated with a deletion in the dystrophin gene. *Neurology* **39**: 1277–1280.

Gowers, W.R. (1879a) Clinical lecture on pseudo-hypertrophic muscular paralysis. *Lancet* **ii**: 1, 37, 73, 113.

Gowers, W.R. (1879b) *Pseudohypertrophic Muscular Paralysis. A Clinical Lecture.* London: J. and A. Churchill.

Gowers, W.R. (1902) A lecture on myopathy and a distal form. *British Medical Journal* **2**: 89–92.

Granata, C., Giannini, S., Ballestrazzi, A. *et al.* (1994) Early surgery in Duchenne muscular dystrophy: experience at Istituto Ortopedico Rizzoli, Bologna, Italy. *Neuromuscular Disorders* **4**: 87–88.

Griggs, R.C. and Karpati, G. (eds) (1990) *Myoblast Transfer Therapy.* New York: Plenum Press, 1990.

Griggs, R.C., Moxley, R.T., Mendell, J.R. *et al.* (1991a) Prednisone in Duchenne dystrophy: a randomized, controlled trial defining the time course and dose response. *Archives of Neurology* **48**: 383–388

Griggs, R.C., Moxley, R.T., Mendell, J.R. *et al.* (1991b) Randomized, controlled trial of prednisone and azathioprine in Duchenne dystrophy. *Neurology* **41**: 166.

Griggs, R.C., Moxley, R.T., Mendell, J.R. *et al* (1993) Duchenne dystrophy: randomised, controlled trial of prednisone (18 months) and azathioprine (12 months). *Neurology* **43** 520–527.

Gussoni, E., Pavlath, G.K., Lanctot, A.M. *et al.* (1992) Normal dystrophin transcripts detected in Duchenne muscular dystrophy patients after myoblast transplantation. *Nature* **356**: 435–438.

Hara, H., Nagara, H., Mawatari, S. *et al.* (1987) Emery-Dreifuss muscular dystrophy – an autopsy case. *Journal of the Neurological Sciences* **79**: 23–31.

Hassan, Z., Fastabend, C.P., Mohanty, P.K. *et al.* (1979) Atrioventricular block and supraventricular arrhythmias with X-linked muscular dystrophy. *Circulation* **60**: 1365–1369.

Heckmatt, J.Z. and Dubowitz, V. (1987) Ultrasound imaging and direct needle biopsy in the diagnosis of selective involvement in neuromuscular disease. *Journal of Child Neurology* **2**: 205–213.

Heckmatt, J.Z., Leeman, S. and Dubowitz, V. (1982) Ultrasound imaging in the diagnosis of muscle disease. *Journal of Pediatrics* **101**: 656–660.

Heckmatt, J.Z., Dubowitz, V., Hyde, S.A. *et al.* (1985) Prolongation of walking in Duchenne muscular dystrophy with lightweight orthoses – Review of 57 cases. *Developmental Medicine and Child Neurology* **27**: 149–154.

Heckmatt, J.Z., Hyde, S.A., Gabain, A. *et al.* (1988) Therapeutic trial of isaxonine in Duchenne muscular dystrophy. *Muscle and Nerve* **11**: 836–847.

Heckmatt, J., Rodillo, E. and Dubowitz, V. (1989) Management of children – Pharmacological and physical. *British Medical Bulletin* **45**: 788–801.

Heckmatt, J.Z., Loh, L. and Dubowitz, V. (1990) Night-time nasal ventilation in neuromuscular disease. *Lancet* **335**: 579–582.

Hobbins, J.C. and Mahoney, M.J. (1974) *In utero* diagnosis of hemoglobinopathies: technic for obtaining fetal blood. *New England Journal of Medicine* **290**: 1065–1067.

Hodgson, S.V. and Bobrow, M. (1989) Carrier detection and prenatal diagnosis in Duchenne and Becker muscular dystrophy. *British Medical Bulletin* **45**: 719–744.

Hodgson, S., Hart, K., Walker, A. *et al.* (1986a) DNA deletion in boy with Becker muscular dystrophy. *Lancet* **i**: 918

Hodgson, S.V., Boswinkel, E., Cole, C. *et al.* (1986b) A linkage study of Emery-Dreifuss muscular dystrophy. *Human Genetics* **74**: 409–416.

Hodgson, S.V., Hart, K.H., Abbs, S. *et al.* (1989) Correlation of clinical and deletion data in Duchenne and Becker muscular dystrophy. *Journal of Medical Genetics* **26**: 682–693.

Hoffman, E.P., Brown, R.H. and Kunkel, L.M. (1987a) Dystrophin: the protein product of the Duchenne muscular dystrophy locus. *Cell* **51**: 919–928.

Hoffman, E.P., Monaco, A.P., Feener, C.C. *et al.* (1987b) Conservation of the Duchenne muscular dystrophy gene in mice and humans. *Science* **238**: 347–350.

Hoffman, E.P., Fishbeck, K.H., Brown, R.H. *et al.* (1988) Characterization of dystrophin in muscle-biopsy specimens from patients with Duchenne's or Becker's muscular dystrophy. *New England Journal of Medicine* **318**: 1363–1368.

Hoffman, E., Arahata, K., Minetti, C. *et al.* (1992) Dystrophinopathy in isolated cases of myopathy in females. *Neurology* **42**: 967–975.

Howard, R. (1908) A case of congenital defect of the muscular system (dystrophia muscularis congenita) and its accociation with congenital talipes equino-varus. *Proceedings of the Royal Society of Medicine* **1**: 157–166.

Hillaire, D., Leclerc, A., Fauré, S. *et al.* (1994) Localisation of merosin-negative congenital muscular dystrophy to chromosome 6q by homozygosity mapping. *Human Molecular Genetics* **3**: 1657–1661.

Huard, J., Bouchard, J.P., Ruy, R. *et al.* (1992) Human myoblast transplantation: preliminary results of 4 cases. *Muscle and Nerve* **15**: 550–560.

Huvos, A.G. and Pruzanski, W. (1967) Smooth muscle involvement in primary muscle disease. II. Progressive muscular dystrophy. *Archives of Pathology* **83**: 234–240.

Inkley, S.R., Oldenburg, F.C. and Vignos, P.J. (1974) Pulmonary function in Duchenne and muscular dystrophy related to stage of disease. *American Journal of Medicine* **56**: 297–306.

Ionasescu, V.V., Searby, C., Ionasescu, R. *et al.* (1989) Duchenne muscular dystrophy in monozygotic twins: deletion of 5 fragments of the gene. *American Journal of Medical Genetics* **33**: 113–116.

Jackson, C.E. and Strehler, D.A. (1968) Limb-girdle muscular dystrophy: clinical manifestations and detection of preclinical disease. *Pediatrics* **41**: 495–502.

Karagan, N.J. and Sorensen, J.P. (1981) Intellectual functioning in non-Duchenne muscular dystrophy. *Neurology* **31**: 448–452.

Karagan, N.J. and Zellweger, H.U. (1978) Early verbal disabiity in children with Duchenne muscular dystrophy. *Developmental Medicine and Child Neurology* **20**: 435–441.

Karpati, G., Ajdukovic, D., Arnold, D. *et al.* (1993) Myoblast transfer in Duchenne muscular dystrophy. *Annals of Neurology* **34**: 8–17.

Khan, Y. and Heckmatt, J.Z. (1994) Obstructive apnoeas in Duchenne muscular dystrophy. *Thorax* **49**: 157–161.

Kissel, J.T., Burrow, K.L., Rammohan, K.W. *et al.* (1991) Mononuclear cell analysis of muscle biopsies in prednisone-treated and untreated Duchenne muscular dystrophy. *Neurology* **41**: 667–672.

Kissel, J.T., Lynn, D.J., Rammohan, K.W. *et al.* (1993) Mononuclear cell analysis of muscle biopsies in azathioprine-treated Duchenne dystrophy. *Neurology* **43**: 532–536.

Koenig, M., Hoffmann, E.P., Bertelson, C.K. *et al.* (1987) Complete cloning of the Duchenne muscular dystrophy (DMD) cDNA and preliminary genomic organisation of the DMD gene in mouse and affected individuals. *Cell* **50**: 509–517.

Koenig, M., Beggs, A.H., Moyer, M. *et al.* (1989) The molecular basis for Duchenne versus Becker muscular dystrophy: correlation of severity with type of deletion. *American Journal of Human Genetics* **45**: 498–506.

Kovick, R.B., Fogelman, A.M., Abbasi, A.S. *et al.* (1975) Echocardiographic evaluation of posterior left ventricular wall motion in muscular dystrophy. *Circulation* **52**: 447–454

Kozicka, A., Prot, J. and Wasilewski, R. (1971) Mental retardation in patients with Duchenne progressive muscular dystrophy. *Journal of the Neurological Sciences* **14**: 209–213.

Khurana, T.S., Watkins, S.C., Chafey, P. *et al.* (1991) Immunolocalization and developmental expression of dystrophin related protein in skeletal muscle. *Neuromuscular Disorders* **1**: 185–194.

Kuhn, E. and Schröder, J.M. (1981) A new type of distal myopathy in two brothers. *Journal of Neurology* **226**: 181–185.

Kuhn, E., Fiehn, W., Schröder, J.M. *et al.* (1979) Early myocardial disease and cramping myalgia in Becker-type muscular dystrophy: a kindred. *Neurology* **29**: 1144–1149.

Kunkel, L.M., Monaco, A.P., Middlesworth, W. *et al.* (1985) Specific cloning of DNA fragments absent from the DNA of a male patient with an X-chromosome deletion. *Proceedings of the National Academy of Sciences, USA* **82**: 4778–4782.

Landouzy, L. and Déjerine, J. (1884) De la myopathie atrophique progressive (myopathie héréditaire) débutant, dans l'enfance, par la face, sans altération du système nerveux. *Compte Rendu hebdomadaire des Séances de l'Académie des Sciences (Paris)* **98**: 53.

Lapresle, J., Fardeau, M. and Godet-Guillain, M.J. (1972) Myopathie distale congenitale, avec hypertrophie des mollets. *Journal of the Neurological Sciences* **17**: 87–102.

Law, P., Goodwin, T., Fang, Q. *et al.* (1991) Pioneering development of myoblast transfer therapy. In: Angelini C. *et al.*, eds, *Muscular Dystrophy Research: From Molecular Diagnosis Toward Therapy*. Amsterdam: Excerpta Medica.

Law, P., Goodwin, T.G., Fang, Q. *et al.* (1992) Feasibility, safety, and efficacy of myoblast transfer therapy on Duchenne muscular dystrophy boys. *Cell Transplantation* **1**: 235–244.

Lazzeroni, E., Favaro, L. and Botti, G. (1989) Dilated cardiomyopathy with regional myocardial hypoperfusion in Becker's muscular dystrophy. *International Journal of Cardiology* **22**: 126–129.

Ledley, F.D. (1987) Somatic gene therapy for human disease: a problem of eugenics? *Trends in Genetics* **3**: 112–115.

Lee, C.C., Pearlman, J.A., Chamberlain, J.S. *et al.* (1991) Expression of recombinant dystrophin and its localization to the cell membrane. *Nature* **349**: 334–336.

Leibowitz, D. and Dubowitz, V. (1981) Intellect and behaviour in Duchenne muscular dystrophy. *Developmental Medicine and Child Neurology* **23**: 577–590.

Leon, S.H., Schuffler, M.D., Kettler, M. *et al.* (1986) Chronic intestinal pseudo-obstruction as a complication of Duchenne's muscular dystrophy. *Gastroenterology* **90**: 455–459.

Levison, H. (1951) Dystrophia Musculorum Progressiva. *Clinical and Diagnostic Criteria; Inheritance.* Copenhagen: Moller.

Leyden, E. (1876) *Klinik der Ruchenmarks – Krankheiten*. Berlin: Hirschwald, 2: 447.

Love, D.R., Hill, D.F., Dickson, G. *et al.* (1989) An autosomal transcript in skeletal muscle with homology to dystrophin. *Nature* **339**: 55–58.

Lunt, P.W. (1994) Report of the 6th International Workshop on Facioscapulohumeral Muscular Dystrophy (San Francisco, 11 November 1992) and current guidelines for clinical application of DNA rearrangements at locus D4S810. *Neuromuscular Disorders* **4**: 83–86.

Lunt, P.W. and Harper, P.S. (1991) Genetic counselling in

facioscapulohumeral muscular dystrophy. *Journal of Medical Genetics* **28**: 655–664.

Lupski, J.R., Garcia, C.A., Zoghbi, H.Y. *et al.* (1991) Discordance of muscular dystrophy in monozygotic female twins. *American Journal of Medical Genetics* **40**: 354–364.

Madrid, R.E., Jaros, E., Cullen, M.J. *et al.* (1975) Genetically determined defect of Schwann basement membrane in dystrophic mouse. *Nature* **257**: 319–321.

Magee, K.R. and DeJong, R.N. (1965) Hereditary distal myopathy with onset in infancy. *Archives of Neurology* **13**: 387–390.

Malhotra, S.B., Hart, K.A., Klamut, H.J. *et al.* (1988) Frame-shift deletions in patients with Duchenne and Becker muscular dystrophy. *Science* **242**: 755–759.

Manni, R., Ottolini, A., Cerveri, I. *et al.* (1989) Breathing patterns and HbSaO2 changes during nocturnal sleep in patients with Duchenne's muscular dystrophy. *Journal of Neurology* **236**: 391–394.

Manzur, A.Y., Hyde, S.A., Rodillo, E. *et al.* (1992) A randomized controlled trial of early surgery in Duchenne muscular dystrophy. *Neuromuscular Disorders* **2**: 379–387.

Marconi, G., Pizzi, A., Arimondi, C.G. *et al.* (1991) Limb girdle muscular dystrophy with autosomal dominant inheritance. *Acta Neurologica Scandinavica* **83**: 234–238.

Markesbery, W.R., Griggs, R.C., Leach, R.P. *et al.* (1974) Late onset hereditary distal myopathy. *Neurology (Minneapolis)* **24**: 127–134.

Marsh, G.G. and Munsat, T.L. (1974) Evidence for early impairment of verbal intelligence in Duchenne muscular dystrophy. *Archives of Disease in Childhood* **49**: 118.

Matsumura, K. and Campbell, K.P. (1993) Deficiency of dystrophin-associated proteins: a common mechanism leading to muscle cell necrosis in severe childhood muscular dystrophies. *Neuromuscular Disorders* **3**: 109–118.

Matsumura, K. and Campbell K.P. (1994) Dystrophin-glycoprotein complex: its role in the pathogenesis of muscular dystrophy. *Muscle and Nerve* **17**: 2–15.

Matsumura, K., Tomé, F.M.S., Collin, H. *et al.* (1992) Deficiency of the 50K dystrophin-associated glycoprotein in severe childhood autosomal recessive muscular dystrophy. *Nature* **359**: 320–322.

Matsumura, K., Nonaka, I. and Campbell, K.P. (1993) Abnormal expression of dystrophin-associated proteins in Fukuyama-type congenital muscular dystrophy. *Lancet* **341**: 521–522.

Matsumoto, T., Mitsudome, A. and Nagayama, T. (1970) Progressive muscular dystrophy in infancy. *Acta Paediatrica Japonica* **12**: 4–8.

Maunder–Sewry, C.A. and Dubowitz, V. (1981) Needle muscle biopsy for carrier detection in Duchenne muscular dystrophy. Part 1. Light microscopy – histology, histochemistry and quantitation. *Journal of the Neurological Sciences* **49**: 305–324.

Mawatari, S. and Katayama, K. (1973) Scapuloperoneal muscular atrophy with cardiomyopathy: An X-linked recessive trait. *Archives of Neurology (Chicago)* **28**: 55–59.

Melacini, P., Fanin, M., Danieli, G.A. *et al.* (1993) Cardiac involvement in Becker muscular dystrophy. *Journal of the American College of Cardiology* **22**: 1927–1934.

Mendell, J.R., Moxley, R.T., Griggs, R.C. *et al.* (1989) Randomized double-blind six-month trial of prednisone in Duchenne's muscular dystrophy. *New England Journal of Medicine* **320**: 1592–1597.

Merchut, M.P., Zdonczyk, D. and Gujrati, M. (1990) Cardiac transplantation in female Emery-Dreifuss muscular dystrophy. *Journal of Neurology* **237**: 316–319.

Merlini, L., Morandi, L., Granata, C. *et al.* (1994) Bethlem myopathy: early-onset benign autosomal dominant myopathy with contractures. Description of two new families. *Neuromuscular Disorders* **4**: 503–511.

Meryon, E. (1852) On granular and fatty degeneration of the voluntary muscles. *Medico-Chirurgical Transactions* **35**: 73.

Meryon, E. (1864) *Practical and Pathological Researches on the Various Forms of Paralysis.* London: Churchill.

Mesa, L.E., Dubrovsky, A.L., Corderi, J. *et al.* (1991) Steroids in Duchenne muscular dystrophy – deflazacort trial. *Neuromuscular Disorders* **4**: 503–511.

Miller, F., Moseley, C.F. and Koreska, J. (1992a) Spinal fusion in Duchenne muscular dystrophy. *Developmental Medicine and Child Neurology* **34**: 775–786.

Miller, G., Beggs, A.H. and Towfighi, J. (1992b) Early onset autosomal dominant progressive muscular dystrophy presenting in childhood as a Becker phenotype – the importance of dystrophin and molecular genetic analysis. *Neuromuscular Disorders* **2**: 121–124.

Miller, R.G., Chalmers, A.C., Dao, H. *et al.* (1991) The effect of spine fusion on respiratory function in Duchenne muscular dystrophy. *Neurology* **41**: 38–40.

Miyoshi, K., Tada, Y., Iwasa, M. *et al.* (1974) Genetico-clinical features of distal myopathy: personal observations of 14 cases in 7 families and other cases in Japan. *Clinical Neurology, Tokyo* (in Japanese) **14**: 963.

Miyoshi, K., Kawai, H., Iwasa, M. *et al.* (1986) Autosomal recessive distal muscular dystrophy as a new type of progressive muscular dystrophy: seventeen cases in eight families including an autopsied case. *Brain* **109**: 31–54.

Mizuno, Y., Nonaka, I., Hirai, S. *et al.* (1993) Reciprocal expression of dystrophin and utrophin in muscles of Duchenne muscular dystrophy patients, female DMD-carriers and control subjects. *Journal of the Neurological Sciences* **119**: 43–52.

Mizuno, Y., Yoshida, M., Nonaka, I. *et al.* (1994) Expression of utrophin (dystrophin-related protein) and dystrophin-associated glycoproteins in muscles from patients with Duchenne muscular dystrophy. *Muscle and Nerve* **17**: 206–216.

Möbius, P.J. (1879) Ueber die hereditären Nervenkrankheiten. *Sammlung klinischer Vorträge* **171**: 1505.

Mohire, M.D., Tandan, R., Fries, T.J. *et al.* (1988) Early-onset benign autosomal dominant limb-girdle myopathy with contractures (Bethlem myopathy). *Neurology* **38**: 573–580.

Monaco, A.P., Bertelson, C.J., Liechti-Gallati, S. *et al.* (1988) An explanation for the phenotypic differences between patients bearing partial deletions of the DMD locus. *Genomics* **2**: 90–95.

Morrow, R.S. and Cohen, J. (1954) The psycho-social factors in muscular dystrophy. *Journal of Child Psychiatry (New York)* **3**: 70.

Moser, H. (1984) Duchenne muscular dystrophy: pathogenetic aspects and genetic prevention. *Human Genetics* **66**: 17–40.

Müller, E., Siciliano, B., Mostacciuolo, M.L. *et al.* (1991) Linkage analysis in one family with recurrence of Emery-Dreifuss muscular dystrophy. In: Angelini, C., Danieli, G.A. and Fontanari, D. eds, *Muscular Dystrophy Research: From Molecular Diagnosis Toward Therapy.* Amsterdam: Excerpta Medica, p. 239.

Muntoni, F., Cau, M., Ganau, A. *et al.* (1993) Deletion of the dystrophin muscle-promoter region associated with X-linked dilated cardiomyopathy. *New England Journal of Medicine* **329**: 921–925.

Murphy, E.G., Corey, P.N.J. and Conen, P.E. (1964) Varying manifestations of Duchenne muscular dystrophy in a family with affected females. In: Paul, W.M., Daniel, E.E., Kay, C.M. *et al.* eds, *Muscle* (Proceedings of Symposium at Faculty of Medicine, University of Alberta). New York: Pergamon, pp. 529–546.

Murray, J.M., Davies, K.E., Harper, P.S. *et al.* (1982) Linkage relationship of a cloned DNA sequence on the short arm of the X-chromosome to Duchenne-muscular dystrophy. *Nature* **300**: 69–71.

Neumeyer, A.M., DiGregorio, D.M. and Brown, R.H. Jr. (1992) Arterial delivery of myoblasts to skeletal muscle. *Neurology* **42**: 2258–2262.

Nicholson, L.V.B., Johnson, M.A., Gardner–Medwin, D. *et al.* (1990) Heterogeneity of dystrophin expression in patients with Duchenne and Becker muscular dystrophy. *Acta Neuropathologica Berlin* **80**: 239–250.

Nigro, G. (1986) Conte or Duchenne? *Cardiomyology* **5**: 3–6.

Nonaka, I., Miyoshino, S., Miike, T. *et al.* (1972) An electron microscopical study of the muscle in congenital muscular dystrophy. *Kumamoto Medical Journal* **25**: 68–75.

Nonaka, I., Sunohara, N., Ishiura, S. *et al.* (1981) Familial distal myopathy with rimmed vacuole and lamellar (myeloid) body formation. *Journal of the Neurological Sciences* **51**: 141–155.

Nonaka, I., Sunohara, N., Satoyoshi, E. *et al.* (1985) Autosomal recessive distal muscular dystrophy: a comparative study with distal myopathy with rimmed vacuole formation. *Annals of Neurology* **17**: 51–59.

Norman, A., Thomas, N., Coakley, J. *et al.* (1989) Distinction of Becker from limb-girdle muscular dystrophy by means of dystrophin cDNA probes. *Lancet* **1**, 466–468.

Nudel, U., Zuk, D., Einat, P. *et al.* (1989) Duchenne muscular dystrophy gene product is not identical in muscle and brain. *Nature* **337**: 76–78.

Oliveira, A.S., Gabbai, A.A., Kiyomoto, B.H. *et al.* (1990) Distrofia muscular congenita. Apresentacao de oito casos com evidencia de comprometimento do SNC. *Revista Paulista de Medicina* **108**: 139–141.

Orfanos, A.P. and Naylor, E.W. (1984) A rapid screening test for Duchenne muscular dystrophy using dried blood specimens. *Clinica Chimica Acta* **138**: 267–274.

Oswald, A., Goldblatt, J., Horak, A. *et al.* (1987) Lethal cardiac conduction defects in Emery-Dreifuss muscular dystrophy. *South African Medical Journal* **72**: 567–570.

Padberg, G.W., Lunt, P.W., Koch, M. *et al.* (1991) Diagnostic criteria for facioscapulohumeral muscular dystrophy. *Neuromuscular Disorders* **1**: 231–234.

Partridge, T.A., Morgan, J.E., Coulton, G.R. *et al.* (1989) Conversion of *mdx* myofibres from dystrophin-negative to positive by injection of normal myoblasts. *Nature* **337**: 176–179.

Passos-Bueno, M.R., Vainzof, M., Pavenello, R.de C. *et al.* (1991a) Limb-girdle syndrome: a genetic study of 22 large Brazilian families. *Journal of the Neurological Sciences* **103**: 65–75.

Passos-Bueno, M.R., Terwilliger, J., Ott, J. *et al.* (1991b) Linkage analysis in families with autosomal recessive limb-girdle muscular dystrophy (LGMD) and 6q probes flanking the dystrophin-related sequence. *American Journal of Medical Genetics* **38**: 140–146.

Passos-Bueno, M.R., Oliveira, J.R., Bakker, E. *et al.* (1993) Genetic heterogeneity for Duchenne-like muscular dystrophy (DLMD) based on linkage and 50 DAG analysis. *Human Molecular Genetics* **2**: 1946–1947.

Pearson, C.M., Fowler, W.M. and Wright, S.W. (1963) X-chromosome mosaicism in females with muscular dystrophy. *Proceedings of the National Academy of Sciences of the USA* **50**: 24.

Pena, S.D., Karpati, G., Carpenter, S. *et al.* (1987) The clinical consequences of X-chromosome inactivation: Duchenne muscular dystrophy in one of monozygotic twins. *Journal of the Neurological Sciences* **79**: 337–344.

Penn, A.S., Lisak, R.P. and Rowland, L.P. (1970) Muscular dystrophy in young girls. *Neurology* **20**: 147–159.

Penrose, L.S. (1946) Phenylketonuria, a problem of eugenics. *Lancet* **i**, 949–954.

Perloff, J.K., Roberts, W.C., de Leon, A.C. Jr and O'Doherty, D. (1967) The distinctive electrocardiogram of Duchenne's progressive muscular dystrophy. *American Journal of Medicine* **42**: 179.

Philpot, J., Topaloglu, H., Pennock, J. *et al.* (1995a) Familial concordance of brain magnetic resonance imaging changes in congenital muscular dystrophy. *Neuromuscular Disorders* **5**: in press.

Philpot, J., Sewry, C., Pennock, J. *et al.* (1995b) Clinical phenotype in congenital muscular dystrophy: correlation with expression of merosin in skeletal muscle. *Neuromuscular Disorders* **5**: (in press).

Pinelli, G., Dominici, P., Merlini, L. *et al.* (1987) Valutazione cardiologica in una famiglia affetta da distrofia muscolare di Emery-Dreifuss. *Giornale Italiano di Cardiologia* 17: 589–593.

Prosser, E.J., Murphy, E.G. and Thompson, M.W. (1969) Intelligence and the gene for Duchenne muscular dystrophy. *Archives of Disease in Childhood* 44: 221–230.

Quinlivan, R.M. and Dubowitz, V. (1992) Cardiac transplantation in Becker muscular dystrophy. *Neuromuscular Disorders* 2: 165–167.

Ragot, T., Vincent, N., Chafey, P. *et al.* (1993) Efficient adenovirus-mediated transfer of a human mini-dystrophin gene to skeletal muscle of *mdx* mice. *Nature* 361: 647–650.

Ray, P.N., Belfall, B., Duff, C. *et al.* (1985) Cloning of the breakpoint of an X;21 translocation associated with Duchenne muscular dystrophy. *Nature* 318: 672–675.

Richards, C.S., Watkins, S.C., Hoffman, E.P. *et al.* (1990) Skewed X inactivation in a female MZ twin results in Duchenne muscular dystrophy. *American Journal of Human Genetics* 46: 672–681.

Rideau, Y. (1984) Treatment of orthopaedic deformity during the ambulatory stage of Duchenne muscular dystrophy. In: Serratrice, G. *et al.* eds, *Neuromuscular Diseases*. New York: Raven Press, pp. 557–564.

Rideau, Y., Duport, G. and Delaubier, A. (1986) Premieres remissions reproductibles dans l'evolution de la dystrophie musculaire de Duchenne. *Bulletin de l'Academie Nationale de Medecine* 170: 605–610.

Ringel, S.P., Carroll, J.E. and Schold, C. (1977) The spectrum of mild X-linked recessive muscular dystrophy. *Archives of Neurology (Chicago)* 34: 408–416.

Roberds, S.L., Ervasti, J.M., Anderson, R.D. *et al.* (1993) Disruption of the dystrophin-glycoprotein complex in the cardiomyopathic hamster. *Journal of Biological Chemistry* 268: 11496–11499.

Roberds, S.L., Leturcq, F., Allamand, V. *et al.* (1994) Missense mutations in the adhalin gene linked to autosomal recessive muscular dystrophy. *Cell* 78: 1–20.

Roberts, R.G., Barby, T.F.M., Manners, E. *et al.* (1991) Direct detection of dystrophin gene rearrangements by analysis of dystrophin mRNA in peripheral blood lymphocytes. *American Journal of Human Genetics* 49: 298–310.

Rodillo, E.B., Fernandez-Bermejo, E., Heckmatt, J.Z. *et al.* (1988) Prevention of rapidly progressive scoliosis in Duchenne muscular dystrophy by prolongation of walking with orthoses. *Journal of Child Neurology* 3: 269–275.

Rodillo, E., Noble-Jamieson, C.M., Aber, V. *et al.* (1989) Respiratory muscle training in Duchenne muscular dystrophy. *Archives of Disease in Childhood* 64: 736–738.

Rosman, N.P. and Kakulas, B.A. (1960) Mental deficiency associated with muscular dystrophy – a neuropathological study. *Brain* 89: 769–787.

Romero, N.B., Tomé, F.M.S., Leturcq, F. *et al.* (1994) Genetic heterogeneity of severe childhood autosomal recessive muscular dystrophy with adhalin (50 kDa dystrophin-associated glycoprotein) deficiency. *Comptes Rendus de l'Academie des Sciences (Paris)* 317: 70–76.

Rotthauwe, H.W., Kowalewski, S. and Mumenthaler, M. (1969) Kongenitale Muskeldystrophie. *Zeitschrift für Kinderheilkunde* 106: 131–162.

Rotthauwe, H.W., Mortier, W. and Beyer, H. (1972) Neuer Typ einer recessive X-Chromosomal vererbten Muskeldystrophie: scapulo-humero-distale Muskeldystrophie mit fruhzeitigen Kontrakturen und Herzyrthmusstorungen. *Humangenetik* 16: 181.

Rowland, L.P. (1975) Progressive external ophthalmoplegia. In: Vinken, P.J. and Bruyn, G.W. eds, *Handbook of Clinical Neurology* Vol.22 (System Disorders and Atrophies, part II). Amsterdam: North Holland Publishing Co., pp. 177–202.

Sakata, C., Yamada, H., Sunohara, N. *et al.* (1990) Cardiomyopathy in Becker muscular dystrophy (in Japanese). *Rinsho Shinkeigaku* 30: 952–955.

Salih, M.A.M., Omer, M.I.A., Bayoumi, R.A. *et al.* (1983) Severe autosomal recessive muscular dystrophy in an extended Sudanese kindred. *Developmental Medicine and Child Neurology* 25: 43–52.

Sansome, A., Royston, P. and Dubowitz, V. (1993) Steroids in Duchenne muscular dystrophy; pilot study of a new low-dosage schedule. *Neuromuscular Disorders* 3: 567–569.

Santavuori, P., Leisti, J. and Kruus, S. (1977) Muscle, eye and brain disease: a new syndrome. *Neuropädiatrie* 8(suppl.): 553.

Santavuori, P., Somer, H., Sainio, K. *et al.* (1989) Muscle-eye-brain disease (MEB). *Brain and Development* 11: 147–153.

Santavuori, P., Pihko, H., Sainio, K. *et al.* (1990) Muscle-eye-brain disease and Walker–Warburg syndrome. *American Journal of Medical Genetics* 36: 371–374.

Schmidt, C.C. (1839) Krankhafte Hypertrophie des Muskelsystems. *C.C. Schmidts Jahrbücher der in- und aüslandischen gesamten Medizin* 24: 176.

Scopetta, C., Vaccario, M.L., Casali, C. *et al.* (1988) Distal muscular dystrophy with autosomal recessive inheritance. *Muscle and Nerve* 7: 478–481.

Segawa, M. (1970) Clinical studies of congenital muscular dystrophy. Arthrogrypotic type congenital muscular dystrophy with mental retardation and facial muscle involvement. *Brain and Development* 2: 439–451.

Segawa, M., Fukuyama, Y., Itoh, K. and Uono, M. (1970) Congenital muscular dystrophy (with progressive development of joint contracture, mental retardation and facial involvement). I. Clinical studies. *Brain and Development (Tokyo)* 2: 67.

Sewry, C.A. and Dubowitz, V. (1994) Histochemical and immunocytochemical studies in neuromuscular diseases. In: Walton, J.N. and Karpati, G., eds, *Disorders of Voluntary Muscle*. Edinburgh: Churchill Livingstone, pp. 261–318.

Sewry, C.A., Sansome, A., Clerk, A. *et al.* (1993) Manifesting carriers of Xp21 muscular dystrophy; lack of correlation between dystrophin expression and clinical weakness. *Neuromuscular Disorders* 3: 141–148.

Sewry, C.A., Sansome, A., Matsumura, K. *et al.* (1994a) Deficiency of the 50 kDa dystrophin-associated glycoprotein and abnormal expression of utrophin in two South Asian cousins with variable expression of severe childhood autosomal recessive muscular dystrophy. *Neuromuscular Disorders* 4: 121–129.

Sewry, C.A., Matsumura, K., Campbell, K.P. *et al.* (1994b) Expression of dystrophin-associated glycoprotein and utrophin in carriers of Duchenne muscular dystrophy. *Neuromuscular Disorders* 4: 401–409.

Shapiro, F., Sethna, N., Colan, S. *et al.* (1992) Spinal fusion in Duchenne muscular dystrophy: a multidisciplinary approach. *Muscle and Nerve* 15: 604–614.

Sharma, K.R., Mynhier, M.A. and Miller, R.G. (1993) Cyclosporine increases muscular force generation in Duchenne muscular dystrophy. *Neurology* 43: 527–532.

Sharp, N.J., Kornegay, J.N., Van Camp, S.D. *et al.* (1992) An error in dystrophin mRNA processing in golden retriever muscular dystrophy, an animal homologue of Duchenne muscular dystrophy. *Genomics* 13: 115–121.

Sherratt, T.G., Vulliamy, T., Dubowitz, V. *et al.* (1993) Exon skipping and translation in patients with frameshift deletions in the dystrophin gene. *American Journal of Human Genetics* 53: 1007–1015.

Sicinski, P., Geng, Y., Ryder-Cook, A.S. *et al.* (1989) The molecular basis of muscular dystrophy in the mdx mouse: A point mutation. *Science* 244: 1578–1580.

Siegel, I.M. (1977) Prolongation of ambulation through early percutaneous tenotomy and bracing with plastic orthoses. *Israel Journal of Medical Sciences* 13: 192–196.

Siegel, I.M., Miller, J.E. and Ray, R.D. (1968) Subcutaneous lower limb tenotomy in the treatment of pseudohypertrophic muscular dystrophy. *Journal of Bone and Joint Surgery* 50A: 1437.

Smith, P.E.M., Calverley, P.M.A. and Edwards, R.H.T. (1988) Hypoxaemia during sleep in Duchenne muscular dystrophy. *American Review of Respiratory Diseases* 137: 884–888.

Smith, P.E.M., Edwards, R.H.T. and Calverley, P.M.A. (1989) Oxygen treatment of sleep hypoxaemia in Duchenne muscular dystrophy. *Thorax* 44: 997–1001.

Somer, H., Laulumaa, V., Paljarvi, L. *et al.* (1989) Adult onset limb-girdle muscular dystrophy with autosomal dominant inheritance. *Progress in Clinical Biological Research* 306: 69–71.

Speer, M.C., Yamaoka, L.H., Gilchrist, J.H. *et al.* (1992) Confirmation of genetic heterogeneity in limb-girdle muscular dystrophy: linkage of an autosomal dominant form to chromosome 5q. *American Journal of Human Genetics* 50: 1211–1217.

Spencer, G.E. and Vignos, P.J. (1962) Bracing for ambulation in childhood progressive muscular dystrophy. *Journal of Bone and Joint Surgery* 44A: 234.

Steare, S.E., Dubowitz, V. and Benatar, A. (1992) Subclinical cardiomyopathy in Becker muscular dystrophy. *British Heart Journal* 68: 304–308.

Stern, L.M., Martin, A.J., Jones, N. *et al.* (1989) Training inspiratory resistance in Duchenne dystrophy using adapted computer games. *Developmental Medicine and Child Neurology* 31: 494–500.

Stevenson, A.C. (1953) Muscular dystrophy in Northern Ireland. 1. An account of the condition in fifty-one families. *Annals of Eugenics* 18: 50–93.

Sumner, D., Crawfurd, M.d'A. and Harriman, D.G.F. (1971) Distal muscular dystrophy in an English family. *Brain* 94: 51–60.

Sunada, Y., Bernier, S.M., Kozak, C.A. *et al* (1994) Deficiency of merosin in dystrophic *dy* mice and genetic linkage of laminin M chain gene to *dy* locus. *Journal of Biological Chemistry* 269: 13729–13732.

Suzuki, A., Yoshida, M., Hayashi, K. *et al.* (1994) Molecular organization at the glycoprotein-complex-binding site of dystrophin: three dystrophin-associated proteins bind directly to the carboxy-terminal portion of dystrophin. *European Journal of Biochemistry* 220: 283–292.

Swinyard, C.A., Deaver, G.G. and Greenspan, L. (1957) Gradients of functional ability of importance in *Journal of Bone and Joint Surgery* 50A: 1437.

Tachi, N., Tachi, M., Sasaki, K. *et al.* (1989) Early-onset benign autosomal dominant limb-girdle myopathy with contractures (Bethlem myopathy). *Pediatric Neurology* 5: 323–236.

Tanaka, H., Ishiguro, T., Eguchi, C. *et al.* (1991) Expression of a dystrophin-related protein associated with the skeletal muscle cell membrane. *Histochemistry* 96: 1–5.

Thomas, N.S.T., Williams, H., Elsas, L.J. *et al.* (1986) Localization of the gene for Emery-Dreifuss muscular dystrophy to the distal long arm of the X-chromosome. *Journal of Medical Genetics* 23: 596–598.

Thomas, P.K., Calne, D.B. and Elliott, C.F. (1972) X-linked scapuloperoneal syndrome. *Journal of Neurology, Neurosurgery and Psychiatry* 35: 208–215.

Thompson, L. (1992) Cell-transplant results under fire. *Science* 257: 472–474.

Tinsley, J.M., Blake, D.J., Roche, A. *et al.* (1992) Primary structure of dystrophin-related protein. *Nature* 360: 591–593.

Toda, T., Segawa, M., Nomura, Y. *et al.* (1993) Localization of a gene for Fukuyama type congenital muscular dystrophy to chromosome 9q31–33. *Nature Genetics* 5: 283–286.

Tomé, F.M.S. and Fardeau, M. (1980) Nuclear inclusions in oculopharyngeal dystrophy. *Acta Neuropathologica (Berlin)* 49: 85.

Tomé, F.M.S., Evangelista, T., Leclerc, A. *et al.* (1994) Congenital muscular dystrophy with merosin deficiency. *Life Sciences* 317: 351–357.

Tremblay, J.P., Bouchard, J.P., Malouin, F. *et al.* (1993) Myoblast transplantation between monozygotic twin girl carriers of Duchenne muscular dystrophy. *Neuromuscular Disorders* **3**: 583–592.

Truitt, C.J. (1955) Personal and social adjustments of children with muscular dystrophy. *American Journal of Physical Medicine* **34**: 124.

Udd, B. (1992) Limb-girdle type muscular dystrophy in a large family with distal myopathy: homozygous manifestation of a dominant gene? *Journal of Medical Genetics* **29**: 383–389.

Udd, B., Kääriäinen, H. and Somer, H. (1991) Muscular dystrophy with separate clinical phenotypes in a large family. *Muscle and Nerve* **14**: 1050–1058.

Ullrich, O. (1930) Kongenitale, atonish-sklerotische Muskeldystrophie, ein Weiterer Typus der heredo-degenerativen Erkrankungen des neuromuskularen Systems. *Zeitschrift für die Gesamte Neurologie und Psychiatrie* **126**: 171.

Upadhyaya, M., Lunt, P.W., Sarfarazi, M. *et al.* (1990) DNA marker applicable to presymptomatic and prenatal diagnosis of facioscapulohumeral disease. *Lancet* **336**: 1320–1321.

Utsunomiya, T., Mori, H., Shibuya, N. *et al.* (1990) Long-term observation of cardiac function in Duchenne's muscular dystrophy: evaluation using systolic time intervals and echocardiography. *Japanese Heart Journal* **31**: 585–597.

Valentine, B.A. and Cooper, B.J. (1991) Canine X-linked muscular dystrophy: selective involvement of muscles in neonatal dogs. *Neuromuscular Disorders* **1**: 31–38.

Valentine, B.A., Cooper, B.J., Cummings, J.F. *et al.* (1986) Progressive muscular dystrophy in a golden retriever dog: light microscope and ultrastructural features at 4 and 8 months. *Acta Neuropathologica* **7**: 301–310.

van der Does de Willebois, A.E.M., Bethlem, J., Meyer, A.E.F.H. *et al.* (1968) Distal myopathy with onset in early infancy. *Neurology* **18**: 383–390.

van Ommen, G.J.B. and Scheuerbrandt, G. (1993) Neonatal screening for muscular dystrophy. Consensus recommendation of the 14th Workshop sponsored by the European Neuromuscular Center (ENMC). *Neuromuscular Disorders* **3**: 231–239.

van Wijngaarden, G.K. and Bethlem, J. (1971) The facio-scapulohumeral syndrome. In: Kakulas, B.A. ed. *The Second International Congress on Muscle Diseases*, Perth, Australia, 1971. Abstracts. Amsterdam: Excerpta Medica, I.C.S. No. 237, p. 54.

Vassella, F., Mumenthaler, M., Rossi, E., Moser, H. and Weismann, U. (1967) Congenital muscular dystrophy. *Deutsche Zeitschrift für Nervenheilkunde* **190**: 349.

Verellen-Dumoulin, C., Freund, M., De Meyer, R. *et al.* (1984) Expression of an X-linked muscular dystrophy in a female due to translocation involving Xp21 and non-random inactivation of the normal X chromosome. *Human Genetics* **67**: 115–119.

Victor, M., Hayes, R. and Adams, R.D. (1962) Oculopharyngeal muscular dystrophy. *New England Journal of Medicine* **267**: 1267–1272.

Vilozni, D., Bar-Yishay, E., Gur, I. *et al.* (1994) Computerized respiratory muscle training in children with Duchenne muscular dystrophy. *Neuromuscular Disorders* **4**: 249–255.

Voit, T., Krogmann, O., Lennard, H.G. *et al.* (1988) Emery-Dreifuss muscular dystrophy: disease spectrum and differential diagnosis. *Neuropediatrics* **19**: 62–71.

Walton, J.N. and Gardner-Medwin, D. (1974) Progressive muscular dystrophy and the myotonic disorders. In: Walton, J.N. ed., *Disorders of Voluntary Muscle* 3rd edn. Edinburgh and London: Churchill Livingstone, pp. 561–613.

Walton, J.N. and Nattrass, F.J. (1954) On the classification, natural history and treatment of the myopathies. *Brain* **77**: 169.

Waters, D.D., Nutter, D.O., Hopkins, L.D. *et al.* (1975) Cardiac features of an unusual X-linked humeroperoneal neuromuscular disease. *New England Journal of Medicine* **293**: 1017–1022.

Wehnert, M., Machill, G., Grimm, T. *et al.* (1991) Evidence supporting tight linkage of X-linked Emery-Dreifuss muscular dystrophy to the factor VIII:C gene. In: Angelini, C., Danieli, G.A. and Fontanari, D., eds, *Muscular Dystrophy Research: From Molecular Diagnosis Toward Therapy.* Amsterdam: Excerpta Medica, pp. 260–261.

Welander, L. (1951) Myopathia distalis tarda hereditaria. *Acta Medica Scandinavica* **141** (Suppl 265): 1–124.

Wells, D.J., Wells, K.E., Walsh, F.S. *et al.* (1992) Human dystrophin expression corrects the myopathic phenotype in transgenic *mdx* mice. *Human Molecular Genetics* **1**: 35–40.

Wijmenga, C., Frants, R.R., Brouwer, O.F. *et al.* (1990) The facioscapulohumeral muscular dystrophy gene maps to chromosome 4. *Lancet* **2**: 651–653.

Wijmenga, C., Padberg, G.W., Moerer, P. *et al.* (1991) Mapping of facioscapulohumeral muscular dystrophy gene to chromosome 4q35-qter by multipoint linkage analysis and *in situ* hybridization. *Genomics* **9**: 570–575.

Wijmenga, C., Hewitt, J., Sandkuijl, L. *et al.* (1992) Chromosome 4q DNA rearrangements associated with facioscapulohumeral muscular dystrophy. *Nature Genetics* **2**: 26–30.

Winand, N.J., Pradhan, D. and Cooper, B.J. (1994a) Molecular characterization of severe Duchenne-type muscular dystrophy in a family of Rottweiler dogs. Poster presentation at MDA Symposium in Tuczon, Arizona, 24–25 January.

Winand, N.J., Edwards, M., Pradhan, D. *et al.* (1994b) Deletion of the dystrophin muscle promoter in feline muscular dystrophy. *Neuromuscular Disorders* **4**: 433–455.

Witt, T.N., Garner, C.G., Pongratz, D. *et al.* (1988) Autosomal dominant Emery-Dreifuss syndrome: evidence of a neurogenic variant of the disease. *European Archives of Psychiatry and Neurological Sciences* **237**: 230–236.

Wolff, J.A., Malone, R.W., Williams, P. *et al.* Direct gene transfer into mouse muscle *in vivo*. *Science* **247**: 1465–1468.

Worden, D.K. and Vignos, P.J. Jr (1962) Intellectual function in childhood progressive muscular dystrophy. *Pediatrics* **29**: 968–977.

Worton, R.G., Duff, C., Sylvester, J.E. *et al.* (1984) Duchenne muscular dystrophy involving translocation of the dmd gene next to ribosomal RNAP gene. *Science* **224**: 1447–1449.

Yamanouchi, Y., Mizuno, Y., Yamamoto, H. *et al.* (1994) Selective defect in dystrophin-associated glycoproteins 50DAG (A2) and 35DAG (A4) in the dystrophic hamster: an animal model for severe childhood autosomal recessive muscular dystrophy (SCARMD). *Neuromuscular Disorders* **4**: 49–54.

Yamaoka, L.H., Westbrook, C.A., Speer, M.C. *et al.* (1994) Development of a microsatellite genetic map spanning 5q31-q33 and subsequent placement of the LGMD1 locus between D5S178 and IL9. *Neuromuscular Disorders* **4**: 471–475.

Yates, J.R.W. (1991) Report on European Workshop on Emery-Dreifuss Muscular Dystrophy, 1991. *Neuromuscular Disorders* **1**: 393–396.

Yates, J.R.W., Affara, N.A., Jamieson, D.M. *et al.* (1986) Emery–Dreifuss muscular dystrophy: localisation to Xq27.3 → qtr confirmed by linkage to the factor VIII gene. *Journal of Medical Genetics* **23**: 587–590.

Yoshioka, M., Okuno, T., Honda, Y. *et al.* (1980) Central nervous system involvement in progressive muscular dystrophy. *Archives of Disease in Childhood* **55**: 589–594.

Yoshioka, M., Saida, K., Itagaki, Y. *et al.* (1989) Follow up study of cardiac involvement in Emery-Dreifuss muscular dystrophy. *Archives of Disease in Childhood* **64**: 713–715.

Young, K., Foroud, T., Williams, P. *et al.* (1992) Confirmation of linkage of limb-girdle muscular dystrophy, type 2, to chromosome 15. *Genomics* **13**: 1370–1371.

Zellweger, H. and Antonik, A. (1975) Newborn screening for Duchenne muscular dystrophy. *Pediatrics* **55**: 30.

Zellweger, H. and Hanson, J.W. (1968) Psychometric studies in muscular dystrophy type IIIa (Duchenne). *Developmental Medicine and Child Neurology* **9**: 576–581.

Zellweger, H. and Niedermeyer, E. (1965) Central nervous system manifestations in childhood muscular dystrophy. I. Psychometric and electroencephalographic findings. *Annales Paediatrici (Basel)* **205**: 25.

Zellweger, H., Afifi, A., McCormick, W.F. and Mergner, W. (1967a) Benign congenital muscular dystrophy: a special form of congenital hypotonia. *Clinica Pediatrica* **6**: 655.

Zellweger, H., Afifi, A., McCormick, W.F. and Mergner, W. (1967b) Severe congenital muscular dystrophy. *American Journal of Disease of Children* **114**: 591.

Zneimer, S.M., Schneider, N.R. and Richards, C.S. (1993) *In situ* hybridization shows direct evidence of skewed X inactivation in one of monozygotic twin females manifesting Duchenne muscular dystrophy. *American Journal of Medical Genetics* **45**: 601–605.

Zubrzycka-Gaarn, E.E., Bulman, D.E., Karpati, G. *et al.* (1988) The Duchenne muscular dystrophy gene product is localised in the sarcolemma of human skeletal muscle. *Nature* **333**: 466–469.

CHAPTER 3

The Congenital Myopathies

With the advent in the 1950s and 1960s of histochemistry and electron microscopy and the more enthusiastic investigation of muscle biopsies, there emerged, out of the morass of non-specific clinical diagnoses such as 'amyotonia congenita', 'universal muscular hypoplasia' and 'benign congenital hypotonia', a series of clearly delineated myopathies, with specific structural changes within the muscle. This also helped to unravel the floppy infant syndrome; much of the confusion in the early literature had been compounded by the chaos in terminology (Dubowitz, 1969).

Historically this group of 'new myopathies' probably dates from Shy and Magee's description in 1956 of 'a new congenital non-progressive myopathy', subsequently named central core disease. The generic term 'congenital myopathy' for the group as a whole is probably a reasonable one, and worth retaining, although not all cases are strictly 'congenital' with symptoms at birth, and many may indeed present much later. In the absence of any structural abnormality in the central nervous system or peripheral nerves they can be looked upon as primary myopathies. These myopathies tend as a rule to be relatively non-progressive but there are exceptions with unequivocal and sometimes fairly rapid progression of weakness.

There is also frequently a genetic element and the inheritance may be autosomal dominant or autosomal recessive, and occasionally X-linked, and indeed some syndromes such as nemaline myopathy and myotubular myopathy may have more than one mode of inheritance.

CLINICAL FEATURES

From a clinical point of view one cannot readily distinguish between the various congenital myopathies, since they all tend to present in a somewhat similar, non-specific way. This may take the form of a floppy infant syndrome at birth or in early infancy, or may present later with features of muscle weakness. In some children this weakness will be predominantly proximal and of girdle distribution, thus resembling a limb girdle muscular dystrophy or a mild spinal muscular atrophy; in others it may be more generalized and may also affect the facial muscles. In some, such as myotubular myopathy, ocular muscles are frequently affected. Some myopathies, such as nemaline myopathy, have a higher incidence of associated 'dysmorphic' features e.g. skeletal deformity, but this is not consistent. Some, like nemaline myopathy, are particularly prone to respiratory deficit, possibly as a result of diaphragmatic involvement, and may present features of nocturnal hypoventilation. On the basis of the associated features one can often arrive at a fairly accurate diagnosis of individual myopathies.

INVESTIGATIONS

Investigations such as serum creatine kinase and electromyography are not likely to be of much help in diagnosis. The serum enzyme levels are frequently normal and the EMG may be normal or may show mild, non-specific changes, usually of a myopathic character (small amplitude, polyphasic potentials) but sometimes even 'neuropathic', as in some cases of nemaline myopathy. Ultrasound imaging may show increased echo in the muscle in some cases such as central core disease, and especially if there is associated disruption of the normal bundle architecture or proliferation of adipose or connective tissue. Muscle biopsy is the only certain way of making an accurate diagnosis and a full histochemical analysis of the muscle, supplemented selectively by immunocytochemistry and electron microscopy, is essential.

There is also an overlap clinically between these congenital myopathies and some of the metabolic myopathies such as mitochondrial myopathies, glycogenoses and lipid storage myopathies, which may also present as a floppy infant syndrome or with generalized or localized muscle weakness of variable severity. Perhaps the demarcation between the 'structural' and 'metabolic' myopathies is to an extent an artificial one and, just as the mitochondrial myopathies were initially recognized because of the morphological changes in the muscle biopsy, others may also prove to have a specific biochemical abnormality.

This chapter will be confined to the congenital myopathies which have a structural abnormality; the recognized metabolic myopathies will be discussed in the following chapters.

The following is a list of the conditions that have been recognized to date. The names in general are descriptive titles reflecting the underlying structural change. The list is bound to grow longer as more conditions are recognized in the future, or perhaps shorten if individual disorders become transferred to specific biochemical or other compartments.

'Structural' Congenital Myopathies

1. Central core disease
2. Minicore disease (multicore disease)
3. Nemaline myopathy ('rod body' myopathy)
4. Myotubular myopathy (centronuclear myopathy)
5. Myotubular myopathy with type 1 fibre hypotrophy
6. Severe congenital X-linked myotubular myopathy
7. Congenital fibre type disproportion (not an entity)
8. Myopathies with abnormality of other subcellular organelles
9. Non-specific congenital myopathies; 'minimal change myopathy'

CENTRAL CORE DISEASE

HISTORICAL ————————————————

In 1956 Shy and Magee described a 'new congenital non-progressive myopathy' affecting five patients, four male and one female, in three generations of the same family. Their ages ranged from 2 to 65 years. The disease was present at birth or shortly after and in one case there was a history of reduced fetal movements. Early features were delay in motor milestones and bizarre postures. The older patients had not walked till 4 or 5 years of age and still had residual difficulty in climbing stairs, running or rising from a supine or sitting posture. The two affected children, aged 2 and 4 years, walked at 14 and 20 months respectively but still had difficulty

going up stairs, running or rising from the supine, which they did with the Gowers' manoeuvre. There was associated hypotonia. In the older patients the condition remained fairly static over the years.

Histologically, the muscle was characterized by amorphous-looking central areas within the muscle fibres composed of compact myofibrils giving a blue stain with Gomori's trichrome, in contrast to the normal red-staining outer fibrils. Greenfield *et al.* (1958) suggested the name 'central core disease'.

A second case was documented by Engel *et al.* (1961). A 19-year-old male had been 'double-jointed' in infancy but not floppy. His motor milestones were delayed and although he walked at 2 years he preferred to crawl or shuffle on his bottom till about 4 years. He had difficulty keeping up with his fellows at school and still had difficulty getting up from the supine or sitting position or going up steps. He was able to walk an unlimited distance on the level without fatigue or cramps.

Histochemical studies of this case showed the cores to be devoid of enzyme activity and presumably a non-functioning part of the muscle (Dubowitz and Pearse, 1960). The cores were not necessarily central and many fibres had multiple cores. The muscle also showed the presence of only type 1 fibres. In longitudinal section the cores ran the length of the fibre. The parents of this patient showed a normal subdivision of their muscle into fibre types and had no cores. Electron microscopy showed a virtual absence of mitochondria and sarcoplasmic reticulum in the core region, a marked reduction in the interfibrillary space and an irregular zig-zag pattern (streaming) of the Z lines (Engel *et al.*, 1961; Seitelberger *et al.*, 1961).

CLINICAL FEATURES ————————————

There have been many reports of central core disease since the initial cases and over 100 cases have now been documented. Some have shown a dominant inheritance but others have been sporadic. In most cases the clinical pattern has been very similar to the initial reports. In an unusual family described by Bethlem *et al.* (1966) three affected females from three successive generations showed a similar clinical pattern of a mild non-progressive proximal weakness and painless, or almost painless, muscle cramps after exercise. They had not been floppy in infancy and had walked at a normal age. The predominance of high oxidative, low glycolytic type 1 fibres in central core disease, and the relative paucity of type 2 fibres, might result in a relative deficiency of glycolytic enzymes. Armstrong *et al.* (1971) and Ramsey and Hensinger (1975) drew attention to the frequent association of congenital dislocation of the hip.

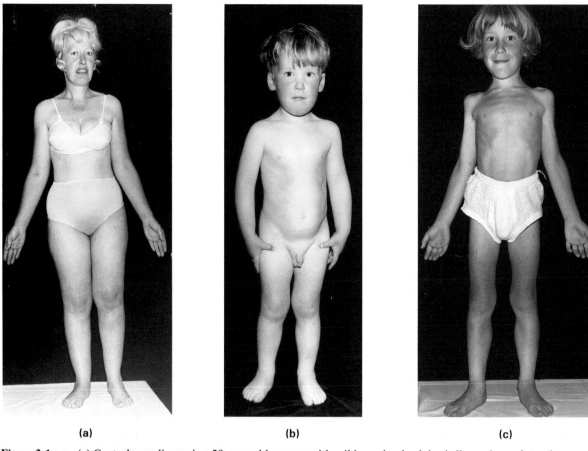

(a)   (b)   (c)

Figure 3-1a-c   (a) Central core disease in a 29-year-old woman with mild proximal pelvic girdle weakness from the age of 5 years. (b) Her 3-year-old son had normal motor milestones and walked at 14 months. Despite his mother's anxiety that he was not up to the standard of his older sib, no suggestion of difficulty was medically apparent until after the age of 3 years, when he supported a hand on the knee when getting up from the floor. EMG and CK were normal. (c) At follow-up he showed no apparent deterioration although his posture was more lordotic when assessed at 7 years (c). He subsequently continued to progress well and had practically no disability or handicap. He did retain a somewhat lordotic posture and he (and his mother) were conscious of a slightly abnormal gait when running.

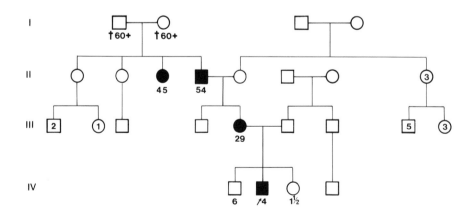

Figure 3-2   Pedigree chart of family in Figure 3-1, showing dominant inheritance. Interview with maternal grandmother revealed that her estranged husband (II,4) and his sister (II,3) had experienced a similar mild weakness.

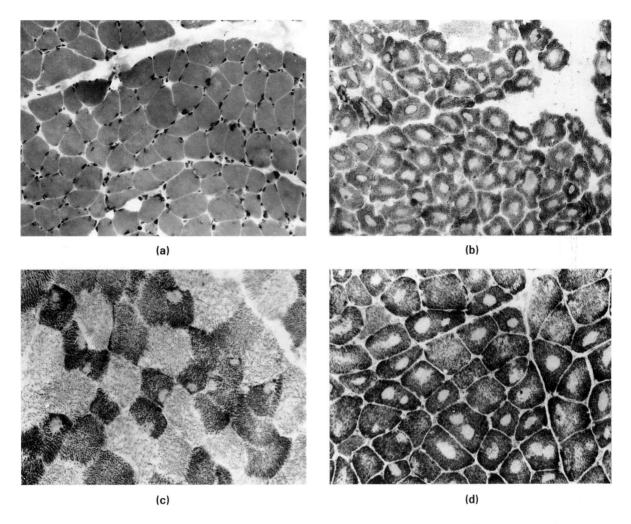

(a) (b)

(c) (d)

Figure 3-3a-d Muscle biopsy (rectus femoris) of mother in Figure 3-1, showing (a) normal looking histological picture apart from some variation in fibre size and a few atrophic fibres. (b) Histochemical reaction for oxidative enzyme shows a striking picture of undifferentiated fibres (all uniformly strong-reacting) and a single central core in every fibre. (c) Biopsy from child in Figure 3-1 shows a normal subdivision into light and dark fibres and a group of type 1 (dark-staining) fibres with eccentric cores in them (about 3% of total fibres). A second (needle) biopsy of his quadriceps at the age of 16 showed a remarkable change. The picture looked identical to his mother's with almost all the fibres being type 1 and having a centrally placed core, usually single, occasionally multiple (d).

The usual clinical presentation is thus one of a mild and relatively non-progressive muscle weakness, either proximal or generalized, and presenting either in early infancy or later. There is usually a mild degree of associated facial weakness with inability to screw the eyes up tightly and completely bury the eyelashes. Illustrative cases are shown in Figures 3-1 to 3-5.

HISTOPATHOLOGY ——————————————————

The cores seem to have a predilection for type 1 fibres. In some cases the muscle is composed totally or almost entirely of type 1 fibres (Dubowitz and Pearse, 1960; Gonatas *et al.*, 1965; Dubowitz and Roy, 1970); in others the muscle may be differentiated into two fibre types with the type 1 fibres selectively affected (Dubowitz and Platts, 1965; Bethlem et al., 1966; Dubowitz and Roy, 1970).

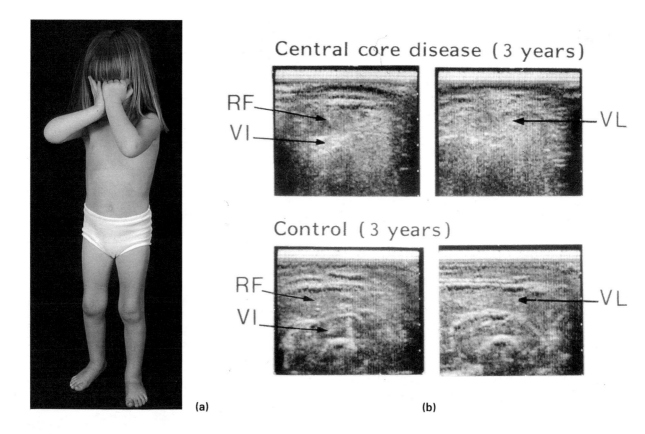

(a)   (b)

Figure 3-4a-i (*continued on facing page*) Central core disease; selective 'dystrophic' change. This 3-year-old girl presented with a history of delayed walking at 2 years and a waddling gait, with instability on rough surfaces (a). There was gradual improvement. She got up from the floor with a minimal Gowers' manoeuvre and had difficulty climbing steps. Ultrasound imaging showed normal appearance of rectus femoris (RF) but increased echo in the vasti (VI,VL) (b). Needle biopsy of both muscles showed normal architecture in the rectus femoris and loss of muscle fibres and proliferation of adipose tissue in the vastus lateralis (c,d, H & E). In both about 50% of fibres had central cores (e,f, NADH-TR). Ultrasound imaging of both parents was normal. Two siblings were also normal. When reviewed at 4 years and 9 months there was further improvement in motor function (g) and a normal facial expression but some limitation of full eye closure and burying of eyelashes (h,i).

In most cases of central core disease the cores are 'structured' so that they retain a myofibrillar pattern and the myofibrillar ATPase reaction is normal and does not show up the cores. In 'unstructured cores' the ultrastructural pattern of the cores is lost (Gonatas *et al.*, 1965; Neville and Brooke, 1973) and, in addition to the absence of oxidative and glycolytic enzymes, the myofibrillar ATPase is also deficient. This is comparable with the unstructured minicores of minicore disease (see below).

Core-like structures have been described in the muscle of patients with long-standing neurogenic atrophy (Engel, 1961) and the name 'target' fibres was suggested to distinguish them from central core fibres.

CENTRAL CORES AND MALIGNANT HYPERTHERMIA

The important association between central cores and malignant hyperthermia was first noted by Denborough *et al.* (1973) and further cases documented by several authors (Isaacs and Barlow, 1974; Eng *et al.*, 1978; Frank *et al.*, 1980). It is still difficult to know what proportion of cases of malignant hyperthermia have cores in their muscle and, conversely, what proportion of cases of central core disease are likely to be sensitive to anaesthetic agents.

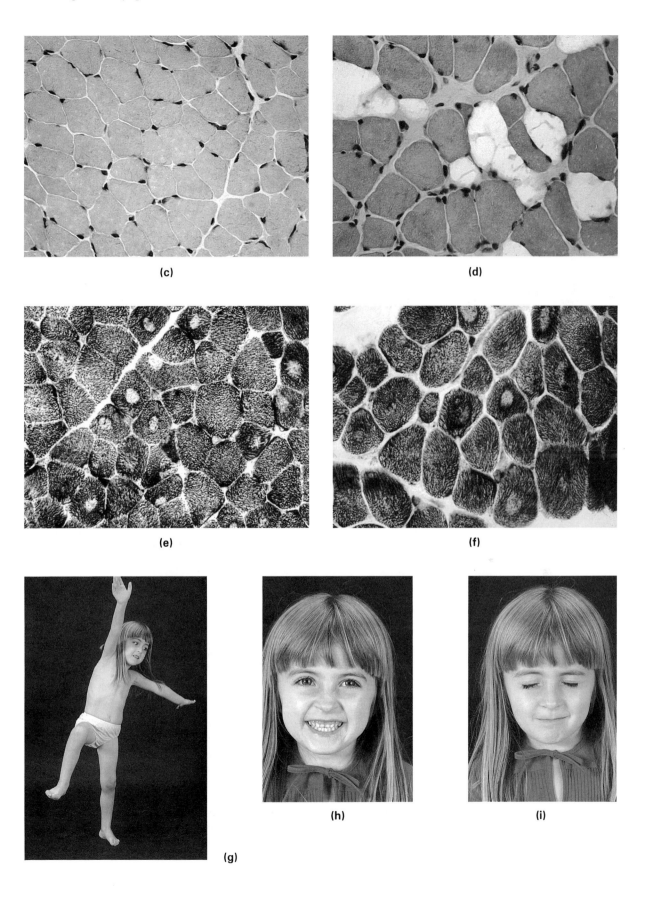

(c)

(d)

(e)

(f)

(g)

(h)

(i)

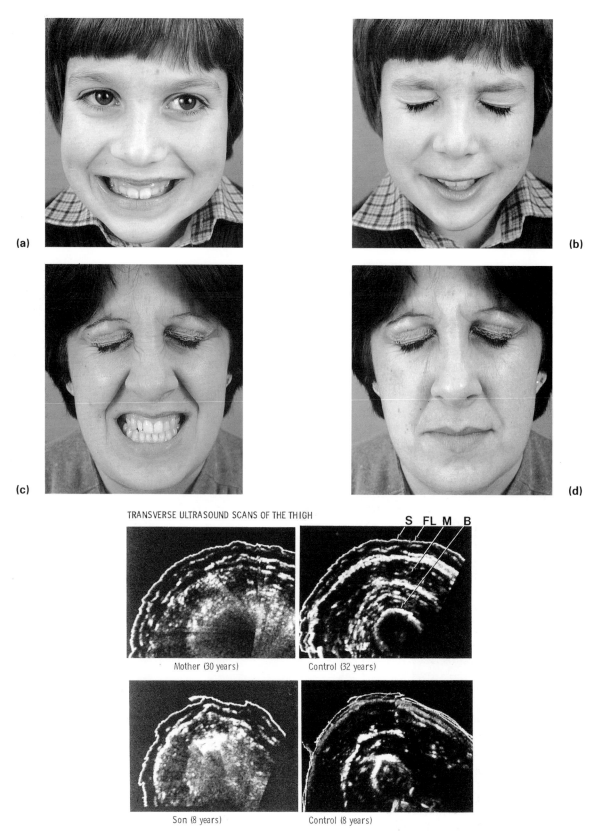

(a)

(b)

(c)

(d)

TRANSVERSE ULTRASOUND SCANS OF THE THIGH

S FL M B

Mother (30 years)   Control (32 years)

Son (8 years)   Control (8 years)

(e)

S=Skin FL=Fascia Lata M=Muscle B=Bone

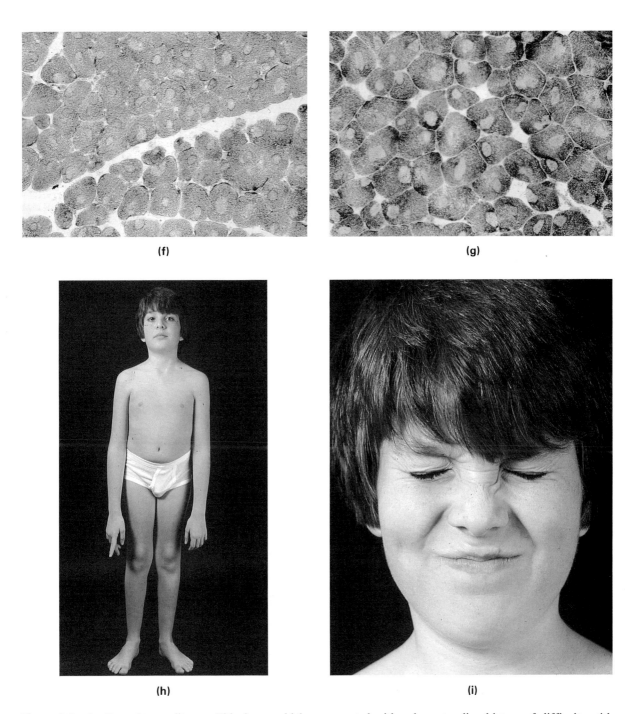

(f)

(g)

(h)

(i)

Figure 3-5 a-i Central core disease. This 8-year-old boy presented with a long-standing history of difficulty with strenuous activities such as running, a tendency to falling, and some difficulty getting up, but there was no progression. Milestones were delayed: he sat at 10 months, stood at 16 months and walked at 19 months. On examination there was minimal weakness of the pelvic girdle muscles. He got up without a Gowers' sign but had difficulty hopping. His face appeared normal and he had good expressive movements but was unable to bury his eyelashes (a,b). His mother showed similar facial features (c,d) and on questioning said she had also experienced some motor difficulties over the years. She was more severely affected, did not walk until 4 years of age and still had difficulty climbing steps. Ultrasound imaging showed increased echo in both their quadriceps (e). Needle biopsy of the quadriceps revealed a classic picture of central core disease with uniformity of fibre type and single prominent cores devoid of oxidative activity in almost all fibres in both mother and son (f,g). On subsequent follow-up his clinical status remained unchanged (h,i), but recently at 24 years he has been having more difficulty with stairs and walking, tending to walk on his toes and to lock his knees.

GENETICS

The inheritance is usually dominant. The close association with malignant hyperthermia, which is also dominantly inherited, suggested the two conditions might be allelic, and the location of the central core disease gene at the same locus as malignant hyperthermia (19q13.1) (Kausch *et al.*, 1991) has now provided an explanation for the overlap. A recent study by Mulley *et al.* (1993) of a large kindred with central core disease showed a very close linkage of the gene for central core disease with the ryanodine receptor, with a lod score of 11.8 and no recombinants, suggesting that the gene for central core disease is allelic with the ryanodine receptor gene, which in turn has been considered to be the gene for malignant hyperthermia (MacLennan *et al.*, 1990) (see Chapter 4).

Romero *et al.* (1994) did a combined gene linkage and muscle biopsy study in two families, the proband in the first presenting with malignant hyperthermia after anaesthesia, and in the second with non-progressive weakness since infancy and found to have central core disease and marked type 1 predominance on muscle biopsy. Additional open biopsy samples were obtained for histochemical detection of central cores and contracture test for malignant hyperthermia susceptibility in eight members of family 1 and two members of family 2. There was no consistent relationship between the presence of the malignant hyperthermia phenotype, the central core disease phenotype and the presence of the genetic haplotype. Thus in family 2 one asymptomatic individual had the same haplotype as his two symptomatic brothers, and in family 1 one individual showed central cores in his muscle but a normal contracture test and had a different haplotype from the malignant hyperthermia-affected members of this family.

Quane *et al.* (1993) and Zhang *et al.* (1993) have recently reported mutations in the ryanodine receptor gene in relation to central core disease.

MINICORE DISEASE (MULTICORE DISEASE)

HISTORICAL

In 1971 Engel *et al.* documented two unrelated children with a benign, congenital, non-progressive myopathy, associated with multifocal areas of degeneration in the muscle fibres. The first case, a boy of 13, had experienced non-progressive weakness of the trunk and extremities all his life. His motor development was slow: he sat at 9 months, walked at 18 months and was unable to climb stairs until 9 years. No other members of the family were affected. Examination revealed weakness of the trunk muscles and moderate proximal and mild distal weakness of the limbs. The second case, an 11-year-old girl, had a non-progressive weakness since infancy. When first seen at 4 months with congestive cardiac failure due to atrial and ventricular septal defects, the muscle weakness was ascribed to the heart problem. After cardiac surgery the heart function was normal but the weakness persisted. She sat at 9 months but had poor head control. She walked at 22 months but could not get up after falling. When assessed at 7 years she had diffuse weakness affecting upper limbs more than lower and proximal muscles more than distal. In addition there was ptosis, thoracic scoliosis, tight heel cords and slight elbow contractures. Although a maternal grandmother became chairbound at 18 years and a maternal uncle had tight Achilles tendons, the child's parents and two siblings had no weakness.

In both cases the serum enzymes were normal and electromyography showed marginal myopathic changes. Biopsy showed similar changes in both cases, with multiple small randomly distributed areas in the muscle with focal decrease in mitochondrial oxidative enzyme activity and focal myofibrillar degenerative change. These focal areas were circumscribed, both in transverse and longitudinal section. At ultrastructural level the lesions were characterized by a decrease in mitochondria, with or without sarcomere disintegration beginning in the Z-disc. Intramuscular nerves and motor endplates were normal.

These two cases seemed sporadic, but the subsequent recording of affected twin males by Heffner *et al.* (1976), affected siblings by Lake *et al.* (1977) and Ricoy *et al.* (1980), and of three affected siblings with symptom-free parents who were first cousins (Dubowitz, 1978) (see Figures 3-6, 3-7) suggested an autosomal recessive pattern of inheritance.

Currie *et al.* (1974) suggested the term 'minicore', which I have also adopted as a more descriptive term for the actual abnormality, since the classical central cores can also be multiple.

CLINICAL FEATURES

The presentation is usually one of a mild, relatively non-progressive weakness, but some cases are more severe (Figures 3-6 to 3-9). There is usually a mild facial weakness with inability to bury the eyelashes fully. There is often associated diaphragmatic weakness which may cause nocturnal hypoventilation. This is important to recognize as it can be life-threatening and is easily treated with nocturnal ventilation by nasal mask. Some cases may manifest disturbed sleep and early morning headaches and drowsiness; others may be symptom-free.

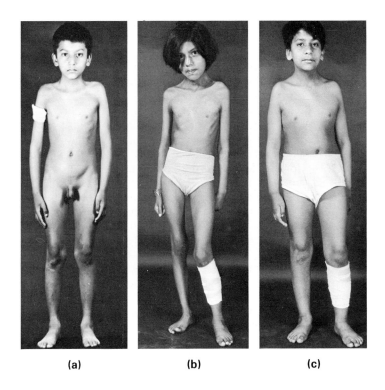

(a) (b) (c)

Figure 3-6a-c Minicore disease in three siblings presenting with mild non-progressive proximal weakness. The parents were first cousins. The family history was negative. CK normal; EMG myopathic.

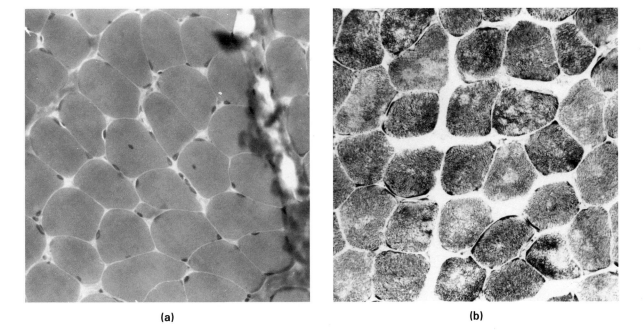

(a) (b)

Figure 3-7a,b Biopsy of deltoid from oldest child (shown in Figure 3-6a), aged 10 years, showing (a) normal histological appearance apart from internal nuclei and some atrophic fibres (trichrome × 225). (b) Histochemical preparation showing undifferentiated muscle with almost entirely type 1 fibres and multiple small cores in many fibres (NADH-TR × 225).

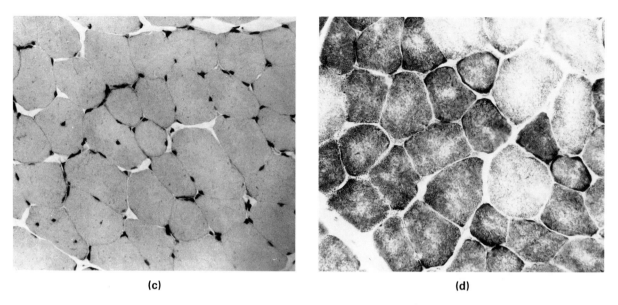

(c)   (d)

Figures 3-7c,d Biopsy of gastrocnemius from second child (shown in Figure 3-6b), aged 9 years, showing (c) fairly normal histological picture apart from internal nuclei (H & E × 225). (d) Oxidative enzyme reaction shows a predominance of type 1 (dark-staining) fibres and minicores in many fibres (NADH-TR × 225).

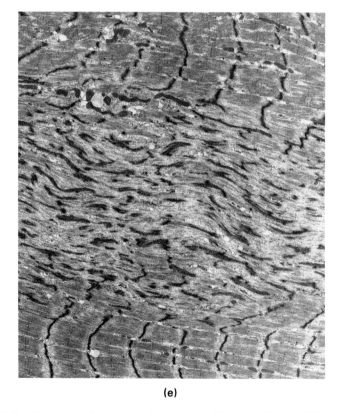

(e)

Figure 3.7e Electron microscopy of biopsy in Figure 3-8c (× 6000) showing circumscribed minicores with loss of myofibrillar structure, surrounded by normally structured muscle.

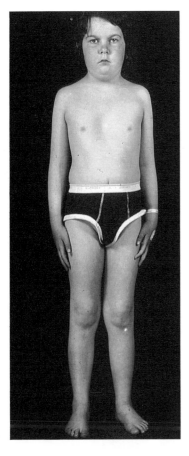

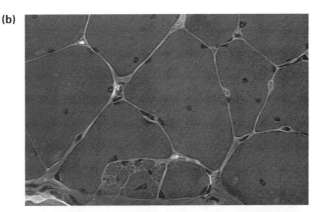

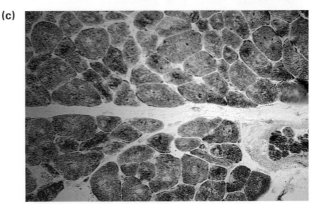

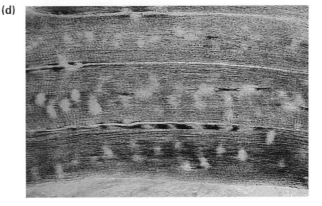

Figure 3-8a-d Minicore disease. This 8-year-old boy presented with non-progressive mild muscle weakness (a). Biopsy of the rectus femoris showed variation in fibre size, frequent internal nuclei and splitting of fibres on routine stains, and characteristic minicores with the oxidative enzyme reactions (b-d). The focal circumscribed nature of the minicores was well illustrated in longitudinally oriented fibres, and contrasts with central cores which tend to be cylindrical and run the length of the fibre. At subsequent follow-up his condition remained unchanged and 10 years later, after leaving school, he was working full time in a clothes shop.

HISTOPATHOLOGY

On routine staining the muscle may be well preserved and show little change apart from variation in fibre size and often a striking tendency to internal nuclei. There is usually a predominance of type 1 fibres for which the minicores have a selectivity. The main structural distinction from central core disease is the finite, oval-shaped cores, both in transverse and longitudinal section, with loss of structure in the cores, whereas the cores in central core disease are tubular structures, running the length of the fibre and usually retaining their structure.

This condition seems to be genetically distinct from central core disease, in spite of some similarity between minicores, and the less frequent variant of unstructured central core disease. There is probably more tendency towards disintegration of the myofibrillar pattern in the minicores (Figure 3-8).

Minicores may also be associated with other structural abnormalities in the muscle.

GENETICS

Inheritance is autosomal recessive. The gene location has not yet been established.

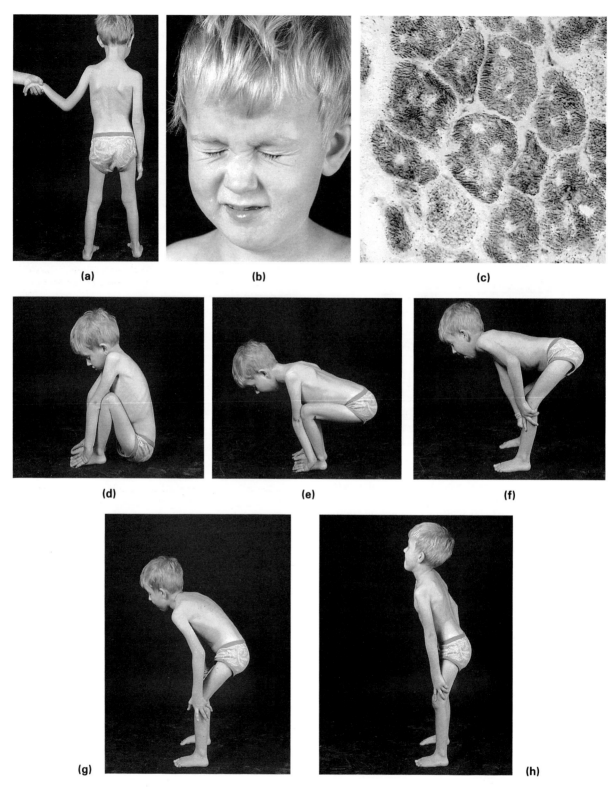

(a) **(b)** **(c)**

(d) **(e)** **(f)**

(g) **(h)**

Figure 3-9a-h Minicore disease. This 6-year-old boy had hypotonia and delay in motor milestones associated with general muscle wasting and weakness and mild facial weakness (a,b). Needle biopsy of the quadriceps showed typical minicores with the oxidative enzyme stains (c). Note unusual Gowers' manoeuvre getting up from the floor, going from a sitting to a squatting position before pushing his hands up his thighs (d-h).

NEMALINE MYOPATHY ('ROD BODY' MYOPATHY)

In 1963 Shy *et al.* described 'nemaline myopathy, a new congenital myopathy' in a 4-year-old girl who had been a floppy infant and had muscle weakness affecting her upper limbs more than the lower. Because they were uncertain whether the rod-like structures in the muscle were separate rods or possibly an undulating thread-like structure, they suggested the name nemaline myopathy (Greek: *nema* – thread). Conen *et al.* (1963) independently observed 'myogranules' in the biopsy of a 4-year-old boy with hypotonia and non-progressive weakness.

CLINICAL FEATURES

There have been several subsequent reports. Most cases have presented with a mild, non-progressive myopathy and indeed one of the cases of Gonatas *et al.* (1966) was a symptom-free sibling of the index case. In contrast, however, some cases have been severely affected, with early death (Engel, 1967; Shafiq *et al.*, 1967). On clinical examination, these patients usually have reduced muscle bulk, and it is of particular interest that the cases of Krabbe's 'universal muscular atrophy' included by Ford in the earlier edition of his textbook of paediatric neurology (Ford, 1960) were subsequently shown to have nemaline myopathy (Hopkins *et al.*, 1966).

Associated features

Many reported cases have shown associated skeletal dysmorphism, with kyphoscoliosis, pigeon chest, pes cavus, high arched palate and unusually long face (Conen *et al.*, 1963; Engel *et al.*, 1964; Price *et al.*, 1965; Spiro *et al.*, 1966; Hudgson *et al.*, 1967).

Kuitonnen *et al.* (1972) drew attention to the high incidence of respiratory problems which occurred in three of their four cases and which also seemed to be a consistent feature of early-onset cases previously recorded in the literature. This probably reflects diaphragmatic involvement, and sleep studies for nocturnal hypoxia are important in order to intervene with nasal mask ventilation at night. In addition, their review of the literature suggested a high incidence of the disease in females. In my experience swallowing difficulty in the neonatal period (or later) is also a common feature and in some cases may be the only prominent symptom apart from general hypotonia.

Tremor of the hands ('minipolymyoclonus') similar to that seen in spinal muscular atrophy (see Chapter 6) was documented by Colamaria *et al.* (1991) in a 7-month-old boy with nemaline myopathy, and we have occasionally noted tremor of the baseline of the electrocardiogram, as in spinal muscular atrophy.

Cardiac involvement

Ishibashi Ueda *et al.* (1990) documented the autopsy features of a 3-year-old boy with congenital nemaline myopathy who had suffered generalized muscle weakness and hypotonia since birth. He developed cardiac symptoms at 2 years of age and died from congestive heart failure. The heart was markedly dilated, involving both ventricles, and rod bodies were noted not only in the skeletal muscle but also in the cardiac muscle on light and electron microscopy. Desmin and α-actinin, which constitutes Z-line protein, were shown to localize in the rod structures in both skeletal and myocardial cell muscle fibres. The authors reviewed seven cases of nemaline myopathy with cardiomyopathy reported in the literature, all of which were over 20 years old and seemed to relate more to the late-onset forms of nemaline myopathy. This is the first record of an infantile case with a dilated cardiomyopathy.

Illustrative case histories showing the wide range in clinical presentation are included in Figures 3-10 to 3-12.

PROGNOSIS

Whilst it may be difficult to prognosticate in such variable clinical severity, it does seem that the cases of congenital or early infantile onset are at risk of early death, which probably relates to their respiratory deficiency. Adequate monitoring of respiratory function, and particularly nocturnal hypoventilation, may allow appropriate early intervention with nocturnal mask ventilation and improve the prognosis. This of course also applies to the milder cases with late onset of respiratory failure.

HISTOPATHOLOGY

The rods are easily overlooked on routine H & E staining. They can be readily demonstrated, however, with the Gomori trichrome stain, with which they stain a red colour in contrast to the blue-green of the muscle fibres (Figures 3-10 to 3-12). The rods do not show up with any of the histochemical enzyme reactions. With the ATPase reaction, the rods are negative, and aggregates of rods may thus appear as clear areas in the fibres.

Studies on the distribution of the rods in several muscles from an autopsied case which I had the opportunity of examining showed a tremendous variation in the proportion of affected fibres, not only from one muscle to another but even in

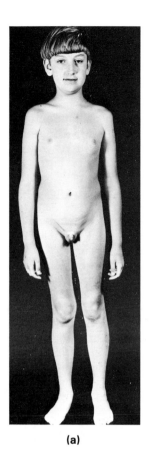
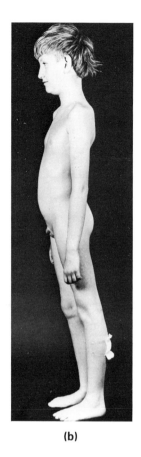

(a)   **(b)**

Figure 3-10a,b Nemaline (rod body) myopathy in a 12-year-old boy who went into respiratory failure when climbing Mount Snowdon while competing for the Duke of Edinburgh award. Subsequently he was noted to have mild proximal pelvic girdle weakness. EMG showed a denervation pattern suggesting a spinal muscular atrophy. CK 14 iu/litre.

different parts of the same muscle (Shafiq *et al.*, 1967). The extent of involvement in a random muscle biopsy is thus no index of the general extent of the disease process.

In many cases the muscle looks normal apart from the presence of the rods. Some may show variability in fibre size and others a population of small fibres with selective involvement by rods. There is usually no necrosis or degenerative change. The fibre type distribution may also be normal but some cases may show a selective involvement of type 1 or type 2 fibres.

The rods are readily demonstrated on electron microscopy as dense structures, usually of rectangular shape, with a lattice pattern of consistent periodicity, and in continuity with the Z lines. They are thought to be abnormal depositions of Z band material of a protein nature and possibly α-actinin. Immunocytochemical techniques with antibodies to α-actinin can also be used to identify the rods in sections.

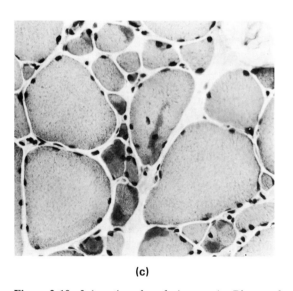
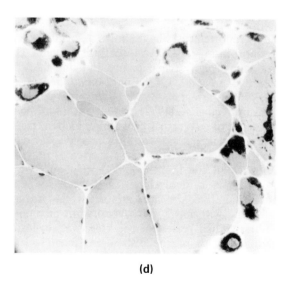

(c)   **(d)**

Figure 3-10c-f (*continued on facing page*) Biopsy of gastrocnemius. (c) On routine stain there are two populations of fibres with abnormally large and abnormally small diameter, and a granularity is apparent in some fibres (Verhoeff-van Gieson × 225). (d) In serial section with trichrome stain the rods show up very clearly as red-staining bodies, confined mainly to the atrophic fibres. (e) With the ATPase reaction the majority of fibres are type 1 and the rod areas show up as clear unstained areas (ATPase pH 4.3 × 225, serial section). (f) Electron microscope section shows the electron dense rods in an atrophic fibre adjacent to a normal fibre (× 4900). Needle biopsies from both parents were devoid of rods.

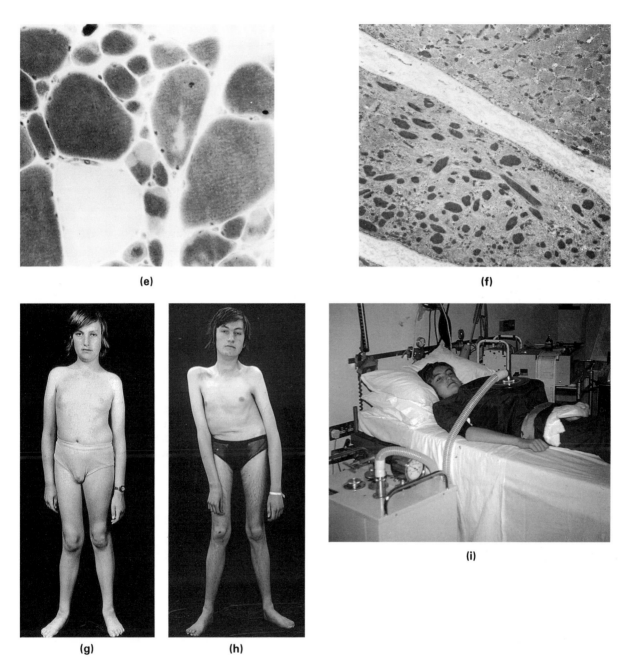

(e)

(f)

(g) **(h)**

(i)

Figure 3-10g-i His skeletal muscle power over the next 12 years of follow-up remained fairly steady and he continued to be ambulant; at 25 years of age he is currently fully employed and drives a car (with appropriate adaptations). However, he has recurrent bouts of respiratory failure with associated life-threatening right heart failure. At 16 years he was admitted with pneumonia and heart failure and had become progressively drowsy, confused and complained of headaches. He was cyanosed but could improve his colour by voluntary hyperventilation, suggesting that he was chronically underbreathing. Provision of a cuirass ventilator at night produced a dramatic symptomatic improvement and resolution of his daytime drowsiness and headache (i). During his growth spurt he also developed a progressive S-shaped scoliosis which had reached 55° at 15 years and 80° by 17 years (g,h). It was difficult to control with a brace but internal fixation was repeatedly deferred because of anxiety by anaesthetists about his poor respiratory function. This was finally outweighed by our anxiety at the progression without operation and a spinal fusion was done with a double Harrington rod at 18 years of age, which successfully stabilized the scoliosis that had already reached 120°. Over the past 10 years he has remained relatively symptom-free and has been able to hold down a full-time job as a clerk. Recently he has made use of a cuirass-type ventilator to tide him over respiratory infections; and also used it for an added boost of better ventilation once a week. He has now been provided with a mask ventilator and a small portable ventilator at night.

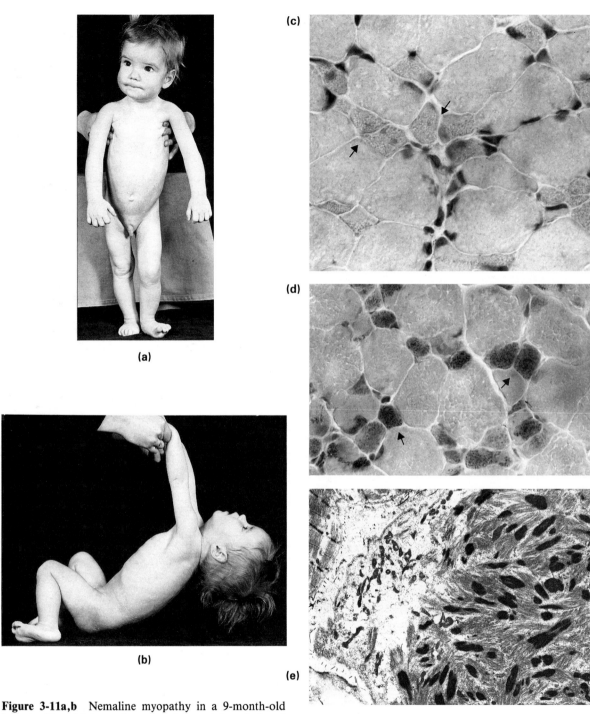

(a)

(b)

(c)

(d)

(e)

Figure 3-11a,b Nemaline myopathy in a 9-month-old infant with a history of a normal neonatal period and development of hypotonia from 2 months, and subsequent weakness of limbs. On examination he was able to stand with support (a), but was unable to sit without support, and still had poor head control (b) with diminished tone and power. CK 39 iu/litre. EMG showed spontaneous potentials at rest and polyphasic fasciculation potentials on activity suggestive of denervation. His condition remained fairly static but at 18 months he died suddenly after a mild respiratory infection.

Figure 3-11c-e Needle muscle biopsy from rectus femoris of this child showing (c) two populations of fibre size on routine stain (H & E × 580) and some granularity of small fibres. (d) The rods are readily apparent on trichrome stain and mainly occur in the small fibres (trichrome × 580). Compare with Figure 3-10. Electron microscopy (e) showed numerous rods in association with loss of fibre structure. Needle biopsy of both parents was normal.

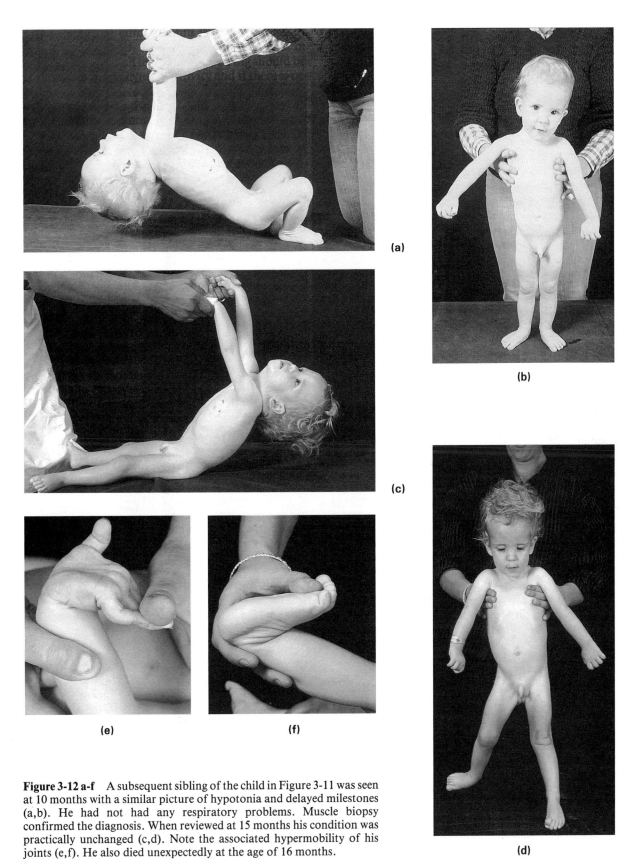

Figure 3-12 a-f A subsequent sibling of the child in Figure 3-11 was seen at 10 months with a similar picture of hypotonia and delayed milestones (a,b). He had not had any respiratory problems. Muscle biopsy confirmed the diagnosis. When reviewed at 15 months his condition was practically unchanged (c,d). Note the associated hypermobility of his joints (e,f). He also died unexpectedly at the age of 16 months.

SEVERE CONGENITAL NEMALINE MYOPATHY WITH INTRANUCLEAR RODS

In contrast to the usually benign course in infants with nemaline myopathy, even of neonatal onset, occasional cases have been reported with very severe weakness at birth and a fatal outcome (Jenis *et al.*, 1969; Norton *et al.*, 1983; Rifai *et al.*, 1993). In addition to the usual small sarcoplasmic nemaline rods, there were also large intranuclear rods, with similar staining on Gomori trichrome and positively reacting immunocytochemically to antibodies to α-actinin.

GENETICS

The familial nature of the disease was established by Spiro and Kennedy (1965) in their study of an affected mother and daughter, and the two siblings reported by Gonatas *et al.* (1966) turned out to be cousins of the patient in Spiro and Kennedy's index case. Hopkins *et al.* (1966) also documented an affected mother and daughter. These affected families conform to a dominant inheritance pattern with variable clinical expression. On the other hand, the muscle biopsy was normal in both parents of the patient of Shafiq *et al.* (1967), two patients of Kuitonnen *et al.* (1972) and in six families we examined. There have also been numerous other reports of sporadic cases (Conen *et al.*, 1963; Engel *et al.*, 1964; Price *et al.*, 1965; Hudgson *et al.*, 1967). It would thus appear that the recessive form of inheritance is much more common than the dominant.

Some confusion has been produced by some authors, who have over-interpreted minor pathological changes, such as variation in fibre size or alterations in distribution of fibre type, without overt nemaline rods, in one or other parent, and implied that these were manifestations of a dominant gene. Thus Kondo and Yuasa (1980) concluded from a review of 50 published cases that the most likely pattern of inheritance was autosomal dominant and that the lower than expected ratio for affected siblings (0.3 against 0.5) could be due to asymptomatic rod-bearing heterozygotes.

Wallgren-Pettersson *et al.* (1990) recently reviewed the genetics of congenital nemaline myopathy in 10 Finnish families, including three families with two affected children. Of the parents, 15 showed deficiency of type 2B fibres and all except one father showed some other minor neuromuscular abnormality on biopsy. These probably represented heterozygous manifestations of a recessive gene. All the Finnish families seemed compatible with recessive mode of inheritance and this is also the situation in most of the published cases in the literature, with only a few instances documented of dominant inheritance.

Laing *et al.* (1992) assigned a gene (NEM1) for autosomal dominant nemaline myopathy to chromosome 1q21-q23 in one large kindred with ten living affected family members using a candidate gene approach. They found no close linkage to the α-actinin gene on chromosome 1, but a close linkage to APOA2. The locus for the more common autosomal recessive form has not yet been located.

MIXED MYOPATHIES

Coexistence of nemaline myopathy and cores in the same patient

Since the rods in nemaline myopathy appear to arise from the Z lines and streaming of the Z lines is a feature of the cores in central core disease, it is perhaps not surprising that an overlap of the conditions has been observed. Afifi *et al.* (1965) observed both central cores and rods in the same muscle, whereas Karpati *et al.* (1971) found central cores and 'targets' in the diaphragm of a fatal case of nemaline myopathy. Bethlem *et al.* (1978) documented 12 cases with a combination of rods with cores or minicores, and Vallat *et al.* (1982) observed unstructured cores, minicores and rods in the same biopsy. In an experimental study Shafiq *et al.* (1969) produced both cores and rods in the soleus of the rat after tenotomy.

A patient in whom coexistence of nemaline myopathy with minicores was found is illustrated in Figure 3-13.

Coexistence of minicores with whorled fibres

Two siblings with a congenital myopathy showed the coexistence of minicores with extensive whorled fibres (Figure 3-14). The parents, who are unrelated, and one other sibling were normal, suggesting an autosomal recessive inheritance. This appears to be a genetically determined congenital myopathy in which the whorled fibres are probably a significant feature. Although whorled fibres do occur as an isolated phenomenon in many other neuromuscular disorders, and particularly in slowly progressive limb girdle dystrophy, they only usually affect a few scattered fibres and it is unusual to see such a large concentration of them. This suggests they may be an integral component of this myopathy in addition to the minicores. The condition appears to be a relatively mild one in this particular family, with a tendency to gradual improvement.

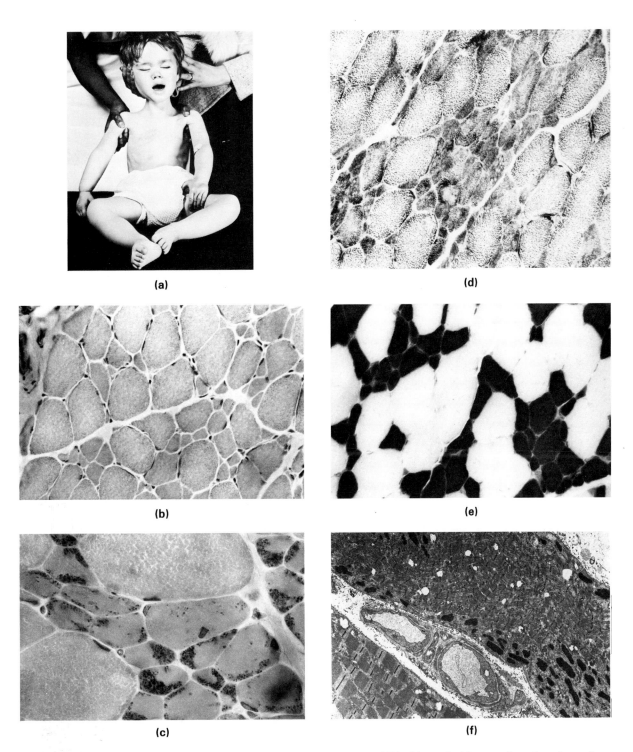

Figure 3-13a-f Nemaline myopathy plus minicores in an 18-month-old child with marked hypotonia and weakness from birth and subsequent deterioration. Recurrent pneumonia. Previous biopsy (formalin fixation) reported as normal. CK 21 iu/litre; EMG normal. (b) Biopsy of rectus femoris from this child showing two populations of large and small fibres but no other abnormality on routine stain (Verhoeff-van Gieson × 230). (c) With the trichrome stain the rods are clearly visible and confined mainly to the small fibres (trichrome × 580). (d) With the oxidative enzyme reaction the small fibres are predominantly type 1 (dark-staining) and also show minicores (NADH-TR × 230). (e) With ATPase the small fibres were type 1 (ATPase pH 4.3 × 230. Type 1 fibres dark). (f) Electron microscopic section showing coincident rods and minicore in same fibre. Adjacent fibre (lower left) normal (× 3400).

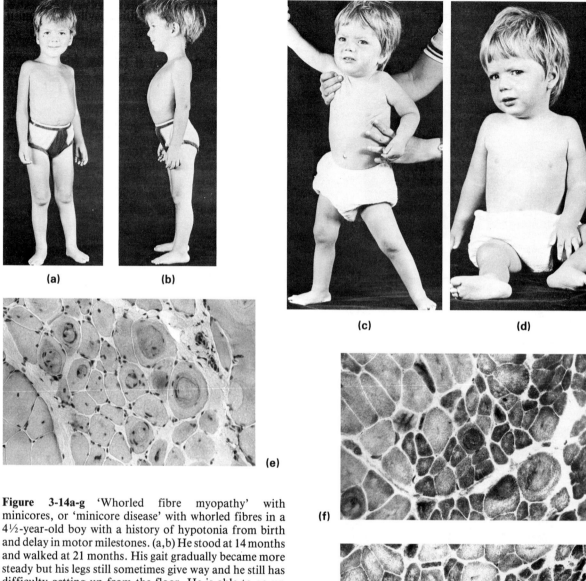

(a)

(b)

(c)

(d)

(e)

(f)

(g)

Figure 3-14a-g 'Whorled fibre myopathy' with minicores, or 'minicore disease' with whorled fibres in a 4½-year-old boy with a history of hypotonia from birth and delay in motor milestones. (a,b) He stood at 14 months and walked at 21 months. His gait gradually became more steady but his legs still sometimes give way and he still has difficulty getting up from the floor. He is able to go up steps one at a time. There is no apparent weakness of the facial or external ocular muscles. Mild proximal weakness affects the lower limbs more than the upper. Nerve conduction velocities normal; EMG myopathic. Previous muscle biopsy, processed only by routine histology, showed no abnormality. (c,d) The 2-year-old sister had a similar history of hypotonia from birth and delayed motor milestones, and also initial feeding difficulty in the newborn period. She sat unsupported at 9 months, but was still not walking unaided at 2 years. She walked well with the support of one hand, and during the ensuing months took a few steps unsupported. There was no facial or ocular involvement. There was general hypotonia and a mild proximal weakness affecting the legs as well as the arms. She had difficulty sustaining the arms against gravity. Nerve conduction normal; EMG myopathic. (e,f) Needle biopsy of quadriceps from girl in (c,d) showing a striking picture of numerous whorled fibres which were particularly obvious on the oxidative enzyme reactions in addition to the routine stains (e, H & E × 230; f, NADH-TR × 150). (g) In addition, many fibres appeared to have minicores (NADH-TR × 150). A similar pattern was present in her brother's biopsy, but was less marked.

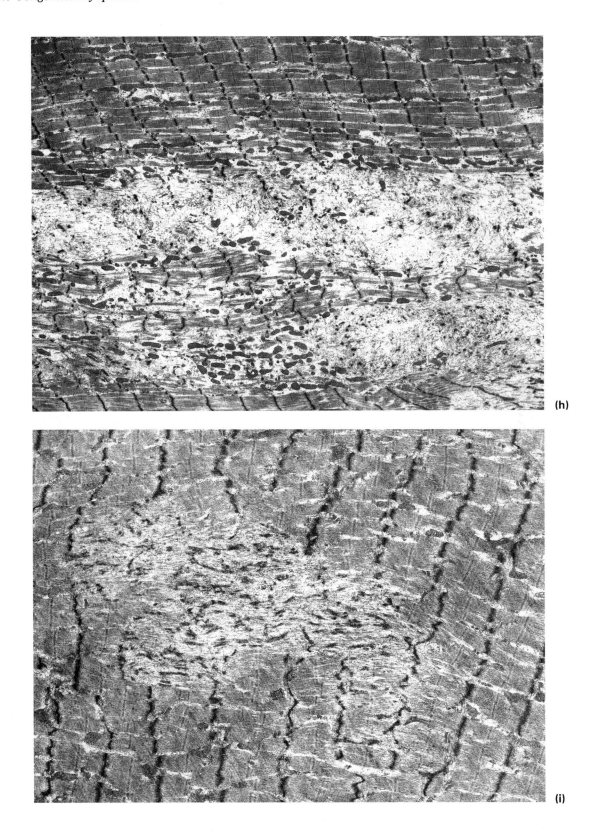

Figure 3-14h,i Electron micrograph of biopsy showing (h) central 'unstructured' core running the length of the fibre and (i) a minicore which is circumscribed and has normal muscle around it.

MYOTUBULAR MYOPATHY (CENTRONUCLEAR MYOPATHY)

HISTORICAL

In 1966, Spiro *et al.* suggested the name 'myotubular myopathy' for the histological changes observed in the biopsies from a 12-year-old boy, because of the striking resemblance to the myotubes of fetal muscle. The clinical history was somewhat complex. The child had experienced delay in early motor milestones and was still unable to raise his head in the prone position at 3 months. Bilateral subdural haematomas were evacuated surgically at 6 months. Although he walked by 17 months he was never able to run. From the age of 5 years he also developed convulsions. There was generalized weakness, which appeared to be progressive, and associated ptosis, external ophthalmoplegia and facial diplegia. On biopsy of the gastrocnemius, the muscle fibres were normal in size, but in about 85% of fibres there were one to four centrally placed nuclei, surrounded by an area devoid of myofibrils. Similar changes were noted in about 45% of fibres in a second biopsy.

Histochemical studies showed normal oxidative enzyme activity in unaffected fibres, but in affected fibres there was a central (or eccentric) zone either devoid of enzyme activity or with increased enzyme activity. Amylophosphorylase and PAS activity also showed either an increase or a decrease in the central zone of respective fibres. The ATPase reaction, on the other hand, showed a consistent absence of activity in these central areas. On electron microscopy the perinuclear zone contained aggregates of mitochondria and myelin figures, which may have resulted from prior freezing of the muscle. There were no ribosomal aggregates.

Spiro *et al.* considered these abnormal fibres to be comparable with the myotubes of developing muscle and postulated an arrest in the development of the muscle at cellular level. The fact that the fibres in the patient were normal in size suggested continued growth of the cell in spite of the developmental arrest.

Sher and her colleagues (1967) subsequently observed similar pathological changes in the muscle of two Negro sisters, aged 18 and 16 years, and their symptom-free mother. The first sister had delay in early motor milestones, generalized atrophy of the musculature, a slowly progressive weakness of the skeletal muscles, ptosis, external ophthalmoplegia and facial weakness. The clinical photograph with the long, thin face shows a striking resemblance to the case of Spiro *et al.* and also to the 'dysmorphic' features of some reported cases of nemaline myopathy. The younger sister, who had not been floppy as an infant and had no delay in motor milestones, showed a fairly diffuse wasting and weakness of the limbs and bilateral ptosis, but no facial weakness or ophthalmoplegia.

Biopsy of the rectus femoris and gastrocnemius in both sisters showed central nuclei in the majority of fibres. In the mother's gastrocnemius, about a third of the fibres had internal nuclei. Sher *et al.* suggested the alternative descriptive title 'centronuclear myopathy'.

Since these initial reports, a number of further cases have been documented, with variability both in clinical manifestations and in muscle morphology.

CLINICAL FEATURES

In general the clinical picture in these patients has been one of varying degrees of weakness, often including ptosis and weakness of the external ocular muscles as well as weakness of the axial musculature. Although most of these cases had symptoms of weakness from infancy, occasionally the disease did not present symptomatically until later in childhood, and in some of them extraocular weakness was not prominent. The disease seemed to be either non-progressive or only slowly progressive in most cases. One child, who also had convulsions or apnoeic spells, died at 8 years of age. The majority of recorded cases have been children under 10 years of age, but at least three adults have been reported (Bethlem *et al.*, 1968; Karpati *et al.*, 1970; Vital *et al.*, 1970).

MYOTUBULAR MYOPATHY WITH TYPE 1 FIBRE HYPOTROPHY

In another, probably related, condition profuse central nuclei are seen in association with type 1 fibre atrophy. Engel *et al.* (1968) recorded an 11-month-old boy with a severe and progressive weakness of the limbs and respiratory muscles but no ocular or facial weakness. The child died at 18 months and at autopsy there was no abnormality in the nervous system. Although agreeing that the small fibres in their patient did have some resemblance to embryonic myotubes, Engel *et al.* were not convinced that these were true myotubes or that they had any unique significance in the context of this child's disease process. They attached more importance to the histochemical pattern and thus suggested calling it 'type 1 fibre hypotrophy with central nuclei', implying a maturational arrest rather than an atrophy of type 1 fibres. Further case reports (Bethlem *et al.*, 1969; Karpati *et al.*, 1970) suggested that this entity was clinically different from the typical myotubular myopathy and not necessarily a progressive and fatal disease.

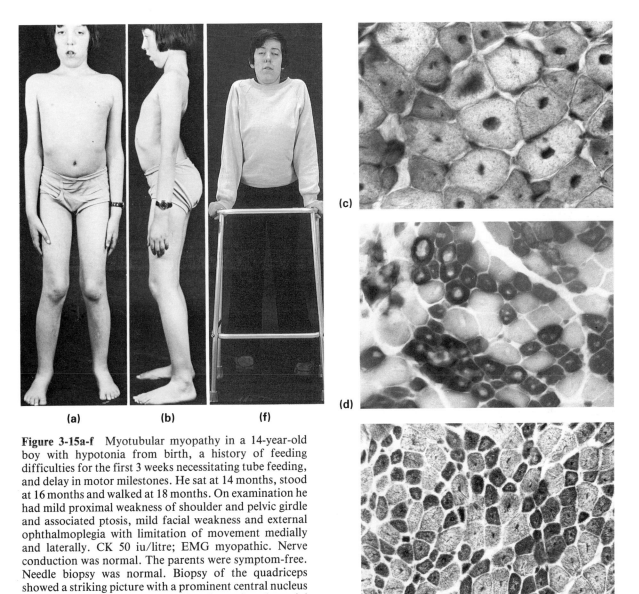

Figure 3-15a-f Myotubular myopathy in a 14-year-old boy with hypotonia from birth, a history of feeding difficulties for the first 3 weeks necessitating tube feeding, and delay in motor milestones. He sat at 14 months, stood at 16 months and walked at 18 months. On examination he had mild proximal weakness of shoulder and pelvic girdle and associated ptosis, mild facial weakness and external ophthalmoplegia with limitation of movement medially and laterally. CK 50 iu/litre; EMG myopathic. Nerve conduction was normal. The parents were symptom-free. Needle biopsy was normal. Biopsy of the quadriceps showed a striking picture with a prominent central nucleus in almost all fibres and proliferation of endomysial connective tissue (c). There was a normal distribution of fibre types, a central clear area devoid of myofibrils with the ATPase reaction (d), and central aggregation of oxidative activity (e). He remained fairly stable in ambulation over the ensuing years but developed increasing breathlessness and even during speech took frequent breaths. At 18 years of age he fractured his femur and had difficulty with remobilization (f). He died unexpectedly after a mild respiratory infection at 19 years. He may well have had nocturnal hypoventilation.

It is, however, difficult to draw a dividing line on clinical grounds between cases of myotubular myopathy with and without type 1 fibre atrophy (or hypotrophy), and whether these will turn out to be distinct entities or variants of the same condition will have to await the gene location. Pongratz *et al.* (1976) described a family in which the mother had centronuclear myopathy and her two daughters a selective type 1 fibre involvement and atrophy in addition.

As regards nomenclature it is likely that the term 'myotubular myopathy' will remain, even though it may prove a misnomer and less accurate than 'centronuclear myopathy', simply because it got there first and has become entrenched in the neuromuscular nomenclature.

For case histories, see Figures 3-15 to 3-17.

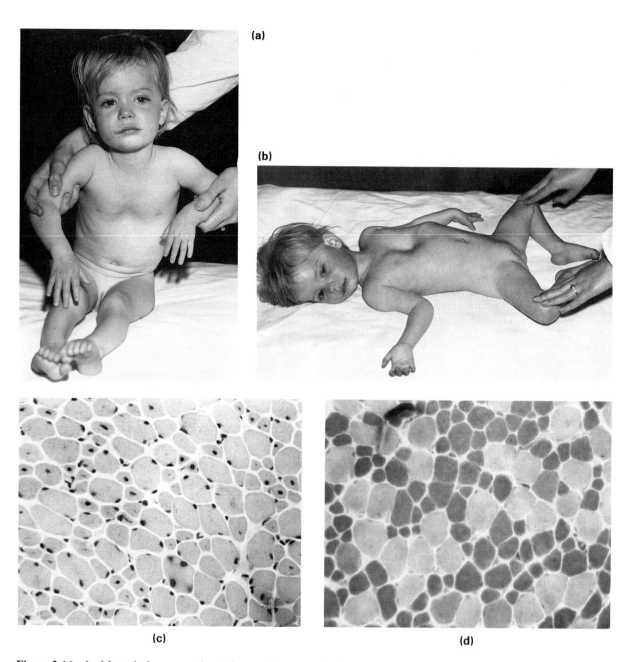

Figure 3-16a-d Myotubular myopathy with type 1 hypotrophy in an 18-month-old infant with general hypotonia and delay in motor milestones. She was unable to sit unsupported; there was associated ptosis and mild facial weakness. There was marked pectus excavatum. She suffered recurrent respiratory infections. CK 24 iu/litre; EMG myopathic. (c,d) Biopsy of rectus femoris showed (c) two-fibre population of large and small fibres and prominent internal nuclei, particularly in the small fibres (H & E × 255). (d) ATPase reactions show small fibres to be mainly type 1 and large fibres a mixture of types 1 and 2 (ATPase pH 4.3 × 255).

Figure 3-16e-j (*facing page*) She subsequently had a remarkable improvement in muscle power and was able to walk unaided by 2½ years of age. Her pectus excavatum also became less prominent. She remained ambulant (e,f aged 4½ years) but developed an increasingly lordotic posture. The facial weakness and ptosis persisted but there was improvement in the eye movements (g,h). She never noted diplopia. She had a number of life-threatening respiratory infections, one of which needed ventilator support. She experienced increasing difficulty with walking and showed progressive lordosis, fixed hip flexion and equinovarus deformity of the feet (i, j). Operative release of the hip flexors improved her posture but not her function. By 15 years of age she was essentially chairbound. She died unexpectedly at 18 years, presumably of respiratory failure.

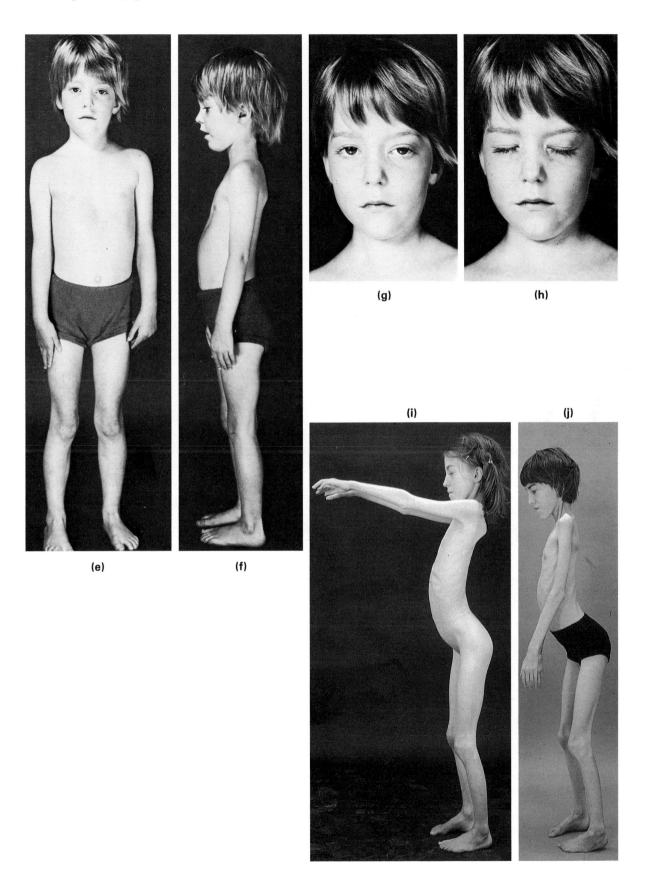

(e)

(f)

(g)

(h)

(i)

(j)

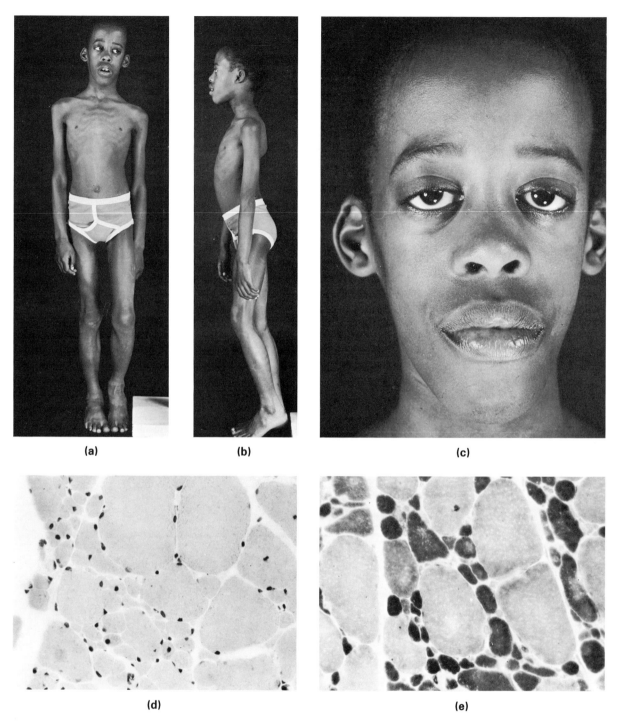

(a)   **(b)**   **(c)**

(d)   **(e)**

Figure 3-17a-e Myotubular myopathy with type 1 hypotrophy in a 10-year-old boy with a history of delay in motor milestones, sitting at 1 year, and not walking until after 2 years. He still had mild residual weakness and fixed flexion of the left knee (a,b). He had a lanky build and a long thin face (c). His face looked expressionless, with associated ptosis present but he was able voluntarily to raise eyelids fully. Nerve conduction was normal. EMG of deltoid showed mixed pattern of large polyphasic potentials suggesting denervation, and small polyphasic potentials suggesting myopathy. EMG of first dorsal interosseous showed spontaneous fibrillation at rest and positive sharp waves, suggesting denervation. CK 36 iu/litre. (d,e) Biopsy from gastrocnemius showing a striking variation in fibre size on routine staining with prominent internal nuclei in many fibres, especially the small ones. (d, H & E × 225.) Histochemical reactions showed most of the small fibres to be type 1 (e, ATPase pH 4.3 × 225).

GENETICS

It would appear from the number of instances already recorded of multiple cases within a family that the condition is certainly genetically determined. Sher *et al.* (1967) suggested an autosomal recessive inheritance for the two affected female cases and their clinically normal but histologically affected mother. An alternative genetic mechanism in this family could be an autosomal dominant gene with variable clinical severity. This mode of inheritance would also be compatible with the familial cases of Munsat *et al.* (1969) and Ortiz de Zarate and Maruffo (1970). It seems likely that, as in the cases of Sher *et al.*, investigation of apparently normal relatives will reveal subclinically affected subjects, a common phenomenon in dominantly inherited conditions.

De Angelis *et al.* (1991) reviewed the pattern of inheritance in 288 cases of myotubular myopathy reported in the literature. Autosomal dominant inheritance occurred in 14 families with 65 patients, X-linked recessive inheritance in 14 families with 84 affected males, and in 54 familial cases and 85 isolated cases the mode of inheritance was uncertain. Clinical genetic analysis of these unclassified cases suggested that most of them fitted in either autosomal dominant or X-linked recessive form and it would appear that an autosomal recessive form of inheritance was relatively infrequent, if it occurred at all.

SEVERE X-LINKED (CONGENITAL) MYOTUBULAR MYOPATHY

HISTORICAL

The Dutch family described by van Wijngaarden *et al.* (1969) had an X-linked pattern of inheritance and a 25% mortality of affected males (two of eight) in the neonatal period. Two of the clinically healthy female carriers also had myotubes in their muscle biopsy. Barth *et al.* (1975) subsequently documented another large Dutch family, unrelated to the previous one, which also had an X-linked pattern of inheritance. There was a 100% mortality of affected males (13 of 13) in the early newborn period due to associated respiratory insufficiency. In some there was an associated history of diminished fetal movements *in utero*, or hydramnios. Muscle biopsies from five clinically normal female carriers showed the presence of mild pathological changes, with the presence of myotubes in four of them.

Since these early descriptions a large number of cases have been documented. The condition is often fatal in the neonatal period and the cardinal manifesting features are severe generalized hypotonia with associated muscle weakness, swallowing difficulty and respiratory deficit (Figures 3-18 to 3-20). They may need ventilator support at birth to sustain their respiratory function. There is a trend to gradual improvement and if they can be weaned off the ventilator support they may cope with independent breathing but are still at risk of respiratory arrest and failure in the face of any precipitating factor such as inhalation of a feed or superadded infection. Two of the infants I followed were doing well and able to go home but died following an acute aspiration following a feed. This risk may possibly be averted by providing a gastrostomy for feeding but one has to weigh all this supportive intervention against the severity of the initial disease and the prospects of any degree of reasonable function.

Additional clinical features may be contractures of the limbs (arthrogryposis), a mild degree of facial weakness and weakness of the external ocular muscles. On cranial ultrasonography, there may also be an associated ventricular dilatation, with or without evidence of germinal layer haemorrhage, affecting those born preterm as well as full term.

GENETICS

The gene for the X-linked myotubular myopathy has been located to Xq28 (Darnfors *et al.*, 1990; Lehesjoki *et al.*, 1990; Starr *et al.*, 1990; Thomas *et al.*, 1987, 1990). Work is currently in progress in several laboratories to try to isolate and characterize the gene, and a European Consortium has been established to co-ordinate collaborative studies (Wallgren-Pettersson and Thomas, 1994).

Liechti-Gallati *et al.* (1993) recently reported prenatal diagnostic studies with the use of four available DNA markers on chorionic villus samples from four families with X-linked myotubular myopathy. The four fetuses, three male and one female, were all carrying the myotubular associated maternal allele. Two male fetuses were aborted and one showed histological evidence of myotubular myopathy. In the other male fetus the pregnancy was continued and the infant was affected at birth.

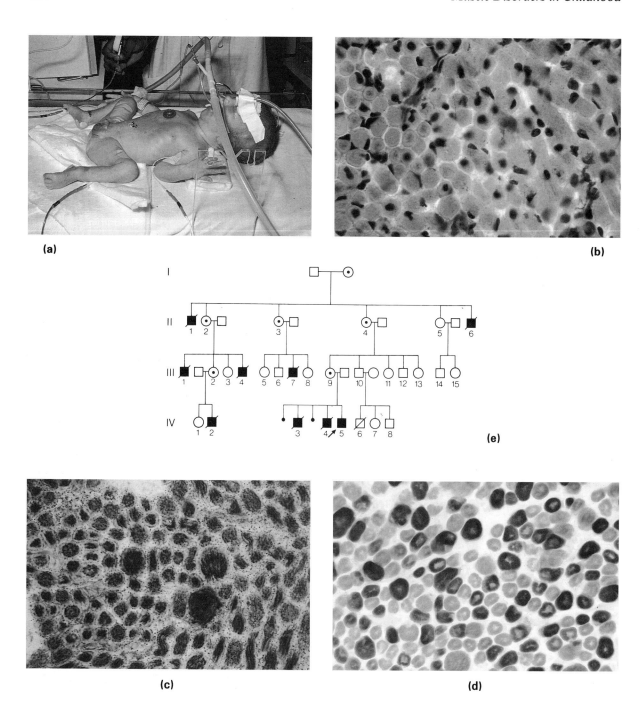

Figure 3-18a-e X-linked myotubular myopathy. This 36-week gestation infant was referred to our newborn intensive care unit with respiratory difficulties from birth, requiring ventilator support. He also had swallowing difficulty needing tube feeding and marked hypotonia (a). On examination there was facial weakness and possible external ophthalmoplegia. The clinical diagnosis of myotubular myopathy was confirmed by needle biopsy of the quadriceps which showed prominent central nuclei in about 15% of fibres in transverse section (b) with central aggregation of oxidative enzyme activity with NADH-TR (c) and central areas devoid of activity with the ATPase reactions (d). He showed gradual improvement and could be weaned off the ventilator but needed a tracheostomy to cope with his inability to swallow pharyngeal secretions, which produced choking episodes. He also began to take food by mouth. However, he died suddenly from cardiorespiratory arrest following an oral feed at 3 months. The remarkable family history showed nine perinatal deaths of male infants on the maternal side in the previous two generations, which was consistent with an X-linked inheritance (e).

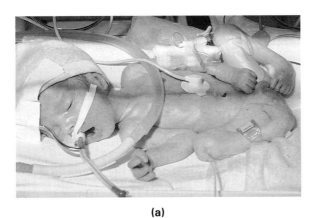

(a)

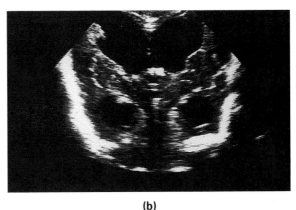

(b)

Figure 3-19a-b X-linked myotubular myopathy. This 32-week gestation infant was referred to our newborn intensive care unit at 8 days with severe respiratory distress needing ventilator support, generalized hypotonia, bilateral severe talipes equinovarus, dislocated hips and mild facial weakness (a). Fetal movements had been poor and there was associated polyhydramnios, which was probably a factor in the premature onset of labour. There was no evidence of myotonic dystrophy in the mother. The family history was negative but the maternal grandmother had suffered four spontaneous abortions of male infants between 15 and 25 weeks gestation. A clinical diagnosis of myotubular myopathy was confirmed by needle biopsy of the quadriceps at 12 days, while the infant was still on the ventilator. Cranial ultrasonography showed remarkable ventricular dilatation (b) presumed to be posthaemorrhagic from a periventricular haemorrhage in the perinatal period. This infant could not be weaned off the ventilator and died at 5 weeks. Autopsy revealed extensive skeletal muscle and diaphragmatic involvement.

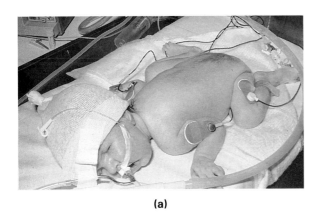

(a)

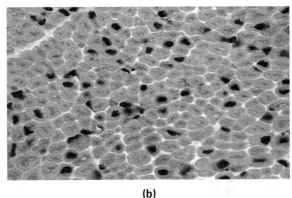

(b)

Figure 3-20a-c X-linked myotubular myopathy. This full-term male infant had marked hypotonia at birth and severe respiratory distress requiring ventilator support. During pregnancy, fetal movements were poor and there was polyhydramnios. He had additional facial weakness and swallowing difficulty (a). The family history was said to be negative, and his mother previously had suffered four spontaneous abortions between 10 and 22 weeks gestation and one near-term stillbirth, said to have hypoplastic lungs. A maternal uncle had died 3 days before delivery and there had been reduced fetal movements and possibly hydramnios. A clinical diagnosis of myotubular myopathy was confirmed by needle biopsy of the quadriceps at 4 weeks of age (b). Cranial ultrasonography showed periventricular haemorrhage and posthaemorrhagic ventricular dilatation, which is unusual in a term baby. He was subsequently weaned off the ventilator, began taking feeds by mouth and showed increased

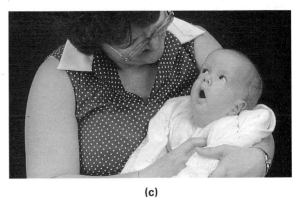

(c)

mobility of his limbs (c). He was allowed home at 3 months but subsequently had a cardiorespiratory arrest, requiring ventilator support at a local hospital, which continued until he died at 13 months.

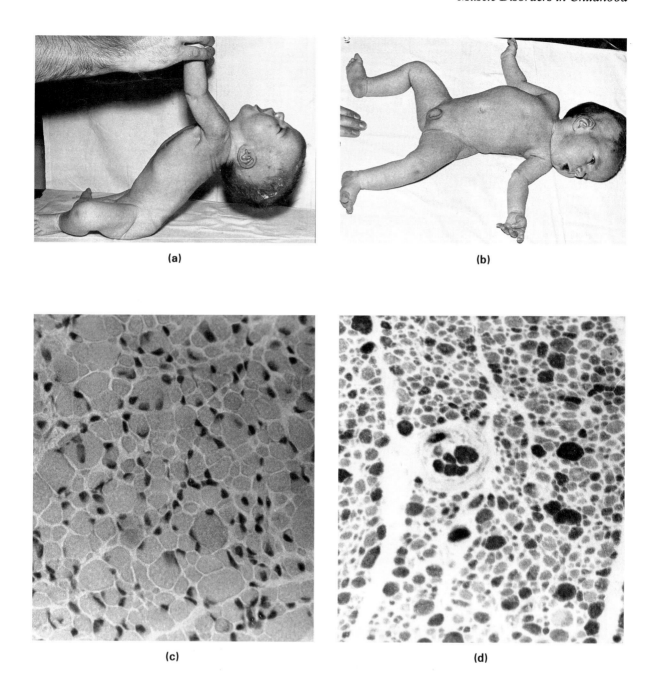

(a)

(b)

(c)

(d)

Figure 3-21 a-d   Congenital fibre type disproportion in 4-week-old infant who had been born by elective caesarean section because of transverse lie and previous caesarean section. There had been diminished fetal movements. He was extremely hypotonic and immobile at birth. There was associated right parietal cephalohaematoma (unusual with non-vaginal delivery). He had difficulty with sucking and swallowing for 2 months and was tube-fed. There was also mild facial weakness. At 4 weeks (a,b) he was still very hypotonic with marked head lag. (c,d) A biopsy was obtained from rectus femoris at 4 weeks of age. (c) Routine stains showed universally small fibres (under 15 μm) and subdivision into two populations. A small proportion of the small fibres had internal nuclei (H & E × 650). (d) Histochemical preparation showed two-fibre type pattern with the larger fibres being mainly type 2 and the very small ones a combination of types 1 and 2 (ATPase pH 9.4 × 325). Note that the intrafusal fibres in the muscle spindle (centre of (d)) are about the same size as the extrafusal fibres. It was thought at the time that this biopsy excluded a spinal muscular atrophy and was compatible with fibre type disproportion, with a better prognosis.

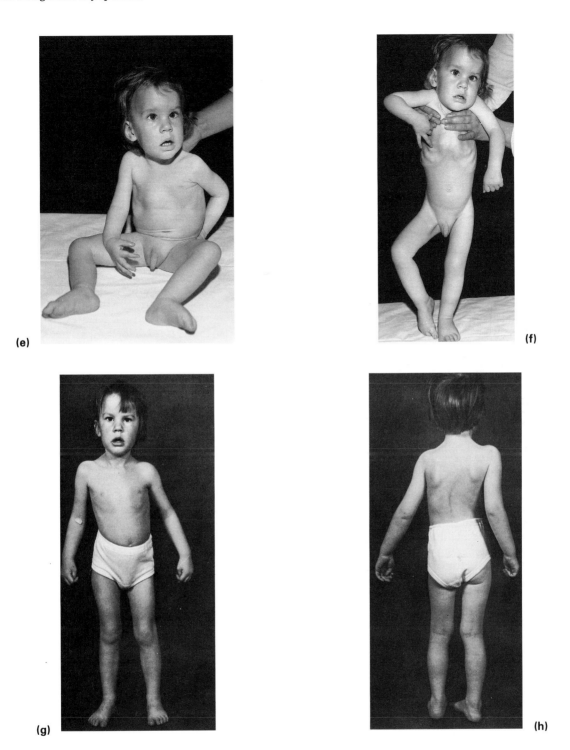

Figure 3-21e-h At 14 months he was showing steady improvement with ability to sit with slight support (e), and to take some weight on his legs (f). Note the deformity of his chest. He subsequently sat unsupported at 17 months. He walked unaided at 2 years. When assessed at 4 years he had developed an associated scoliosis (g,h). CK and EMG were normal. A further biopsy was not done, but would have been of interest to see whether the muscle had become normal or reflected a more striking fibre type disproportion due to type 2 fibre hypertrophy.

CONGENITAL FIBRE TYPE DISPROPORTION – A PATHOLOGY IN SEARCH OF A DISEASE

This condition was initially delineated by Brooke (1973) purely on the basis of the consistent muscle biopsy picture. The type 1 fibres were smaller than the type 2 fibres by a margin of more than 12% of the diameter of the type 2 fibres, in contrast to normal muscle in children where the type 1 and type 2 fibres were of approximately equal size. Brooke then recognized a fairly consistent clinical picture in these cases. All the children were floppy infants, the condition being noted at or shortly after birth. In half of the cases contractures of various muscles of either the hands or feet were noted. One patient had a torticollis due to a contracted sternomastoid. Half of the patients also had congenital dislocation of the hip, either bilaterally or unilaterally. The degree of weakness varied quite considerably. It seemed to involve all the muscles of the trunk and extremities, although in some patients the legs appeared to be more involved than the arms. It was so severe in one patient that little voluntary movement of the arms or legs was possible until almost 2 years of age. In other cases the weakness was mild enough to cause only a delay in the development of the motor milestones, rather than any obvious paralysis. In some there appeared to be an initial progression of the weakness during the first year of life, but in no case did Brooke see any progression once the child had attained 2 years of age. As the child grew older, the disease became static or improvement took place.

Recurrent respiratory infections were frequently a problem during the first year of life. There was an associated abnormality in stature, and 12 of the 14 patients were below the 3rd percentile in weight, even though the birthweight was normal in most cases. The height was below the 10th percentile in eight of the patients. Eight patients had a high arched palate, and a kyphoscoliosis was seen in six patients as the children grew older. Deformities of the feet, including either flat feet or occasionally high arched feet, were common.

Although the genetic basis of this disease has not been determined, about half of the patients had a relative with a similar clinical condition. In some there were only affected siblings, suggesting an autosomal recessive pattern of inheritance, but one patient had both a father and brother affected, suggesting a dominant mechanism.

It is important to make the diagnosis for prognostic reasons. Some of these cases had been diagnosed as Werdnig–Hoffmann's disease and given an erroneously poor prognosis. Because patients with congenital fibre type disproportion frequently improve after the first 2 years of life, it is important that this condition should not be confused with Werdnig–Hoffmann's disease. There is also clinical overlap with congenital myotonic dystrophy (see Chapter 6).

The question arises as to whether this is indeed a single entity or possibly just a pathological pattern in search of a disease. Most of Brooke's cases showed no change other than the variation in fibre size but some did show a more striking pathological picture with degenerative changes and internal nuclei, which suggests that these were possibly variants of congenital muscular dystrophy. Cases of myotonic dystrophy, which can also be associated with small type 1 fibres, should be excluded. Diagnostic problems may arise in early cases of severe spinal muscular atrophy, where one may find universally small fibres but with the type 1 fibres significantly smaller than type 2 (see Chapter 8). To avoid this it is advisable for a diagnosis of congenital fibre type disproportion to be made only in the presence of normal sized or enlarged type 2 fibres and not in cases where both type 1 and type 2 fibres are small (Figure 3-21).

Fardeau *et al.* (1975) studied two sisters with neonatal hypotonia and congenital fibre type disproportion. The type 1 fibres were at the lower limit of normal size, the type 2 fibres larger than normal. No abnormality was found on electron microscopy. The father's biopsy also showed small type 1 fibres with a bimodal distribution. These authors considered that the small size of type 1 fibres was more likely to be due to lack of development rather than an atrophy, but the mechanism of this hypotrophy remains unknown.

It is possible that the clinical condition is not a uniformly benign one; Lenard and Goebel (1975) documented a case with fairly severe weakness and associated respiratory deficit necessitating tracheostomy. This child subsequently survived into adolescence (Figure 3-22).

The pathogenesis of congenital fibre type disproportion is not known. There is a possibility that early on in the disease process the type 2 fibres may also be small and that, with time, they are able to hypertrophy and thus compensate for the weakness and account for the tendency to improvement. This could explain the very marked hypertrophy of type 2 fibres which one may see in some of the older children. Possibly it may even reflect different underlying disease processes and in some cases may reflect the early stages of pathological change in congenital dystrophy, comparable with the 'prepathological' picture in severe infantile spinal muscular atrophy.

It is also essential before making this diagnosis to measure fibre diameters carefully and to prepare a histogram or graph of the size distribution of the fibre types. While initially suggesting a 12% difference in the mean fibre diameter of the type 1 fibres compared with the type 2, Brooke subsequently thought this was perhaps too narrow a range and suggested 25%. I have felt more comfortable with making the diagnosis in muscle biopsy sections where the fibre type distinction in size was strikingly obvious rather than having to depend on the variability shown up by the statistics. It is also important that this diagnosis is not made in the face of obvious clinical pictures such as myotonic dystrophy, Prader–Willi syndrome or congenital muscular dystrophy, as has been done in several cases included in the literature. Perhaps in the future, with a more accurate recognition of underlying diseases or possible genetic disorders, this non-specific diagnosis will also fade into oblivion, comparable with some of the earlier descriptive diagnoses in relation to the floppy infant syndrome such as universal muscle hypoplasia.

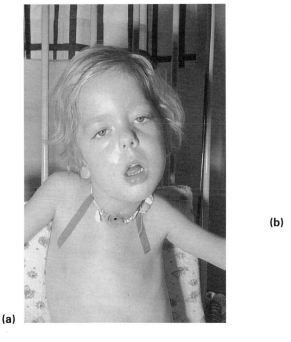

(a)

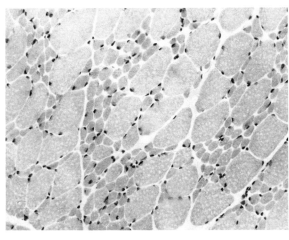

(b)

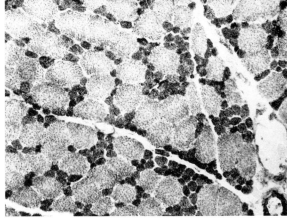

(c)

Figure 3-22a-c Congenital fibre type disproportion. This 4½-year-old boy was documented by Lenard and Goebel (1975). He had marked hypotonia from birth with associated respiratory distress needing ventilator support. He was subsequently left with a permanent tracheostomy. He also had facial weakness and ptosis (a). He could stand with support. His muscle biopsy showed the typical picture with two populations of fibres, one normal-sized or enlarged and type 2 in histochemical reactions, and the other atropic and type 1 (b,c). There was no other pathological change in the fibres. His condition subsequently remained stable. He achieved the ability to walk unaided, and currently at 18 years of age is in a residential school for the handicapped. He occasionally needs ventilator support. (Courtesy Professor Lenard.)

MYOPATHIES WITH ABNORMALITY OF OTHER SUBCELLULAR ORGANELLES

Apart from the well-recognized abnormalities of the mitochondria a number of cases have been reported in which other organelles have shown abnormality. Since most of these involve single case reports they will be discussed collectively. Some of these may be congenital, others possibly acquired.

'FINGERPRINT' MYOPATHY

Engel *et al.* (1972) found abundant subsarcolemmal inclusions consisting of complex lamellae resembling fingerprints on electron microscopic examination of the muscle from a 5-year-old girl with generalized weakness and hypotonia from birth, and also subnormal intelligence and static tremor. Fardeau *et al.* (1976) subsequently reported fingerprint bodies in the muscle of two half brothers with muscle weakness from birth.

'SARCOTUBULAR' MYOPATHY

Jerusalem *et al.* (1973) described two brothers, aged 15 and 11 years, with a congenital non-progressive myopathy in whom the muscle showed a vacuolar myopathy on light microscopy and the presence of dilated and coalesced sarcotubular systems on electron microscopy.

'ZEBRA-BODY' MYOPATHY

Lake and Wilson (1975) found rod-shaped bodies on electron microscopy of the muscle from a 15-year-old boy with a congenital myopathy. Light microscopy showed variation in fibre size, vacuolation, calcification and fibre splitting.

REDUCING BODY MYOPATHY

Brooke and Neville (1972) reported two infants with a progressive neuromuscular disorder from birth, who died at 2½ years, and 9 months respectively.

The muscle showed small inclusions on light microscopy capable of reducing tetrazolium salts histochemically, hence the suggested name. The bodies also contained RNA and glycogen and on electron microscopy had a distinctive appearance, with a round or oval shape, composed of densely packed, moderately osmiophilic particles, in the midst of which were non-membrane limited holes containing glycogen granules. The origin of these particles is uncertain but they resemble inclusions found with Coxsackie virus infections. Similar inclusions were found in the biopsy of a previously healthy 4½-year-old girl with progressive symmetrical weakness thought to be of possible viral origin (Dubowitz and Brooke, 1973). Her muscle biopsy showed more marked destructive changes in the fibres than the earlier cases, but the electron microscopic appearance of the reducing bodies was identical. She had a steadily progressive downhill course and died 3 years later (see Chapter 10). A number of additional cases have been documented with similar structural abnormalities. A 14-year-old boy reported by Tomé and Fardeau (1975) had a milder course with relatively non-progressive proximal weakness.

CYTOPLASMIC BODY MYOPATHY (SPHEROID BODY MYOPATHY)

Cytoplasmic bodies are unusual structures which can be suspected in a muscle biopsy on light microscopy and show as very striking features on electron microscopy, with a central granular core surrounded by a halo of radiating filaments 7–10 nm in diameter. They are relatively non-specific and may be found on occasion in the biopsies of a wide range of disorders (MacDonald and Engel, 1969; Dubowitz, 1985). A number of cases of mainly congenital myopathy have been documented in which the cytoplasmic bodies have been the predominant feature (Nakashima *et al.*, 1970; Kinoshita *et al.*, 1975; Jerusalem *et al.*, 1979; Goebel *et al.*, 1981; Wolburg *et al.*, 1982; Mizuno *et al.*, 1989; Halbig *et al.*, 1991). There have also been a number of familial cases, with autosomal dominant inheritance (Clark *et al.*, 1978; Goebel *et al.*, 1978; Patel *et al.*, 1983; Chapon *et al.*, 1989).

In some families, biopsies from clinically normal individuals have also shown the presence of cytoplasmic bodies (Clark *et al.*, 1978; Caron *et al.*, 1993).

Immunocytochemical studies have shown the presence of desmin in the filaments, and also actin, and recently Caron *et al.* (1994) have shown the presence of dystrophin in the cytoplasmic bodies.

HYALINE BODY MYOPATHY

Ceuterick *et al.* (1993) found subsarcolemmal hyaline bodies in the skeletal muscle biopsy of a 10-year-old boy with a mild non-progressive muscle weakness from early childhood. The hyaline bodies were present in about 10% of fibres, stained a light pink with H & E and had a green hyaline appearance with the Gomori trichrome. They seemed to be restricted to type 1 fibres and stained negatively for PAS, oil Red O, oxidative enzymes and standard ATPase (pH 9.4) but stained intensely with the myosin ATPase reaction at pH 4.2. They immuno-stained strongly with polyclonal anti-skeletal myosin and monoclonal anti-skeletal fast myosin. Additionally, immunoreactive deposits to anti-desmin were observed at the border of some bodies. At the ultra-structural level, these bodies were not surrounded by a limiting membrane and were only localized in subsarcolemmal areas. They contained moderately dense and disorganized filaments which appeared to be in continuity with thick myosin filaments of intact adjacent myofibrils. They stained negatively for polysaccharides.

Similar subsarcolemmal deposits were previously reported by Cancilla *et al.* (1971), under the descriptive title of focal lysis of myofibrils, in the type 1 fibres of 5- and 2-year-old siblings with a slowly progressive congenital myopathy, and by Sahgal and Sahgal (1977) in a 50-year-old patient with a non-progressive myopathy.

Recently Barohn *et al.* (1994) documented two further cases with identical changes in the muscle in a 40-year-old man with non-progressive lower limb weakness from childhood and a 3-year-old girl with decreased fetal movements during pregnancy, delayed motor milestones and a subsequent mild motor disability, which did not change substantially during 16 years of follow-up assessment.

X-LINKED MYOPATHY WITH AUTOPHAGIC VACUOLES

A large Finnish family has been described with an X-linked, mild, slowly progressive weakness affecting mainly the lower limbs and characterized by lysosomal autophagic vacuoles on electron micro-scopy (Kalimo *et al.*, 1988). Linkage studies have localized the gene to distal Xq (Saviranta *et al.*, 1988). We have observed similar pathological changes in a mother and son with a periodic paraly-sis-like problem in the mother and a mild weakness in the son and presumed that the mother might be a manifesting carrier of the X-linked condition in view of the similarity to the Finnish cases.

NON-SPECIFIC CONGENITAL MYOPATHIES; 'MINIMAL CHANGE MYOPATHY'?

Even after the full battery of investigations one has a residue of patients with muscle weakness of presumptive congenital origin in whom one finds no evidence of any specific abnormality in the muscle, and the serum enzymes and electromyography may frequently be normal as well. In some of these subjects the muscle is completely normal on histo-chemical as well as electron microscopic assessment. Others show relatively minor changes such as variation in fibre size without overt evidence of degeneration, or some non-specific changes on electron microscopic assessment such as loss of myofibrils. It is possible that these patients may have a more localized muscle involvement which may be missed in the particular muscle biopsied.

For want of a better alternative, these cases can be collectively categorized as congenital myopathy (non-specific) and one can follow their clinical course. With the advent of needle biopsy as a routine procedure one can probably justify a repeated muscle biopsy at a later date if the muscle weakness persists or deteriorates, whereas one might have been reluctant to subject the child to a second open biopsy.

In many of these cases patients seem initially to have a good prognosis with a tendency to improve with time (Figures 3-23, 3-24). However, they may die unexpectedly, presumably from respiratory failure, and it is important to check for nocturnal hypoventilation. I have used the term 'minimal change myopathy' for describing the pathological changes in this group, somewhat analogous to the minimal change nephropathy in association with the nephrotic syndrome in childhood. This helps to categorize this group of patients more specifically until such time as we have a better understanding of the underlying pathogenesis. It at least provides a pathological label in a biopsy which one cannot pass as normal.

It is possible that in some of these cases patients may be found to have a metabolic myopathy without overt structural change such as, for example, the myopathy associated with deficiency of carnitine palmitoyl transferase. The next stage in the analysis of these biopsies may well entail a routine bio-chemical screen for several enzyme systems, even in the absence of excess lipid or glycogen store, as a supplement to the routine histochemical and electron microscopic assessment.

With the routine use of ultrasound imaging of muscle as a diagnostic screen in our Muscle Clinic, we have identified several patients with selective

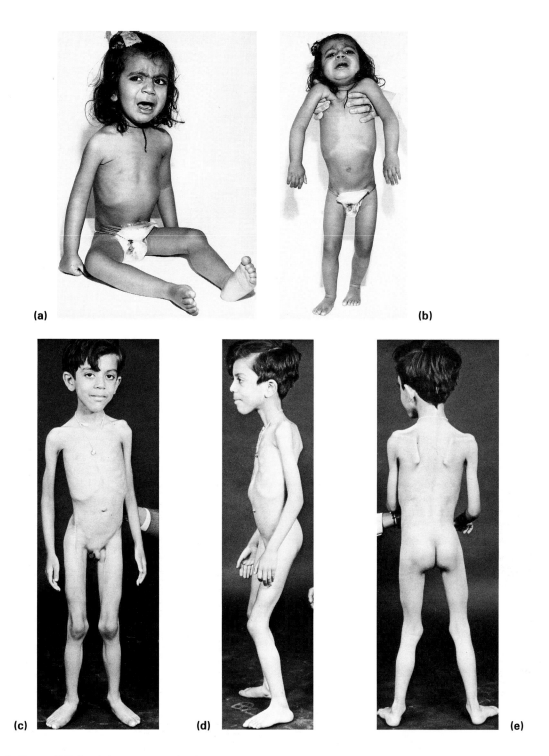

(a)

(b)

(c)

(d)

(e)

Figure 3-23a-e 'Minimal change myopathy' in (a,b) a 20-month-old infant, able to sit unaided since 18 months but not yet able to stand. He had probably been floppy from birth. At 4 months he was noted to have poor mobility of arms and legs. CK was normal; EMG was essentially normal. There were occasional polyphasic potentials. Muscle biopsy of the quadriceps showed abnormal variation in fibre size but no evidence of degeneration and no structural abnormality on histochemistry or electron microscopy. There was no selective type atrophy. There was a subsequent improvement and operative treatment of fixed flexion deformities of both hips. (c,d,e) At 6 years of age he was able to stand but not yet able to walk. Subsequently he started walking with the aid of callipers. He remained reasonably stable but died unexpectedly in his early teens presumably from respiratory failure.

involvement of one muscle, or part of a muscle, and sparing of others. Thus some cases of congenital dystrophy have shown selective involvement of the vastus muscles and sparing of the rectus femoris and double needle biopsies of these muscles (through the same incision) have shown 'minimal change myopathy' in the rectus and overt dystrophic change in the vastus (Heckmatt and Dubowitz, 1987) (see Figure 3-25). Once the gene and its product are identified for these various different muscle disorders such as congenital dystrophy, it will be possible to more accurately define whether these cases of 'minimal change myopathy' are variants of one or other recognized muscle disorder.

Some patients with fairly severe disability and weakness apparently localized initially to certain muscles such as the neck muscles may also show minimal change on biopsy (Figure 3-24). Further documentation of such cases may in the future help to clarify whether they conform to specific syndromes or are merely variations of a more generalized non-specific type of myopathy, or indeed of congenital muscular dystrophy.

(a) **(b)** **(c)**

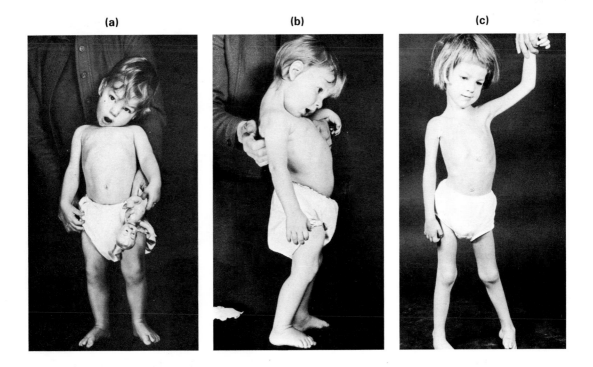

Figure 3-24a-c Weakness of neck muscles in a 14-month old boy (a,b) who initially presented at 10 months because of inability to hold head erect. Muscle weakness seemed confined to neck flexors and extensors. Nerve conduction was normal (ulnar 50 m/s), EMG (left deltoid) normal. Muscle biopsy showed minimal change with variation in fibre size and scattered atrophic fibres but no correlation with fibre type. There was no evidence of any abnormal structure, at either light or electron microscopic level. His neck showed gradual improvement but he developed a marked equinovarus deformity of his feet (c, aged 4 years). He subsequently died unexpectedly following a minor respiratory infection.

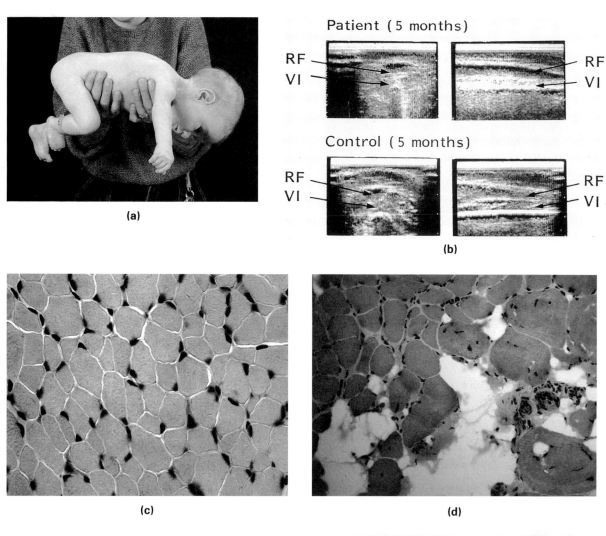

Patient (5 months)

RF
VI

RF
VI

(a)

RF
VI

Control (5 months)

RF
VI

(b)

(c)

(d)

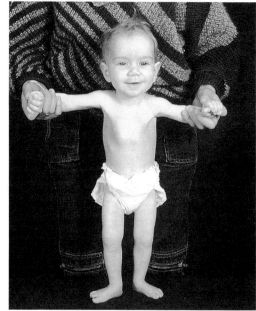

Figure 3-25a-e Minimal change myopathy/congenital muscular dystrophy (differential involvement). This 5-month-old floppy infant presented with delay in motor milestones (a). Ultrasonography of the quadriceps showed a striking differential involvement with (b) sparing of rectus temoris (RF) and involvement of vasti (VI). Selective needle biopsy of both components through the same incision confirmed this with an essentially normal picture in the rectus (minimal change myopathy) (c) and a striking dystrophic picture in the vastus lateralis (d). The pathology would have been completely missed by a standard open biopsy of the rectus. At subsequent follow-up she showed marked improvement in muscle function and was able to stand well with support by 8 months (e).

(e)

REFERENCES

Afifi, A.K., Smith, J.W. and Zellweger, H. (1965) Congenital non-progressive myopathy. Central core and nemaline myopathy in one family. *Neurology (Minneapolis)* **15**: 371–381.

Armstrong, R.M., Koenigsberger, R., Mellinger, J. and Lovelace, R.E. (1971) Central core disease with congenital hip dislocation: study of two families. *Neurology (Minneapolis)* **21**: 369.

Barohn, R.J., Brumback, R.A. and Mendell, J.R. (1994) Hyaline body myopathy. *Neuromuscular Disorders* **4**: 257–262.

Barth, P.G., van Wijngaarden, G.K. and Bethlem, J. (1975) X-linked myotubular myopathy with fatal neonatal asphyxia. *Neurology* **25**: 531–536.

Bethlem, J., van Gool, J., Hülsmann, W.C. and Meijer, A.E.F.H. (1966) Familial non-progressive myopathy with muscle cramps after exercise. A new disease associated with cores in the muscle fibres. *Brain* **89**: 569–588.

Bethlem, J., Meijer, A.E.F.H., Schellens, J.P.M. and Vroom, J.J. (1968) Centronuclear myopathy. *European Neurology* **1**: 325.

Bethlem, J., van Wijngaarden, G.K., Meijer, A.E.F.H. and Hülsmann, W.C. (1969) Neuromuscular disease with type 1 fibre atrophy, central nuclei, and myotube-like structures. *Neurology (Minneapolis)* **19**: 705–710.

Bethlem, J., Arts, W.F. and Dingermans, K.P. (1978) Common origin of rods, miniature cores and focal loss of cross-striation. *Archives of Neurology (Chicago)* **35**: 555–566.

Brooke, M.H. (1973) A neuromuscular disease characterized by fibre type disproportion. In: Kakulas, B.A. ed., *Clinical Studies in Myology*. Proceedings of the Second International Congress on Muscle Diseases, Perth, Australia, 1971. Part 2, Amsterdam: Excerpta Medica, I.C.S. No. 295.

Brooke, M.H. and Neville, H.E. (1972) Reducing body myopathy. *Neurology (Minneapolis)* **22**: 829.

Cancilla, P.A., Kalyanaraman, K., Verity, M.A. *et al.* (1971) Familial myopathy with probable lysis of myofibrils in type 1 fibers. *Neurology* **21**: 579–585.

Caron, A., Chapon, F., Berthelin, C. *et al.* (1993) Inclusions in familial cytoplasmic body myopathy are stained by anti-dystrophin antibodies. *Neuromuscular Disorders* **3**: 541–546.

Ceuterick, C., Martin, J.J. and Martens, C. (1993) Hyaline bodies in skeletal muscle of a patient with a mild chronic non-progressive congenital myopathy. *Clinical Neuropathology* **12**: 79–83.

Chapon, F., Viader, F., Fardeau, M. *et al.* (1989) Myopathi familiale avec inclusions de type 'corps cytoplasmiques' (ou 'sphéroides') révélée par une unsuffisance respiratoire. *Revue Neurologique*, **145**: 460–465.

Clark, J.R., d'Agostino, A.N., Wilson, J. *et al.* (1978) Autosomal dominant myofibrillar inclusion body myopathy: clinical, histologic, histochemical and ultrastructural characteristics. *Neurology* **28**: 399.

Colamaria, V., Zanetti, R., Simeone, M. *et al.* (1991) Minipolymyoclonus in congenital nemaline myopathy: a nonspecific clinical marker of neurogenic dysfunction. *Brain and Development* **13**: 358–362.

Conen, P.E., Murphy, E.G. and Donohue, W.L. (1963) Light and electron microscopic studies of 'myogranules' in a child with hypotonia and muscle weakness. *Canadian Medical Association Journal* **45**: 661.

Currie, S., Noronha, M. and Harriman, D.G.F. (1974) 'Minicore' disease. In: *The Third International Congress on Muscle Diseases, Newcastle-upon-Tyne, 1974*. Amsterdam: Excerpta Medica, I.C.S. No. 334, Abstracts, p. 12.

Darnfors, C., Larsson, H.E.B., Oldfors, A. *et al.* (1990) X-linked myotubular myopathy: a linkage study. *Clinical Genetics* **37**: 335–340.

De Angelis, M.S., Palmucci, L., Leone, M. *et al.* (1991) Centronuclear myopathy: clinical, morphological and genetic characters. A review of 288 cases. *Journal of the Neurological Sciences* **103**: 2–9.

Denborough, M.A., Dennett, X. and Anderson, R.McD. (1973) Central core disease and malignant hyperpyrexia. *British Medical Journal* i: 272.

Dubowitz, V. (1969) *The Floppy Infant*. Clinics in Developmental Medicine, No. 31. London: Spastics International/Heinemann.

Dubowitz, V. (1978) *Muscle Disorders in Childhood*. London and Philadelphia: W.B. Saunders.

Dubowitz, V. (1985) *Muscle Biopsy: A Practical Approach* 2nd edn. London: Baillière Tindall, pp.152–155.

Dubowitz, V. and Brooke, M.H. (1973) *Muscle Biopsy: A Modern Approach*. London and Philadelphia: W.B. Saunders.

Dubowitz, V. and Pearse, A.G.E. (1960) Oxidative enzymes and phosphorylase in central core disease of muscle. *Lancet* ii: 23–24.

Dubowitz, V. and Platts, M. (1965) Central core disease of muscle with focal wasting. *Journal of Neurology, Neurosurgery and Psychiatry* **28**: 432–437.

Dubowitz, V. and Roy, S. (1970) Central core disease of muscle: clinical, histochemical and electron microscopic studies of an affected mother and child. *Brain* **93**: 133–146.

Eng, G.D., Epstein, B.S., Engel, W.K. *et al.* (1978) Malignant hyperthermia and central core disease in a child with congenital dislocating hips. *Archives of Neurology (Chicago)* **35**: 189–197.

Engel, A.G., Gomez, M.R. and Groover, R.V. (1971) Multicore disease. *Mayo Clinic Proceedings* **10**: 666.

Engel, A.G., Angelini, C. and Gomez, M.R. (1972) Fingerprint body myopathy. *Mayo Clinic Proceedings* **47**: 377.

Engel, W.K. (1961) Muscle target fibres, a newly recognized sign of denervation. *Nature (London)* **191**: 389–390.

Engel, W.K. (1967) A critique of congenital myopathies and other disorders, In: Milhorat, A.T. eds, *Exploratory Concepts in Muscular Dystrophy and Related Disorders*. Amsterdam: Excerpta Medica, I.C.S. No. 147, pp. 27–40.

Engel, W.K., Foster, J.M., Hughes, B.P., Huxley, H.E. and Mahler, R. (1961) Central core disease – an investigation of a rare muscle cell abnormality. *Brain* **84**: 167–185.

Engel, W.K., Wanko, T. and Fenichel, G.M. (1964) Nemaline myopathy. A second case. *Archives of Neurology (Chicago)* **11**: 22–39.

Engel, W.K., Gold, G.N. and Karpati, G. (1968) Type 1 fibre hypotrophy and central nuclei. A rare congenital muscle abnormality with a possible experimental model. *Archives of Neurology* **18**: 435–444.

Fardeau, M., Harpey, J.-P. and Caille, B. (1975) Disproportion congénitales des différents types de fibre musculaire avec petitesse relative des fibres de type 1 – documents morphologiques concernant les biopsies musculaires prélevées chez trois membres d'une même famille. *Revue Neurologique (Paris)* **131**: 745–766.

Fardeau, M., Tomé, F.M.S. and Derambure, S. (1976) Familial fingerprint body myopathy. *Archives of Neurology* **33**: 724–725.

Ford, F.R. (1960) *Diseases of the Nervous System in Infancy, Childhood and Adolescence* 4th edn. Springfield, Illinois: Charles C. Thomas, p. 1259.

Frank, J.P., Harati, Y., Butler, I.J. *et al.* (1980) Central core disease and malignant hyperthermia syndrome. *Annals of Neurology* **7**: 11–17.

Goebel, H.H., Muller, J., Gillen, H.W. *et al.* (1978) Autosomal dominant 'spheroid body myopathy'. *Muscle and Nerve* **1**: 14–16.

Goebel, H.H., Schloon, H., Lenard, H.G. (1981) Congenital myopathy with cytoplasmic bodies. *Neuropediatrics* **12**: 166–180.

Gonatas, N.K., Perez, M.C., Shy, G.M. and Evangelista, I. (1965) Central core disease of skeletal muscle. Ultrastructural and cytochemical observations in two cases. *American Journal of Pathology* **47**: 503–524.

Gonatas, N.K., Shy, G.M. and Godfrey, E.H. (1966) Nemaline myopathy. The origin of nemaline structures. *New England Journal of Medicine* **274**: 535–539.

Greenfield, J.G., Cornman, T. and Shy, G.M. (1958) The prognostic value of the muscle biopsy in the floppy infant. *Brain* **81**: 461.

Halbig, L., Goebel, H.H., Hopf, H.C. *et al.* (1991) Spheroid-cytoplasmic complexes in a congenital myopathy. *Revue Neurologique* **147**: 300–307.

Heckmatt, J.Z. and Dubowitz, V. (1987) Ultrasound imaging and directed needle biopsy in the diagnosis of selective involvement in muscle disease. *Journal of Child Neurology* **2**: 205–213.

Heffner, R., Cohen, M., Duffner, P. and Daigler, G. (1976) Multicore disease in twins. *Journal of Neurology, Neurosurgery and Psychiatry* **39**: 602–606.

Hopkins, I.J., Lindsey, J.R. and Ford, F.R. (1966) Nemaline myopathy. A long-term clinicopathologic study of affected mother and daughter. *Brain* **89**: 299–310.

Hudgson, P., Gardner-Medwin, D., Fulthorpe, J.L. and Walton, J.N. (1967) Nemaline myopathy. *Neurology (Minneapolis)* **17** 1125–1142.

Isaacs, H. and Barlow, M.B. (1974) Central core disease associated with elevated creatine phosphokinase levels: two members of a family known to be susceptible to malignant hyperpyrexia. *South African Medical Journal* **48**: 640–642.

Ishibashi Ueda, H., Imakita, M., Yutani, C. *et al.* (1990) Congenital nemaline myopathy with dilated cardiomyopathy: an autopsy study. *Human Pathology* **21**: 77–82.

Jenis, E.H., Lindquist, R.R. and Lister, R.C. (1969) New congenital myopathy with crystalline intranuclear inclusions. *Archives of Neurology* **20**: 281–287.

Jerusalem, F., Engel, A.G. and Gomez, M.R. (1973) Sarcotubular myopathy: a newly recognized benign, congenital, familial muscle disease. *Neurology* **23**: 897–906.

Jerusalem, F., Ludin, H., Bischoff, A. *et al.* (1979) Cytoplasmic body neuromyopathy presenting as respiratory failure and weight loss. *Journal of the Neurological Sciences* **41**: 1–9.

Kalimo, H., Savontaus, M.L., Lang, H. *et al.* (1988) X-linked myopathy with excessive autophagy: a new hereditary muscle disease. *Annals of Neurology* **23**: 258–265.

Karpati, G., Carpenter, S. and Nelson, R.F. (1970) Type 1 muscle fibre atrophy and central nuclei. A rare familial neuromuscular disease. *Journal of the Neurological Sciences* **10**: 489–500.

Karpati, G., Carpenter, S. and Andermann, F. (1971) A new concept of childhood nemaline myopathy. *Archives of Neurology* **24**: 291–304.

Kausch, K., Lehmann-Horn, F., Janka, M. *et al.* (1991) Evidence for linkage of the central core disease locus to the proximal long arm of human chromosome 19. *Genomics* **10**: 765–769.

Kinoshita, M., Satoyoshi, E. and Suzuki, Y. (1975) Atypical myopathy with myofibrillar aggregates. *Archives of Neurology* **32**: 417–420.

Kondo, K. and Yuasa, T. (1980) Genetics of congenital nemaline myopathy. *Muscle and Nerve* **3**: 308.

Kuitonnen, P., Rapola, J., Noponen, A.L. and Donner, M. (1972) Nemaline myopathy. Report of 4 cases and review of literature. *Acta Paediatrica Scandinavica* **61**: 353.

Laing, N.G., Majda, B.T., Akkari, P.A. *et al.* (1992) Assignment of a gene (NEM1) for autosomal dominant nemaline myopathy to chromosome 1. *American Journal of Human Genetics* **50**: 576–583.

Lake, B.D. and Wilson, J. (1975) Zebra body mypathy: clinical, histochemical and ultrastructural studies. *Journal of the Neurological Sciences* **24**: 437–446.

Lake, B.D., Cavanagh, N. and Wilson, J. (1977) Myopathy with minicores in siblings. *Neuropathology and Applied Neurobiology* **3**: 159.

Lehesjoki, A-E., Sankila, E-M., Miao, J. *et al.* (1990) X-linked neonatal myotubular myopathy: one recombination detected with four polymorphic DNA markers from Xq28. *Journal of Medical Genetics* **27**: 288–291.

Lenard, H.G. and Goebel, H.H. (1975) Congenital fibre type disproportion. *Neuropädiatrie* **6**: 220–231.

Liechti-Gallati, S., Wolff, G., Ketelsen, U.-P. *et al.* (1993) Prenatal diagnosis of X-linked centronuclear myopathy by linkage analysis. *Pediatric Research* **33**: 201–204.

MacDonald, R.D. and Engel, A.G. (1969) The cytoplasmic body: another structural anomaly of the Z disk. *Acta Neuropathologica (Berlin)* **14**: 99–107.

MacLennan, D.H., Duff, C., Zorato, F. *et al.* (1990) Ryanodine receptor gene is a candidate for predisposition to malignant hyperthermia. *Nature* **343**: 559–561.

Mizuno, Y., Nakamura, Y. and Komiya, K. (1989) The spectrum of cytoplasmic body myopathy: report of a congenital severe case. *Brain and Development* **11**: 20–25.

Mulley, J.C., Kozman, H.M., Phillips, H.A. *et al.* (1993) Refined genetic localization for central core disease. *American Journal of Human Genetics* **52**: 398–405.

Munsat, T.L., Thompson, L.R. and Coleman, R.F. (1969) Centronuclear ('myotubular') myopathy. *Archives of Neurology* **20**: 120–131.

Nakashima, N., Tamura, Z., Okamoto, S. *et al.* (1970) Inclusion bodies in human neuromuscular disorder. *Archives of Neurology* **22**: 270–278.

Neville, H.E. and Brooke, M.H. (1973) Central core fibers: structured and unstructured. In: Kakulas, B.A. ed., *Basic Research in Myology.* Proceedings of 2nd International Congress on Muscle Diseases, Perth, Australia, November 1971. Part 1. Amsterdam: Excerpta Medica, I.C.S. No. 294, pp. 497–511.

Norton, P., Ellison, P., Sulaiman, A.R. *et al.* (1983) Nemaline myopathy in the neonate. *Neurology* **33**: 351–356.

Ortiz de Zarate, J.C. and Maruffo, A. (1970) The descending ocular myopathy of early childhood. Myotubular or centronuclear myopathy. *European Neurology* **3**: 1–12.

Patel, H., Berry, K., MacLeod, P. *et al.* (1983) Cytoplasmic body myopathy: report on a family and review of the literature. *Journal of the Neurological Sciences* **60**: 281–292.

Pongratz, D., Weindl, A., Reichl, W., Koppenwallner, C., Heuser, M. and Hübner, G. (1976) Congenitale centronucleäre Myopathie. Zwei morphologische Varianten in einer Familie. *Klinische Wochenschrift* **54**: 423–430.

Price, H.M., Gordon, G.B., Pearson, C.M., Munsat, T.L. and Blumberg, J.M. (1965) New evidence for excessive accumulation of Z-band material in nemaline myopathy. *Proceedings of the National Academy of Sciences of the USA* **54**: 1398–1406.

Quane, K.A., Healy, J.M.S., Keating, K.E. *et al.* (1993) Mutations in the ryanodine receptor gene in central core disease and malignant hyperthermia. *Nature Genetics* **5**: 51–55.

Ramsey, P.L. and Hensinger, R.N. (1975) Congenital dislocation of the hip associated with central core disease. *Journal of Bone and Joint Surgery* **57A**: 648–651.

Ricoy, J.R., Cabello, A. and Goizueta, G. (1980) Myopathy with multiple minicores: report of two

siblings. *Journal of the Neurological Sciences* **48**: 81.

Rifai, Z., Kazee, A.M., Kamp, C. *et al.* (1993) Intranuclear rods in severe congenital nemaline myopathy. *Neurology* **43**: 2372–2377.

Romero, N.B., Nivoche, Y., Lunardi, J. *et al.* (1995) Malignant hyperthermia and central core disease: analysis of two families with heterogeneous clinical expression. *Neuromuscular Disorders* **5**: in press.

Sahgal, V. and Sahgal, S. (1977) A new congenital myopathy: a morphological, cytochemical and histochemical study. *Acta Neuropathologica (Berlin)* **37**: 225–230.

Saviranta, P., Lindlöf, M., Lehesjoki, A-E. *et al.* (1988) Linkage studies in a new X-linked myopathy, suggesting exclusion of DMD locus and tentative assignment to distal Xq. *American Journal of Human Genetics* **42**: 84–88.

Seitelberger, F., Wanko, T. and Gavin, M.A. (1961) The muscle fiber in central core disease. Histochemical and electron microscopic observations. *Acta Neuropathologica* **1**: 223–237.

Shafiq, S.A., Dubowitz, V., Peterson, H. de C. and Milhorat, A.T. (1967) Nemaline myopathy: report of a fatal case with histochemical and electron microscopic studies. *Brain* **90**: 817–828.

Shafiq, S.A., Gorycki, M.A., Asiedu, S.A. and Milhorat, A.T. (1969) Tenotomy. Effect on the fine structure of the soleus of the rat. *Archives of Neurology (Chicago)* **20**: 625–633.

Sher, J.H., Rimalovski, A.B., Athanassiades, T.J. and Aronson, S.M. (1967) Familial centronuclear myopathy: a clinical and pathological study. *Neurology (Minneapolis)* **17**, 727–742.

Shy, G.M. and Magee, K.R. (1956) A new congenital non-progressive myopathy, *Brain* **79**: 610

Shy, G.M., Engel, W.K., Somers, J.E. and Wanko, T. (1963) Nemaline myopathy. A new congenital myopathy. *Brain* **86**: 793.

Spiro, A.J. and Kennedy, C. (1965) Hereditary occurrence of nemaline myopathy. *Archives of Neurology* **13**: 155–159.

Spiro, A.J., Shy, G.M. and Gonatas, N.K. (1966) Myotubular myopathy. *Archives of Neurology* **14**: 1–14.

Starr, J., Lamont, M., Iselius, J. *et al.* (1990) A linkage study of a large pedigree with X-linked centronuclear myopathy. *Journal of Medical Genetics* **27**: 2881–283.

Thomas, N.S.T., Sarfarazi, M., Roberts, K. *et al.* (1987) X-linked myotubular myopathy (MTM1): evidence for linkage to Xq28 DNA markers. (Abstract). *Cytogenetics and Cell Genetics* **46**: 704.

Thomas, N.S.T., Williams, H., Cole, G. *et al.* (1990) X-linked neonatal centronuclear/myotubular myopathy: evidence for linkage to Xq28 DNA marker loci. *Journal of Medical Genetics* **27**: 284–287.

Tomé, F.M.S. and Fardeau, M. (1975) Congenital myopathy with 'reducing bodies' in muscle fibres. *Acta Neuropathologica (Berlin)* **24**: 62.

Vallat, J.M., de Lumley, L., Loubet, A. *et al.* (1982) Coexistence of minicores, cores, and rods in the same muscle biopsy. *Acta Neuropathologica (Berlin)* **58**: 229–232.

van Wijngaarden, G.K., Fleury, P., Bethlem, J. and Meijer, A.E.F.H. (1969) Familial 'myotubular' myopathy. *Neurology (Minneapolis)* **19**: 901–908.

Vital, C., Vallat, J.M., Martin, F., Le Blanc, M. and Bergouignan, M. (1970) Étude clinique et ultrastructurale d'un cas de myopathie centronucleaire (myotubular myopathy) de l'adulte. *Revue Neurologique* **123**: 117–130.

Wallgren-Pettersson, C. and Thomas, N.S.T. (1994) Report on 20th ENMC-Sponsored International Workshop: Myotubular/centronuclear myopathy. *Neuromuscular Disorders* **4**: 71–74.

Wallgren-Pettersson, C., Kaariainen, H., Rapola, J. *et al.* (1990) Genetics of congenital nemaline myopathy: a study of 10 families. *Journal of Medical Genetics* **27**: 480–487.

Wolburg, H., Schlote, W., Langohr, H.D. *et al.* (1982) Slowly progressive congenital myopathy with cytoplasmic bodies: report of two cases and a review of the literature. *Clinical Neuropathology* **1**: 55–66.

Zhang, Y., Chen, H.S., Khanna, V.K. *et al.* (1993) A mutation in the human ryanodine receptor gene associated with central core disease. *Nature Genetics* **5**: 46–50.

CHAPTER 4

Metabolic Myopathies I
Glycogenoses

INTRODUCTION

At the time of the first edition of this book, a number of glycogenoses affecting muscle were already well established, disorders of lipid metabolism were being recognized and the bubble was about to burst on the mitochondrial myopathies. The advances in this area have been nothing short of spectacular.

A number of new glycolytic enzyme deficiencies affecting muscle have been added to the list, and the genes that encode several of these enzymes have been located and isolated. Several new disorders affecting the metabolism of long chain fatty acids have been discovered.

The mitochondrial myopathies have mushroomed beyond recognition on several fronts, with the definition of a number of clinical syndromes, the recognition of a number of metabolic abnormalities in the various complexes of the respiratory chain and the discovery of specific mutations in the mitochondrial or nuclear DNA associated with some of these. Moreover, and perhaps more important from the viewpoint of the clinician, some order is beginning to appear in this chaos, with the correlation of the clinical syndromes with some of the biochemical abnormalities and with the mutations in the genome, plus some understanding of the tremendous variability in the clinical phenotype that may occur within the same family.

Another major advance has been the elucidation of specific ion channel disorders in relation to the myotonias and periodic paralyses, followed rapidly by the location and cloning of the relevant genes and the recognition of a number of different mutations within a particular gene. The common denominator of voltage-sensitive ion channels has brought together this somewhat diverse group of disorders ('ion channel disorders'), and, perhaps predictably, our colleagues across the Atlantic have already coined the term 'channelopathies'.

As in the case of the muscular dystrophies, there is a strong temptation to try and view all these disorders through the eyes of the biochemist or the molecular geneticist. However, the clinician has to keep his feet firmly on the ground in order to recognize the clinical phenotypes and to relate to the patient and his problems, and I have decided to retain the classical descriptions of the various clinical syndromes, appropriately updated in relation to recent clinical advances, and to try and relate these to the remarkable advances at the biochemical or molecular level. Not surprisingly, the original single chapter has now expanded into three separate chapters, to accommodate all these advances.

GLYCOGENOSES

The discovery by the Coris of deficient glucose-6-phosphatase in von Gierke's disease (Cori and Cori, 1952) heralded the recognition of a number of inborn errors of glycogen metabolism. The numerical classification suggested by Cori (1958) found wide acceptance, although some confusion occurred in recent times when different authors were staking a claim for a different new metabolic defect at the same time.

To date there are nine documented enzyme defects affecting muscle, either alone or in conjunction with other tissues (Table 4-1).

Table 4-1 Glycogenoses affecting muscle

Type	Enzyme deficiency	Eponymous or other names	Subunit; Isozyme	Gene location	Clinical features	Other tissues/ systems affected
II	α-1,4-glucosidase (acid maltase)	Pompe's disease	—	17(q23 – q25)	(a) Severe form: generalized resembles infantile spinal muscular atrophy (b) Mild form: resembles limb girdle dystrophy	Heart, nervous system, leucocytes, liver, kidneys ? Heart
III	Amylo-1,6-gluco-sidase ('debranching enzyme')	Limit dextrinosis Forbes' disease Cori's disease	—	NK	Infantile hypotonia Mild weakness	Hepatic Hypoglycaemia Ketosis Leucocytes Cardiac
IV	α-1,4-glucan: α1,4-glucan 6-glycosyl transferase ('branching enzyme'; amylo (1,4→1,6) transglucosidase)	Amylopectinosis	—	NK	Usually no muscle symptoms In some wasting or weakness	Hepatomegaly Cirrhosis Liver failure Cardiac
V	Muscle phosphorylase	McArdle's disease	M	11q13	Exercise intolerance Muscle cramps Fatigue Myoglobinuria	None
VII	Phosphofructokinase	Tarui's disease	M	1(cen – q32)	Exercise intolerance Muscle cramps Fatigue Myoglobinuria	Haemolytic anaemia
VIII	Phosphorylase *b* kinase		α β	Xq12 – q13 16q12 – q13	Exercise intolerance Muscle stiffness Weakness	Liver Cardiac
IX	Phosphoglycerate kinase		A	X(q13)	Exercise intolerance Muscle cramps Fatigue Myoglobinuria	Haemolytic anaemia Central nervous system
X	Phosphoglycerate mutase		M	7	Exercise intolerance Muscle cramps Fatigue Myoglobinuria	
XI	Lactate dehydrogenase		M	11	Exercise intolerance Muscle cramps Fatigue Myoglobinuria	

NK = Not known

These are:

Type II   alpha-1,4-glucosidase (acid maltase) deficiency

Type III   amylo-1,6-glucosidase (debranching enzyme) deficiency

Type IV   amylo (1,4→1,6) transglucosidase (branching enzyme) deficiency

Type V   myophosphorylase deficiency

Type VII   phosphofructokinase deficiency

Type VIII   phosphorylase b kinase deficiency

Type IX   phosphoglycerate kinase deficiency

Type X   phosphoglycerate mutase deficiency

Type XI   lactate dehydrogenase deficiency

One of these enzymes (branching enzyme) involves the synthesis of glycogen, one (acid maltase) involves the intralysosomal degradation of glycogen, the remaining seven are cytoplasmic enzymes acting at different levels of glycogen breakdown and glycolysis (see Figure 4-1).

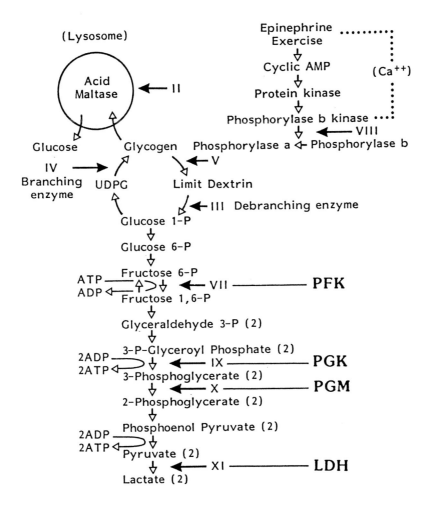

Figure 4-1 Glycogenoses affecting skeletal muscle. (Courtesy Dr S. di Mauro.)

Some enzymes, such as acid maltase, exist in a single molecular form and a deficiency is thus likely to involve many different tissues. Others, such as phosphorylase, have tissue-specific isoforms, encoded by separate genes, so that a deficit in muscle phosphorylase selectively affects muscle only, whereas deficit of the liver enzyme causes hepatomegaly and hypoglycaemia but does not involve muscle. Enzymes with multiple isoforms may also show a different isoform in immature muscle, compared with the muscle specific form in mature muscle, which accounts, for example, for the presence of phosphorylase-positive, regenerating fibres in the muscle in McArdle's disease, or in its cultured myotubes.

Some enzymes, such as phosphofructokinase, have different, genetically distinct, subunits occurring in different combinations in different tissues, so that the clinical manifestations are dependent on which subunit is affected by the genetic defect. In many of these single enzyme defects, heart muscle is probably protected by the presence of alternative isozymes or subunits of the particular enzyme.

The clinical presentation may be with hypotonia or muscle weakness (e.g. types II and III) or with cramps on exertion (e.g. types V and VII). Those forms with other systems involved (e.g. type IV) may present with hypoglycaemia or hepatic failure, or with other specific features (see Table 4-1).

The muscle biopsy picture varies from a very striking vacuolar myopathy with marked glycogen deposit in type II glycogenosis, to a relatively normal looking muscle, with only minor pathological change, in which the excess glycogen may still be apparent with the PAS stain or on electron microscopy in, for example, type V. The diagnosis is confirmed by the demonstration biochemically of the excess glycogen content of the muscle and the specific enzyme defect.

The particular glycogenosis can usually be suspected clinically from the clinical presentation. However, there are still a number of cases on record with excess glycogen in the muscle in which no specific enzyme abnormality has yet been delineated, as well as other cases of glycogenosis with more than one enzyme deficit occurring concurrently. For details of the biochemical and molecular aspects of the glycogenoses the recent excellent review of DiMauro and Servidei (1993) should be consulted.

TYPE II GLYCOGENOSIS (ACID MALTASE DEFICIENCY)

This is the most severe form of glycogenosis and the classical form, Pompe's disease (Pompe, 1933), is usually fatal in infancy (Figures 4-2 to 4-4). It is a generalized disease with involvement not only of heart and skeletal muscle, but also of many other tissues such as the liver, central nervous system, kidneys and leucocytes. In fact, demonstration of droplets of PAS-positive glycogen in the lymphocytes in a peripheral blood smear is a useful diagnostic screen for type II glycogenosis.

Affected infants present either with severe hypotonia and weakness, or with symptoms of cardiac or respiratory failure. They may be floppy from birth (Figure 4-2) or there may be a period of apparent normal motor development in the first weeks or months of life before clinical onset (Figures 4-3, 4-4), which sometimes seems to follow after a respiratory infection. The muscle weakness is due mainly to direct involvement of the muscle itself, but there may also be involvement of the anterior horn cells of the cord. These severely affected infants may look similar clinically to cases of infantile spinal muscular atrophy (SMA). There are, however, a number of distinguishing features. Unlike the severe intercostal weakness and sparing of the diaphragm in SMA, the diaphragm is involved as well in Pompe's disease and one does not see the same pattern of breathing and chest deformity as in SMA (see Chapter 8). In contrast to the sparing of the facial muscles in SMA, there is frequently some facial weakness in Pompe's disease (Figures 4-3, 4-4) and there may be associated enlargement of the tongue, in contrast to the normal sized or atrophic tongue with possible fasciculation in SMA. The heart is spared in SMA, whereas there is usually gross cardiomegaly in Pompe's disease.

Since the same enzyme deficiency has been demonstrated in the heart, liver and skeletal muscle (Hers, 1963), the traditional 'cardiac glycogenosis' is no longer regarded as a separate entity, and similarly the later onset, milder form that tends to be confined to the skeletal muscle without overt cardiomyopathy is also due to the same enzyme deficiency.

MILDER FORMS

Over the past few years a number of cases of type II glycogenosis have been documented in which there has been a much milder myopathy, often resembling a limb girdle dystrophy (Figure 4-5). Although some have had evidence of associated cardiac involvement, other systems do not appear to have been significantly involved. These cases include a 14-year-old boy reported by Courtecuisse *et al.* (1965) with clinical features of limb girdle dystrophy, a 12-fold rise in serum creatine phosphokinase and a myopathic EMG tracing, who had no clinical, radiological or electrocardiographic evidence of cardiac involvement and no hepatomegaly; two brothers aged 15 and 4½ years respectively with mild myopathy (Zellweger *et al.*, 1965); a 6-year-old girl (Isch *et al.*, 1966); a 3½-year-old girl with associated cardiac involvement who subsequently died at 4 years and showed autopsy evidence of glycogen deposition in the heart and central nervous system but not in other organs (Smith *et al.*, 1966); a boy with delay in motor milestones with a non-progressive weakness till 8 years and then deterioration with loss of ability to walk, and death at 10 years (Smith *et al.*, 1967); two unrelated adult female cases aged respectively 19 years (with onset of symptoms at 15 months) and 44 years (with onset at 31 years) (Hudgson *et al.*, 1968); a 3-year-old boy with mild muscle weakness (Swaiman *et al.*, 1968); and the four adult cases studied by Engel (1970).

The clinical picture in type II glycogenosis is thus a very variable one and the prognosis is probably dependent on the presence or absence of cardiac involvement, and the associated involvement of the respiratory muscles, and particularly the diaphragm, which may cause nocturnal hypoventilation and apnoea and unexpected death. This type of case stresses once again the importance of muscle biopsy even in apparently typical 'limb girdle muscular dystrophy' with a myopathic electromyographic pattern and raised serum enzyme levels, or with late-onset syndromes (Figures 4.5, 4.6).

DIAGNOSIS

In the severe form the diagnosis may be suspected if cardiomegaly and hepatomegaly are found in association with a clinical picture resembling severe spinal muscular atrophy (Werdnig–Hoffmann disease), in which cardiomegaly is not a feature.

The *electrocardiogram* shows a characteristic abnormality with gigantic QRS complexes and a very short P–R interval (Figure 4-2).

Electromyography may show a predominantly myopathic or a predominantly denervation pattern but may demonstrate in addition a feature characteristic of type II glycogenosis, namely pseudomyotonic bursts, resembling the spontaneous myotonic bursts seen in myotonic syndromes (see Chapter 5) but not showing the characteristic waning of the action potentials.

Muscle biopsy

The excess glycogen is readily apparent on muscle biopsy, even in mild cases. On light microscopy there is a marked vacuolar myopathy with complete distortion of the muscle pattern, and PAS-positive glycogen can be demonstrated in the vacuoles (Figures 4-2 to 4-6). The staining intensity is often very marked. There is also a very strong reaction in the vacuoles for acid phosphatase, a lysosomal enzyme. On electron microscopy the sequestration of glycogen in membrane bound spaces in type II glycogenosis is further evidence for the lysosomal location of the glycogen (see Figure 4-2f).

BIOCHEMISTRY

There is a marked increase in glycogen in skeletal muscle and heart, as well as in all other tissues, in the infantile form of type II glycogenosis, but this is less marked and very variable in the later onset, milder clinical phenotypes. In the infantile form acid maltase is absent in all tissues. In the milder forms the enzyme deficiency also occurs in all tissues, although the clinical manifestations may be restricted to skeletal muscle. The enzyme deficiency can be demonstrated in a muscle biopsy sample or in lymphocytes. The marked clinical heterogeneity is explained by the presence of a small but crucial residual acid maltase activity in the childhood and adult forms, but not in the infantile (Mehler and DiMauro, 1977).

THERAPEUTIC POSSIBILITIES

Enzyme replacement

A number of attempts have been made to replace the missing enzyme by use of alpha-glucosidase prepared from bacteria, fungi or human placenta, but without success (Lauer *et al.*, 1968; Hug, 1974; De Barsy *et al.*, 1973). Alpha-glucosidase in lipid envelopes (liposomes), was given intravenously in the case described in Figure 4-2 (Tyrrell *et al.*, 1976). Although there was a reduction in the liver size clinically and there may have been some possible reduction in liver glycogen storage, the therapy did not influence the fatal outcome for the child, who was already in a terminal stage of cardiac failure. Attempts have also been made to improve the delivery of the enzyme to cardiac or skeletal muscle by binding to low-density lipoproteins, but without success (Williams and Murray, 1980). A number of experimental studies with an acid maltase precursor have been of interest. The precursor isolated from human urine was taken up by cultured muscle cells from patients with acid maltase deficiency, with reduction in intralysosomal glycogen content (van der Ploeg *et al.*, 1988), whilst intravenous administration into mice of the precursor obtained from bovine testis was taken up by muscle and heart, but not by brain (van der Ploeg *et al.*, 1991).

text continues, p.188

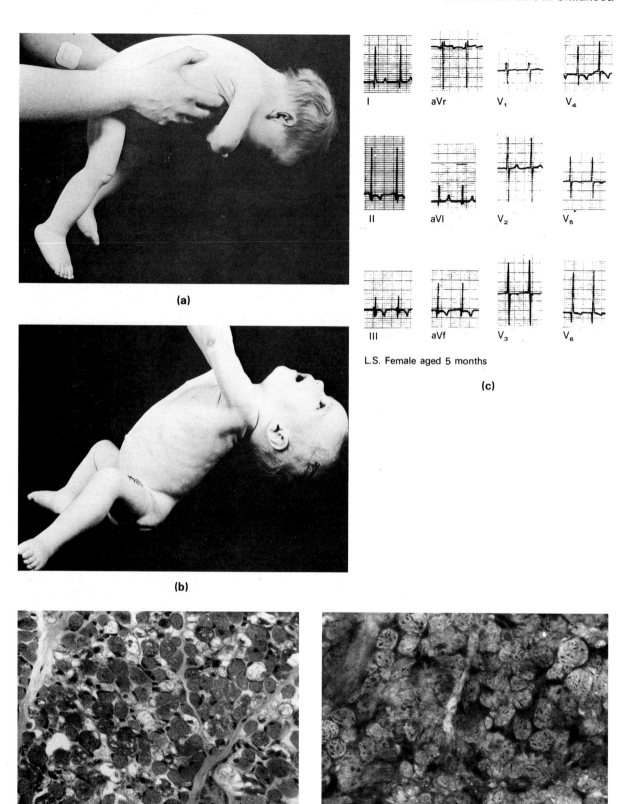

(a)

(b)

I   aVr   V₁   V₄

II   aVl   V₂   V₅

III   aVf   V₃   V₆

L.S. Female aged 5 months

(c)

(d)   (e)

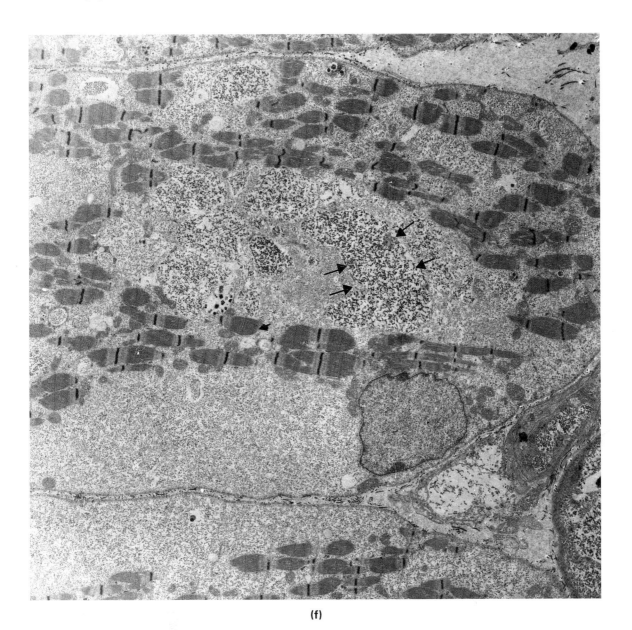

(f)

Figure 4-2 a-e (*facing page*) Type II glycogenosis (Pompe's disease) in a 4-month-old infant (a,b) with marked hypotonia from birth and associated congenital dislocation of the hip, who presented with feeding difficulty and respiratory infection. There was associated hepatomegaly and gross cardiomegaly. CK 290 iu/litre; EMG (deltoid and rectus femoris): pseudomyotonic bursts present. Her ECG (c) showed characteristic giant complexes and short P-R interval. (Tracings done at half sensitivity.) The patient died of heart failure at 8 months. A quadriceps biopsy (d) showed a striking vacuolar myopathy (Verhoeff-van Gieson × 265). (e) The vacuoles were strongly PAS positive for glycogen (PAS × 265).

Figure 4-2f Electron microscopy showed extensive replacement of myofibrils by glycogen, some of which is membrane bound and presumably lysosomal (arrows) (× 4500). Biochemical assay showed about 15 times normal glycogen content and complete absence of acid maltase.

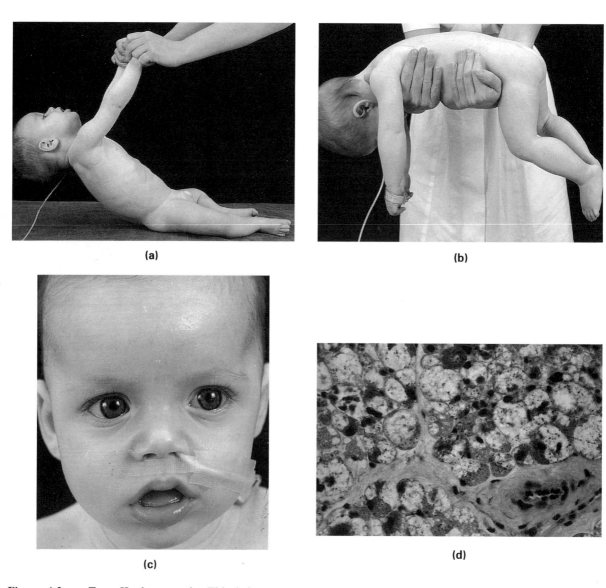

(a)

(b)

(c)

(d)

Figure 4-3a-e Type II glycogenosis. This infant was referred at 6 months of age, 2 weeks after limb hypotonia was noted at his routine clinic attendance. He had seemed well since birth, but his mother had always thought his legs were less active and mobile than his arms. On examination he was extremely floppy and generally weak (a,b). He had antigravity movements in the arms but not the legs. He was overtly tachypnoeic and breathless and had cardiomegaly and a 4cm hepatomegaly. He had needed tube feeding since a respiratory infection 2 months earlier (c). A clinical diagnosis of type II glycogenosis was supported by profuse myotonic discharges on EMG and confirmed on needle biopsy showing a remarkable vacuolar myopathy with almost total loss of underlying myofibrillar structure (d), and intense PAS stain for glycogen (e). Biochemical analysis showed a 30-fold increase in glycogen and low acid maltase activity. On follow-up he had persistent swallowing and breathing difficulties and increasing weakness in the arms. He died after a respiratory infection at 9 months of age.

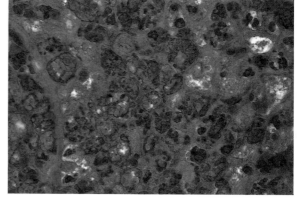

(e)

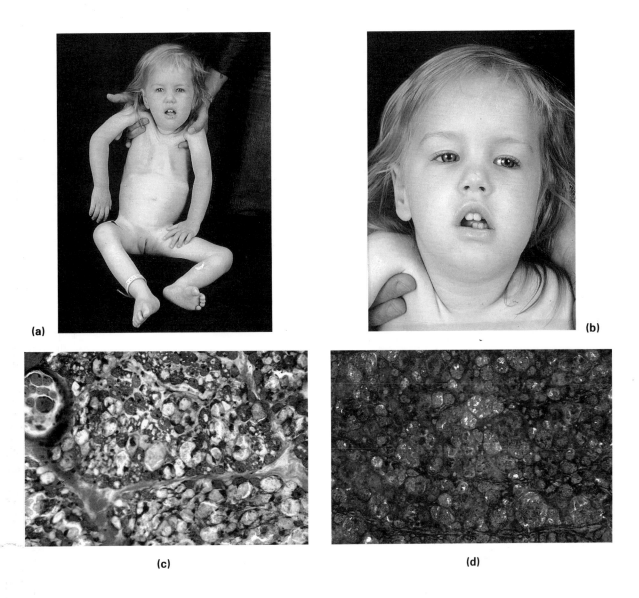

(a)

(b)

(c)

(d)

Figure 4-4a-d   Type II glycogenosis. This child presented at 21 months with generalized weakness, inability to raise the arms or legs against gravity (a) and associated facial weakness (b). Her early development had been normal but at 9 months she was slow to recover from a respiratory infection, and her muscles seemed to become weak. She sat unsupported at 11 months but lost this ability by 13 months and was never able to stand or walk. She became much weaker between 13 and 15 months and then stabilized. An EMG showed myotonic bursts; the ECG had giant QRS complexes and a short P-R interval, and echocardiography revealed thickening of the anterior wall and septum. The CK was raised at 580 iu/litre. Needle biopsy of the quadriceps showed a remarkable vacuolar myopathy with apparent sparing of the intrafusal fibres of a muscle spindle present (top left) (c). There was intense PAS stain for glycogen (d). Biochemical assay showed a 20-fold increase in glycogen and absence of acid maltase. The patient died of cardiac failure at 23 months of age.

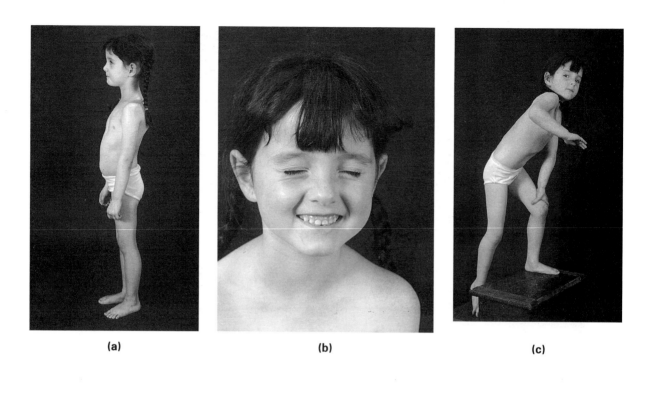

(a)   (b)   (c)

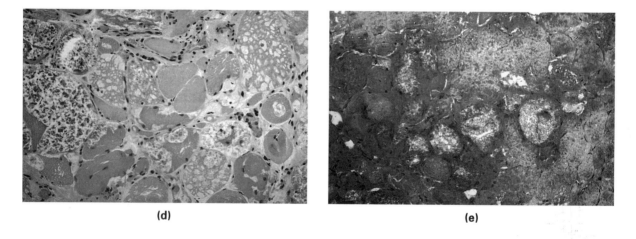

(d)   (e)

Figure 4-5a-e   Type II glycogenosis. This 5-year-old child presented with a history of frequent falls, inability to run normally, tiring with walking and the inability to climb stairs (a-c). Early milestones were normal; she sat at 6 months, stood at 12 months and walked at 16 months. Abnormality was noted from the time she started walking, with no apparent deterioration over the years. She was unable to hop or jump. She got up from the floor with Gowers' manoeuvre. She had a waddling gait on a narrow base, accentuated by trying to run. CK 2000 iu/litre; EMG myopathic. Needle biopsy of the quadriceps showed remarkable vacuolar myopathy (d) with excess glycogen (e). Glycogen droplets in lymphocytes were present on PAS staining of peripheral blood smear. Her liver and heart were not enlarged. An ECG showed short P-R interval. The family history was negative. The parents were unrelated and a female sibling was normal.

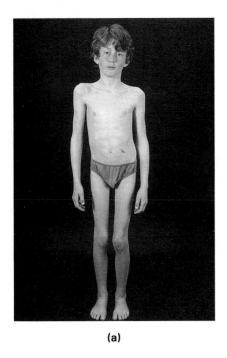

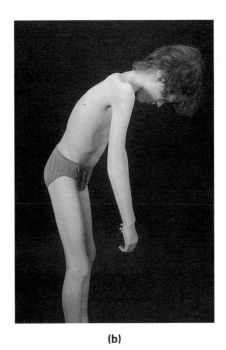

(a)

(b)

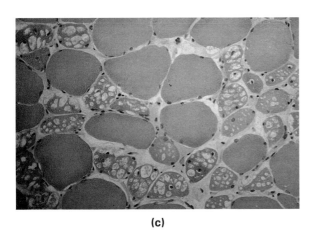

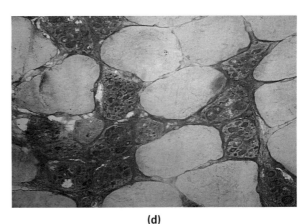

(c)

(d)

Figure 4-6a-d Type II glycogenosis: mild, with unusual Emery–Dreifuss-like presentation. This 11-year-old boy presented with a long-standing history of motor difficulties and delay in early motor milestones. He sat at 2 years and walked at 3 years. He could walk up to 2 miles but got tired. He was unable to run and had difficulty climbing steps. He had always had a stiff spine with limited flexion and inability to touch his knees. Neck flexion was full. He had experienced progressive scoliosis for 1 year. On examination he was found to be generally of thin build (a). He also had mild weakness in limb muscles and marked limitation of trunk flexion (b). No elbow contractures were evident. He was unable to sit up from the supine position without rolling over. The clinical picture was somewhat suggestive of Emery–Dreifuss dystrophy or rigid spine syndrome. His parents were not related. A female sibling was normal. His maternal grandfather had died unexpectedly at 33 years of age, 3 months after passing a physical examination for the army! This suggested a possible cardiomyopathy and X-linked inheritance. CK was elevated at 2180 iu/litre; EMG and ultrasound were normal; ECG was also normal. Needle biopsy of quadriceps showed (c; H&E) a striking vacuolar myopathy with excess glycogen (d, PAS). On EM glycogen was membrane bound (lysosomal). Glycogen droplets were present in lymphocytes on blood smear, which is characteristic of type II glycogenosis. He continued to be stable but went into respiratory failure from nocturnal hypoventilation, presumably from diaphragmatic involvement. He responded well to mask ventilation at night.

Dietary

Low-carbohydrate and ketogenic diets have proved ineffective, but a number of reports have claimed a beneficial effect of a high protein diet (Slonim *et al.*, 1983; Isaacs *et al.*, 1986; Umpleby *et al.*, 1987). The beneficial effect is thought to compensate for the increased protein catabolism in type II glycogenosis.

Marrow transplantation

A number of attempts to treat Pompe's disease by bone marrow transplantation did not produce any benefit (Hug *et al.*, 1984; Harris *et al.*, 1986; Hoogerbrugge *et al.*, 1986; Watson *et al.*, 1986).

Respiratory

The milder, ambulant cases are prone to respiratory failure, usually due to diaphragmatic weakness, and this can be life-threatening. Supportive mask ventilation at night can be extremely beneficial and improve the well-being of the patient by day as well (Figure 4-6). Later onset, adult cases are also prone to respiratory failure (Rosenow and Engel, 1978; Trend *et al.*, 1985; Margolis and Hill, 1986).

ANIMAL MODELS

Acid maltase deficiency has been diagnosed in a number of animals, including a Lapland dog (Walvoort *et al.*, 1982), Japanese quail (Suhara *et al.*, 1989) and Australian cattle, which manifested both an infantile and a late-onset type, comparable with the human disease (Howell *et al.*, 1981). A recent interesting study of chimaeric twin cattle with type II glycogenosis, producing a natural experiment comparable with a bone marrow transplant, failed to produce any benefit for the affected calf (Howell *et al.*, 1991). This bovine model could provide a valuable resource for potential therapeutic trials.

GENETICS

The inheritance of type II glycogenosis is autosomal recessive and the gene has been localized to 17q23-q25, the location of the gene for acid maltase (Solomon *et al.*, 1979; D'Ancona *et al.*, 1979; Weil *et al.*, 1979; Nickel *et al.*, 1982; Martiniuk *et al.*, 1985). The infantile and later onset forms are considered to be allelic.

The gene has been cloned and sequenced (Hoefsloot *et al.*, 1988; Martiniuk *et al.*, 1990a), and studies of the mRNA in a series of patients have shown the same diversity as at the clinical and biochemical level (van der Ploeg *et al.*, 1989;

Martiniuk *et al.*, 1990a). Martiniuk *et al.* (1990b) postulated at least six different mutations of the acid maltase gene in their 14 cases.

Prenatal diagnosis can be offered by measuring acid maltase activity in cultured amniotic fluid fibroblasts (Niermeijer *et al.*, 1975).

TYPE III GLYCOGENOSIS (DEBRANCHER ENZYME DEFICIENCY)

In 1952, Illingworth and Cori discovered an abnormal glycogen with very short side chains (limit dextrin) in the liver and muscle of the 12-year-old girl recorded by Forbes (1953). They postulated that the deficient enzyme was probably amylo-1,6-glucosidase (the debranching enzyme) and this was subsequently confirmed (Illingworth *et al.*, 1956; Hers, 1959).

Skeletal muscle is usually only mildly affected in type III glycogenosis, which can present with hypotonia and weakness (see Figure 4.7). However, the effects of hepatic involvement are likely to be more serious and the clinical presentation is often with hypoglycaemia and ketosis. Hepatomegaly and delayed development may be present in early infancy but the hepatomegaly can resolve spontaneously by adolescence with eventual normal development, despite the persistence of the underlying enzymic defect.

Several reports have documented a definite myopathy in association with type III glycogenosis, usually in adult cases. Oliner *et al.* (1961) described a chronic progressive myopathy in a man of 51 years, and Brunberg *et al.* (1971) a man of 43 with an 8-month history of progressive muscle weakness and a previous long-standing mild muscle disability. Further cases have been documented by DiMauro *et al.* (1979) and Cornelio *et al.* (1984). In some of the early reports there was a suggestion of muscle involvement from such clinical features as 'flaccidity' (Pearson, 1968) or 'weak tone' (van Creveld and Huijing, 1964) but in others no clinical features of muscle involvement were apparent despite the presence of excessive glycogen deposition in the muscle (Brombacher *et al.*, 1964; Brandt and DeLuca, 1966; Hug *et al.*, 1966). It is noteworthy that in a recent review of 16 cases of type III glycogenosis, aged 2–27 years, Moses *et al.* (1986) found no weakness in 11.

CARDIAC INVOLVEMENT

Most of the documented cases of myopathy have shown abnormality on ECG or echocardiography,

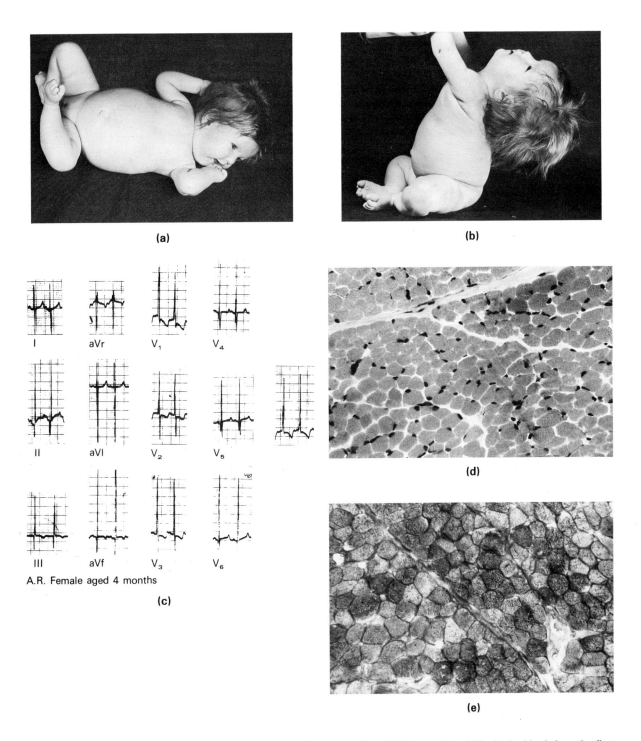

(a)

(b)

I aVr V₁ V₄

II aVl V₂ V₅

III aVf V₃ V₆

A.R. Female aged 4 months

(c)

(d)

(e)

Figure 4-7a-e Type III glycogenosis in a 4-month-old infant presenting with hypotonia which she had had since the first week of life (a). She had good spontaneous movement of limbs but (b) poor head control. She also had associated gross hepatomegaly and mild cardiomegaly. Fasting blood sugar was low. Clinical diagnosis of type III glycogenosis was made on combination of hypoglycaemia with muscle, liver and cardiac involvement. CK 64 iu/litre; EMG borderline myopathic. No pseudomyotonia was found. (c) The ECG showed massive complexes and short P-R interval. (Compare with Figure 4-2.) (Tracings done at half sensitivity.) Muscle biopsy from the quadriceps showed (d) a reasonably normal looking histology (H & E × 225) apart from a few isolated vacuolar fibres and (e) a suggestion of excess glycogen in comparison with control sections (PAS × 225), with retention of the variation between fibres. Biochemical assessment revealed glycogen levels of about 20 times normal and complete absence of amylo-1,6-glucosidase (debrancher enzyme).

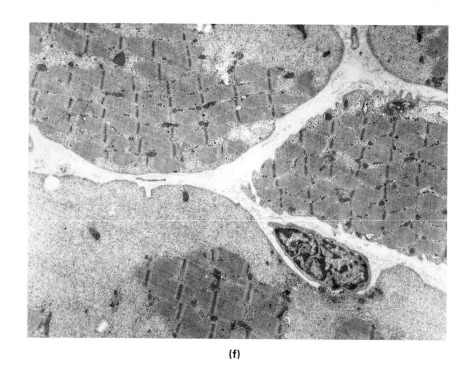

(f)

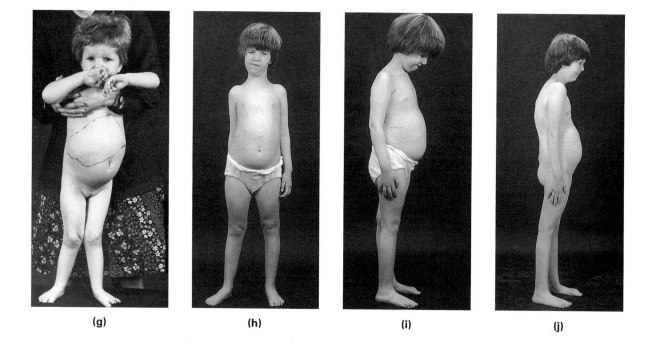

(g)   **(h)**   **(i)**   **(j)**

Figure 4-7f-j   (f) Electron microscopy of the biopsy showed extensive replacement of myofibrils by cytoplasmic, non-membrane bound, glycogen (× 5000). Her hypoglycaemia was controlled with frequent small carbohydrate feeds. She showed steady improvement in her motor ability, sat unsupported at 20 months, stood with support at 3½ years (g) and subsequently walked unsupported (h,i, 7½ years; j, 12 years). The hepatomegaly persisted but gradually reduced in size (g-j). She had mild intellectual retardation. She also had laxity of her joints with hyperextension of the knees and a somewhat unusual posture with associated abdominal protrusion (i,j).

with evidence of left ventricular or biventricular hypertrophy, but symptoms of cardiac insufficiency are uncommon and were present in only one of the 20 patients of Moses *et al.* (1989) and two of the five cases of DiMauro *et al.* (1979), though Miller *et al.* (1972), in contrast, reported a child who died of cardiac failure at 4 years of age.

DIAGNOSIS

Serum enzymes are variable and the CK may be normal or elevated. EMG may also be normal, or may show a myopathic pattern and at times also additional features of denervation. The motor nerve conduction velocity may also be slowed.

Muscle biopsy may also show a fairly normal histological appearance but the excess glycogen may be suspected on the PAS staining and confirmed by electron microscopy (see Figure 4-7). Although the glycogen has an abnormal structure on biochemical analysis, the appearances of the glycogen granules on electron microscopy are similar to those seen in conditions with deposition of normally structured glycogen. The distribution is intrasarcoplasmic and subsarcolemmal and there is no suggestion of any lysosomal accumulation. There have also been reports of glycogen storage in motor and sensory peripheral nerves (Powell *et al.*, 1985; Ugawa *et al.*, 1986).

The definitive diagnosis may be confirmed by demonstrating the enzyme deficiency in muscle or liver biopsy or in the leucocytes.

MANAGEMENT

Frequent small feeds and a high protein intake may help to prevent hypoglycaemia (Fernandes and van de Kamer, 1968; Fernandes and Huijing, 1968). Slonim *et al.* (1982) claimed a remarkable improvement in muscle function in a seven-year-old boy with severe diffuse weakness after 6 months of high protein intake by nocturnal intragastric therapy. Slonim *et al.* (1984) subsequently studied seven patients with debrancher enzyme deficiency associated with childhood or adolescent onset myopathy, four of whom also had growth failure. They gave long-term treatment with high-protein enteral infusion overnight and high protein feeds during the day for periods varying from 8 to 24 months. All patients demonstrated improved physical activity and endurance, with improvement in muscle strength documented in five patients. In addition, all four patients with growth failure showed dramatic improvement in growth rate. They suggest that this positive response to high-protein therapy supports their thesis that the myopathy in

debrancher enzyme deficiency is at least partly the result of reversible muscle amino acid depletion. In contrast, Cornelio *et al.* (1984) found no benefit in an adult with myopathy after 6 months of high protein diet.

GENETICS

Inheritance is autosomal recessive. Although a full-length cDNA for human debrancher enzyme has been cloned by Ding *et al.* (1989), chromosomal location has not yet been achieved. Studies of the mRNA suggest that there is genetic heterogeneity, which will probably explain the marked variability in clinical phenotype.

Prenatal diagnosis is possible on assay of cultured amniocytes (Yang *et al.*, 1990).

TYPE IV GLYCOGENOSIS (BRANCHER ENZYME DEFICIENCY)

This is a rare form of glycogenosis, characterized by liver dysfunction with hepatosplenomegaly, progressive cirrhosis and chronic hepatic failure, followed by early death from liver failure or gastrointestinal bleeding. The muscle involvement is relatively insignificant and overshadowed by the liver problem.

The first case (Andersen, 1952, 1956) was a boy with normal nutrition and development, who presented at 11 months of age with liver and spleen enlargement and ascites, and subsequently died at 17 months. There was glycogen deposition in the cirrhotic liver and the reticulo–endothelial system but no excess in striated muscle. The glycogen was found to be of abnormal structure with unusual chain length, characteristic of amylopectin. Illingworth and Cori (1952) speculated that deficiency of the branching enzyme (α-1,4-glucan: α-1,4-glucan 6-glycosyl transferase; amylo (1,4$\rightarrow$1,6) transglucosidase) might produce a glycogen of this structure, but Hers (1964) pointed out several difficulties in explaining the presence of some branching in the amylopectin in the absence of branching enzyme alone.

A second case was reported by Sidbury *et al.* (1962). This 12-month-old child also presented with hepatic failure and subsequently died at 32 months; PAS-positive material with delayed digestion by salivary diastase, suggestive of an abnormal glycogen, was present in the liver as well as skeletal and cardiac muscle, but the total glycogen content of these tissues was low.

The patient reported by Holleman *et al.* (1966) was ill from birth and died at 6½ months. In addition to gross liver and spleen enlargement, he also had muscle weakness, and autopsy examination of the tissues showed mixtures of various amylopectin-like polysaccharides in the liver, spleen, heart and striated muscle.

On the other hand, Brown and Brown (1966, 1968) found that the glycogen in the skeletal muscle was normal, both in amount and in structure, in a 2-year-old child with type IV glycogenosis. The liver contained glycogen of abnormal structure and they were also able to demonstrate for the first time the postulated deficiency of branching enzyme in the liver and leucocytes of this child. The 25-month-old child described by Reed *et al.* (1968) also showed no abnormal glycogen deposition in the skeletal muscle. A sibling of the patient reported by Holleman *et al.* (1966) was reported by Fernandes and Huijing (1968). This 5-month-old child made few spontaneous movements, muscle tone was poor and tendon reflexes depressed. They were able to demonstrate a deficiency of the branching enzyme in his leucocytes but did not study the muscle. The patient reported by Schochet *et al.* (1970) had generalized muscle wasting and associated muscle weakness, and there was biopsy as well as autopsy evidence of deposits of polysaccharide in the skeletal muscle. Autopsy also revealed deposits in the tongue and heart and in the central nervous system. Biochemical assay of the muscle biopsy gave a normal value for the glycogen content (0.5%).

In some reports cardiomyopathy has been a predominant feature in older children with less severe hepatic disease (Farrans *et al.*, 1966; Servidei *et al.*, 1987). The patient reported by Servidei *et al.*, who died, had deficiency of branching enzyme in the muscle, heart, liver and brain, confirming that this was still a generalized disorder. Further evidence for clinical heterogeneity comes from patients with later (juvenile) onset of liver dysfunction (Guerra *et al.*, 1986) or without apparent evidence of liver dysfunction, despite documented deficiency of brancher enzyme in liver, muscle and fibroblasts (Greene *et al.*, 1988a). Moreover, branching enzyme deficiency has recently been demonstrated by Lossos *et al.* (1991) in the leucocytes, but not in the muscle, of two patients with adult polyglucosan body disease, a neurological disorder with onset in the fifth or sixth decade, characterized by progressive upper and lower motor neurone involvement (Cafferty *et al.*, 1991).

DIAGNOSIS

In the classical form presenting with hepatic failure, the diagnosis is readily established by demonstration of abnormal polysaccharide deposit in the muscle biopsy and confirmed by enzyme assay. It also needs to be kept in mind as a possibility in the milder, late onset cases, or those presenting with cardiomyopathy.

GENETICS

Inheritance is autosomal recessive. The gene for branching enzyme has not yet been isolated or sequenced, and the chromosome location not known. As branching enzyme is thought to be a monomeric protein (Caudwell and Cohen, 1980) further resolution of the molecular genetics will be necessary before one can understand the clinical heterogeneity.

THERAPY

No specific therapy is available and attempts to influence the course of the disease with steroids, high protein, low carbohydrate diet, or administration of α-1,4-glucosidase and α-1,6-glucosidase have failed. Greene *et al.* (1988b) reported an improvement in liver function and prolonged survival in two children by careful dietary control of their fasting hypoglycaemia. Beneficial results were reported following liver transplantation in ten children, which seemed a reasonable approach in a condition with a consistently fatal outcome from hepatic failure (Selby *et al.*, 1991). However, their hope that following the liver transplant the enzyme might be transported to other tissues, such as the heart, has not been fulfilled, and indeed one such child developed progressive cardiac failure 2 years after a successful orthotopic liver transplant (Sokal *et al.*, 1992).

TYPE V GLYCOGENOSIS (PHOSPHORYLASE DEFICIENCY)

Type V glycogenosis (McArdle's disease, muscle phosphorylase deficiency) is entirely restricted to striated muscle. In 1951 McArdle demonstrated a failure of blood lactic acid to rise after ischaemic exercise in a 30-year-old man suffering from muscle cramps on exertion, and he postulated an enzymic defect along the glycolytic pathway. It was not until 8 years later that the deficient enzyme was shown to be phosphorylase in two separately studied cases (Mommaerts *et al.*, 1959; Schmid and Mahler, 1959). McArdle's disease holds historical pride of place as the first myopathy in which a single enzyme defect was demonstrated.

CLINICAL FEATURES ——————————

The main clinical features of McArdle's disease are cramps on exertion, but these may not be present in the early stages. Schmid and Mahler (1959) recognized three phases of symptoms in their 52-year-old patient. In childhood and adolescence the only symptom was easy fatiguability. From the age of 20 there were severe cramps and weakness on exertion, and transient myoglobinuria. Subsequently he developed weakness and wasting of proximal muscles. There is, however, marked variation in severity from one patient to another.

Most index cases have not been diagnosed until adult life, although symptoms could often be traced back to childhood. At the time of his diagnosis the patient in Figure 4-8 was the youngest index case on record. It is of interest that his presenting symptom was stiffness on sustained exertion, rather than actual cramps, and any form of discomfort on exertion, relieved by rest, should raise suspicion of a possible phosphorylase deficiency, or other glycolytic disorder, particularly if associated with normal muscle power. Williams and Hosking (1985) subsequently reported three children with type V glycogenosis. The first, an 8-year-old girl, presented with a 4-year history of reluctance to walk more than short distances, particularly uphill, and needing frequent rests. She had been considered clumsy and frequently fell but had never complained of any cramps on exercise. The other two were 10-year-old girls who had limited exercise tolerance and associated cramps. Some cases may have associated myoglobinuria, and this may be severe enough to cause acute renal failure.

Cardiac muscle does not appear to be affected although there is one report of ECG changes in a case of McArdle's disease (Ratinov *et al.* 1965).

DIAGNOSIS ——————————————

An accurate history is essential for diagnosis, since between attacks clinical examination may prove completely normal (see Figure 4-9). Some subjects may have myoglobinuria after the exertion and cramps. The cramps can be produced by exercising a forearm under ischaemic conditions, by occlusion of the circulation with a sphygmomanometer cuff. This causes shortening and stiffness of the muscle and true contracture in the physiological sense, with electrical silence on electromyography. The contracture and cramp may persist for some time after the circulation is re-established, and may be associated with severe discomfort and pain (Figure 4-9).

Following ischaemic exercise there is no rise in the blood lactate or pyruvate levels in contrast to a two- to five-fold elevation in a normal subject. This is measured in the venous blood from the ischaemic area, according to the technique described by McArdle (1951), Pearson *et al.* (1959), Rimer and Mommaerts (1959) and Mellick (1962). This in itself is not pathognomonic of phosphorylase deficiency, since a similar result could be produced by absence of other enzymes along the glycolytic pathway.

Muscle biopsy

The diagnosis of McArdle's disease may be confirmed on biopsy. The absence of phosphorylase can be clearly demonstrated histochemically and the excess of glycogen may be suspected on light microscopy (PAS stain) and confirmed on electron microscopy. Biochemical study of the muscle will confirm the excess of muscle glycogen of normal structure and the deficiency of phosphorylase. Most patients completely lack immunologically reactive enzyme protein in the muscle; Servidei *et al.* (1988a) found virtually no protein in 41 of 48 cases, and McConchie *et al.* (1991) no protein in 10 of 11 cases. The enzymes necessary for the interconversion of the inactive phosphorylase *b* and the active phosphorylase *a* are present in normal amounts.

BIOCHEMISTRY ——————————

Mature human muscle has a single phosphorylase isoenzyme. In contrast, both cardiac muscle and brain show three separate bands on gel electrophoresis: a minor, slow-migrating isozyme identical to muscle phosphorylase, comprising about 13% of total activity in heart and 8% in brain; a fast-moving 'brain' isozyme comprising 58% of total activity in heart and 64% in brain; and an intermediate band, a hybrid muscle and brain isozyme, forming 29% of total in heart and 28% in brain (Bresolin *et al.*, 1983a). In McArdle's disease, phosphorylase activity is normal in erythrocytes, leucocytes, platelets, skin and cultured skin fibroblasts, suggesting that these tissues contain non-muscle isozymes.

GENETICS ——————————————

A number of familial cases have been reported suggesting an autosomal recessive pattern of inheritance (Schmid and Hammaker, 1961; Rowland *et al.*, 1963, 1966; Sidbury, 1965, Tobin and Coleman, 1965; Salter *et al.* 1967). However, the possibility of a dominant inheritance was raised by Schimrigk *et al.* (1967) to explain the possible involvement of the mother of their patient and

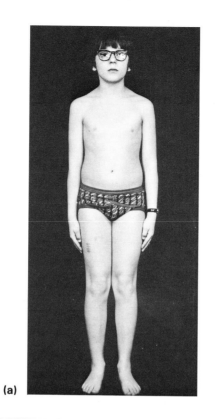

(a)

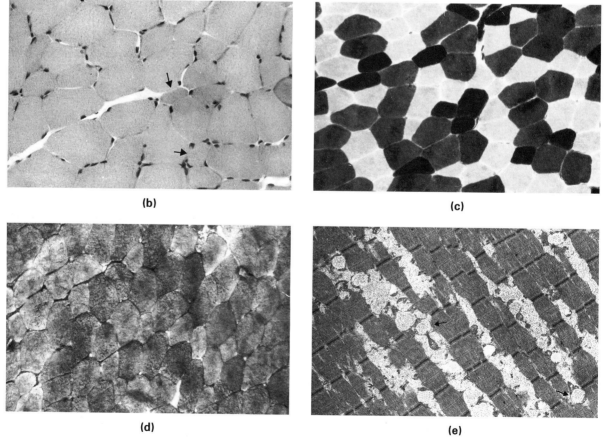

(b)

(c)

(d)

(e)

subsequently also by Chui and Munsat (1976). An alternative explanation may be the occurrence of homozygotes and manifesting heterozygotes of the same recessive gene within the same family (Schmidt *et al.*, 1987; Papadimitriou *et al.*, 1990).

The genes for the three phosphorylase isoenzymes have been cloned and sequenced and assigned to individual chromosome loci: chromosome 11q13 for the muscle (M) isozyme (Lebo *et al.*, 1984, 1990), chromosome 14 for the liver (L) isozyme and chromosomes 10 and 20 for the brain (B) form. Immature, developing and regenerating muscle contain the brain isozyme, which would explain the positive phosphorylase reaction in regenerating fibres and cultured myotubes from McArdle muscle (Roelofs *et al.*, 1967; Sato *et al.*, 1977; DiMauro *et al.*, 1978; Crerar *et al.*, 1988).

A series of studies of the mRNA in the muscle from McArdle patients has shown striking variability, suggesting genetic heterogeneity (Servidei *et al.*, 1988a; McConchie *et al.*, 1991). This has now been confirmed by the demonstration of a number of different mutations in the DNA. Tsujino *et al.* (1993a) sequenced complementary DNA in four patients and studied by restriction-endo-nuclease analysis 40 patients with McArdle's disease, including six children and an infant with the severe infantile form. Sequence analysis revealed three distinct point mutations: the substitution of thymine for cytosine at codon 49 in exon 1, changing an encoded arginine to a stop codon; the substitution of adenine for guanine at codon 204 in exon 5, changing glycine to serine; and the substitution of cytosine for adenine at codon 542 in exon 14, changing lysine to threonine. Analysis of restriction-fragment-length polymorphisms of appropriate fragments of genomic DNA after amplification with the polymerase chain reaction showed that 18 patients (including the infant with the fatal infantile form) were homozygous for the stop-codon mutation, six had different mutations in the two alleles (compound heterozygotes), and 11 were presumed to be compound heterozygotes for a known mutation plus an unknown one; only five patients had none of the three mutations. All three mutations were present in various combinations in five members of a family with an apparently autosomal dominant transmission. This exciting advance opens the way for making a diagnosis of McArdle's disease on the basis of the mutations in the DNA in their leucocytes in about 90% of patients.

THERAPEUTIC POSSIBILITIES ————

Most patients learn to restrict their activities within limits — short of producing muscle cramps or discomfort. The ingestion of glucose or fructose has been shown to increase acute exercise tolerance but has not proved of practical value. Pearson *et al.* (1961) also noted the disappearance of subjective symptoms with sustained exercise, which they looked upon as a 'second wind' phenomenon and ascribed to the delayed mobilization and utilization of free fatty acids as a secondary source of energy during muscle exercise. They were also able to demonstrate a beneficial effect of continuous infusion of emulsified fat in 4% glucose in a patient with McArdle's disease. Viskoper *et al.* (1975) followed up this possibility and demonstrated a subjective increase in physical fitness and a shorter recovery period after an acute workload in a patient on a high fat diet, but no apparent objective improvement in muscle function. In line with his contention that the weakness in several different glycogenoses may relate to an associated amino acid deficiency (see type II and type III above), Slonim treated a patient with fixed weakness with a high protein diet and noted an improvement in muscle endurance and strength, both after a single protein-rich meal and after a prolonged dietary regimen (Slonim and Goans, 1985). Argov *et al.* (1987) were unable to demonstrate an acute effect of a protein load on energy metabolism by ^{31}P magnetic resonance spectroscopy, but Jensen *et al.* (1990) were able to demonstrate a change, both on ^{31}P-MRS and with formal exercise testing following an isocaloric high-protein diet for 6 weeks.

Figure 4-8a-e (*facing page*)   Type V glycogenosis (McArdle's disease) in a 12-year-old boy (a) presenting with stiffness of his muscles with exercise, noted during a 10-mile charity walk, forcing him to stop after 5 miles and at frequent intervals after that. After a 100-yard sprint his legs stiffened and swelled up. Any long-distance swimming caused his arms and shoulders to stiffen. There was no history of myoglobinuria. An ischaemic lactate test had to be abandoned after 2 minutes because of his marked discomfort by contracture of the hand for 15 minutes. There was no weakness or physical disability. The family history was negative. CK 276 iu/litre; EMG normal; ECG normal. (b) Biopsy of rectus femoris showed a normal looking muscle apart from some isolated atrophic fibres (arrows) (H & E × 230), (c) a normal two-fibre pattern (ATPase pH 9.4 × 140), and (d) a suggestion of excess glycogen (PAS × 140). The phosphorylase reaction was completely negative in contrast to the control. (e) The phosphofructokinase reaction was normal. Biochemical assay showed 15 times the normal glycogen level and an absence of phosphorylase. Electron microscopy of biopsy showed focal areas of replacement of myofilaments by glycogen. Some appeared to be in distended mitochondria (arrows) (× 5300).

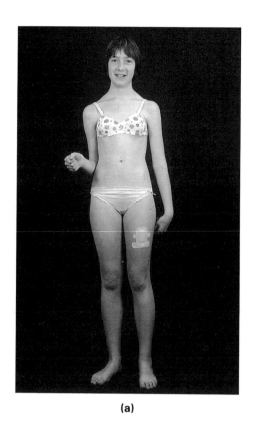

(a)

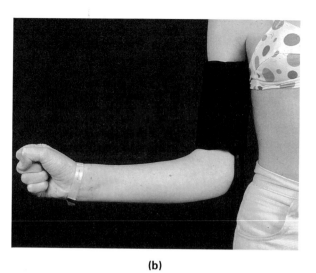

(b)

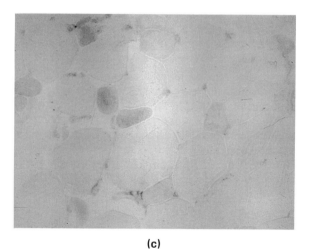

(c)

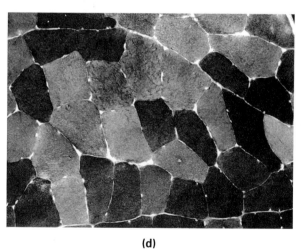

(d)

Figure 4-9a-d Type V glycogenosis. This 13-year-old girl (a) presented with a history of cramps on exercise with no weakness between attacks, which suggested phosphorylase deficiency. An ischaemic lactate test on the forearm produced a marked painful spasm of the muscles with tight contraction of the hand which persisted for 30 minutes (b). A needle biopsy of the quadriceps showed a normal looking muscle with absent phosphorylase activity (c), apart from weakly positive reaction in isolated atrophic fibres, presumably regenerating, in contrast to the control muscle (d).

PHOSPHORYLASE DEFICIENCY: SEVERE INFANTILE FORM ————————

DiMauro and Hartlage (1978) reported an infant with progressive generalized weakness, starting at 4 weeks, and dying of respiratory insufficiency at 13 weeks. Muscle biopsy showed increased glycogen content and complete absence of phosphorylase. This presentation with a floppy infant syndrome contrasts with the classical presentation in later childhood and the distinction between the two clinical syndromes is difficult to understand in the face of the same enzymatic defect.

Miranda *et al.* (1979) subsequently studied the phosphorylase isoenzymes in the heart muscle of an affected sister of the above child who died at 4 months of age. Two of the three normal isoenzymes were absent in the heart, only the fast cardiac type isoenzyme remaining. The inheritance in this family with two affected siblings was autosomal recessive. It still remains to be seen whether this severe infantile form of phosphorylase deficiency is biochemically and genetically similar to the more usual, late onset, more benign form of McArdle's disease, or genetically completely distinct. The clinical situation is somewhat analogous to the benign and severe forms of type II glycogenosis, but somewhat compounded by the involvement of more than one isoenzyme.

A further case of the fatal infantile type was documented by Milstein *et al.* (1989) in a 33-week gestation, premature female infant, of consanguineous parents, who had birth asphyxia and required ventilator support. She was generally weak and flaccid and had associated contractures of the knees, hips and elbows. A muscle biopsy at 14 days showed a myopathic pattern and glycogen storage on light and electron microscopy preparations, and absence of phosphorylase. She died at 16 days, and autopsy studies on various muscles gave the same results. There was no glycogen storage in the heart or liver but the myocardium showed fibrosis.

Cornelio *et al.* (1983) reported another clinical variant in a 4-year-old boy, born at 32 weeks gestation, with delayed motor milestones and psychomotor delay. After starting to walk at 20 months he fell frequently and had difficulty rising, and developed a waddling gait. Muscle biopsy was histologically normal, but phosphorylase was absent and the glycogen twice normal.

TYPE VII GLYCOGENOSIS (PHOSPHOFRUCTOKINASE DEFICIENCY) ————————————

This muscle glycogenosis with a specific enzyme defect was first identified by Tarui and his associates in 1965. They described three siblings, a female of 20 years and her 23- and 27-year-old brothers, with clinical features identical to McArdle's syndrome. All three had experienced easy fatiguability and intolerance of exercise since childhood. Vigorous exertion produced marked weakness and stiffness. In the ischaemic exercise test there was no rise in venous lactate. Muscle biopsy showed raised glycogen levels in all three. The glycogen was normal in structure. Phosphorylase activity was normal but phosphofructokinase (PFK) practically zero (1–3% of normal) in all three. The levels of PFK in the parents, who were first cousins, were normal. Tarui *et al.* also observed a lowered level of phosphofructokinase in the erythrocytes of their three patients and a slight but definite reduction in the mother.

A further case with identical features was described by Layzer *et al.* (1967). This 18-year-old male had also been intolerant of exercise since childhood but his two siblings were normal. Ischaemic exercise produced contracture of the forearm muscles and no rise in venous lactate or pyruvate. On muscle biopsy the PFK was practically zero (less than 2%) and immmunological studies, using an antibody to purified normal human muscle PFK, failed to reveal the presence of a structurally related but inactive protein, thus confirming the absence of PFK. The small amount of activity of PFK present in this and the previous patients is compatible with contamination of the muscle by blood and other non-muscle tissues. As in Tarui's cases, there was a marked reduction in the PFK of the erythrocytes in this case and also a similar reduction in both parents. Muscle biopsy was not performed on the parents. Additional cases conforming to the typical clinical pattern were subsequently documented by Tobin *et al.* (1973) and Dupond *et al.* (1977). The absence of the muscle isozyme in the erythrocytes probably accounts for the commonly associated mild haemolytic anaemia (Tarui *et al.*, 1978). Some cases of phosphofructokinase deficiency may present with haemolytic anaemia without myopathy.

ATYPICAL CASES ————————

Phosphofructokinase deficiency has also been found in a number of cases with somewhat atypical presentation. Serratrice *et al.* (1969) reported a 37-year-old man with a slowly progressive scapuloperoneal wasting and weakness since the age of 15 and an associated hepatomegaly. A number of severe infantile cases have also been diagnosed. Guibaud *et al.* (1978) reported two Moroccan siblings with severe congenital weakness and contractures. The boy died of respiratory infection at six months, the girl was still unable to sit unsupported at 14 months. Danon *et al.* (1981a) documented a fatal infantile glycogen storage disease in a girl with weakness of the limbs from birth, mental retardation and corneal opacities, who died at 4 years of respiratory insufficiency. The muscle biopsy showed non-specific changes on light microscopy but excessive glycogen at the electron microscopic level. Biochemical studies revealed an increased glycogen content, lack of PFK and a reduction in phosphorylase *b* kinase to about 30% of normal. Another child presented in the neonatal period with weakness, seizures, cortical blindness and corneal opacities and died of respiratory failure at 7 months (Servidei *et al.*, 1986).

DIAGNOSIS

As in phosphorylase deficiency, there is no rise in lactate on the forearm ischaemic exercise test. The spectra obtained with ^{31}P-magnetic resonance spectroscopy differ from those in McArdle's disease, with an increase after exercise of glycolytic intermediates as phosphorylated monoesters (PME) which produce a discrete peak (Argov and Bank, 1991). The muscle biopsy is similar to that of phosphorylase deficiency with focal necrotic or regenerating fibres and focal increase in glycogen. The deficiency in PFK can be demonstrated histochemically (Bonilla and Schotland, 1970) and confirmed by biochemical analysis.

BIOCHEMISTRY

Phosphofructokinase is a tetrameric enzyme under the control of three structural loci that encode three different subunits, muscle (M), liver (L), and platelet (P), of similar molecular size, which are variably expressed in different tissues. Mature muscle expresses only the M subunit and contains the homotetramer M4. Erythrocytes express both the M and L subunits, producing five isozymes, the homotetramers M4 and L4 and three hybrids (M3L1, M2L2, M1L3). Immature muscle expresses all three subunits, whilst the M subunit is the main component in heart and brain (Davidson *et al.*, 1983a, b).

GENETICS

Inheritance of phosphofructokinase deficiency is autosomal recessive, and the three genes encoding the M, P and L subunits have been localized to chromosomes 1(cen→q32), 10p and 21q22.3 respectively. The full-length cDNA for the M-subunit has been isolated and sequenced (Nakajima

et al., 1978), and the genetic lesion in the original family of Tarui has been identified (Nakajima *et al.*, 1990): a G-to-T transversion at the splice site of intron 13 activated a cryptic 5'-splice site 75 bases upstream, resulting in a 75-base in-frame deletion between nucleotides 422 and 446.

ANIMAL MODELS

Phosphofructokinase deficiency has been found in English springer spaniel dogs with chronic haemolytic anaemia, with hyperventilation-induced haemolysis (Giger *et al.*, 1985), but no obvious weakness, exercise intolerance or myoglobinuria, despite the complete lack of the M subunit of PFK in erythrocytes and muscle (Vora *et al.*, 1985). In contrast to affected humans, the dogs have about 10% of residual PFK activity in their muscle, due to anomalous expression of the L subunit. Nevertheless, ^{31}P-MRS showed a rise in PME in dog muscle during exercise and an acute depletion of phosphocreatine and ATP after isometric muscle stimulation (Giger *et al.*, 1988).

THERAPY

The approach to therapy is similar to that of phosphorylase deficiency, except that glucose cannot provide an alternative substrate (see Figure 4-1). A high protein intake should provide the same benefit as in McArdle's.

TYPE VIII GLYCOGENOSIS (PHOSPHORYLASE *b* KINASE DEFICIENCY)

In 1967 Strugalska-Cynowska described an 8-year-old boy with cramps on exercise, who was thought to have a deficiency of phosphorylase *b* kinase, which converts inactive phosphorylase *b* into the active *a* form.

An X-linked form of phosphorylase kinase deficiency has been documented which only affects the liver enzyme and is normal in muscle. However, several cases have been reported suggesting that there may be a syndrome with deficiency of muscle phosphorylase kinase as well as of the liver enzyme and inherited through an autosomal recessive mechanism.

Hug *et al.* (1970) documented a 5-year-old girl with increasing hepatomegaly from early infancy and no associated deficit in muscle bulk or function and no hypoglycaemia. Two needle biopsies of the liver and four of the gastrocnemius were assayed for glycogen and for various glycolytic and associated enzymes. The glycogen was increased in the liver and muscle and there was no detectable phosphorylase *a* in the muscle and it comprised less than 1% of the total phosphorylase in the liver. In both muscle and liver the total phosphorylase was normal. Normally 60% of the phosphorylase would be in the active *a* form.

Bashan *et al.* (1981) studied a 4-year-old boy found to have incidental hepatomegaly when admitted for a respiratory infection. The family history disclosed that two sisters were similarly affected, whereas an older brother was healthy. Biopsy of the patient's liver and muscle showed excess glycogen in both and a deficiency of phosphorylase kinase, the liver having 20% of the normal level and no detectable phosphorylase *a* activity, and the muscle 25% of normal and a marked decrease in phosphorylase *a* activity. Biopsy of the liver and muscle in the two affected sisters gave similar results, whereas the glycogen and enzyme levels in the healthy brother were normal. They concluded that this family were suffering from an autosomal recessive form of phosphorylase kinase deficiency involving both liver and muscle.

Ohtani *et al.* (1982) documented a 19-month-old girl who presented with hypotonia and delayed walking but had no associated hepatomegaly, cardiomegaly or other system involvement. Biopsy of the quadriceps showed small vacuoles with PAS-positive material in many fibres. Histochemical preparations revealed a marked reduction in phosphorylase *a* activity, normal total phosphorylase, and a deficiency of phosphorylase kinase activity. Biochemical analysis showed a four-fold increase in muscle glycogen, normal total phosphorylase and a reduction of phosphorylase to 10% of control values. They suggested that this case might represent a new form of phosphorylase kinase deficiency and that the variability in clinical expression might relate to the fact that the enzyme is composed of four subunits, which probably have separate genetic control.

A comprehensive review of phosphorylase kinase deficiency in man has recently been provided by van der Berg and Berger (1990). Four clinical syndromes can be recognized:

(1) Liver disease, a benign condition in infancy and childhood, usually with X-linked recessive inheritance. In the two large pedigrees documented by Huijing and Fernandes (1969), many of the 26 patients with liver phosphorylase deficiency also had mild muscle weakness but no muscle biopsies were performed. Some cases have also been described with an autosomal recessive inheritance.

(2) Liver and muscle disease. This also has an autosomal recessive inheritance, the myopathy is non-progressive and the hepatomegaly may resolve with age.

(3) Muscle disease. Some cases, such as that of Ohtani above, present with weakness in infancy, but the majority of the eight cases documented to date have presented with exercise intolerance, usually in childhood.

(4) Heart disease. Two patients with a cardio-myopathy and absence of heart phosphorylase *b* kinase have been described (Mizuta *et al.*, 1984; Servidei *et al.*, 1988b). Both, a boy and a girl, died within 6 months of birth and were diagnosed at autopsy. Phosphorylase kinase in liver, muscle and kidney was normal.

BIOCHEMISTRY

Phosphorylase *b* kinase is a multimeric enzyme composed of four different subunits, alpha and beta, which have regulatory funtion, gamma, which is catalytic, and delta, which is identical to the calcium binding protein, calmodulin. Two isoforms of the alpha subunit have been described, α and α', the latter occurring in heart and type 1 muscle fibres.

MOLECULAR GENETICS

Francke and colleagues (1989) found a single locus for the (muscle) α subunit on the X-chromosome at Xq12-q13. They presumed that the α isoforms originate from the α gene by tissue specific splicing, so that the α gene is most likely affected in the X-linked form of isolated liver phosphorylase *b* kinase deficiency. This hypothesis implies that the α subunits of the muscle and liver enzymes are different, and does not explain the commonly observed muscle hypotonia in the majority of these cases (Willems *et al.*, 1990). Francke *et al.* assigned the β subunit to chromosome 16q12-q13. Mutations leading to the autosomal recessive phosphorylase *b* kinase deficiency in both liver and muscle must be in a gene coding for a common subunit. The β gene could be a candidate provided that the mutations occur in exons common to the liver and muscle mRNAs.

The human γ gene has not yet been assigned, but animal studies suggest that the γ subunit is tissue specific so it is unlikely to be a candidate for the muscle disease.

ANIMAL MODELS

An autosomal recessive form of phosphorylase *b*

kinase deficiency has been described in the rat (Malthus *et al.*, 1980); there was enzyme deficiency and glycogen storage in the liver but the muscle was unaffected.

THERAPY

Given the clinical and biochemical similarities to phosphorylase deficiency, high protein diet might be potentially beneficial but has not yet been documented.

NEWCOMER GLYCOGENOSES

Three new glycogenoses have been recognized in recent years, all three presenting with intolerance of intense exercise and associated myoglobinuria and due to defiency of enzymes of terminal glycolysis.

TYPE IX GLYCOGENOSIS (PHOSPHOGLYCERATE KINASE DEFICIENCY)

Phosphoglycerate kinase (PGK) deficiency is an X-linked trait usually causing a non-spherocytic haemolytic anaemia but may have an associated enzyme deficit in the leucocytes and also neurological deficits, including mental retardation (Valentine *et al.*, 1969; Konrad *et al.*, 1973). No associated myopathy was recorded.

However, DiMauro *et al.* (1983) documented a deficiency of PGK in the muscle of a 14-year-old boy who developed severe pain and weakness of the calves and thighs after running for 15 minutes in the snow, followed within 2 hours by pigmenturia and 24 hours later by renal shutdown. He gradually recovered over a period of 3 weeks. From the age of 5 years he had experienced myalgia and weakness after sustained activities such as running or cycling, and at 13 years of age he had a similar but milder episode, with cramps, weakness and pigmenturia following intense exercise.

Muscle biopsy of the biceps 10 days after the episode was histologically normal, apart from some regenerating fibres, and showed no obvious excess glycogen on PAS staining. The glycogen content was also normal. A second biopsy (quadriceps) 4 months later was histologically and histochemically normal. There was marked deficiency of PGK (5% of normal mean) and the enzyme deficit was also expressed in his erythrocytes and in fibroblast and muscle cultures. All the other glycolytic enzymes were normal. Muscle biopsies (quadriceps) from his parents showed a partial deficiency in his mother (54%) but a normal level in his father, confirming an X-linked inheritance; PGK was slightly reduced in the mother's erythrocytes (about 75%) but was normal in her fibroblast and muscle cultures.

A similar case was also recorded by Rosa *et al.* (1982) in a 31-year-old man with recurrent episodes of rhabdomyolysis and acute renal failure with no associated haemolysis. He had a history since childhood of painful cramps in the legs with exercise, associated with abdominal pain, vomiting and seizures. An ischaemic exercise test produced no pain or contracture and a normal rise in venous lactate. Muscle biopsy showed no obvious abnormality or excess glycogen storage under light microscopy, but a moderate accumulation of glycogen granules under electron microscopy. A marked decrease in PGK activity (25% of normal) was found in the muscle and a deficiency down to 3% of normal in the red cells despite absence of haemolysis. The enzyme was also very low in his platelets and about 25% of the normal level in his leucocytes. All other glycolytic enzymes were normal. The patient's father had normal PGK in his red cells, whereas his mother and two daughters had intermediate levels compatible with an X-linked inheritance.

Two further cases have been documented, a 37-year-old man with muscle cramps and myoglobinuria and also a mild, slowly-progressive muscle weakness (Tonin *et al.*, 1989) and an 11-year-old boy with recurrent myoglobinuria as well as haemolytic anaemia and mental retardation (Sugie *et al.*, 1989).

BIOCHEMISTRY

PGK is a single polypeptide and there is no evidence of tissue-specific isoenzymes (except for sperm) – thus genetic mutations of this enzyme would be expected to affect all tissues. In addition, a single molecular form is expressed throughout muscle development (Miranda *et al.*, 1982), which would explain the deficit of the enzyme in cultured muscle from affected patients.

GENETICS

A full-length cDNA clone for the normal human X-linked gene has been isolated and sequenced (Michelson *et al.*, 1983) and using this cDNA as a probe Tonin *et al.* (1993) have recently documented genetic heterogeneity in two cases.

TYPE X GLYCOGENOSIS (PHOSPHOGLYCERATE MUTASE DEFICIENCY)

DiMauro *et al.* (1981) identified a deficit of phosphoglycerate mutase (5% of lowest control value) in the muscle of a 52-year-old man with intolerance for strenuous exercise and recurrent pigmenturia since adolescence. All other enzymes of glycolysis, as well as the glycogen concentration, were normal. A second case was subsequently documented by Bresolin *et al.* (1983b) in a 17-year-old girl with recurrent myoglobinuria after intense exercise. Muscle biopsy showed increased PAS staining, a glycogen level twice normal and a markedly decreased phosphoglycerate mutase activity (6% of normal mean). Intermediate enzyme levels were found in muscle biopsies from the patient's asymptomatic parents, suggesting an autosomal recessive inheritance.

Two further cases have since been reported, with patients showing similar intolerance to intense exercise, abnormally low lactate response to ischaemic forearm exercise, and a normal or moderately increased muscle glycogen together with a marked deficit of PGAM (Kissel *et al.*, 1985; Vita *et al.*, 1990).

BIOCHEMISTRY

Human PGAM is a dimeric enzyme composed of a muscle-specific (M) and brain-specific (B) subunit. Normal mature muscle contains predominantly the MM homodimer, comprising about 95% of the total activity. Cardiac muscle shows three bands of PGAM activity, a slow-migrating MM isozyme, a fast-migrating BB isozyme, and an intermediate hybrid MB band (DiMauro *et al.*, 1981, 1982; Bresolin *et al.*, 1983a). The small residual activity found in muscle biopsy specimens of all patients was exclusively BB isozyme, suggesting a genetic defect of the M subunit. The predominance of the BB isozyme in non-muscle tissues explains why symptoms of PGAM-M deficiency are confined to skeletal muscle. In heart, where the MM and MB isozymes together account for about 50% of total activity, the residual BB isozyme must be sufficient to prevent the clinical expression of cardiopathy.

GENETICS

PGAM-M deficiency is transmitted by autosomal recessive inheritance; all patients were isolated cases,

but partial PGAM deficiency was documented in the parents of Bresolin's patient (Bresolin *et al.*, 1983b). A full-length cDNA (Shanske *et al.*, 1987) and the genomic clone containing the entire gene for PGAM-M (Tsujino *et al.*, 1989) have been isolated and sequenced, and the gene has been localized to chromosome 7 (Edwards *et al.*, 1989). In three patients, Tsujino *et al.* (1993b) found a G-to-A transition at codon position 78 of PGAM-M, converting an encoded tryptophan (TGG) to a stop codon (TAG).

TYPE XI GLYCOGENOSIS (LACTATE DEHYDROGENASE DEFICIENCY)

Kanno *et al.* (1980) documented a complete absence of the M subunit of lactate dehydrogenase (LDH) in an 18-year-old male with a 2-year history of fatiguability after hard exercise and pigmenturia 10 to 12 hours later. Serum enzyme levels during a period of myoglobinuria after exercise showed a marked increase in CK (26290 iu/litre) as well as aspartate and alanine aminotransferase, but only a slight elevation of LDH. Electrophoretic separation of LDH isoenzymes from serum, erythrocytes, leukocytes and vastus intermedius muscle showed a similar pattern, with only one band present (H_4, LDH_1) in place of the usual five bands. A similar single band was shown in the serum and erythrocytes of three symptom-free siblings of the propositus and a partial absence of the M subunit in two remaining siblings and the parents, suggesting a heterozygote state in them and an autosomal recessive inheritance. Ischaemic exercise of the forearm produced fatiguability within 25 seconds and a contracture after 60 seconds. There was only a slight transitory rise in lactate (well below the normal response) immediately after the ischaemia but a very marked rise in pyruvate, and after 5–12 hours a marked rise in serum CK and associated myoglobinuria.

A second, similar case has recently been reported by Bryan *et al.* (1990).

BIOCHEMISTRY

LDH is a tetrameric enzyme composed of two subunits, one (M) predominant in skeletal muscle, the other (H) predominant in heart muscle. Random tetramerization results in the formation of five isozymes, the two homotetramers M4 and H4, and three heterotetramers, M3H, M2H2, and MH3. In tissues from patients, only the homotetramer H4 was detected, suggesting a defect of LDH-M. The small residual LDH activity (about 5% of normal) present in muscle of patients corresponds to the proportion of LDH-H4 present in normal muscle. Bicycle ergometer studies in the second patient showed that maximal exercise raised blood pyruvate but not lactate, with a paradoxical fall of the lactate to pyruvate ratio.

GENETICS

Biochemical studies in the family members of Kanno's patient showed that the defect was inherited as an autosomal recessive trait. The location of the gene for the human LDH-M subunit has been established on chromosome 11 (Boone *et al.*, 1972).

OTHER GLYCOGENOSES

There have been several reports in the literature of glycogenoses with possible muscle involvement, in which the enzyme defect has not been clearly delineated.

LYSOSOMAL GLYCOGEN STORAGE WITH CARDIOMYOPATHY, MENTAL RETARDATION, VACUOLAR MYOPATHY AND NORMAL ACID MALTASE

Danon *et al.* (1981b) documented two unrelated 16-year-old boys with mental retardation, cardio-megaly and proximal myopathy, whose muscle showed lysosomal glycogen storage resembling acid maltase deficiency but with normal acid maltase levels and no other demonstrable enzyme deficiency associated with glycogen storage. A number of similar cases have subsequently been published (Riggs *et al.*, 1983; Bergia *et al.*, 1986; Byrne *et al.*, 1986; Hart *et al.*, 1987; Bru *et al.*, 1988; Tachi *et al.*, 1989). The syndrome seems to be of childhood onset, affecting predominantly males and characterized by a severe hypertrophic cardiomyopathy, a mild and relatively stable myopathy and mental retardation of variable degree. Affected female relatives appear to have only cardiomyopathy.

In the recently reported family of Dworzak *et al.* (1994) the patient had toe-walking and difficulty running since infancy, and fatigue and cramps after exercise. He never attended school and was unable to read or write. At 23 years he had two bouts of syncope, which revealed an underlying hypertrophic cardiomyopathy with arrhythmia and heart block. A pacemaker was inserted. Skeletal muscle biopsy showed a vacuolar myopathy with PAS-positive material and acid phosphatase activity and on electron microscopy resembled autophagic vacuoles with membranous bodies and degraded organelles, plus high levels of lysosomal and free glycogen. He subsequently went into cardiac failure again and needed a heart transplant. The explanted heart showed similar histological changes to the skeletal muscle but with more severe tissue disruption. His mother died of heart disease at 41 years, an older brother was said to be similarly affected to him and died suddenly at the age of 20 years, and one of his sisters was also found to have a cardiomyopathy, after her 10-year-old son was found to have a cardiomyopathy, mild mental retardation and a mild myopathy with biopsy changes similar to his uncle.

In another family recently documented by Muntoni *et al.* (1994), the patient presented at 23 years with cardiac failure and had associated mental retardation and a clumsy gait, bilateral pes cavus plus rigidity of the lumbar spine and mild thoracic scoliosis. A similarly affected brother had been investigated previously for advanced cardiac failure and had died suddenly at 24 years. The mother, grandmother, great-grandmother and a maternal aunt had died suddenly at 46, 61, 58 and 57 years of age, and had no mental retardation, whereas three maternal male cousins had the full-blown syndrome and died suddenly at 24, 22 and 23 years respectively. The muscle biopsy of the patient showed vacuoles in about 30% of fibres, but only a minority were weakly positive for PAS and, unlike lysosomes, they were acid phosphatase negative. Moreover, the vacuoles were positively stained by anti-dystrophin and anti-spectrin antibodies, suggesting that the vacuoles may have derived from splitting of fibres or invagination of the sarcolemmal membrane. This was supported by electron microscopic observations of continuity of the membrane forming the vacuole with the plasma membrane. They also found desmin-type intermediate filaments in the vacuoles. Similar changes were found in a cardiac muscle biopsy.

The inheritance in these families seems X-linked dominant, but an autosomal dominant with variable expression in the sexes cannot be completely excluded, although there are no recorded cases of male to male transmission.

It is also still questionable whether this is a glycogenosis at all, or whether the underlying pathology may be a vacuolar myopathy and the glycogen accumulation a secondary component. The clinical picture seems very different from the X-linked myopathy with autophagic vacuoles (see Chapter 3).

MYOADENYLATE DEAMINASE DEFICIENCY (AMP DEAMINASE DEFICIENCY)

This sarcoplasmic enzyme catalyses the irreversible deamination of adenosine monophosphate (AMP) to inosine monophosphate (IMP) and leads to the production of ammonia in muscle, which accompanies the rise of lactic acid during muscle contraction. Its function in muscle may be the removal of AMP to maintain a high ratio of adenosine triphosphate (ATP) to adenosine diphosphate (ADP) during strenuous muscular activity.

Fishbein *et al.* (1978) first drew attention to the absence of myoadenylate deaminase activity by histochemical reaction in five of 250 muscle biopsies. Four of these patients had some intolerance of exercise with cramps, stiffness or pain. Shumate *et al.* (1979) subsequently confirmed the fairly common occurrence of the enzyme defect in six of 256 of their biopsies examined. However, they questioned its pathogenetic significance since only two of the six patients had exercise-related symptoms, whereas three had apparently unrelated myopathic or neurogenic disorders and one had myoglobinuria after a viral illness. The significance of the biochemical abnormality thus seemed uncertain and it was difficult to know whether it reflected a genuine and possibly genetically determined disorder or was merely an enzyme deficiency in search of a disease.

Kelemen *et al.* (1982) studied four families with exertional myalgia and found histochemical and biochemical absence of AMP deaminase in the muscle biopsies of five of eight symptomatic individuals, normal activity (biochemically) in two and intermediate activity in the remaining one. Asymptomatic relatives had normal histochemical activity but three had intermediate biochemical levels. In a separate analysis of 302 routine biopsies, three of the 36 patients presenting with myalgia had absence of AMP deaminase compared with three of the 266 patients biopsied for other conditions. They concluded that, despite the inconsistencies, AMP deaminase deficiency does seem to have some relevance to the syndrome of exertional myalgia. Fishbein *et al.* (1984) subsequently produced evidence for a possible carrier state of adenylate deaminase deficiency. They compared by histochemistry and quantitative biochemical assay muscle biopsies from three putative carriers and 34 control biopsies without notable abnormalities. The carriers had a 2.5 to 5.7 times lower adenylate deaminase level than the mean control level but were still at least 20 times higher than their enzyme-deficient kinsfolk.

Since Fishbein's original report, some 180 additional cases have been recorded in the literature, with varying amounts of useful clinical data on individual cases. Whilst a substantial proportion had exertional myalgia and fatigue, comparable with the original cases, more than half had other associated neuromuscular disorders, or non-neuromuscular disorders. The subject has recently been exhaustively reviewed and critically analysed by Sabina (1993). Of the 187 documented cases with AMP deaminase deficiency, 85 (45%) had no other identifiable laboratory abnormality in their muscle, and in 77 of these there was exertional myalgia and fatigue. This suggested a cause and effect relationship between these two findings.

In contrast, associated or secondary AMP deaminase deficiency has been found in the biopsies of a wide range of neuropathies, myopathies, dystrophies, collagen vascular diseases and also other metabolic myopathies, which have dominated the clinical picture.

BIOCHEMISTRY

Three isoforms of AMP deaminase have been identified, muscle (M), liver (L) and erythrocyte (E1,E2) (Ogasawara *et al.*, 1982). The M isozyme is confined to skeletal muscle, where it is developmentally regulated.

GENETICS

There is circumstantial evidence for an autosomal recessive inheritance of AMP deaminase deficiency. The gene (AMPD1) for the muscle isozyme (mAMPD) has been localized to chromosome 1p13-p21 (Sabina *et al.*, 1990) and comprises 16 exons. Southern blot analysis in 10 cases of mAMPD deficiency has demonstrated a normal restriction pattern (Hind III), thus excluding large structural abnormalities in the AMPD1 gene as a basis for the defect (Gross *et al.*, 1990) and suggesting that a point mutation is more likely. Recently Morisaki *et al.* (1992) found a single nonsense mutation in 11 unrelated families.

REFERENCES

Andersen, D. H. (1952) Studies on glycogen disease with report of a case in which the glycogen was abnormal. In: Najjar, V. A. ed., *Carbohydrate Metabolism*. Baltimore: Johns Hopkins Press, pp. 28–42.

Andersen, D. H. (1956) Familial cirrhosis of the liver with storage of abnormal glycogen. *Laboratory Investigation* **5**: 11.

Argov, Z. and Bank, W.J. (1991) Phosphorus magnetic resonance spectroscopy (^{31}P MRS) in neuromuscular disorders. *Annals of Neurology* **30**: 90–97.

Argov, Z., Bank, W.J., Maris, J. *et al.* (1987) Muscle energy metabolism in McArdle's syndrome by *in vivo* phosphorus magnetic resonance spectroscopy. *Neurology* **37**: 1720–1724.

Bashan, N., Iancu, T.C., Lerner, A. *et al.* (1981) Glycogenosis due to liver and muscle phosphorylase kinase deficiency. *Pediatric Research* **15**: 299–303.

Bergia, B., Sybers, H.D. and Butler, I.J. (1986) Familial lethal cardiomyopathy with mental retardation and scapuloperoneal muscular dystrophy. *Journal of Neurology, Neurosurgery and Psychiatry* **49**: 1423–1426.

Bonilla, E. and Schotland, D.L. (1970) Histochemical diagnosis of muscle phosphofructokinase deficiency. *Archives of Neurology* **22**: 8–12.

Boone, C.M., Chen, T.R. and Ruddle, F.H. (1972) Assignment of three human genes to chromosomes (LDH-A to 11, TK to 17, and IDH to 20) and evidence for translocation between human and mouse chromosomes in somatic cell hybrids. *Proceedings of the National Academy of Sciences of the USA* **69**: 510–514.

Brandt, I. K. and DeLuca, V. A. Jr (1966) Type III glycogenosis. A family with an unusual tissue distribution of the enzyme lesion. *American Journal of Medicine* **40**: 779–784.

Bresolin, N., Miranda, A.F., Jacobson, M.P. *et al.* (1983a) Phosphorylase isoenzymes of human brain. *Neurochemical Pathology* **1**: 171–178.

Bresolin, N., Ro, Y., Reyes, M. *et al.* (1983b) Muscle phosphoglycerate mutase (PGAM) deficiency: A second case. *Neurology* **33**: 1049–1053.

Brombacher, P. J., van Creveld, S., Damme, J. P., Huijing, F. and Ploem, J. E. (1964) A report on two adult patients with glycogen storage disease. *Acta Medica Scandinavica* **176**: 269–276.

Brown, B. I. and Brown, D. H. (1966) Lack of an alpha-1, 4-glucan: alpha-1, 4-glucan 6-glycosyl transferase in a case of type IV glycogenosis. *Proceedings of the National Academy of Sciences of the USA* **56**: 725.

Brown, B. I. and Brown, D. H. (1968) Glycogen-storage diseases. Types I, III, IV, V, VII and unclassified glycogenoses. In: Dickens, F., Randle, P. J. and Whelan, W. J. eds, *Carbohydrate Metabolism and its Disorders* Vol. 2. London and New York: Academic Press, p. 123.

Bru, P., Pellissier, J.F., Gatau-Pelanchon, J. *et al.* (1988) Glycogenose lysosomiale cardio-musculaire de l'adulte sans déficit enizmatique connu. *Archives des Maladies du Coeur* **1**: 109–114.

Brunberg, J.A., McCormick, W.F. and Schochet, S.S. Jr. (1971) Type III glycogenosis: an adult with diffuse weakness and muscle wasting. *Archives of Neurology (Chicago)* **25**: 171–178.

Bryan, W., Lewis, S.F., Bertocci, I. *et al.* (1990) Muscle lactate dehydrogenase deficiency: A disorder of anaerobic glycogenolysis associated with exertional myoglobinuria. *Neurology* **40** (Suppl 1): 203.

Byrne, E., Dennett, X., Crotty, B. *et al.* (1986) Dominantly inherited cardioskeletal myopathy with lysosomal glycogen storage and normal acid maltese levels. *Brain* **109**: 523–536.

Cafferty, M.S., Lovelace, R.E., Hays, A.P. *et al.* (1991) Polyglucosan body disease. *Muscle and Nerve*, **14**: 102–107.

Caudwell, F.B. and Cohen, P. (1980) Purification and subunit structure of glycogen-branching enzyme from rabbit skeletal muscle. *European Journal of Biochemistry* **109**: 391–394.

Chui, L.A. and Munsat, T.L. (1976) Dominant inheritance of McArdle syndrome. *Archives of Neurology* **33**: 636–641.

Cori, G. T. (1958) Biochemical aspects of glycogen deposition disease. In: Hottinger, A., Hauser, F. and Berger, H. eds, *Modern Problems in Paediatrics* Vol. 3. Bibliotheca Paediatricia, Fascicle No. 66. Basel: Karger, pp. 344–358.

Cori, G. T. and Cori, C. F. (1952) Glucose-6-phosphatase of the liver in glycogen storage disease. *Journal of Biological Chemistry* **199**: 661–667.

Cornelio, F., Bresolin, N., DiMauro, S. *et al.* (1983) Congenital myopathy due to phosphorylase deficiency. *Neurology* **33**: 1383–1385.

Cornelio, F., Bresolin, N., Singer, P.A. *et al.* (1984) The clinical varieties of neuromuscular disease in debrancher deficiency. *Archives of Neurology* **41**: 1027–1032.

Courtecuisse, V., Royer, P., Habib, R., Monnier, C. and Demos, J. (1965) Glycogénose musculaire par déficit d'alpha-1, 4-glucosidase simulant une dystrophie musculaire progressive. *Archives Françaises de Pédiatrie* **22**: 1153.

Crerar, M.M., Hudson, J.W., Matthews, K.E. *et al.* (1988) Studies on the expression and evolution of the glycogen phosphorylase gene family in the rat. *Genome* **30**: 582–590.

D'Ancona, G.G., Wurm, J. and Croce, C. (1979) Genetics of type II glycogenosis: Assignment of the human gene for acid alpha-glucosidase to chromosome 17. *Proceedings of the National Academy of Sciences of the USA* **76**: 4526–4529.

Danon, M.J., Carpenter, S., Manaligod, J.R. *et al.* (1981a) Fatal infantile glycogen storage disease: deficiency of phosphofructokinase and phosphorylase b kinase. *Neurology* **31**: 1303–1307.

Danon, M.J., Oh, S.J., DiMauro, S. *et al.* (1981b) Lysosomal glycogen storage disease with normal acid maltase. *Neurology* **31**: 51–57.

Davidson, M., Miranda, A.F., Bender, A. *et al.* (1983a) Muscle phosphofructokinase deficiency: Biochemical and immunological studies of phosphofructokinase isoenzymes in muscle culture. *Journal of Clinical Investigation* **72**: 545–550.

Davidson, M., Collins, M., Byrne, J. *et al.* (1983b) Alterations in phosphofructokinase isoenzymes during early human development. *Biochemical Journal* **214**: 703–710.

De Barsy, Th., Jacquemin, P., Van Hoof, F. *et al.* (1973) Enzyme replacement in Pompe's disease. An attempt with purified human acid alpha-glucosidase. *Birth Defects* **9**: 184–190.

DiMauro, S. and Hartlage, P.L. (1978) Fatal infantile form of muscle phosphorylase deficiency. *Neurology* **28**: 1124–1129.

DiMauro, S. and Servidei, S. (1993) Disorders of carbohydrate metabolism: glycogen storage diseases. In: Rosenberg, R.N., Prusiner, S.B., DiMauro, S. *et al.* eds, *The Molecular and Genetic Basis of Neurological Disease.* Boston: Butterworth-Heinemann, pp. 93–119.

DiMauro, S., Arnold, S., Miranda, A.F. *et al.* (1978) McArdle disease: The mystery of reappearing phosphorylase activity in muscle culture. A fetal isoenzyme. *Annals of Neurology* **3**: 60–66.

DiMauro, S., Hartwig, G.B., Hays, A.P. *et al.* (1979) Debrancher deficiency: Neuromuscular disorder in five adults. *Annals of Neurology* **5**: 422–436.

DiMauro, S., Miranda, A.F., Khan, S. *et al.* (1981) Human muscle phosphoglycerate mutase deficiency: A new cause of recurrent myoglobinuria. *Science* **212**: 1277–1279.

DiMauro, S., Miranda, A.F., Olarte, M. *et al.* (1982) Muscle phosphoglycerate mutase deficiency. *Neurology* **32**: 548–591.

DiMauro, S., Dalakas, M. and Miranda, A.F. (1983) Phosphoglycerate kinase deficiency: another cause of recurrent myoglobinuria. *Annals of Neurology* **13**: 11–19.

Ding, J-H., Harris, D.A., Yang, B-Z. *et al.* (1989) Cloning of cDNA for human glycogen debrancher, the enzyme deficient in type III glycogen storage disease (GSD-III). *Pediatric Research* **25**: 140A.

Dupond, J.L., Robert, M., Carbillet, J.P. *et al.* (1977) Glycogénose musculaire et anémie hémolytique par déficit enzymatique chez deux germains. Forme familiale de maladie de Tarui, par déficit en phosphofructokinase musculaire et érythrocytaire. *Nouvelle Presse Médicale* **6**: 2665.

Dworzak, F., Casazza, F., Mora, M. *et al.* (1994) Lysosomal glycogen storage with normal acid maltase: a familial study with successful heart transplant. *Neuromuscular Disorders* **4**: 243–247.

Edwards, Y.H., Sakoda, S., Schon, E.A. *et al.* (1989) The gene for human muscle-specific phosphoglycerate mutase, PGAMM, mapped to chromosome 7 by polymerase chain reaction. *Genomics* **5**: 948–951.

Engel, A.G. (1970) Acid maltase deficiency in adults: studies in four cases of a syndrome which may mimic muscular dystrophy or other myopathies. *Brain* **93**: 599–616.

Farrans, V.J., Hibbs, R.G., Walsh, J.J. *et al.* (1966) Cardiomyopathy, cirrhosis of the liver and deposits of a fibrillar polysaccharide. *American Journal of Cardiology* **17**: 457–469.

Fernandes. J. and Huijing, F. (1968) Branching enzyme-deficiency glycogenosis. Studies in therapy. *Archives of Disease in Childhood* **43**: 347–352.

Fernandes. J. and van de Kamer, J. H. (1968) Hexose and protein tolerance tests in children with liver glycogenosis caused by a deficiency of the debranching enzyme system. *Pediatrics* **41**: 935.

Fishbein, W.N., Armbrustmacher, V.W. and Griffin, J.L. (1978) Myoadenylate deaminase deficiency: A new disease of muscle. *Science* **200**: 545–548.

Fishbein, W.N., Armbrustmacher, V.W., Griffin, J.L. *et al.* (1984) Levels of adenylate deaminase, adenylate kinase, and creatine kinase in frozen human muscle biopsy specimens relative to type 1/type 2 fiber distribution: evidence for a carrier state of myoadenylate deaminase deficiency. *Annals of Neurology* **15**: 271–277.

Forbes, G. B. (1953) Glycogen storage disease. Report of a case with abnormal glycogen structure in liver and skeletal muscle. *Journal of Pediatrics* **42**: 645.

Francke, U., Darras, B.T., Zander, N.F. *et al.* (1989) Assignment of human genes for phosphorylase kinase subunits α (PHKA) to Xq12-q13 and β (PHKB) to 16q12-q13. *American Journal of Human Genetics* **45**: 276–282.

Giger, U., Harvey, J.W., Yamaguchi, R.A. *et al.* (1985) Inherited phosphofructokinase deficiency in dogs with hyperventilation-induced hemolysis: Increased *in vitro* and *in vivo* alkaline fragility of erythrocytes. *Blood* **65**: 345–351.

Giger, U., Argov, Z., Schnall, M. *et al.* (1988) Metabolic myopathy in canine muscle-type phospho-fructokinase deficiency. *Muscle and Nerve* **11**: 1260–1265.

Greene, H.L., Brown, B.I., McClenathan, D.T. *et al.* (1988a) A new variant of type IV glycogenosis: Deficiency of branching enzyme activity without apparent progressive liver disease. *Hepatology* **8**: 302–306.

Greene, H.L., Ghishan, F.K., Brown, B.I. *et al.* (1988b) Type IV glycogenosis: Improvement in two patients treated by maintenance of normal blood glucose levels. *Journal of Pediatrics* **112**: 55–58.

Gross, M., Morisaki, T., Pongratz, D. *et al.* (1990) Normal restriction pattern (Hind III) of the myoadenylate deaminase gene in enzyme deficient patients. *Klinische Wochenschrift* **68**: 1084.

Guerra, A.S., van Diggelen, O.P., Carneiro, F. *et al.* (1986) A juvenile variant of glycogenosis IV (Andersen disease). *European Journal of Pediatrics* **145**: 179–181.

Guibaud, P., Carrier, H., Mathieu, M. *et al.* (1978) Observation familiale de dystrophie musculaire congénitale par déficit en phosphofructokinase. *Archives Françaises de Pédiatrie* **35**: 1105.

Harris, R.E., Hannon, D., Vogler, C. *et al.* (1986) Bone marrow transplantation in type IIa glycogen storage disease. *Birth Defects* **22**: 119–132.

Hart, Z.H., Servidei, S., Peterson, P.L. *et al.* (1987) Cardiomyopathy, mental retardation and autophagic vacuolar myopathy. *Neurology* **37**: 1065–1068.

Hers, H. G. (1959) Etudes enzymatiques sur fragments hepatiques: application à la classification des glycogénoses. *Revue Internationale d'Hepatologie* **9**: 35.

Hers, H. G. (1963) α-Glucosidase deficiency in generalised glycogen-storage disease (Pompe's disease). *Biochemical Journal* **86**: 11.

Hers, H. G. (1964) Glycogen storage disease. *Advances in Metabolic Diseases* **1**: 1.

Hoefsloot, L.H., Hoogeveen-Westerveld, M., Kroos, M.A. *et al.* (1988) Primary structure and processing of lysosomal alpha-glucosidase: Homology with the intestinal sucrase-isomaltase complex. *EMBO Journal* 7: 1697–1704.

Holleman, L. W. J., van der Haar, J. A. and de Vaan, G. A. M. (1966) Type IV glycogenosis. *Laboratory Investigation* 15: 357.

Hoogerbrugge, P.M., Wagemaker, G., van Bekkum, D.W. *et al.* (1986) Bone marrow transplantation for Pompe's disease. *New England Journal of Medicine* 315: 65–66.

Howell, J.McC., Dorling, P.R., Cook, R.D. *et al.* (1981) Infantile and late-onset form of generalised glycogenosis type II in cattle. *Journal of Pathology* 134: 266–267.

Howell, J.McC., Dorling, P.R., Shelton, J.N. *et al.* (1991) Natural bone marrow transplantation in cattle with Pompe's disease. *Neuromuscular Disorders* 1: 449–454.

Hudgson, P., Gardner-Medwin, D., Worsfold, M., Pennington, R. J. T. and Walton, J. N. (1968) Adult myopathy from glycogen storage disease due to acid maltase deficiency. *Brain* 91: 435–462.

Hug, G. (1974) Enzyme therapy and prenatal diagnosis in glycogenosis type II. *American Journal of Diseases of Children* 128: 607–609.

Hug, G., Garancis, J.C., Schubert, W.K. *et al.* (1966) Glycogen storage disease, types II, III, VIII and IX. A biochemical and electron microscopic analysis. *American Journal of Diseases in Children* 111: 457–474.

Hug, G., Schubert, W.K. and Chuck, G. (1970) Loss of cyclic 3′5′-AMP dependent kinase and reduction of phosphorylase kinase in skeletal muscle of a girl with deactivated phosphorylase and glycogenosis of liver and muscle. *Biochemical and Biophysical Research Communications* 40: 982–988.

Hug, G., Harris, R., Hannon, D. *et al.* (1984) Bone marrow transplant in glycogen storage disease type IIa. *Clinical Research* 32: 560A (abstract).

Huijing, F. and Fernandes, J. (1969) X-Chromosomal inheritance of liver glycogenosis with phosphorylase kinase deficiency. *American Journal of Human Genetics* 21: 275–284.

Illingworth, B. and Cori, G. T. (1952) Structure of glycogens and amylopectins. III. Normal and abnormal human glycogen. *Journal of Biological Chemistry* 199: 653.

Illingworth, B., Cori, G. T. and Cori, C. F. (1956) Amylo-1,6-glucosidase in muscle tissue in generalised glycogen storage disease. *Journal of Biological Chemistry* 218: 123.

Isaacs, H., Savage, N., Badenhorst, M. *et al.* (1986) Acid maltase deficiency: A case study and review of the pathophysiological changes and proposed therapeutic measures. *Journal of Neurology Neurosurgery and Psychiatry* 49: 1011–1018.

Isch, F., Juif, J. G., Sacrez, R. and Thiébaut, F. (1966) Glycogénose musculaire à forme myopathique par déficit en maltase acid. *Pédiatrie* 21: 71–86.

Jensen, K.E., Jakobsen, J., Thomsen, C. *et al.* (1990) Improved energy kinetics following high protein diet in McArdle's syndrome. A ^{31}P magnetic resonance spectroscopy study. *Acta Neurologica Scandinavica* 81: 499–503.

Kanno, T., Sudo, K., Takeuchi, I. *et al.* (1980) Hereditary deficiency of lactate dehydrogenase M-subunit. *Clinica Chimica Acta* 108: 267–276.

Keleman, J., Rice, D.R., Bradley, W.G. *et al.* (1982) Familial myoadenylate deaminase deficiency and exertional myalgia. *Neurology* 32: 857–863.

Kissel, J.T., Beam, W., Bresolin, N. *et al.* (1985) Physiologic assessment of phosphoglycerate mutase deficiency. *Neurology* 35: 828–833.

Konrad, P.M., McCarthy, D.J., Mauer, A.M. *et al.* (1973) Erythrocyte and leukocyte phosphoglycerate kinase deficiency with neurologic disease. *Journal of Pediatrics* 82: 456–460.

Lauer, R.M., Mascarinas, T., Racela, A.S. *et al.* (1968) Administration of a mixture of fungal glucosidases to a patient with type II glycogenosis (Pompe's disease). *Pediatrics* 42: 672–676.

Layzer, R. B., Rowland, L. P. and Ranney, H. M. (1967) Muscle phosphofructokinase deficiency. *Archives of Neurology* 17: 512.

Lebo, R.V., Gorin, F., Fletterick, R.J. *et al.* (1984) High-resolution chromosome sorting and DNA spot-blot analysis assign McArdle's syndrome to chromosome 11. *Science* 225: 57–59.

Lebo, R.V., Anderson, L.A., DiMauro, S. *et al.* (1990) Rare McArdle disease locus polymorphic site on 11q13 contains CpG sequences. *Human Genetics* 86: 17–24.

Lossos, A., Barash, V., Soffer, D. *et al.* (1991) Hereditary branching enzyme dysfunction in adult polyglucosan body disease *Annals of Neurology* 30: 655–662.

Malthus, R., Clark, D.G., Watts, C. *et al.* (1990) Glycogen-storage disease in rats, a genetically determined deficiency of liver phosphorylase kinase. *Biochemical Journal* 188: 99–106.

Margolis, M.L. and Hill, A.R. (1986) Acid maltase deficiency in an adult. *American Review of Respiratory Diseases* 134: 328–331.

Martiniuk, F., Ellenbogen, A., Hirschhorn, K. *et al.* (1985) Further regional localization of the genes for human acid alpha glucosidase (GAA), peptidase D (PEPD), and alpha mannosidase B (MANB) by somatic cell hybridization. *Human Genetics* 69: 109–111.

Martiniuk, F., Mehler, M., Tzall, S. *et al.* (1990a) Sequence of the cDNA and 5′-flanking region from human acid alpha-glucosidase, detection of an intron in the 5′untranslated leader sequence, definition of 18-bp polymorphisms, and differences with previous cDNA and amino acid sequence. *DNA Cell Biology* 9: 85–94.

Martiniuk, F., Mehler, M., Tzall, S. *et al.* (1990b) Extensive genetic heterogeneity in patients with alpha glucosidase deficiency as detected by abnormalities of DNA and mRNA. *American Journal of Human Genetics* 47: 73–78.

McArdle, B. (1951) Myopathy due to a defect in muscle glycogen breakdown. *Clinical Science* 10: 13.

McConchie, S.M., Coakley, J., Edwards, R.H.T. *et al.*

(1991) Molecular heterogeneity in McArdle's disease. *Biochimica et Biophysica Acta* **1096**: 26–32.

Mehler, M. and DiMauro, S. (1977) Residual acid maltase activity in late-onset acid maltase deficiency. *Neurology* **27**: 178–184.

Mellick, R. S., Mahler, R. F. and Hughes, B. P. (1962) McArdle's syndrome. Phosphorylase deficient myopathy. *Lancet* **i**: 1045.

Michelson, A.M., Markham, A.F. and Orkin, S.H. (1983) Isolation and DNA sequence of a full-length cDNA clone for human X chromosome encoded phosphoglycerate kinase. *Proceedings of the National Academy of Sciences of the USA* **80**: 472–476.

Miller, C.G., Alleyne, G.A. and Brooks, S.E.H. (1972) Gross cardiac involvement in glycogen storage disease type III. *British Heart Journal* **34**: 862–864.

Milstein, J.M., Herron, T.M. and Haas, J.E. (1989) Fatal infantile phosphorylase deficiency. *Journal of Child Neurology* **4**: 186–188.

Miranda, A.F., Nette, E.G., Hartlage, P.L. *et al.* (1979) Phosphorylase isoenzymes in normal and myophosphorylase-deficient human heart. *Neurology* **29**: 1538–1541.

Miranda, A.F., Shanske, S. and DiMauro, S. (1982) Developmentally regulated isozyme transitions in normal and diseased muscle. In: Pearson, M.L. and Epstein, H.F. eds, *Muscle Development: Molecular and Cellular Control*. New York: Cold Spring Harbor Laboratory, pp. 515–525.

Mizuta, K., Hashimoto, E., Tsutou, A. *et al.* (1984) A new type of glycogen storage disease caused by deficiency of cardiac phosphorylase kinase. *Biochemical and Biophysical Research Communications* **119**: 582–587.

Mommaerts, W. F. H. M., Illingworth, B., Pearson, C. M., Guillory, R. J. and Seraydarian, K. (1959) A functional disorder of muscle associated with the absence of phosphorylase. *Proceedings of the National Academy of Sciences of the USA* **45**: 791.

Morisaki, T., Gross, M., Morisaki, H. *et al.* (1992) Molecular basis of AMP deaminase deficiency in skeletal muscle. *Proceedings of the National Academy of Sciences of the USA* **89**: 6457–6471.

Moses, S.W., Gadoth, N., Bashan, N. *et al.* (1986) Neuromuscular involvement in glycogen storage disease type III. *Acta Pediatrica Scandinavica* **5**: 289–296.

Moses, S.W., Wanderman, K.L., Myroz, A. *et al.* (1989) Cardiac involvement in glycogen storage disease type III. *European Journal of Pediatrics* **148**: 764–756.

Muntoni, F., Catani, G., Mateddu, A. *et al.* (1994) Familial cardiomyopathy, mental retardation and myopathy associated with desmin-type intermediate filaments. *Neuromuscular Disorders* **4**: 233–241.

Nakajima, H., Noguchi, T., Yamasaki, T. *et al.* (1978) Cloning of human muscle phosphofructokinase cDNA. *FEBS Letters* **223**: 113–116.

Nakajima, H., Kono, N., Yamasaki, T. *et al.* (1990) Genetic defect in muscle phosphofructokinase deficiency. *Journal of Biological Chemistry* **265**: 9292–9395.

Nickel, B.E., Chudley, A.E., Pabello, P.D. *et al.* (1982) Exclusion mapping of the GAA locus to chromosome 17q21-q25. *Cytogenetics and Cell Genetics* **32**: 303–304.

Niermeijer, M.F., Koster, J.F., Jahodova, M. *et al.* (1975) Prenatal diagnosis of type II glycogenosis (Pompe's disease) using microchemical analysis. *Pediatric Research* **9**: 498.

Ogasawara, N., Goto, H., Yamada, Y. *et al.* (1982) AMP deaminase isozymes in human tissues. *Biochimica et Biophysica Acta* **714**: 298–306.

Ohtani, Y., Matsuda, I., Iwamasa, T. *et al.* (1982) Infantile glycogen storage myopathy in a girl with phosphorylase kinase deficiency. *Neurology (NY)* **32**: 833–838.

Oliner, L., Schulman, M. and Larner, J. (1961) Myopathy associated with glycogen deposition resulting from generalized lack of amylo-1, 6-glucosidase. *Clinical Research* **9**: 243.

Papadimitriou, A., Manta, P., Divari, R. *et al.* (1990) McArdle's disease: Two clinical expressions in the same pedigree. *Journal of Neurology* **237**: 267–270.

Pearson, C. M. (1968) Glycogen metabolism and storage diseases of types III, IV and V. *American Journal of Clinical Pathology* **50**: 29–43.

Pearson, C. M., Rimer, D. G. and Mommaerts, W. F. (1959) Defect in muscle phosphorylase: a newly defined human disease. *Clinical Research* **7**: 298.

Pearson, C. M., Rimer, D. and Mommaerts, W. F. H. M. (1961) A metabolic myopathy due to absence of muscle phosphorylase. *American Journal of Medicine* **30**: 502.

Pompe, J. C. (1933) Hypertrophie idiopathique du coeur. *Annales d'Anatomie Pathologique* **10**: 23.

Powell, H.C., Haas, R., Hall, C.H. *et al.* (1985) Peripheral nerve in type III glycogenosis: Selective involvement of unmyelinated fiber Schwann cells. *Muscle and Nerve* **8**: 667–671.

Ratinov, G., Baker, W.P. and Swaiman, K. E. (1965) McArdle's syndrome with previously unreported electrocardiographic and serum enzyme abnormalities. *Annals of Internal Medicine* **62**: 328.

Reed, G.B.Jr, Dixon, J.F.P., Neustein, H.B., Donnell, G.N. and Landing, B. H. (1968) Type IV glycogenosis. Patient with absence of a branching enzyme α-1, 4-glucan: β-1, 4-glucan 6-glycosyl transferase. *Laboratory Investigation* **19**: 546.

Riggs, J.E., Schochet, S.S., Gutman, L. *et al.* (1983) Lysosomal glycogen storage disease without acid maltase deficiency. *Neurology* **33**: 773–877.

Roelofs, R.I., Engel, W.K. and Chauvin, P.B. (1967) Histochemical phosphorylase activity in regenerating muscle fibers from myophosphorylase-deficient patients. *Science* **177**: 795–797.

Rosa, R., George, C., Fardeau, M. *et al.* (1982) A new case of phosphoglycerate kinase deficiency: PGK creteil associated with rhabdomyolysis and lacking hemolytic anemia. *Blood* **60**: 84–91.

Rosenow, E.C. and Engel, A.G. (1978) Acid maltase deficiency in adults presenting as respiratory failure. *American Journal of Medicine* **64**: 485–491.

Rowland, L.P., Fahn, S. and Schotland, D.L. (1963) McArdle's disease: hereditary myopathy due to absence of muscle phosphorylase. *Archives of Neurology* 9: 325.

Rowland, L.P., Lovelace, R.E., Schotland, D.L. Araki, S. and Carmel, P. (1966) The clinical diagnosis of McArdle's disease. Identification of another family with deficiency of muscle phosphorylase. *Neurology (Minneapolis)* 16: 93.

Sabina, R. (1993) Myoadenylate deaminase deficiency. In: Rosenberg, R.N., Prusiner, S.B., DiMauro, S. *et al.* eds, *The Molecular and Genetic Basis of Neurological Disease*. Boston: Butterworth-Heinemann, pp. 261–275.

Sabina, R.L., Morisaki, T., Clarke, P. *et al.* (1990) Characterization of the human and rat myoadenylate deaminase genes. *Journal of Biological Chemistry* 265: 9423–9433.

Salter, R.H., Adamson, D.G. and Pearce, G.W. (1967) McArdle's syndrome (myophosphorylase deficiency). *Quarterly Journal of Medicine* 36: 565.

Sato, K., Imai, F., Hatayama, I. *et al.* (1977) Characterization of glycogen phosphorylase isoenzymes present in cultured skeletal muscle from patients with McArdle's disease. *Biochemical and Biophysical Research Communications* 78: 663-668.

Schimrigk, K., Mertens, H.G., Ricker, K., Führ, J., Eyer, P. and Pette, D. (1967) McArdle-Syndrom (Myopathie bei fehlender Muskelphosphorylase). *Klinische Wochenschrift* 45: 117.

Schmid, R. and Hammaker, L. (1961) Hereditary absence of muscle phosphorylase (McArdle's syndrome). *New England Journal of Medicine* 264: 223.

Schmid, R. and Mahler, R. (1959) Chronic progressive myopathy with myoglobinuria. Demonstration of a glycogenolytic defect in the muscle. *Journal of Clinical Investigation* 38: 2044.

Schmidt, B., Servidei, S., Gabbai, A.A. *et al.* (1987) McArdle's disease in two generations: Autosomal recessive transmission with manifesting heterozygote. *Neurology* 37: 1558-1561.

Schochet, S.S. Jr, McCormick, W.F. and Zellweger, H. (1970) Type IV glycogenosis (amylopectinosis). Light and electron microscopic observations. *Archives of Pathology* 90: 354.

Selby, R., Starzl, T.E., Yunis, E. *et al.* (1991) Liver transplantation for type IV glycogen storage disease. *New England Journal of Medicine* 324: 39–42.

Serratrice, G., Monges, A., Roux, H., Aquatron, R. and Gambarelli, D. (1969) Myopathic forms of phosphofructokinase deficit. *Revue Neurologique* 120: 271.

Servidei, S., Bonilla, E., Diedrich, R.G. *et al.* (1986) Fatal infantile form of phosphofructokinase deficiency. *Neurology* 36: 1465-1470.

Servidei, S., Riepe, R.E., Langston, C. *et al.* (1987) Severe cardiopathy in branching enzyme deficiency. *Journal of Pediatrics* 111: 51–56.

Servidei, S., Shanske, S., Zeviani, M. *et al.* (1988a) McArdle's disease: Biochemical and molecular genetic studies. *Annals of Neurology* 24: 774–781.

Servidei, S., Metlay, L.A., Chodosh, J. *et al.* (1988b) Fatal infantile cardiopathy caused by phosphorylase b

kinase deficiency. *Journal of Pediatrics* 113: 82–85.

Shanske, S., Sakoda, S., Hermodson, M.A. *et al.* (1987) Isolation of a cDNA encoding the muscle-specific subunit of human phosphoglycerate mutase. *Journal of Biological Chemistry* 262: 14612–14617.

Shumate, J.B., Katnik, R., Ruiz, M., *et al.* (1979) Myoadenylate deaminase deficiency. *Muscle and Nerve* 2 213–216.

Sidbury, J.B. Jr: (1965) The genetics of the glycogen storage diseases. In: Steinberg, H.G. and Bearn, J.G. eds, *Progress in Medical Genetics* Vol.4. New York: Grune and Stratton.

Sidbury, J.B. Jr, Mason, J., Burns, W.B. Jr and Ruebner, B.H. (1962) Type IV glycogenosis. Report of a case proven by characterization of glycogen and studied at necropsy. *Bulletin of the Johns Hopkins Hospital* 3: 157.

Slonim, A.E. and Goans, P.J. (1985) Myopathy in McArdle's syndrome: Improvement with a high-protein diet. *New England Journal of Medicine* 312: 355–359.

Slonim, A.E., Weisberg, C., Benke, P. *et al.* (1982) Reversal of debrancher deficiency myopathy by the use of high-protein nutrition. *Annals of Neurology* 11: 420–422.

Slonim, A.E., Coleman, R.A., McElligot, M.A. *et al.* (1983) Improvement of muscle function in acid maltase deficiency by high-protein therapy. *Neurology* 33: 34–38.

Slonim, A.E., Coleman, R.A. and Moses, W.S. (1984) Myopathy and growth failure in debrancher enzyme deficiency: improvement with high-protein nocturnal enteral therapy. *Journal of Pediatrics* 105: 906–911.

Smith H.L., Amick, L.D. and Sidbury, J.B. Jr (1966) Type II glycogenosis. Report of a case with four-year survival and absence of acid maltase associated with an abnormal glycogen. *American Journal of Diseases of Children* 111: 475–481.

Smith, J., Zellweger, H. and Afifi, A.K., (1967) Muscular form of glycogenosis, type II (Pompe). Report of a case with unusual features. *Neurology (Minneapolis)* 17: 537–549.

Sokal, E.M., Van Hoof, F., Alberti, D. *et al.* (1992) Progressive cardiac failure following successful orthotopic liver transplantation for type IV glycogenosis. *European Journal of Pediatrics* 151: 200–203.

Solomon, E., Swallow, D., Burgess, S. *et al.* (1979) Assignment of the human acid alpha-glucosidase gene (αGLU) to chromosome 17 using somatic cell hybrids. *Annals of Human Genetics* 42: 273–281.

Strugalska-Cynowska, M. (1967) Disturbances in the activity of phosphorylase-b-kinase in a case of McArdle myopathy. *Folia Histochemica et Cytochemica (Krakow)* 5: 151.

Sugie, H., Sugie, Y., Nishida, M. *et al.* (1989) Recurrent myoglobinuria in a child with mental retardation: Phosphoglycerate kinase deficiency. *Journal of Child Neurology* 4: 95–99.

Suhara, Y., Ishiura, S., Tsukahara, T. *et al.* (1989) Mature 98,000-dalton acid alpha-glucosidase is deficient in

Japanese quail with acid maltase deficiency. *Muscle and Nerve* 12: 670–678.

Swaiman, K.F., Kennedy, W.R. and Sauls, H.S. (1968) Late infantile acid maltase deficiency. *Archives of Neurology* 18: 642–648.

Tachi, N., Tachi, M., Sasaki, K. *et al.* (1989) Glycogen storage disease with normal acid maltase: skeletal and cardiac muscles. *Pediatric Neurology* 5: 60–63.

Tarui, S., Okuno, G., Ikura, Y. *et al.* (1965) Phospho-fructokinase deficiency in skeletal muscle. A new type of glycogenosis. *Biochemical and Biophysical Research Communications* 19: 517.

Tarui, S., Kono, N., Kuwajima, M. *et al.* (1978) Type VII glycogenosis (muscle and erythrocyte phosphofructokinase deficiency). *Monographs in Human Genetics* 9: 42.

Tobin, R.B. and Coleman, W.A. (1965) A family study of phosphorylase deficiency in muscle. *Annals of Internal Medicine* 62: 313.

Tobin, W.E., Huijing, F., Porro, R.S. *et al.* (1973) A case of muscle phosphofructokinase deficiency. *Archives of Neurology (Chicago)* 28: 128.

Tonin, P., Shanske, S., Brownell, A.K. *et al.* (1989) Phosphoglycerate kinase (PGK) deficiency: A third case with recurrent myoglobinuria. *Neurology* 39 (Suppl 1): 359–360.

Tonin, P., Shanske, S., Miranda, A.F. *et al.* (1993) Phosphoglycerate kinase deficiency: biochemical and molecular genetic studies in a new myopathic variant (PGK Alberta). *Neurology* 43: 387–391.

Trend, P.St.J., Wiles, C.M., Spencer, G.T. *et al.* (1985) Acid maltase deficiency in adults. *Brain* 108: 845–860.

Tsujino, S., Sakoda, S., Mizuno, R. *et al.* (1989) Structure of the gene encoding the muscle-specific subunit of human phosphoglycerate mutase. *Journal of Biological Chemistry* 264: 15334–15337.

Tsujino, S., Shanske, S. and DiMauro, S. (1992a) Molecular genetic heterogeneity of myophosphory-lase deficiency (McArdle's disease). *New England Journal of Medicine* 329: 241–245.

Tsujino, S., Shanske, S., Sakoda, S. *et al.* (1993b) The molecular basis of muscle phosphoglycerate mutase (PGAM-M) deficiency. *American Journal of Human Genetics* 52: 472–477.

Tyrrell, D.A., Ryman, B.E.E., Keeton, B.R. and Dubowitz, V. (1976) Use of liposomes in treating type II glycogenosis. *British Medical Journal* iii: 88.

Ugawa, Y., Inoue, K., Takemura, T. *et al.* (1986) Accumulation of glycogen in sural nerve axons in adult-onset type III glycogenosis. *Annals of Neurology* 19: 294–297.

Umpleby, A.M., Wiles, C.M., Trend, P.St.J. *et al.* (1987) Protein turnover in acid maltase deficiency before and after treatment with a high protein diet. *Journal of Neurology, Neurosurgery and Psychiatry* 50: 587–592.

Valentine, W.N., Hsieh, H., Paglia, D.E. *et al.* (1969) Hereditary hemolytic anemia associated with phosphoglycerate kinase deficiency in erythrocytes and leukocytes: a probable X-chromosome-linked syndrome. *New England Journal of Medicine* 280: 528.

van Creveld, A. and Huijing, F. (1964) Differential diagnosis of the type of glycogen disease in two adult patients with long history of glycogenosis. *Metabolism* 13: 191.

van der Berg, I.E.T. and Berger, R. (1990) Phosphorylase b kinase deficiency in man: A review. *Journal of Inherited Metabolic Diseases* 13: 442–451.

van der Ploeg, A.T., Bolhuis, P.A., Wolterman, R.A. *et al.* (1988) Prospect for enzyme therapy in glycogenosis type II variants: A study on cultured muscle cells. *Journal of Neurology* 235: 392–396.

van der Ploeg, A.T., Hoefsloot, L.H., Hoogeveen-Westerveld, M. *et al.* (1989) Glycogenosis type II: Protein and DNA analysis in five South African families from various ethnic origins. *American Journal of Human Genetics* 44: 787–793.

van der Ploeg, A.T., Kroos, M.A., Willemsen, R. *et al.* (1991) Intravenous administration of phosphorylated acid alpha-glucosidase leads to uptake of enzyme in heart and skeletal muscle of mice. *Journal of Clinical Investigation* 87: 513–518.

Viskoper, R.J., Wolf, E., Chaco, J., Katz, R. and Chowers, I. (1975) McArdle's syndrome: the reaction to a fat-rich diet. *American Journal of the Medical Sciences* 269: 217–221.

Vita, G., Toscano, A., Bresolin, N. *et al.* (1990) Muscle phosphoglycerate mutase (PGAM) deficiency in the first caucasian patient. *Neurology* 40 (Suppl 1): 297.

Vora, S., Giger, U., Turchen, S. *et al.* (1985) Characterization of the enzymatic lesion in inherited phosphofructokinase deficiency in the dog: An animal analogue of human glycogen storage disease type VII. *Proceedings of the National Academy of Sciences of the USA* 82: 8109–8113.

Walvoort, H.C., Slee, R.G. and Koster, J.F. (1982) Canine glycogen storage disease type II: A biochemical study of an acid alpha-glucosidase deficient Lapland dog. *Biochimica et Biophysica Acta* 715: 63–69.

Watson, J.G., Gardner-Medwin, D., Goldfinch, M.E. *et al.* (1988) Bone marrow transplantation for glycogen storage disease type II (Pompe's disease). *New England Journal of Medicine* 314: 385.

Weil, D., Cong, N.V., Gross, M-S. *et al.* (1979) Localisation du gene de l'α-glucosidase acide (αGLUa) sur le segment q21->qter du chromosome 17 par l'hybridation cellulaire interspecifique. *Human Genetics* 52: 249–257.

Willems, P.J., Gerver, W.J.M., Berger, R. *et al.* (1990) The natural history of liver glycogenosis due to phosphorylase b kinase deficiency. A longitudinal study of 41 patients. *European Journal of Pediatrics* 149: 268–271.

Williams, J. and Hosking, G. (1985) Type V glycogen storage disease. *Archives of Disease in Childhood* 60: 1184–1186.

Williams, J.C. and Murray, A.K. (1980) Enzyme replacement in Pompe's disease with an alpha-glucosidase low-density lipoprotein complex. *Birth Defects* 16: 415–420.

Yang, B-Z., Ding, J-H., Brown, B.I. *et al.* (1990) Definitive prenatal diagnosis for type III glycogen storage disease. *American Journal of Human Genetics* **47**: 735–739.

Zellweger, H., Illingworth-Brown, B., McCormick, W.F. and Jun-Bi, T.U. (1965) A mild form of muscular glycogenosis in two brothers with alpha-1, 4-glucosidase deficiency. *Annales Paediatrici (Basel)* **205**: 413.

CHAPTER 5

Metabolic Myopathies II
Lipid Disorders
Mitochondrial Disorders

LIPID DISORDERS

Since lipids provide muscle with an alternative source of energy to carbohydrates and may well be the main source of energy at rest and during sustained exercise, one might anticipate the finding of disorders of muscle to be associated with a defect in lipid metabolism.

In 1970, Engel *et al.* (1970) suggested such a possibility in 18-year-old identical twin sisters who from childhood had muscle cramps associated with myoglobinuria and at times occurring some hours after exercise. Carbohydrate metabolism was normal. Attacks could be provoked by prolonged fasting or by a high fat, low carbohydrate diet. Muscle biopsy was histologically normal but showed excess lipid droplets on oil red O staining. They postulated a defect in the utilization of long-chain fatty acids, and Bressler (1970) predicted a deficiency of either carnitine or carnitine palmitoyl transferase (CPT) to account for this lipid storage myopathy.

Engel and Angelini (1973) were able to demonstrate carnitine deficiency in the muscle of a 24-year-old woman with weakness all her life and progression from the age of 19. Muscle biopsy showed a vacuolar myopathy filled with lipid droplets on histochemical staining. In the same year, DiMauro and DiMauro (1973) reported a 29-year-old man with episodic cramps and myoglobinuria of 16 years' duration but no muscle weakness. Muscle biopsy showed no excess of lipid but a deficiency of the enzyme carnitine palmitoyl transferase.

In the ensuing years, many more cases of patients with carnitine or CPT deficiency have contributed to the definition of the various clinical syndromes and a number of additional metabolic syndromes have been added.

BIOCHEMICAL ASPECTS

Carnitine

Carnitine (β-hydroxy-γ-trimethylaminobutyric acid) is the indispensable carrier of medium- and long-chain fatty acids across the inner mitochondrial membrane into the mitochondrion, where they undergo β-oxidation. There are two sources of carnitine – diet and synthesis. The synthesis of carnitine (which is dependent on two essential amino acids, lysine and methionine) takes place predominantly, if not exclusively, in the liver and it is then transported by the blood to other tissues. The highest concentration of free carnitine is in muscle, followed by liver with about half the concentration, and the heart which is still lower (DiMauro *et al.*, 1980). The concentration of carnitine in muscle is about 40 times that in serum, suggesting an active transport system. The excretion of carnitine takes place mainly in an unchanged form in the urine.

Carnitine deficiency could arise from: (a) defective biosynthesis, (b) abnormal degradation, (c) altered transport into and/or out of cells, or (d) abnormal renal handling. In a study of two children with primary systemic carnitine deficiency and three healthy adult controls, Rebouche and Engel (1981) were unable to detect any defective biosynthesis or abnormal degradation of carnitine. In a separate study of four children with systemic carnitine deficiency, two of their mothers, one patient with muscle carnitine deficiency and seven controls, Engel *et al.* (1981) concluded that a renal defect could not fully account for primary systemic carnitine deficiency but might contribute to the carnitine depletion.

Carnitine palmitoyl transferase (CPT)

The enzyme CPT catalyses the reversible reaction of carnitine and long-chain fatty acyl groups. It exists in two forms, CPT I and CPT II; CPT I acts at the outer face of the inner mitochondrial membrane to form palmitoyl carnitine from carnitine and palmitoyl coenzyme A. Palmitoyl carnitine then crosses to the inner membrane surface where it is converted by CPT II into carnitine and palmitoyl coenzyme A (Hoppel and Tomec, 1972). Acetyl coenzyme A is then formed by β-oxidation of the palmitoyl coenzyme A, and can be utilized in the Krebs' cycle.

CLINICAL FEATURES

The clinical features of lipid disorders of muscle fall into two broad groups: those in which muscle symptoms are the predominant abnormality and those in which muscle involvement is part of a more general systemic illness. In those patients in whom the muscle involvement is the major or only clinical feature, the presenting symptoms and signs may be proximal or diffuse muscle weakness, or muscle pain, particularly on prolonged exertion, which may be associated with muscle necrosis and myoglobinuria. The muscle symptoms seen in children in whom muscle involvement is part of a systemic illness are predominantly hypotonia and generalized muscle weakness. In some, the symptoms may resolve as the clinical condition improves; in others, the hypotonia and muscle weakness persist, and recovery may take several months.

CARNITINE DEFICIENCY

A decreased content of free carnitine in muscle may result from: (a) deficient dietary supply, (b) decreased hepatic synthesis, (c) defective transport into the muscle, (d) increased excretion, or (e) abnormally high proportion of esterified to free carnitine. These may in turn be due to a primary and isolated disorder of carnitine metabolism or transport, or may be secondary to a variety of other disorders (Rebouche and Engel, 1983). These biochemical possibilities still await resolution. Meanwhile, two distinct clinical syndromes have been delineated in association with decreased free carnitine in the muscle – a myopathic form confined to muscle and a systemic form affecting multiple systems.

MYOPATHIC CARNITINE DEFICIENCY

Myopathic carnitine deficiency is characterized by weakness, a lipid storage myopathy, and a decreased concentration of carnitine in the muscle but not in the serum. DiMauro *et al.* (1980) reviewed the nine cases documented in the literature up to that time. Five were female and four male. There was generalized weakness, usually starting in childhood and affecting proximal limb and trunk muscles, but sometimes also facial and pharyngeal muscles. The weakness was usually slowly progressive, but worsened rapidly in two adult women and in one adolescent boy. Cardiac involvement was suggested by abnormal electro-, echo- and vector-cardiography in one patient and by death from cardiac failure in one 2-year-old child. No other patient died.

Investigations

The serum carnitine level was normal or only slightly decreased. Serum creatine kinase (CK) was variably raised in all but one case. Electromyography showed myopathic features.

Muscle biopsy

Muscle biopsy showed striking accumulation of lipid droplets affecting type 1 more than type 2 fibres. On electron microscopy, the lipid spaces, which were not membrane-bound, were often adjacent to mitochondria, which showed no major change in size or number but did show occasional structural changes.

Inheritance

The inheritance seemed to follow an autosomal recessive pattern. Although only one patient had an affected sibling as well as consanguineous parents, the muscle carnitine concentration was decreased in the parents and maternal aunt of one patient and in the mother and father of two others. The relatives had no clinical or histological abnormality.

Because of the normal serum carnitine level, it was suggested that the primary defect may lie in the active transport of carnitine into muscle. However, more than one mechanism may be responsible since Willner *et al.* (1979) documented a case with muscle carnitine deficiency that did not respond to oral replacement therapy. In addition, the carnitine uptake of the muscle *in vitro* was normal and the addition of carnitine did not correct the impaired fatty acid oxidation in muscle homogenates.

SYSTEMIC CARNITINE DEFICIENCY

In addition to the lipid storage myopathy and muscle weakness usually starting in childhood, these patients may also have recurrent episodes of acute hepatic encephalopathy, with nausea, vomiting, confusion or coma (reminiscent of Reye's syndrome) and, in some, associated hypoglycaemia, and a metabolic acidosis caused by increased levels of lactate and ketoacids.

In the eight cases from the literature reviewed by DiMauro *et al.* (1980), six patients had died from cardiorespiratory failure, five of them before the age of 20 years. In two patients, the weakness worsened towards the end of pregnancy or after delivery.

Investigations

The serum carnitine concentration was markedly reduced in all patients tested. The serum CK was elevated in some but not in others and electromyography showed a myopathic pattern.

Muscle biopsy

Muscle biopsy showed severe lipid storage, similar to the myopathic form of carnitine deficiency. A liver biopsy in one case showed only proliferation of endoplasmic reticulum, but in two others there was lipid accumulation and three cases studied at autopsy showed lipid storage in the liver, heart and tubular epithelium of the kidney. Muscle carnitine was deficient in all cases. The liver carnitine level was 12% of normal in one biopsy specimen and ranged from 14% to 55% of normal in three autopsy cases.

The decreased carnitine in liver, serum and muscle suggested a primary defect in hepatic biosynthesis, with resultant inadequate carnitine supply for tissues from dietary sources alone. This still awaits proof. In one study of a liver biopsy, the third stage in carnitine synthesis by the enzyme γ-butyrobetaine hydroxylase was shown to be normal (Karpati *et al.*, 1975), and Rebouche and Engel (1981) were unable to pinpoint any defective biosynthesis in their isotopic studies of two cases and three controls.

Genetics

The evidence available from the few cases with familial incidence suggests an autosomal recessive inheritance (DiMauro *et al.*, 1980; Di Donato *et al.*, 1982; Cruse *et al.*, 1984).

Treatment

With the low level of serum carnitine and the suggestion of defective synthesis by the liver, replacement therapy with oral carnitine would seem to be potentially more logical and therapeutically beneficial than in the myopathic form. Indeed, some subjects have responded well (Karpati *et al.*, 1975), but surprisingly the carnitine concentration in the liver or muscle did not rise in spite of the blood level becoming normal. Other patients have apparently not responded to the same therapy (Cornelio *et al.*, 1977; Cruse *et al.*, 1984), suggesting once again possible varying types of biochemical deficit. Di Donato *et al.* (1984) documented a 20-year-old woman with systemic carnitine deficiency who had a dramatic improvement in her clinical state, accompanied by resolution of the lipid myopathy and elevation of the muscle carnitine from low to normal levels. They suggested the possibility of three distinct clinical variants of systemic carnitine deficiency, depending on the presence or absence of response to replacement therapy and the associated resolution of the tissue deficit in responsive cases.

MIXED FORMS OF CARNITINE DEFICIENCY

While the muscle and systemic forms of carnitine deficiency seem fairly distinct, there are some cases that are not easily compartmentalized and may share features of either form. Thus they may have the clinical features of systemic carnitine deficiency but normal serum carnitine levels, or they may have consistently low serum carnitine but no evidence of hepatic involvement.

CARNITINE PALMITOYL TRANSFERASE DEFICIENCY

MYOPATHIC CPT DEFICIENCY

Di Mauro *et al.* (1980) reviewed 21 documented cases of CPT deficiency. All but one were male. Most remembered having muscle pains since childhood and myoglobinuria appeared earlier than in cases of phosphorylase or phosphofructokinase deficiency. Myalgia and pigmenturia usually followed vigorous exercise of at least a few hours' duration and fasting before exercise was recognized by most patients as a precipitating factor. In about a third of patients, however, there was no apparent cause for at least some of the episodes of myoglobinuria.

During attacks there was swelling, tenderness and weakness of affected muscles, respiratory muscles were often severely involved and assisted ventilation was necessary in three cases. Between attacks the patients were normal.

The diagnosis of CPT deficiency should be considered in any patient with recurrent myoglobinuria, particularly if precipitated by prolonged exercise and fasting.

Two clinical features help to distinguish it from phosphorylase or phosphofructokinase deficiency: 1) there is no intolerance to vigorous exercise of short duration and no second-wind phenomenon, and 2) cramps are unusual and contracture is not induced by ischaemic exercise.

Laboratory diagnosis

Muscle biopsy between attacks usually does not show any structural changes or evidence of lipid storage. When lipid storage is increased this is not marked and certainly not as striking as in carnitine deficiency.

Biochemical estimation shows marked reduction (less than 20% of normal) or complete absence of CPT, depending on the assay technique used. There appears to be no correlation between the degree of residual activity and the number or severity of attacks. The enzyme defect is also expressed in leucocytes, platelets and cultured fibroblasts.

Genetics

Among the 21 cases of DiMauro there were three pairs of brothers; the parents were all clinically normal and one couple was consanguinous. Although the preponderance of males is still not understood, inheritance is considered to be autosomal recessive.

Therapy

A high-carbohydrate, low-fat diet appeared to reduce the frequency of attacks of myoglobinuria in all nine patients so treated.

Amongst further reports in the literature, Sadeh and Gutman (1990) reviewed six personal patients (five male, one female) with CPT deficiency presenting with myoglobinuria following severe exertion, four of whom had associated renal shutdown. Schiffmann *et al.* (1992) recently documented an unusual case in a 7½-year-old girl with recurrent severe myalgia during periodic attacks of fever, vomiting and pharyngitis, but no myoglobinuria or exercise-induced pain. She was found to have CPT deficiency in leucocytes, fibroblasts and muscle.

MIXED FORMS OF CPT DEFICIENCY ——

Occasional cases of CPT deficiency have been recorded with predominantly hepatic involvement (Bougnères *et al.*, 1981) and more recently fatal neonatal cases of CPT2 deficiency with multisystem involvement including liver and muscle (Demaugre *et al.*, 1991; Hug *et al.*, 1991), whilst Land *et al.* (1995) have described a fatal case of a patient presenting as a floppy infant with no evidence of hepatic involvement.

CLINICAL FEATURES ASSOCIATED WITH OTHER SPECIFIC DEFECTS OF LIPID METABOLISM

In recent years a number of additional clinical syndromes have been identified in relation to specific defects in the metabolism of fatty acids (Jackson and Turnbull, 1993).

BIOCHEMISTRY ————————————————

Before the β-oxidation of fatty acids can occur, they have to be converted first to their CoA thioesters, which is catalysed by the acyl-CoA synthetases, of which there are at least three types, classified according to their chain lengths as short-chain, medium-chain and long-chain acyl-CoA synthetases. Long-chain acyl-CoA synthetase is present on the outer mitochondrial membrane, short-chain and medium-chain acyl-CoA synthetases in the mitochondrial matrix.

ACYL-COA DEHYDROGENASE DEFICIENCY

Defects of the acyl-CoA dehydrogenases are the most frequently identified abnormalities of fatty acid oxidation.

SHORT-CHAIN ACYL-COA DEHYDROGENASE DEFICIENCY

This deficiency has been described in two different clinical situations: a myopathic form in which the defect is limited to muscle and presenting with a slowly progressive muscle weakness and exercise-induced pain (Turnbull *et al.*, 1984), and a systemic form with hepatomegaly and microcephaly (Amendt *et al.*, 1987; Coates *et al.*, 1988). The 16-year-old girl documented by Tein *et al.* (1991) had recurrent myoglobinuria, hypoketotic hypoglycaemia, encephalopathy and an associated cardiomyopathy.

MEDIUM-CHAIN ACYL-COA DEHYDROGENASE DEFICIENCY

This may be one of the most commonly inherited metabolic disorders, with an incidence of 1 in 5000 to 10 000 live births (Roe and Coates, 1989). It usually presents in infancy with an episodic illness in which muscle symptoms and signs are not prominent (Stanley *et al.*, 1983), the clinical presentations including sudden infant death, Reye's syndrome and hypoglycaemic episodes. Some cases, however, present in later life and exercise-induced muscle pain may be a feature, and yet others are asymptomatic and are detected only when the disorder is diagnosed in another family member (Duran *et al.*, 1986).

Medium-chain acyl-CoA dehydrogenase deficiency is inherited in an autosomal recessive pattern, with intermediate enzyme activity in fibroblasts from the parents (Coates *et al.*, 1985).

LONG-CHAIN ACYL-COA DEHYDROGENASE DEFICIENCY

These defects can be divided into three different clinical phenotypes (Hale *et al.*, 1990), one group presenting in early life (<6 months) with a severe illness with cardiac involvement and often death (Hale *et al.*, 1985); the second with coma associated with fasting (those surviving this initial insult have no cardiac involvement or muscle weakness); and a third group of children with a later onset with muscle pain when stressed as a prominent feature (Naylor *et al.*, 1980; Amendt *et al.*, 1988), accompanied by myoglobinuria and increased plasma creatine kinase. Between episodes there is no evidence of muscle disease. Long-chain acyl-CoA dehydrogenase deficiency seems to be inherited as an autosomal recessive disorder (Hale *et al.*, 1985).

Several children and adults have also been documented with multiple acyl-CoA dehydrogenase deficiency with a combined defect of the acyl-CoA dehydrogenases. Muscle pain and weakness were prominent features in these patients (Turnbull *et al.*, 1988a; Di Donato *et al.*, 1989).

GLUTARIC ACIDURIA TYPE II

This complex disorder, associated with electron transfer flavoprotein and electron transfer flavoprotein ubiquinone oxidoreductase deficiency, has different clinical presentations. Some patients present in infancy with renal cystic dysplasia and other congenital anomalies, and usually death occurs in the first few weeks (Yamaguchi *et al.*, 1991); other infants and children develop episodic hypoglycaemia, acidosis and hepatomegaly (Loehr *et al.*, 1990); and a third group present with muscle weakness (Turnbull *et al.*, 1988b). Morphological changes in muscle have been observed in all three clinical groups. The child described by Turnbull *et al.* (1988b) presented with severe muscle weakness at 6 months and responded well to treatment with a low-fat diet, riboflavine, carnitine and glycine. Her brother had died at 3 months, probably with the same condition.

LONG-CHAIN 3-HYDROXYACYL-COA DEHYDROGENASE DEFICIENCY

This enzyme deficiency now seems firmly established, with a number of reported cases (Wanders *et al.*, 1990; Rocchiccioli *et al.*, 1990; Jackson *et al.*, 1991). Age of onset ranged from 3 days to 3 years, and clinical manifestations included recurrent episodes of non-ketotic hypoglycaemia, sudden infant death, cardiomyopathy and myopathy. Muscle weakness was prominent in some children and associated with myoglobinuria and respiratory failure. Sensorimotor polyneuropathy and pigmentary retinopathy have also been described.

INVESTIGATION OF LIPID DISORDERS

Muscle biopsy

The major abnormality in these patients is the accumulation of lipid in muscle, particularly in type 1 muscle fibres; but not all defects of fatty acid oxidation are associated with excess lipid. Thus in carnitine palmitoyl transferase deficiency there is usually no lipid accumulation, and in other enzyme defects lipid accumulation in muscle may vary with the metabolic state of the patient. There may also be associated muscle necrosis or regeneration, especially in those patients with severe muscle pain and myoglobinuria. Lipid storage is also seen in other tissues in those patients with systemic involvement.

Biochemical studies

This usually requires the facilities of laboratories specialized in this area of metabolism.

1. Measurement of free fatty acids in the blood may reveal an increase in association with impaired fatty acid oxidation; this may be associated with hypoglycaemia on fasting and no associated increase in ketone bodies.
2. Carnitine. Measurement of the different acyl esters in blood and urine may throw light on individual abnormalities.
3. Measurement of carnitine palmitoyl transferase and acyl-CoA dehydrogenase. Defects of CPT in which muscle symptoms predominate have been shown to involve CPT II biochemically, with an absence of CPT II immunoreactive protein.

Molecular studies have also been initiated in several laboratories in relation to these specific enzyme deficiencies.

ANIMAL MODELS

An inbred mouse strain subline (BALB/CByJ) has been described that has no detectable short-chain acyl-CoA dehydrogenase activity (Wood *et al.*, 1989), and no immunoreactive short-chain acyl-CoA dehydrogenase protein present in muscle and liver. Molecular studies suggest the primary lesion in these mice may involve a deletion in the short-chain acyl-CoA dehydrogenase gene.

On prolonged fasting, the mutant mice become hypoglycaemic and develop fatty changes in liver and kidney but do not show any overt clinical signs. It is possible, therefore that some cases of short-chain acyl-CoA dehydrogenase deficiency in humans may be clinically asymptomatic and go undetected.

TREATMENT

Diet

It is important in all patients with mitochondrial β-oxidation defects to provide sufficient calories to ensure that prolonged fasting does not occur. This is particularly important in infants and young children, who may die suddenly following prolonged fasting. Overnight fasts should be avoided, and there must be adequate carbohydrate intake during intercurrent infections. Episodes of illness with hypoglycaemia must be treated promptly and aggressively with intravenous glucose infusions aimed at completely suppressing lipolysis. A low-fat, high-carbohydrate diet is recommended for most patients, although medium-chain triglycerides may be helpful for patients with defects of long-chain enzymes.

Carnitine

Carnitine therapy (100 mg/kg in children) is effective in the treatment of primary carnitine deficiency, and in some patients with myopathy the muscle strength and cardiac function may return to normal. The benefit of carnitine therapy in other defects of fatty acid oxidation is uncertain.

Riboflavin

Some patients with multiple acyl-CoA dehydrogenase deficiency and some with apparent glutaric aciduria type II have responded to administration of pharmacological doses of riboflavin (100–300 mg/day) (Turnbull *et al.*, 1988a; Di Donato *et al.*, 1989).

MITOCHONDRIAL DISORDERS

Abnormal mitochondria are a feature of a wide range of different clinical syndromes, including a number of encephalomyopathies. In the first edition of this book I placed the mitochondrial myopathies with the congenital myopathies with structural changes within the muscle, as that was the basis on which they were usually diagnosed, fully realising that these structural changes might well be non-specific and secondary to many different bio-chemical abnormalities within the respiratory chain.

Over the past decade the field has mushroomed on a number of fronts – the clinical, with recognition of an ever-increasing variety of presenting disorders, often with overlap of features between different syndromes; the genetic, with recognition of a maternal pattern of inheritance in a number of specific syndromes; the biochemical, with identification of specific biochemical abnormalities within the various complexes of the respiratory chain; and the molecular, with recognition of certain specific mutations in relation to the mitochondrial genome. As if this were not complex enough, the situation has been further compounded by the fact that the same molecular abnormality may produce very divergent clinical features and, in addition, there can also be a wide range in the severity of expression of a mutation within a single family.

The mitochondrial literature is probably one of the biggest growth industries within the neuro-muscular field and in this section I shall try and highlight some of the main features from a clinical, pathological, biochemical and molecular point of view, whilst still trying to keep my feet firmly on the ground in order to produce something digestible and comprehensible for the practising clinician.

One of the major challenges for the clinician has been to try and relate some of the apparently well-defined clinical syndromes to the advances and revelations on the biochemical and the molecular genetic front. Things finally are falling into place and what seemed initially like an irreconcilable jigsaw of disparate and unmatched pieces are now resolving into a coherent, integrated whole, with an explanation for many of the apparent incongruities.

DiMauro (1993) recently suggested a rational approach to the classification and understanding of the mitochondrial disorders, based initially on a genetic distinction between the respective influences of the nuclear and the mitochondrial genome, and then subdividing these broad categories into individual compartments on the basis of their clinical and biochemical features.

Much of the clinical and biochemical hetero-geneity, even within affected sibships and families, has now been resolved with the revelation of the unique characteristics of the mitochondrial genome, which has multiple copies within each cell (in contrast to the single copy of nuclear encoded DNA), and consequently has seemingly endless permutations of the normal and mutated DNA within individual cells and tissues.

HISTORICAL BACKGROUND ——————————

The concept of mitochondrial disease was introduced in 1962, when Luft *et al.* described a young Swedish woman with severe hypermetabolism not due to thyroid dysfunction. This classic piece of clinical investigation was based on three sets of data: 1) morphological evidence of abnormal mito-chondria in muscle, 2) biochemical documentation of loose coupling of oxidation and phosphorylation in isolated muscle mitochondria, and 3) good correlation between biochemical abnormalities and clinical features. During the decade that followed, the attention of clinical scientists was confined to muscle disorders and directed mostly to muscle morphology. Systematic ultrastructural investi-gation of muscle biopsies led to the recognition of different patterns of mitochondrial changes, which were believed to characterize distinct diseases, such as excessive proliferation of normal-looking mito-chondria ('pleoconial myopathy') or greatly en-larged mitochondria with disoriented cristae ('megaconial myopathy') (Shy and Gonatas, 1964; Shy *et al.*, 1966). In 1963, Engel and Cunningham introduced a modification of the Gomori trichrome stain that allowed one to identify abnormal deposits of mitochondria as irregular reddish patches in what they called ragged-red fibres.

During the 1970s, specific biochemical defects were described in increasing number, including pyruvate dehydrogenase complex (PDHC) defi-ciency (Blass *et al.*, 1970), carnitine palmitoyl transferase (CPT) deficiency (DiMauro and DiMauro, 1973), carnitine deficiencies (Engel and Angelini, 1973; Karpati *et al.*, 1975), and defects of individual complexes of the respiratory chain (Spiro *et al.*, 1970; Willems *et al.*, 1977). It was also realized that in many patients with *mitochondrial myo-pathies*, both symptoms and biochemical defects were not confined to skeletal muscle but involved multiple tissues. Because brain and muscle were often most severely affected, Shapira *et al.* (1977) introduced the term *mitochondrial encephalo-myopathies*, whereas others preferred *mitochondrial cytopathies* (Egger *et al.*, 1981) to stress the general-ized nature of these disorders. The multisystem nature of many mitochondrial diseases has generated controversy between 'splitters', who find it both useful and rational to identify distinct syndromes (Rowland *et al.*, 1983), and the 'lumpers', who choose to stress overlapping features and consider individual clinical pictures simply as variations on a common theme (Petty *et al.*, 1986).

In the 1980s, rapid accumulation of biochemical knowledge led to a rational biochemical classification (Morgan-Hughes, 1982). Attention was then directed to mitochondrial DNA (mtDNA) and maternal inheritance, and molecular genetic analysis of patients' tissues led first to the detection of large-scale deletions of mtDNA (Holt *et al.*, 1988) and soon after to the identification of a point mutation in patients with Leber's hereditary optic neuroretinopathy (LHON) (Wallace *et al.*, 1988a), followed by the recognition of three more point mutations associated with mitochondrial diseases and two disorders apparently caused by faulty communication between nuclear and mitochondrial genome.

The genetic classification of the mitochondrial disorders proposed by DiMauro (1993) recognizes three groups: 1) defects of nuclear DNA (nDNA), 2) defects of mtDNA (point mutations, deletions, duplications), and 3) defects of communication between nuclear and mitochondrial genomes (multiple deletions and mtDNA depletion).

HISTOLOGICAL DIAGNOSIS ——————————

The first clue to diagnosis of mitochondrial myopathy is usually the finding in biopsy sections of ragged-red fibres on Gomori trichrome, or of intensely reactive fibres with oxidative enzymes, or of ultrastructural alterations of mitochondria in muscle biopsy specimens from patients with myopathies or multisystem disorders. There are two important cautions – ragged-red fibres may be absent or inconspicuous in some cases of mitochondrial disorder and may also occur in association with other muscle disorders. Longitudinal studies have also shown that the presence of these ragged-red fibres may depend on the stage of the disease. For example, in the benign form of infantile myopathy caused by reversible cytochrome oxidase deficiency (DiMauro *et al.*, 1983), the ragged-red fibres may disappear as the enzyme activity returns to normal. The reverse can also occur; a child reported by Tritschler *et al.* (1992) with mtDNA depletion in muscle had only non-specific changes in a muscle biopsy taken at 1 year, when his symptoms started, but there were abundant ragged-red fibres in a second biopsy at 15 months of age.

Two additional histochemical reactions are useful. Staining for succinate dehydrogenase (SDH) or NADH-tetrazolium reductase activity provides a sensitive indicator of mitochondrial proliferation and helps identify ragged-red fibres by their more intense reaction. Staining for cytochrome oxidase (COX) activity has shown that most ragged-red fibres and also some of the other fibres are COX-negative (Johnson *et al.*, 1983; Müller-Höcker *et al.*, 1983; Byrne *et al.*, 1985). The coexistence of ragged-red fibres and COX-negative fibres has been observed especially in patients with progressive external ophthalmoplegia and mtDNA deletions and in patients with MERRF syndrome, whereas in patients with MELAS syndrome ragged-red fibres are usually COX-positive, suggesting that the biochemical trigger of ragged-red fibres may be different in different diseases.

There may also be excessive storage of lipid or glycogen in some cases with abnormal fibres, the so-called mitochondrial-lipid-glycogen storage diseases (Jerusalem *et al.*, 1973) (see Figures 5-1 to 5-4).

New techniques, such as immunocytochemistry and *in situ* hybridization, are providing useful insights into the pathogenesis of mitochondrial diseases but are currently still essentially a research rather than a diagnostic tool.

text continues, p. 226

Figure 5-1a-f (*facing page*) Mitochondrial-lipid-glycogen storage myopathy. This female infant was noted to be floppy on the first day of life and developed progressive muscle weakness. She also had difficulty with feeding from 2 weeks of age and by 3 weeks needed tube feeding. When referred at 5 weeks, with a diagnosis of severe spinal muscular atrophy, she had general trunk and limb hypotonia and weakness, but her chest movements were considered too good for severe SMA (a,b). An EMG was normal with no evidence of denervation. CK 170iu/litre and blood lactate and pyruvate elevated. Needle biopsy of the quadriceps showed a vacuolar myopathy, with extensive involvement of the fibres throughout (c). There was an increase in oxidative enzymes (d), glycogen (e) and lipid (f), with similar striking changes on electron microscopy, showing abnormal mitochondria and excess lipids. Biochemical assay showed deficiency of cytochrome oxidase and a low level of free carnitine. About a week later she developed respiratory failure needing ventilator support and although it was possible to wean her off the ventilator intermittently, she had a sudden collapse and died 2 weeks later. At autopsy a further sample of quadriceps gave similar histochemical and biochemical results and deficiency of cytochrome oxidase was also demonstrated in the liver. The parents were unrelated Turkish-Cypriots. An older male child was also floppy in the newborn period but this gradually resolved and when examined at 5 years he had no weakness. The parents refused to allow any investigations on him. They later had another female infant whom they did not wish to have investigated, who also became weak and floppy and followed a similar course, with death at 5 weeks.

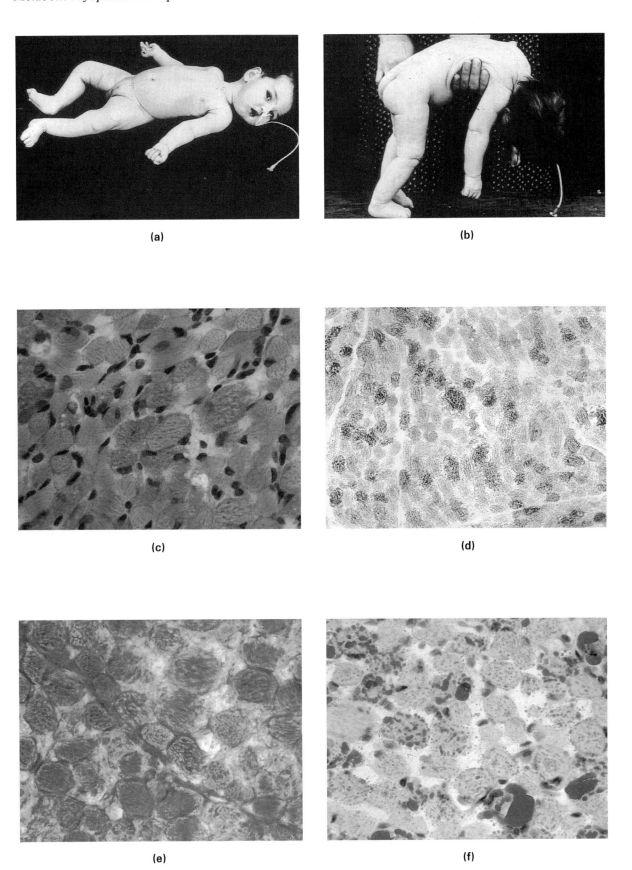

(a)

(b)

(c)

(d)

(e)

(f)

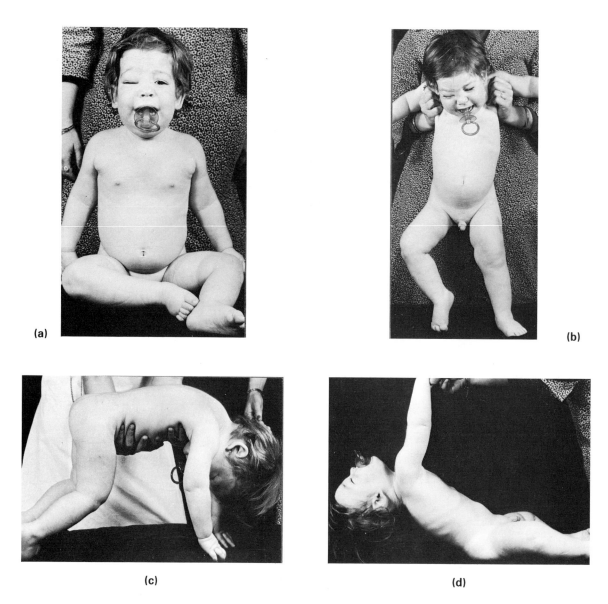

(a)

(b)

(c)

(d)

Figure 5-2a-d Mitochondrial myopathy in 21-month-old infant with normal motor milestones. He sat unsupported at 7 months and walked at 13 months. (a) He had ptosis of the right eye from birth thought to be due to haemangioma of eyelid. He was progressively unsteady from 14 months, with frequent falls and associated poor head control. (b) He lost the ability to walk at 19 months and to stand 2 weeks later. His intellect was normal. (c) Note poor head control and general hypotonia in ventral suspension and (d) when supine. CK 240 iu/litre; ulnar nerve conduction 54 m/s (normal); EMG of deltoid showed myopathic pattern plus reduced interference pattern. Previous biopsy from left quadriceps processed by formalin fixation showed variation in fibre size and increased cellularity and was diagnosed as myositis. Repeat biopsy showed marked mitochondrial abnormalities (e-i).

Figure 5-2e-i (*facing page*) Needle biopsy from quadriceps showed (e,f) almost universal abnormality of fibres with many disintegrating fibres showing typical 'ragged-red' appearance with trichrome stain (Gomori trichrome × 580). (g) Fibres also showed disintegration in the ATPase reaction (ATPase pH 9.4 × 580) and (h) increased glycogen reaction in small vacuoles (PAS × 580). Biochemical studies showed markedly increased glycogen level (0.36%; normal = up to 0.2%) but no deficit of any glycolytic enzymes. (i) Electron microscopy of biopsy showed strikingly abnormal muscle with marked disruption of fibre architecture and many abnormal mitochondria (arrows) (× 12 000).

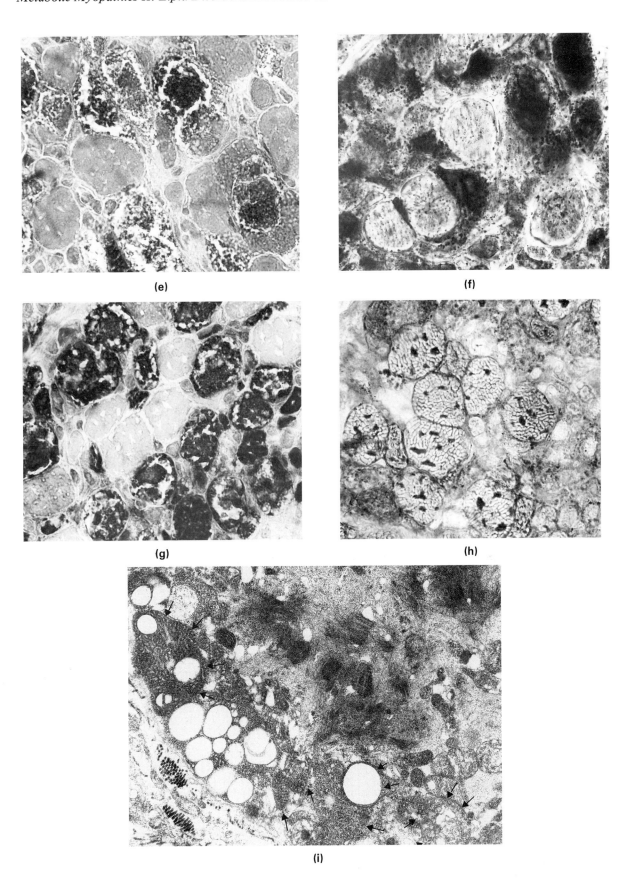

(e)

(f)

(g)

(h)

(i)

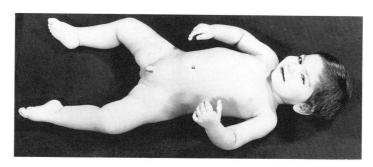

(a)

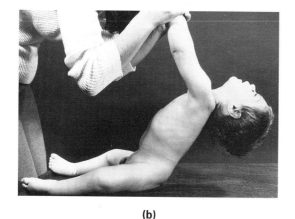

(b)

(c)

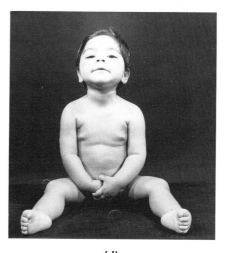

(d)

Figure 5-3a-d Mitochondrial-lipid-glycogen storage myopathy. This child developed normally until 12 months, when he was already taking some independent steps, but then developed an illness with recurrent fever, irritability, cough and vomiting, and associated weakness of legs and loss of ability to walk. At 17 months there was rapid deterioration in power and generalized weakness, with minimal arm or leg movement, weak voice and inability to chew or swallow. Spontaneous improvement followed and by 18 months he was again able to sit unsupported but not able to crawl or walk. When first assessed at 21 months his functional ability had remained unchanged (a,b,c,d) and he was still unable to stand or to roll over when lying, or to raise hands to mouth. There was associated respiratory and bulbar weakness. Weakness of limbs was more marked proximally than distally. CK 635 iu/litre (normal = <125); EMG showed myopathic change; nerve conduction velocity normal. Fasting lactate was raised (3.2 mmol/litre), pyruvate was normal (0.09 mmol/litre).

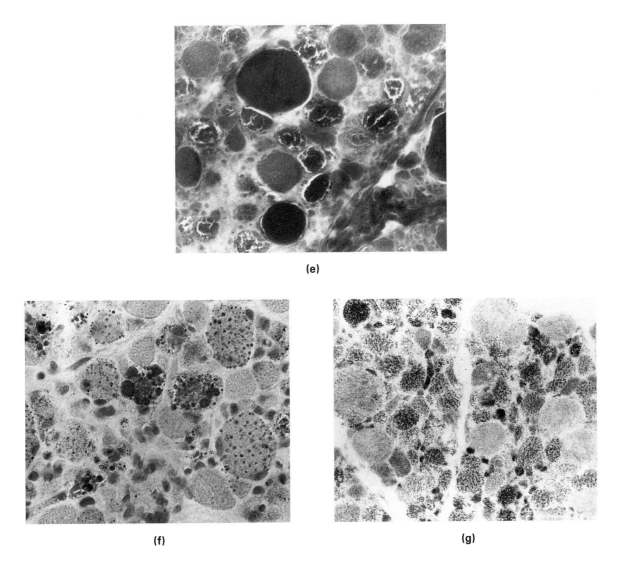

(e)

(f)   (g)

Figure 5-3e-g Needle biopsy of quadriceps showed grossly abnormal muscle with marked loss of muscle tissue and extensive degenerative changes and 'ragged-red' appearance in many fibres on trichrome stain (e). There was marked excess of lipid on oil red 0 stain (f) and also excess of oxidative enzyme activity, suggesting mitochondrial abnormality (g). Electron microscopy showed markedly disorganized muscle with excessive lipid and mitochondria, also mild excess of glycogen. Muscle carnitine was markedly reduced (7.4 nmol/mg NC; normal = 12.5–28), as was serum carnitine (16.5 µmol/litre; normal = 21–53 µmol/litre). He was treated with D-L carnitine, initially 100 mg/kg/day and subsequently raised to 400mg/kg/day, and also prednisone, but his condition did not improve and he subsequently needed tracheostomy because of recurrent aspiration of feeds, progressive respiratory deficit and focal lung collapse. He died as a result of these respiratory complications and also possibly of cardiac involvement (there had been persistent tachycardia and mild hepatomegaly, suggesting early cardiac failure). Autopsy was refused.

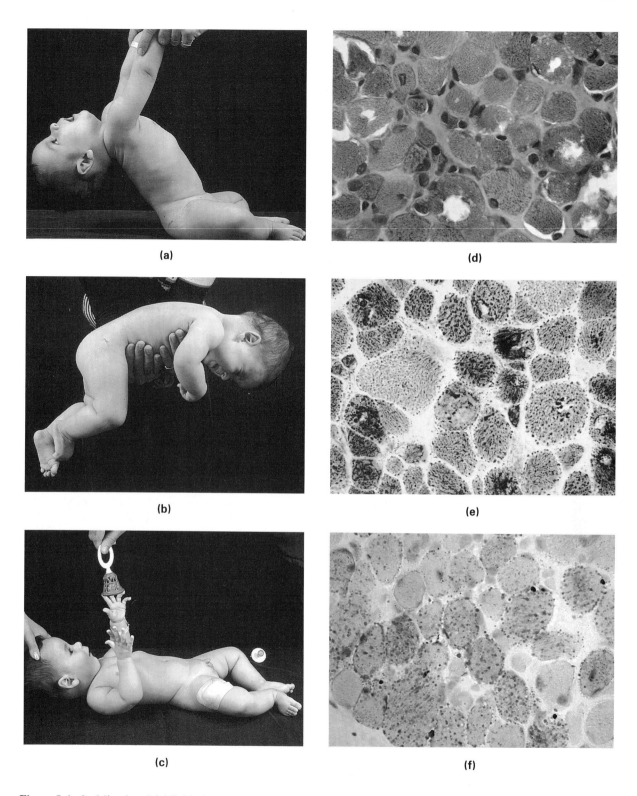

Figure 5-4a-f Mitochondrial-lipid-glycogen storage myopathy. This infant was referred at 7 months with a history of delayed motor milestones. On examination he showed general hypotonia and weakness with poor trunk and head control and more marked weakness in the arms than the legs (a-c). Needle biopsy of the quadriceps showed striking changes with disruption of fibres, proliferation of connective tissue (d) and an increase in oxidative enzyme activity (e), lipid (f) and glycogen, and also marked acid phosphatase activity in degenerating fibres.

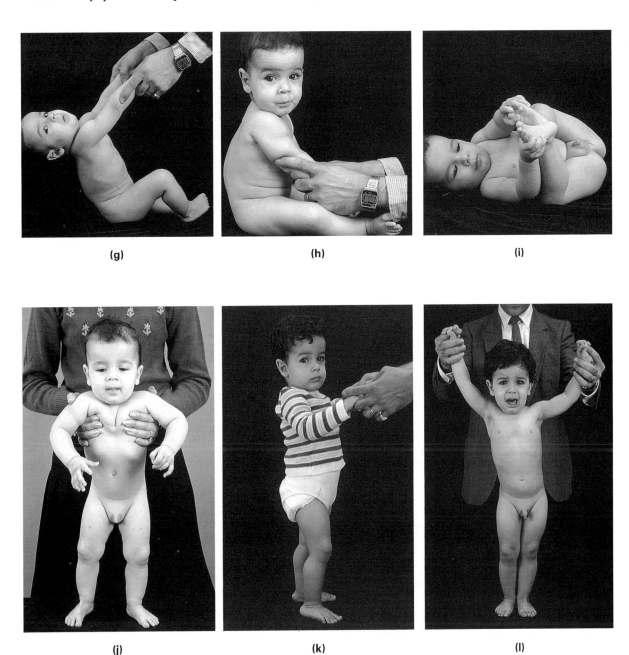

Figure 5-4g-l He subsequently showed steady improvement and was sitting with support by 8 months (g-i) and taking good weight on his legs by 9 months (j), standing well by 18 months (k), and started walking with support at 2 years (l). He was later admitted for observation with a mild respiratory infection and was about to go home after 3 days when he collapsed and had a cardiorespiratory arrest and despite immediate resuscitation and supportive measures died a few hours later. No metabolic or other cause for his collapse could be identified and it was assumed that there might have been an associated cardiomyopathy. Autopsy was refused. The parents were unrelated Turkish-Cypriots.

CLINICAL SYNDROMES ——————

Mitochondrial diseases are clinically heterogeneous. Pure myopathies vary considerably in age at onset (birth to adulthood), course (rapidly progressive, static, or even reversible), and distribution of weak-

ness (generalized with respiratory failure, proximal more than distal, facioscapulohumeral, orbicularis and extraocular muscles with ptosis and progressive external ophthalmoplegia). Besides fixed weakness, patients with mitochondrial myopathies may complain of exercise intolerance and fatigue (see Figures 5-5 to 5-14).

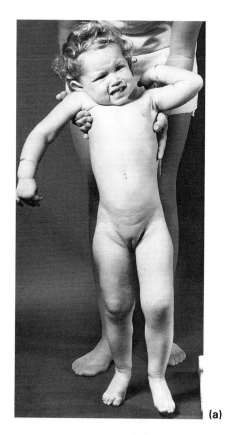

(a)

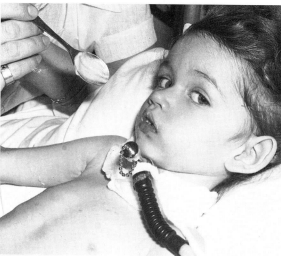

(b)

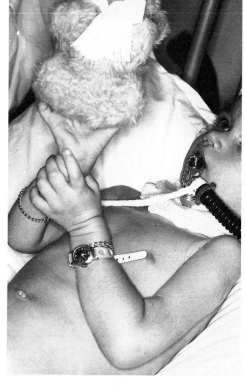

(c)

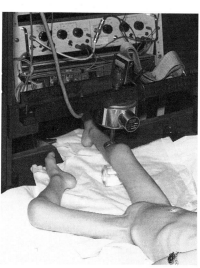

(d)

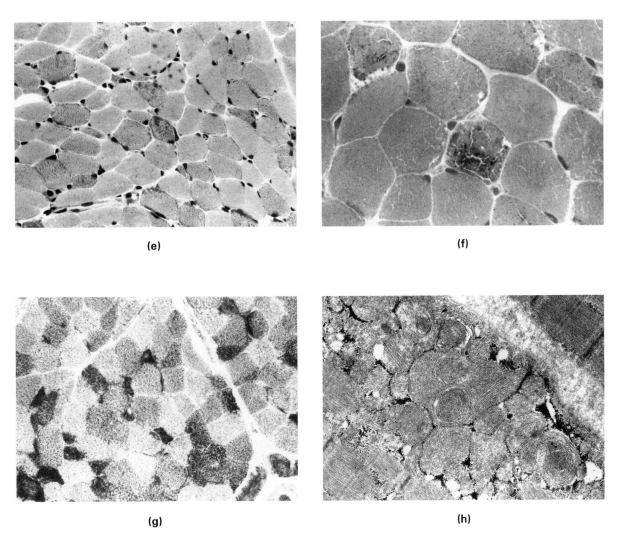

(e)

(f)

(g)

(h)

Figure 5-5e-h Biopsy of rectus femoris showed (e) numerous granular fibres on routine staining (H & E × 230) with (f) the typical 'ragged-red' fibre on trichrome staining (× 560). (g) Oxidative enzyme reaction shows numerous fibres with intense coarsely granular activity (NADH-TR × 230). (h) At electron microscopic level, the grossly enlarged, distorted and bizarre mitochondria are readily apparent (× 17 500).

Figure 5-5a-d *(facing page)* Mitochondrial myopathy in a 2-year-old child (a) with 2 month history of progressive hypotonia and inability to walk. There was subsequent steady deterioration and she was unable to sit unaided after 6 months. CK was initially elevated (200 iu/litre) but subsequently was normal (80; 100iu/litre); EMG normal. At 2½ years of age she went into respiratory failure necessitating tracheostomy and mechanical ventilation (b). The facial and ocular movements were normal. She was unable to raise her limbs against gravity (c). (d) Quantitative assessment by Professor Richard Edwards of quadriceps on stimulation of femoral nerve showed unexpectedly high force of 1.2 kg. This suggests that the inability to move the limbs might have had a volitional element or have been due to a central executive failure. There was a slight general improvement. She was mobilized in a wheelchair and mobile ventilator and subsequently managed at home, but she died suddenly because of mechanical failure of the machine. Her parents were first cousins. One sibling, born prematurely, died in newborn period of respiratory distress syndrome.

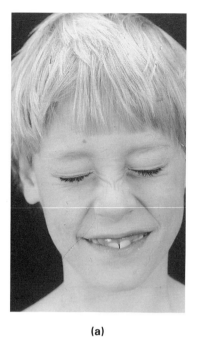
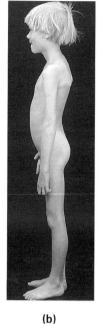

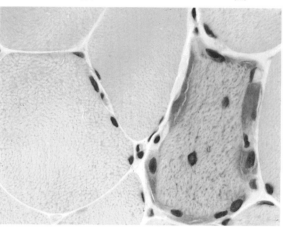
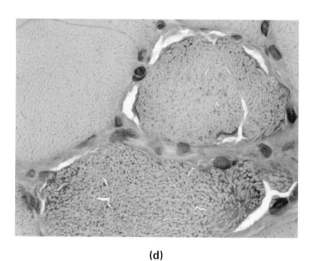

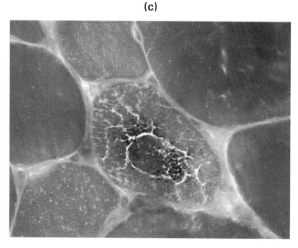
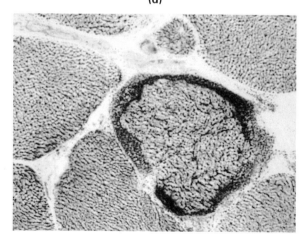

Figure 5-6a-f Mitochondrial myopathy. This 8-year-old boy (a,b) presented with a history of feeding difficulty in the newborn period, poor growth and delay in motor milestones with inability to walk until after 2 years of age. He subsequently improved but fatigued readily and could not participate in competitive sports. On examination he was able to hop, jump and run and rose from the floor without difficulty. There was mild facial weakness but no weakness of the external ocular muscles or fundal changes. CK and ECG normal; EMG of quadriceps mildly myopathic. There was no decrement of response to repetitive nerve stimulation. The family history was negative. His mother had had diabetes since the age of 21 years. Needle biopsy of the quadriceps showed isolated granular fibres throughout the biopsy, readily apparent on H & E and Verhoeff-van Gieson stains (c,d) and ragged-red with the Gomori trichrome (e). These fibres showed intense staining with NADH-TR (f).

(a)　　　　　　　　　　　　(b)

(c)　　　　　　　　　　　　(d)

(e)　　　　　　　　　　　　(f)

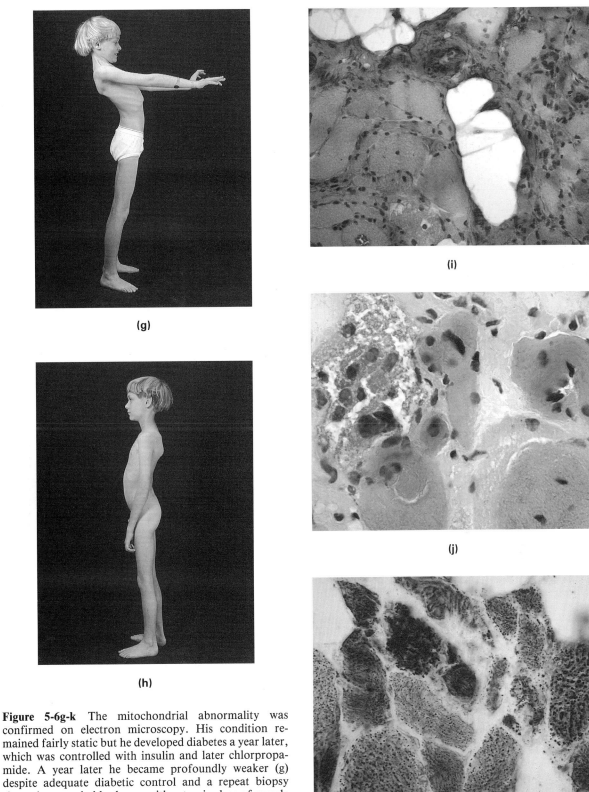

(g)

(h)

(i)

(j)

(k)

Figure 5-6g-k The mitochondrial abnormality was confirmed on electron microscopy. His condition remained fairly static but he developed diabetes a year later, which was controlled with insulin and later chlorpropamide. A year later he became profoundly weaker (g) despite adequate diabetic control and a repeat biopsy showed a remarkable change with extensive loss of muscle fibres and replacement by fat and connective tissue (i-k). The granular fibres were still present. He subsequently regained his strength (h).

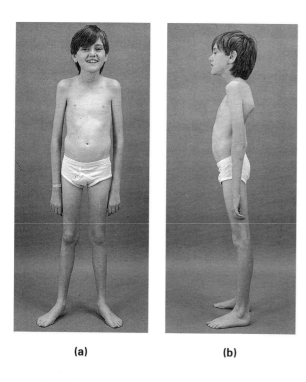

(a)   (b)

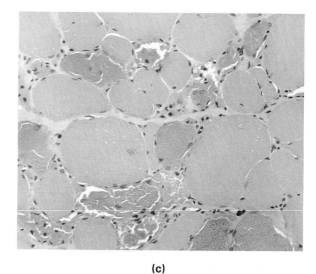

(c)

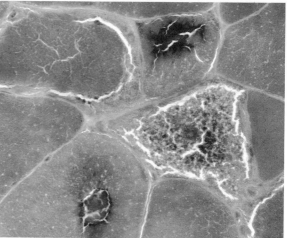

(d)

Figure 5-7a-e This 11-year-old boy had a history of motor weakness from 3 years of age, with a tendency to fall and a reluctance to do things. There was gradual progression and by 7 years he had difficulty climbing stairs, was unable to dress himself and was reluctant to go out playing (a,b). He was investigated at his local hospital and diagnosed as having Duchenne dystrophy. A muscle biopsy was said to be consistent with this diagnosis. From 9 years of age he somewhat surprisingly began to improve. On assessment he was able to run and to jump and almost to hop on one leg; he got up from the floor with a minimal Gowers' manoeuvre. His disability seemed too mild for a Duchenne dystrophy and the original CK of 180 iu/litre (normal = <80), was too low for a Duchenne or even a Becker dystrophy. Current CK was 240 iu/litre (normal = <180); EMG was only marginally abnormal and there was a marked increase of muscle echo on ultrasonography. Needle biopsy of the quadriceps showed marked variation in fibre size and many disrupted fibres with marked granularity on the routine stains (c) and ragged-red fibres with trichrome (d). With NADH-TR there were intensely positive fibres with subsarcolemmal aggregation and vacuolation (e). Electron microscopy confirmed the presence of abnormal mitochondria in most fibres. Biochemical assay showed a partial deficiency of cytochrome oxidase. He was reassured that he did not have muscular dystrophy and that the prognosis was much better. When reassessed 3 months later he was much more active, was able to jump and hop more readily and had also improved markedly in temperament and was participating in games.

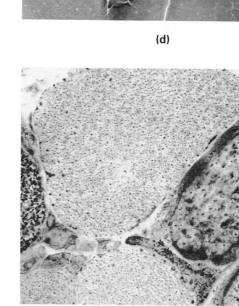

(e)

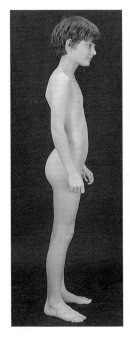
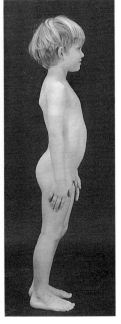

(a)

(b)

Figure 5-8a-f These two brothers, aged 12 and 7 years (a,b) had a similar history of marked tiring with exercise, associated with cramps, and the inability to participate in sport, suggestive of a metabolic disorder. Motor milestones and power were normal. CK was normal. Needle biopsy of their quadriceps showed well-preserved muscle with increased staining around the periphery of individual fibres which stained red with the Gomori trichrome (c-e) and showed increased activity for NADH-TR (f). Electron microscopy confirmed the presence of increased numbers of mitochondria, especially subsarcolemmal. Their blood lactate was elevated and biochemistry of the muscle biopsy showed an almost ten-fold increase in cytochrome oxidase and in succinate oxidation, with no increase in pyruvate oxidation, suggesting a deficit in complex I activity. At follow-up they remained fairly static, and if anything there was some improvement in exercise tolerance. The younger brother had more marked limitation than the older.

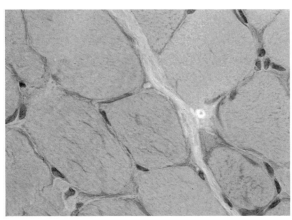

(c)

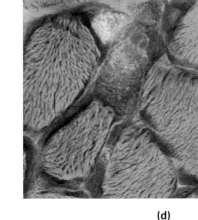

(d)

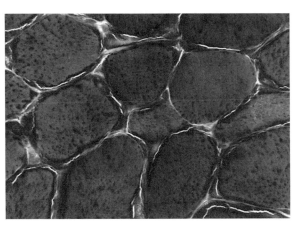

(e)

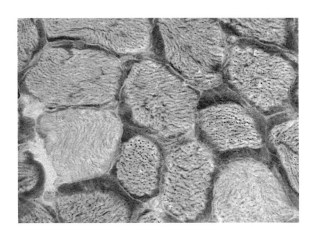

(f)

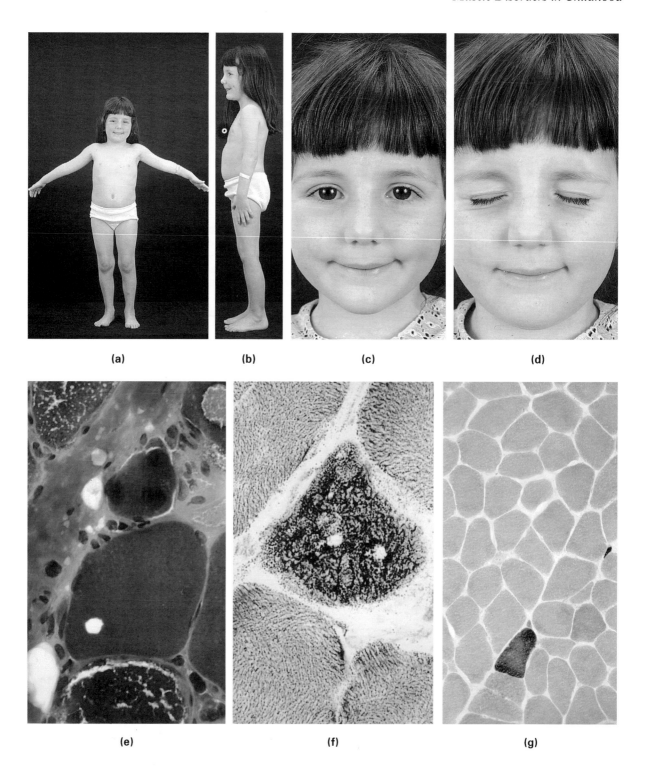

(a) (b) (c) (d)

(e) (f) (g)

Figure 5-9a-g Hypermetabolic myopathy. This child was referred at 5 years of age with a history of weakness from 3 years affecting particularly the arms, but also causing frequent falls and some chewing and swallowing difficulty (a,b). On examination she had limb and trunk weakness and mild facial weakness with inability to bury the eyelashes (c,d), but no ptosis or ophthalmoplegia. Needle biopsy showed well-preserved muscle with isolated disrupted granular fibres, which were ragged-red on trichrome (e) and intensely positive on NADH-TR (f). There was a striking predominance of type 1 fibres with the ATPase reaction (g). The mitochondrial abnormality was confirmed on electron microscopy. No biochemical abnormality could be identified.

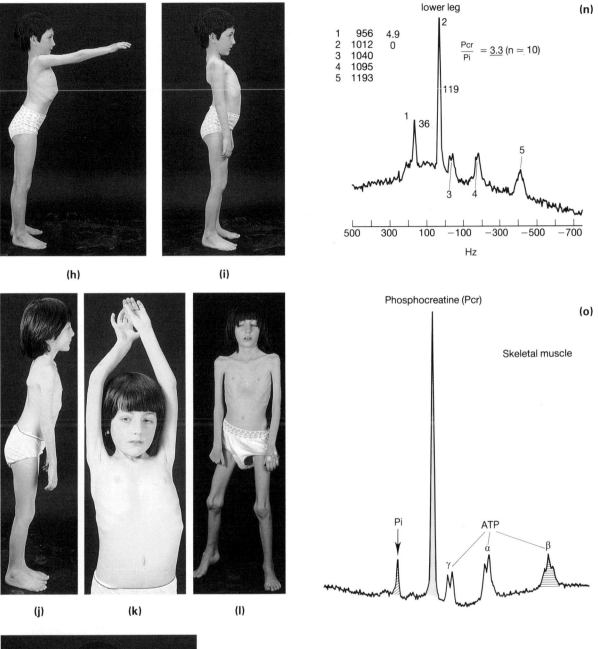

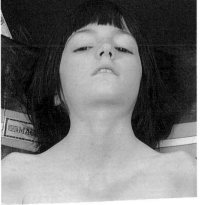

Figure 5-9h-o She remained fairly static for the next 2 years (h,i), but from 8 years of age she showed a marked and progressive increase in weakness, with loss of ability to stand, marked weakness of the neck muscles and associated ptosis and swallowing difficulty, but no ophthalmoplegia (j-m). Her blood lactate was normal; CK elevated at 290 iu/litre. Magnetic resonance spectroscopy (Dr Brian Ross) showed a strikingly abnormal pattern at rest (n), with marked increase in the inorganic phosphate peak and a phosphocreatine/phosphate ratio of 3.3, compared with a norm of about 10 (o). This suggested a hypermetabolic state. She failed to respond to various therapeutic efforts, including thiamine and riboflavin, and subsequently died at 11½ years of age.

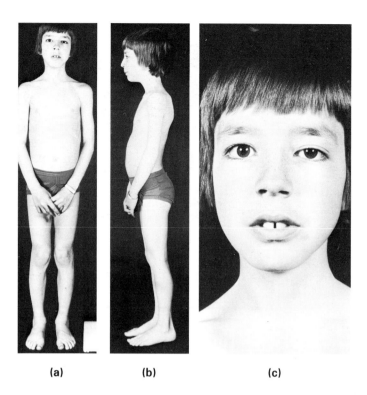

(a) **(b)** **(c)**

Figure 5-10a-c Mitochondrial myopathy in an 11-year-old boy (a) who presented with cardio-myopathy and associated neck and girdle weakness and mild ptosis. Cardiac muscle biopsy at the time of catheterization showed mitochondrial abnormality. Note presence of (b) lumbar lordosis and (c) ptosis. EMG of deltoids and sternomastoid normal.

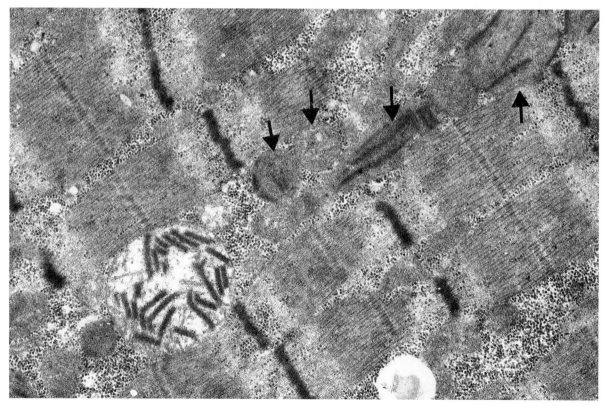

(d)

Figure 5-10d Electron microscopic preparation of biceps biopsy showed grossly abnormal mitochondrion (lower left) with dense inclusions. The other mitochondria lying in the same longitudinal axis are also abnormal (arrows).

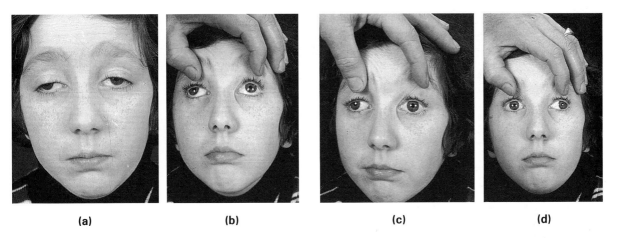

(a)   **(b)**   **(c)**   **(d)**

Figure 5-11a-d Kearns–Sayre syndrome. This 14-year-old girl was referred for investigation of her mild muscle weakness. She had already been referred by her paediatrician to an ophthalmologist for her ptosis and ophthalmoplegia (a-d), to a cardiologist for her heart block and had a pacemaker inserted, and was awaiting consultation with an endocrinologist for growth failure and delayed puberty. A diagnosis of Kearns–Sayre syndrome, made over the telephone, was confirmed by needle biopsy, which showed occasional granular fibres with high oxidative activity in an otherwise normal muscle. There was mild retinopathy and progressive loss of visual acuity and also associated deafness.

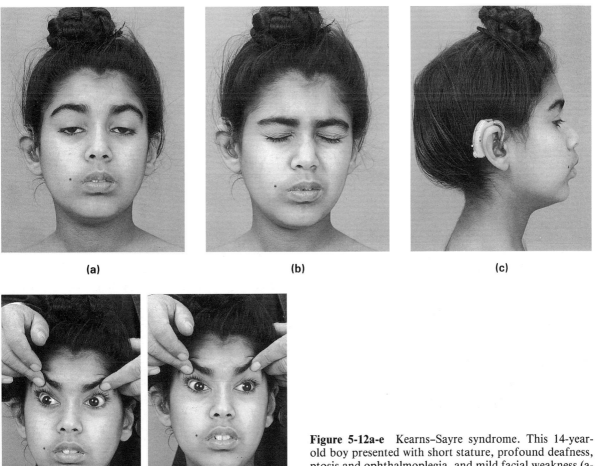

(a)   **(b)**   **(c)**

(d)   **(e)**

Figure 5-12a-e Kearns–Sayre syndrome. This 14-year-old boy presented with short stature, profound deafness, ptosis and ophthalmoplegia, and mild facial weakness (a-e); (d and e) show him looking to right and left respectively. Mitochondrial myopathy was confirmed on needle biopsy.

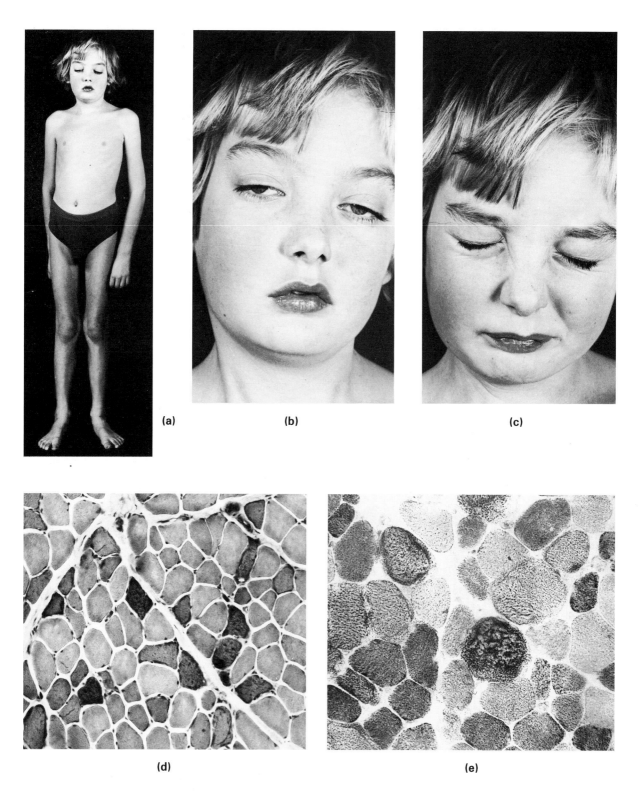

(a)   **(b)**   **(c)**

(d)   **(e)**

Figure 5-13a-e   Kearns–Sayre syndrome. This 11-year-old boy (a) was referred with a 4-year history of proximal weakness of the lower limbs and effort fatigue, with associated ptosis, ophthalmoplegia and mild facial weakness (b,c). Myasthenia was excluded on electro-diagnostic tests and edrophonium. A previous biopsy had been passed as normal. CK was normal. A repeat biopsy showed numerous granular fibres on routine stains (d) and fibres with excessive oxidative enzyme activity (e).

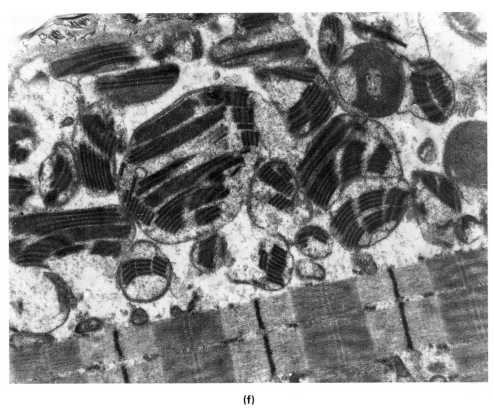

(f)

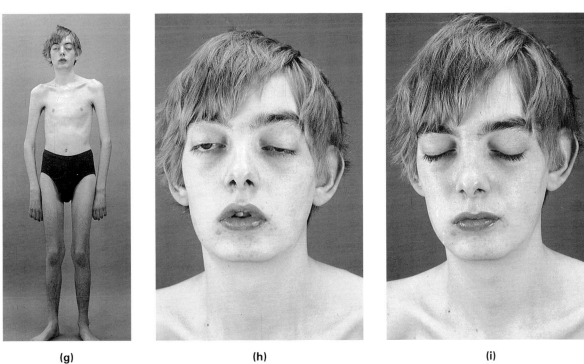

(g)   **(h)**   **(i)**

Figure 5-13f-i   The mitochondrial myopathy was confirmed on electron microscopy (f). There was no retinopathy. On follow-up over the ensuing 12 years his general activity remained fairly steady (g), but there was marked progression of his ptosis and ophthalmoplegia (h), and an increase in the facial weakness (i). He has also had symptoms in the mornings that are suggestive of nocturnal hypoventilation.

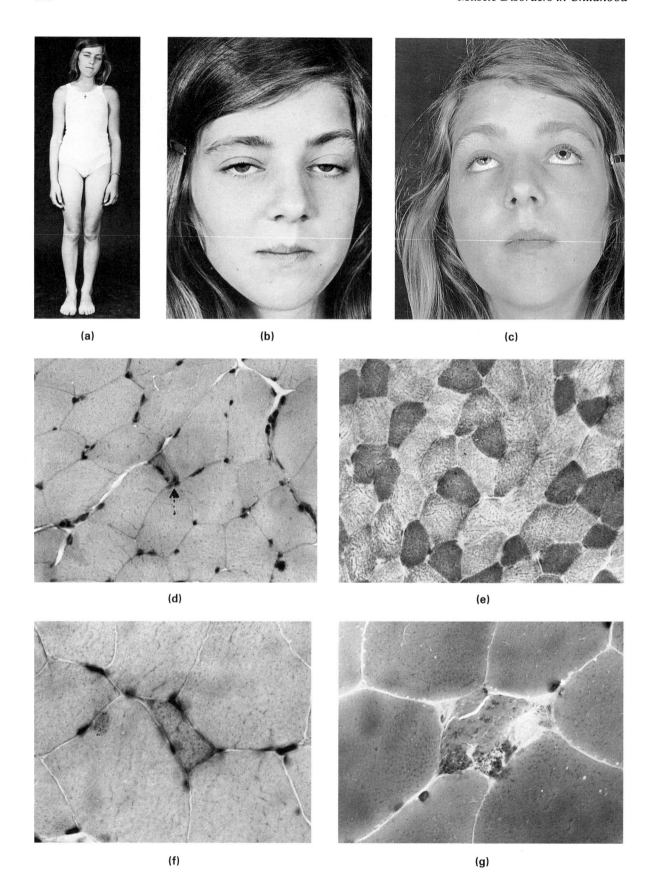

(a)   (b)   (c)

(d)   (e)

(f)   (g)

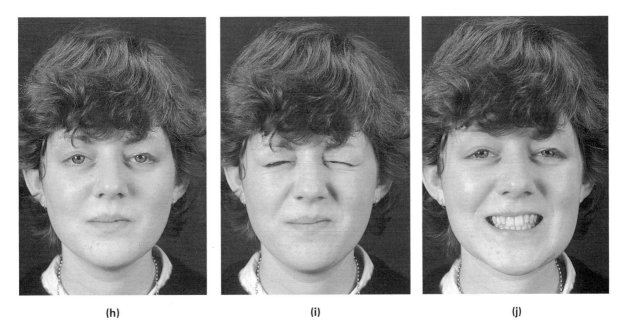

(h) (i) (j)

Figure 5-14a-j Kearns–Sayre syndrome. This girl presented at 14 years of age with a 2-year history of progressive ptosis and ophthalmoplegia (a-c). She had no physical weakness. There was an associated pigmentary retinopathy. Her visual acuity was normal. CK, EMG and ECG were normal. Quadriceps biopsy showed isolated granular fibres with excess oxidative activity in an otherwise normal muscle (d-g). There has been no significant deterioration in the ensuing 17 years (h-j). The ptosis was treated by surgical retraction. Molecular studies of her mitochondrial genome (Dr J. Poulton) showed the common deletion of 4977 base pairs, associated with Kearns–Sayre syndrome. She has recently developed some hearing difficulty.

Multisystem disorders are especially difficult to classify because of the many overlapping symptoms and signs.

The 'lumpers' and 'splitters' have been at loggerheads about the classification of the three best recognized syndromes of mitochondrial encephalomyopathy (see Table 5-1, taken, with permission, from the excellent review of the mitochondrial disorders by DiMauro, 1993). The boxes highlight the distinctive clinical features according to the splitters: for the Kearns–Sayre syndrome (KSS), progressive external ophthalmoplegia, pigmentary retinopathy, heart block, and cerebrospinal fluid protein above 100 mg/dl; for MERRF (myoclonus epilepsy with ragged-red fibres), myoclonus, epilepsy, ataxia and weakness; and for MELAS (mitochondrial encephalomyopathy, lactic acidosis, stroke-like episodes) migrainous headache and vomiting and acute, often reversible, stroke-like manifestations such as cortical blindness, hemian-

opia and hemiparesis. Although they stressed the differential value of these symptoms and signs, the splitters did list a series of non-specific features common to all three syndromes, including short stature, dementia, sensorineural hearing loss, lactic acidosis and ragged-red fibres (DiMauro *et al.*, 1985). In contrast, the lumpers chose to stress the common features and the existence of 'overlap cases', that is, patients in whom the cardinal features of two syndromes coexist.

We now know that all three syndromes are due to mutations of mtDNA. The observation that three distinct mutations underlie the three syndromes has bolstered the position of the splitters by providing a molecular genetic basis to their clinical classification. On the other hand, better understanding of the biochemical consequences of these genetic defects is needed to understand why clinical expression should, in fact, differ in the three syndromes.

Table 5-1 Distinguishing features of mitochondrial encephalomyopathies

Clinical feature	KSS	MERRF	MELAS
Ophthalmoplegia	+	−	−
Retinal degeneration	+	−	−
Heart block	+	−	−
CSF protein >100mg/dl	+	−	−
Myoclonus	−	+	−
Ataxia	+	+	−
Weakness	+	+	+
Episodic vomiting	−	−	+
Cerebral blindness	−	−	+
Hemiparesis, hemianopia	−	−	+
Seizures	−	+	+
Dementia	+	+	+
Short stature	+	+	+
Sensorineural hearing loss	+	+	+
Lactic acidosis	+	+	+
Family history	−	+	+
Ragged-red fibres	+	+	+
Spongy degeneration	+	+	+
mtDNA deletion	+	−	−
mtDNA point mutation	−	tRNA^{lys}	tRNA$^{leu(UUR)}$

KSS, Kearns–Sayre syndrome; MERRF, myoclonus epilepsy and ragged-red fibres; MELAS, mitochondrial encephalomyopathy with lactic acidosis and stroke-like episodes. From DiMauro (1993) with kind permission of the author and the publishers, Butterworth–Heinemann.

BIOCHEMICAL ASPECTS

In a schematic overview of mitochondrial metabolism (Figure 5.15), five main steps can be recognized (DiMauro, 1993):

1. The inner mitochondrial membrane is impermeable to anions and neutral metabolites and these have to be transported across the membranes by a set of carriers or translocases.

2. In the matrix, metabolites are further oxidized, pyruvate by the pyruvate dehydrogenase complex, fatty acids through the β-oxidation pathway.

3. The common product of intramitochondrial oxidation, acetyl-CoA, is oxidized in the Krebs cycle.

4. The reducing equivalents produced by the oxidation of acetyl-CoA are passed along a chain of proteins embedded in the inner mitochondrial membrane (the electron transport or respiratory chain) through a series of oxidation/reduction reactions in which the final hydrogen acceptor is molecular oxygen and the final product is water.

5. The energy released in this series of reactions is harnessed to pump protons from one side of the membrane to the other, and the resulting electrochemical proton gradient is used to synthesize adenosine triphosphate (ATP) at three sites along the respiratory chain, which are the sites of oxidation/phosphorylation coupling.

Mitochondrial encephalomyopathies can be subdivided into five groups, depending on the area of mitochondrial metabolism specifically affected (Table 5-2): 1) defects of transport, 2) defects of substrate utilization, 3) defects of the Krebs cycle, 4) defects of the respiratory chain, and 5) defects of oxidation/phosphorylation coupling.

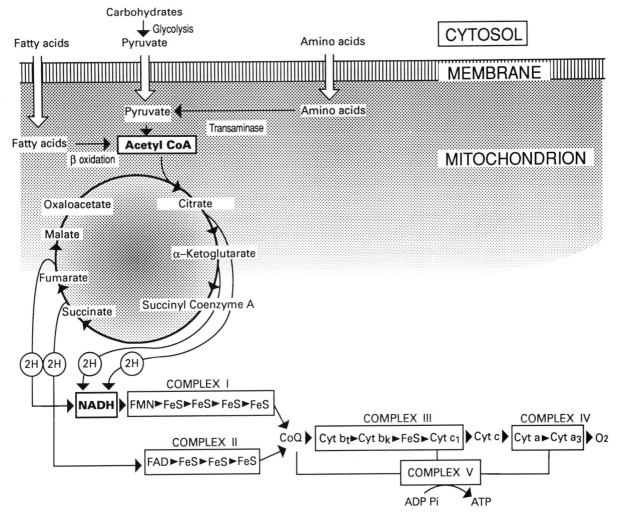

Figure 5-15 Schematic overview of mitochondrial metabolism. NADH, nicotinamide adenine nucleotide, reduced; FMN, flavin mononucleotide; FAD, flavin adenine dinucleotide; FeS, non-haem iron-sulphur protein; CoQ, coenzyme Q; Pi, inorganic phosphate. From DiMauro and DeVivo (1989) with permission of the authors and Raven Press, New York.

Table 5-2 Biochemical classification of the mitochondrial myopathies

Defects of transport
  CPT deficiency
  carnitine deficiency
	Defects of oxidation-phosphorylation coupling
	  Luft's syndrome (loose coupling of muscle
	  mitochondria)

Defects of substrate utilization
  pyruvate carboxylase deficiency
  pyruvate dehydrogenase deficiency
  defects of β-oxidation
	Defects of the respiratory chain
	  complex I deficiency
	  complex II deficiency
	  complex III deficiency
	  complex IV deficiency
	  complex V deficiency

Defects of the Krebs cycle
  fumarase deficiency
  α-ketoglutarate dehydrogenase (dihydrolipoyl
  dehydrogenase deficiency)
	combined defects of respiratory chain components

CPT, carnitine palmitoyl transferase
From DiMauro (1993), with kind permission of the author and the publishers, Butterworth–Heinemann.

Table 5-3 Mitochondrial DNA (mtDNA)-associated clinical syndromes

Clinical syndrome	Inheritance	Ragged-red fibres	mtDNA gene defect
Complete KSS	Sporadic	+	Single deletion/insertion; several genes affected
Incomplete KSS	Sporadic	+	Single deletion; several genes affected
Pearson syndrome	Sporadic	+	Single deletion/insertion; several genes affected
LHON	Maternal	−	Point mutation; ND4, ND1, apocytochrome b
NARP	Maternal	−	Point mutation; ATPase subunit 6
MELAS	Maternal	+	Point mutation; tRNA$^{Leu(UUR)}$
MERRF	Maternal	+	Point mutation; tRNA^{Lys}
MIMyCa	Maternal	+	Point mutation; tRNA$^{Leu(UUR)}$
Multiple deletion syndrome	Autosomal dominant	+	Multiple deletions; several genes affected
Deletion syndrome	Autosomal recessive	+	Reduced mtDNA amount; all genes affected

KSS, Kearns–Sayre syndrome; LHON, Leber's hereditary optic neuropathy; NARP, neuropathy, ataxia, and retinitis pigmentosa; MELAS, mitochondrial encephalomyopathy with lactic acidosis and stroke-like episodes; MERRF, myoclonus epilepsy and ragged-red fibres; MIMyCA, maternally inherited disorder with adult-onset myopathy and cardiomyopathy.
From De Vivo (1993), with kind permission of the author and the publishers, Raven Press.

GENETICS ─────────────────────────

Mitochondrial DNA is maternally inherited, so that a mutant mitochondrial gene can be passed from the mother to her sons and daughters but only the daughters in turn can pass it on to their sons and daughters (Figure 5.16). Maternal inheritance is now well established as the pattern of non-Mendelian inheritance in a number of syndromes, including Leber hereditary optic neuroretinopathy (LHON), neuropathy, ataxia, retinitis pigmentosa (NARP), myoclonus epilepsy with ragged-red fibres (MERRF), mitochondrial encephalomyopathy with lactic acidosis and stroke-like episodes (MELAS), and a maternally inherited disorder with adult-onset myopathy and cardiomyopathy (MIMyCa) (Table 5-3). Inevitably these new disorders have generated their own new acronyms, for rapid reference. Ragged-red fibres are generally present in MELAS, MERRF and MIMyCa, and lactic acidosis often accompanies these clinical syndromes. On the other hand, LHON and NARP do not have ragged-red fibres in biopsied skeletal muscle, and lactic acidosis is absent in LHON and may also be absent in NARP.

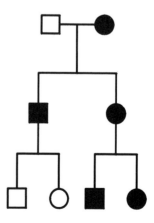

Figure 5-16 Maternal inheritance. Mitochondrial DNA is maternally inherited, so that a mutant mitochondrial gene can be passed from the mother to her sons and daughters but only the daughters in turn can pass it on to their sons and daughters.

Other mtDNA-associated syndromes appear to be sporadic, whereas the recently recognized multiple deletion or depletion syndromes seem to be under nuclear DNA control and thus follow a Mendelian inheritance pattern.

MOLECULAR GENETICS ————————

Mitochondria are unique in being the only sub-cellular organelles endowed with their own DNA (mtDNA) (Nass and Nass, 1963) and thus capable of synthesizing a small but vital set of proteins. Human mtDNA is a small (16.5 kb), circular, double-stranded molecule, and has already been sequenced in its entirety (Anderson *et al.*, 1981). It encodes 13 structural proteins, all of them subunits of respiratory chain complexes, and also two ribosomal RNAs (rRNAs) and 22 transfer RNAs (tRNAs) needed for translation (Figure 5-17).

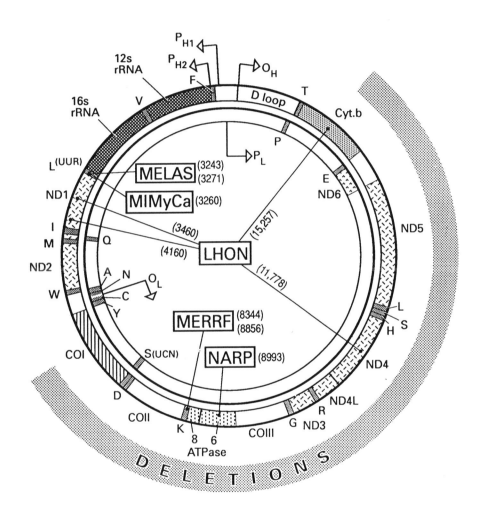

Figure 5-17 Human mtDNA is a small, circular, double-stranded molecule encoding 13 structural proteins, all of them subunits of respiratory chain complexes, and also two ribosomal RNAs (rRNAs) and 22 transfer RNAs (tRNAs) needed for translation. Diagram shows map of human mitochondrial DNA and localization of the molecular lesions. *Outer and inner circles* represent the 'heavy' and the 'light' strand, respectively. *Single capital letters* indicate amino acid-specific tRNA genes. The *shaded circular strip* indicates the major arc between the D-loop and O_L, containing most of the known mitochondrial DNA deletions. The *labelled boxes* refer to the regions of mitochondrial DNA where the point mutations associated with the corresponding syndromes have been identified. CO I-III, cytochrome *c* oxidase subunits; Cyt *b*, cytochrome *b*; LHON, Leber hereditary optic neuropathy; MELAS, mitochondrial myopathy, encephalopathy, lactic acidosis, and stroke-like episodes; MERRF, myoclonic epilepsy with ragged-red fibres; MIMyCa, maternally-inherited, adult-onset myopathy and cardiomyopathy; O_H, origin of heavy strand replication; O_L, origin of light strand replication; P_{H1}, major heavy strand promoter; P_{H2}, minor heavy strand promoter; 12*s* rRNA and 16*s* rRNA, mitochondrial RNAs. Adapted from Wallace and Lott (1993) with permission of the authors and the publishers, Raven Press.

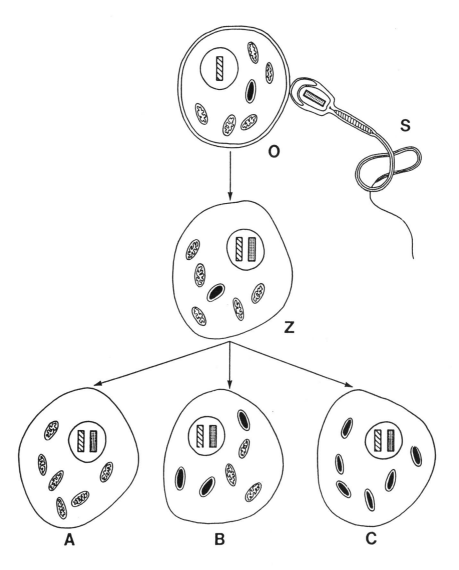

Figure 5-18 Cartoon illustrating the maternal inheritance of mitochondrial genomes and the random distribution of mutant and wild-type genomes in daughter cells of the zygote. For simplicity, the relative sizes of the oocyte and the sperm have not been respected, and it has been assumed that individual mitochondria contain either a single mitochondrial genome or uniform populations of mutant (filled mitochondria) or wild-type (open mitochondria) genomes. O, oocyte; S, sperm; Z, zygote; A, B, C, daughter cells representing stem cells of different tissues. From DiMauro (1993) with permission of the author and the publisher, Butterworth–Heinemann.

mtDNA has several unique features, all relevant to our understanding of mitochondrial diseases: 1) its genetic code differs from that of nuclear DNA (nDNA), 2) it is tightly packed with information because it contains no introns, 3) it is subject to spontaneous mutations at a higher rate than nDNA, 4) it has less efficient repair mechanisms than nDNA, 5) it is present in hundreds or thousands of copies in each cell, and 6) it is transmitted by maternal inheritance.

In the formation of the zygote (Figure 5-18), mtDNA is contributed exclusively by the oocyte (Giles *et al.*, 1980). A mutation affecting some mtDNA in the ovum or in the zygote may be passed on randomly to subsequent generations of cells; some will receive few or no mutant genomes (normal or wild-type homoplasmy), others will receive predominantly or exclusively mutant genomes (mutant homoplasmy), and still others will receive a mixed population of mutant and wild-type mtDNAs (heteroplasmy). Each time a heteroplasmic cell

Table 5-4

Site of defect	Heredity	Clinical features	Biochemistry
Nuclear DNA (nDNA)			
tissue-specific gene	Mendelian	Tissue-specific syndrome	Tissue-specific monoenzymopathy
non-tissue-specific gene	Mendelian	Multisystemic disorder	Generalized monoenzymopathy
Mitochondrial DNA (mtDNA)			
point mutations	Maternal	Multisystemic, heterogeneous	Generalized monoenzymopathy (structural genes) Generalized multienzymopathy (tRNA genes)
deletions or duplications	Sporadic	PEO; KSS; Pearson	Generalized ($\pm$) multienzymopathy
nDNA/mtDNA communication			
multiple mtDNA deletions	Mendelian (AD)	PEO $\pm$ other features	Generalized multienzymopathy
mtDNA depletion	Mendelian (AR)	Myopathy $\pm$ nephropathy; hepatopathy; encephalopathy	Tissue-specific multienzymopathy

KSS, Kearns–Sayre syndrome; PEO, progressive external ophthalmoplegia.
From DiMauro (1993), with kind permission of the author and the publishers, Butterworth–Heinemann

divides, the mutant and normal mtDNAs are randomly distributed into the daughter cells. Thus, over many meiotic or mitotic divisions the percentage of mutant and normal mtDNAs drifts, ultimately generating cells that are pure mutant or pure normal (homoplasmy). This replicative segregation process can thus generate all possible proportions of mutant and normal mtDNAs along cell or family lineages. If the mtDNA mutation illustrated in Figure 5-18 impaired oxidation-phosphorylation and the three cells derived from the zygote were stem cells of distinct tissues, one can see how different tissues can be either spared or affected to a variable degree by a mtDNA mutation.

The concepts of maternal inheritance and heteroplasmy have important implications:

1. Inheritance of the disease is maternal; males and females are equally affected in the next generation, but only females can in turn pass the mutation on to the males and females of the next generation.

2. Because there are multiple copies of mtDNA in each cell, the phenotypic expression of a mtDNA mutation will depend on the relative proportions of mutant and wild-type genomes, a minimum critical number of mutant genomes being necessary for expression (*threshold effect*).

3. At cell division, this proportion may shift in daughter cells (*mitotic segregation*), and the phenotype may change accordingly.

4. Subsequent generations are also affected, as in autosomal dominant transmission, but the number of affected individuals in each generation should be higher than in autosomal dominant diseases. In fact, theoretically all children of an affected mother would be affected, were it not for the threshold effect.

The threshold effect is a relative concept because the critical number of mutant mtDNAs needed to cause cell dysfunction will vary from one tissue to another, depending on the vulnerability of any given tissue to impairment of oxidative metabolism. Thus the central nervous system, being highly oxidative, is more vulnerable, followed by heart and skeletal muscle, kidney and liver. Specific tissues such as the insulin-producing islets of Langerhans are also highly oxidative and thus vulnerable. In addition, this metabolic vulnerability may vary in the same tissue with time. Thus, partial depletion of mtDNA in muscle seems to be well tolerated (and clinically silent) for the first year of life, when metabolic demands are limited, but may result in myopathy when an impaired oxidative metabolism cannot cope with increasing energy requirements (Moraes *et al.*, 1991). Similarly, the same percentage of mtDNA point mutations in muscle may be clinically silent in a young MERRF patient but symptomatic in an older one, owing to the documented decline of oxidative metabolism in muscle with ageing (Wallace *et al.*, 1988b).

Although functionally important, mtDNA-encoded peptides represent only a small proportion of total mitochondrial protein. Most mitochondrial proteins are encoded by nDNA, synthesized in the cytoplasm, and imported into mitochondria. The transport of proteins from the cytoplasm into the mitochondria and the targeting of imported proteins to intra-mitochondrial compartments require a series of post-translational events and a complex trans-location machinery.

The dual genetic control of mitochondrial proteins and the complexity of the process required for the transport and correct assembly of proteins synthesized in the cytoplasm help explain why mitochondrial diseases can be due to diverse genetic errors. Recent advances in understanding the molecular basis of mitochondrial diseases have provided a genetic classification that takes into account defects of nDNA, defects of mtDNA and defects of communication between the two genomes (DiMauro, 1993) (Table 5-4).

Mutations of nuclear genes

One would anticipate that mutations of nuclear genes encoding structural mitochondrial proteins would cause diseases transmitted by mendelian inheritance and most disorders in this group are, in fact, inherited as autosomal recessive traits. One might also expect that defects of structural genes encoding mitochondrial proteins ought to be the most common causes of mitochondrial diseases, but no such defect has yet been documented at the molecular level. These defects could involve either genes encoding tissue-specific proteins producing a specific enzyme defect limited to the same tissue, or genes encoding proteins common to all tissues causing a multisystem disorder characterized biochemically by a generalized defect of a single enzyme.

Another group of nuclear defects involves genes controlling the transport of proteins from cytoplasm into mitochondria.

Defects of the mitochondrial genome

Abnormalities in the mitochondrial genome consist of point mutations, deletions and duplications. The first point mutation of mtDNA was described in 1988 by Wallace et al. (1988a) in patients with Leber's hereditary optic neuroretinopathy (LHON), resulting in the substitution of a highly conserved arginine to histidine in subunit 4 of complex I. Within 2 years, three more point mutations were identified, one affecting a structural gene (Holt et al., 1990) and two affecting tRNA genes (Shoffner et al., 1990; Goto et al., 1990a; Kobayashi et al., 1990).

Large-scale deletions were the first molecular defects of mtDNA described in patients with mitochondrial diseases (Holt et al., 1988) and shortly after, Zeviani et al. (1988) reported the almost invariable presence of such mtDNA deletions in patients with Kearns–Sayre syndrome.

Defects of communication between nuclear and mitochondrial genomes

Although separate, the nuclear and mitochondrial genomes work in tandem, apparently under the overriding control of the nuclear genome. Mutations affecting such control may well occur in humans, as they occur in yeast, and should be transmitted by mendelian inheritance. There is good, if indirect, evidence that two human disorders are due to faulty communications between nuclear and mitochondrial genomes. One is an autosomal dominant disorder dominated by progressive external ophthalmoplegia (PEO) and characterized at the molecular level by multiple deletions of mtDNA (Zeviani et al., 1989), the other an apparently autosomal recessive disorder, usually but not invariably or exclusively affecting muscle and characterized by more or less severe depletion of mtDNA (Moraes et al., 1991).

PHYSIOLOGICAL MEASUREMENTS ———

Alterations of oxidative metabolism, the major source of energy for muscle contraction, can be detected by standardized exercise physiology tests employing cycle ergometers or treadmill protocols (Haller et al., 1989). Maximal oxygen uptake (VO_{2max}) is the most useful indicator of a patient's capacity for oxidative metabolism. In patients with alterations of oxidative phosphorylation there are typical physiological responses:

1. The increase of cardiac output during exercise is greater than normal relative to the rate of oxidative metabolism.

2. There is a gross mismatch between oxygen transport and utilization; oxygen extraction per unit of blood remains almost unchanged, in contrast to the three-fold increase seen in normal subjects from rest to maximal exercise.

3. Ventilation is normal at rest but increases excessively relative to oxygen uptake; hyperpnoea during exercise is greater than normal, relative to the increase in metabolic rate.

4. Venous lactate is usually elevated at rest but increases excessively relative to workload and level of oxygen uptake.

Magnetic resonance spectroscopy

The following cluster of changes detectable on ^{31}P magnetic resonance spectroscopy is thought to be characteristic of mitochondrial myopathies (Argov and Bank, 1991):

1. the PCr to Pi ratio is lower than normal at rest;
2. the PCr to Pi ratio decreases more than normal during exercise, even when patients perform less work than normal;
3. postexercise recovery of the PCr to Pi ratio is much slower than normal, which is probably the most sensitive indicator of mitochondrial dysfunction.

MITOCHONDRIAL DISEASES CLASSIFIED BY GENETIC ABNORMALITIES

DiMauro's (1993) classification subdivides individual mitochondrial diseases on a genetic basis, considering first disorders caused by defects of nDNA, then disorders caused by defects of mtDNA, and finally disorders caused by defects of communication between the two genomes (Table 5-4). The conditions within each group can then be further characterized on the basis of their clinical phenotype and specific biochemical abnormalities.

DISEASES CAUSED BY DEFECTS OF NUCLEAR DNA

A systematic approach to a rational classification of these disorders can be based on biochemical criteria, and five groups of diseases can be identified according to the area of mitochondrial metabolism affected (Table 5-2).

DEFECTS OF SUBSTRATE TRANSPORT

The better known defects of mitochondrial substrate transport affect lipid metabolism and are due to carnitine palmitoyl transferase deficiency and carnitine deficiencies, both primary and secondary (see previous section).

DEFECTS OF SUBSTRATE OXIDATION

Specific enzyme defects have been identified at several steps in the β-oxidation pathway. Defects of

the pyruvate dehydrogenase complex (PDHC) can affect each of the three catalytic components of PDHC, E_1 (pyruvate decarboxylase), E_2 (dihydrolipoyl transacetylase), or E_3 (dihydrolipoyl dehydrogenase), as well as either of the two regulatory components, PDH-kinase, which inactivates the enzyme, and PDH-phosphatase, which activates it. Most of the disorders associated with these enzymes affect the central nervous system, with little 'muscle' component, apart from associated hypotonia in some of the infantile syndromes.

DEFECTS OF THE KREBS CYCLE

There are three known defects in the Krebs cycle, involving α-ketoglutarate dehydrogenase, fumarase and aconitase. Once again these enzyme deficiencies affect predominantly the central nervous system.

DEFECTS OF THE RESPIRATORY CHAIN

Respiratory chain defects may result from genetic errors in either the nuclear or the mitochondrial genome. The following are presumed to be due to defects of nDNA.

COMPLEX I DEFICIENCY

NADH-CoQ reductase, the largest complex of the respiratory chain, contains at least 25 different polypeptides (seven of which are encoded by the mtDNA) and several non-protein components, including flavin mononucleotides (FMN), eight non-heme iron–sulphur clusters, and phospholipid.

From the clinical point of view, complex I deficiencies fall into three broad categories:

Fatal infantile multisystem disorders

These disorders are characterized by severe congenital lactic acidosis, psychomotor delay, diffuse hypotonia and weakness, cardiopathy, and cardiorespiratory failure causing death in the neonatal period. The enzyme defect is present in multiple organs (Moreadith *et al.*, 1984; Hoppel *et al.*, 1987). There is currently no chromosomal assignment for any of the nDNA-encoded human complex I subunits. Therapeutic trials with thiamine, biotin, carnitine and ketogenic diet have been unsuccessful.

Myopathy

Myopathy starts in childhood or in adult life, with exercise intolerance followed by fixed weakness, usually accompanied by lactic acidosis at rest, exaggerated by exercise. The tissue-specific nature of this disorder suggested that one or more of the nDNA-encoded, complex I subunits might exist as tissue-specific isoforms, but immunoblot analysis in a few patients showed a generalized decrease of all bands rather than a selective defect of any one band (Morgan-Hughes *et al.*, 1988; Bet *et al.*, 1990). Family history is usually negative or compatible with mendelian inheritance.

Mitochondrial encephalomyopathy

With onset in childhood or adult life, mitochondrial encephalomyopathy presents with ophthalmoplegia, seizures, dementia, ataxia, neurosensory hearing loss, pigmentary retinopathy, sensory neuropathy, and involuntary movements (Morgan-Hughes *et al.*, 1988). This heterogeneous group, which overlaps clinically with MELAS, is likely to include some patients with nDNA and others with mtDNA defects.

COMPLEX II DEFICIENCY

Biochemical documentation of complex II deficiency has been incomplete and largely based on more or less severe defects of succinate-cytochrome *c* reductase activity in five reported patients with encephalomyopathy (Sengers *et al.*, 1983; Behbehani *et al.*, 1984; Riggs *et al.*, 1984; Sperl *et al.*, 1988). More convincing evidence of an isolated biochemical defect (accompanied by complete lack of SDH stain in muscle biopsies) has been provided in two patients. Haller *et al.* (1991) documented a 22-year-old Swedish man with exercise intolerance and exercise-related myoglobinuria, in whom studies of isolated muscle mitochondria showed impaired succinate but normal glutamate oxidation, in association with deficiency of succinate dehydrogenase on biochemical and histochemical analysis. Similar results were obtained by Garavaglia *et al.* (1990) in a 14-year-old girl with weakness and exercise intolerance but no myoglobinuria.

COENZYME Q_{10} (COQ_{10}) DEFICIENCY

Ogasahara *et al.* (1989) found a marked deficiency of CoQ_{10} in the muscle but not in cultured fibroblasts of two sisters with normal early development followed by exercise intolerance and slowly progressive weakness of axial and proximal limb muscles, sparing facial and extraocular muscles. In addition they both had learning disability, one had seizures, and the other had a cerebellar syndrome. Both sisters had episodes of myoglobinuria following seizures or intercurrent infections. Family history suggested autosomal recessive inheritance. Investigations showed a lactic acidosis, increased serum CK and

myopathic electromyogram. Muscle biopsies showed excessive accumulation of lipid droplets and mitochondria in type 1 fibres. It was thought that the primary defect in this family probably involved a tissue-specific isozyme in the CoQ_{10} synthetic pathway of muscle and brain. Replacement therapy appeared to improve both muscle and brain symptoms.

COMPLEX III DEFICIENCY

Complex III is composed of 11 subunits, and a block at the level of complex III should impair utilization of both NAD-linked and FAD-linked substrates. Enzymatic analyses show defects of both succinate cytochrome *c* reductase and NADH-cytochrome *c* reductase, whereas cytochrome oxidase activity is normal.

Clinical presentation is heterogeneous, but falls into two major groups: multisystem disease (encephalomyopathy) and tissue-specific defects such as myopathy or cardiopathy.

Encephalomyopathies

A fatal infantile form has been described in a child with severe lactic acidosis presenting a few hours after birth with hypotonia, and generalized aminoaciduria, dystonic posturing, seizures and coma, followed by death at 53 hours (Birch-Machin *et al.*, 1989). Muscle biopsy was histochemically normal, but detailed biochemical studies of muscle, heart, liver and kidney showed an isolated defect of complex III and a 75% decrease of cytochrome *b* in muscle. Both parents were asymptomatic and two siblings were normal, suggesting a defect in a nDNA-encoded subunit rather than a mtDNA mutation. Later onset forms (childhood to adult life) manifest various combinations of weakness, short stature, dementia, ataxia, sensorineural deafness, pigmentary retinopathy, sensory neuropathy, and pyramidal signs (Morgan-Hughes *et al.*, 1985; Kennaway, 1988). Family history has been non-informative except for two pairs of patients, one involving a father and son (Kennaway, 1988) and implying a nDNA defect; the other a mother and daughter (Morgan-Hughes *et al.*, 1977), raising the possibility of a mtDNA defect.

Myopathy

This is characterized by exercise intolerance with premature fatigue and hyperpnoea, often followed by fixed weakness. In two patients, measurement of oxygen consumption during incremental exercise showed minimal increase of oxygen uptake despite higher than normal minute ventilation (Morgan-

Hughes *et al.*, 1985; Kennaway, 1988). Low levels of cytochrome *b* were found in most patients (Morgan-Hughes *et al.*, 1977; Hayes *et al.*, 1984; Kennaway *et al.*, 1984) but not all (Reichmann *et al.*, 1986). The existence of tissue-specific isoforms is suggested by the observation of normal complex III activity in fibroblasts and lymphoid cells from a patient with pure myopathy (Darley-Usmar *et al.*, 1983). This and the lack of maternal inheritance suggest that in patients with myopathy the defect may reside in a nDNA gene encoding a muscle-specific subunit.

Cardiopathy

A marked reduction in complex III activity and reducible cytochrome *b* was found in the myocardium from a patient with a rare, invariably fatal, cardiopathy – histiocytoid cardiomyopathy of infancy (Papadimitriou *et al.*, 1984). Absence of a block of the respiratory chain in muscle or liver further supports the existence of tissue-specific isozymes.

COMPLEX IV (CYTOCHROME OXIDASE) DEFICIENCY

Complex IV (cytochrome oxidase; COX), the last component of the respiratory chain, catalyses the transfer of reducing equivalents from cytochrome *c* to molecular oxygen. The apoprotein is composed of 13 polypeptides; the three largest subunits (I,II and III) are encoded by mtDNA and are synthesized in mitochondria; the 10 smaller subunits (IV, Va, Vb, VIa, VIb, VIc, VIIa, VIIb, VIIc and VIII) by nDNA and synthesized in the cytoplasm. Full-length cDNAs have been obtained for all subunits of human COX and Northern analysis using these cDNAs as probes has shown that only subunits VIa and VIIa are tissue-specific (DiMauro *et al.*, 1990).

Clinical phenotypes fall into two groups: one characterized by myopathy, the other involving multiple tissues with predominantly encephalopathy (DiMauro *et al.*, 1990).

Myopathy

Two forms of myopathy have been described, both presenting soon after birth with severe diffuse weakness, respiratory distress and lactic acidosis but with very different outcomes.

1. *Fatal infantile myopathy*. This causes respiratory insufficiency and death before 1 year of age. Heart, liver and brain are clinically spared, but many patients have renal disease with DeToni–Fanconi syndrome. Pedigree analysis in informative families suggests autosomal recessive transmission.

Immunological studies, using antibodies against human heart COX holoenzyme, showed decreased amount of enzyme in muscle of patients, both by enzyme-linked immunosorbent assay (ELISA) and by immunocytochemistry (Bresolin *et al.*, 1985). Moreover, by using antibodies against the individual subunits of cytochrome oxidase, Tritschler *et al.* (1991) showed a selective defect of COX VIIa in four patients, which would support the postulated nuclear and tissue-specific nature of this disorder.

2. *Benign infantile myopathy*. These infants also have severe weakness, which can be life-threatening, and often need assisted ventilation and tube feeding early in life, but then improve spontaneously and are usually normal by two or three years of age (DiMauro *et al.*, 1983; Zeviani *et al.*, 1987; Nonaka *et al.*, 1988; Servidei *et al.*, 1988).

Muscle biopsies from children with this benign COX deficiency lack both subunit VIIa and subunit II. The spontaneous recovery in these children is associated with a gradual return of COX activity in the muscle, which can be demonstrated both histochemically and biochemically (DiMauro *et al.*, 1983). The defect probably involves a nDNA-encoded COX subunit that is not only tissue-specific but also developmentally regulated. Mutations of a fetal or neonatal muscle isozyme would be corrected when the mature isozyme starts to be expressed.

A different clinical presentation, probably not related genetically to the fatal infantile myopathy, is characterized by the association of *myopathy and cardiopathy* with cytochrome oxidase deficiency (Zeviani *et al.*, 1986; Hart and Chang, 1988).

Encephalomyopathies

COX deficiency is the most common biochemical abnormality in Leigh syndrome (DiMauro *et al.*, 1990), thought to be due to the mutation of a nuclear regulatory gene that controls assembly or stability of the complex, rather than to the mutation of a gene encoding a specific COX subunit.

COX deficiency has also been found by Prick *et al.* (1983) in muscle biopsy specimens from two unrelated cases of poliodystrophy (Alpers disease) and by Bardosi *et al.* (1987) in three patients with MNGIE syndrome (myoneurogastrointestinal disorder and encephalopathy), characterized by PEO, limb weakness, peripheral neuropathy, gastroenteropathy with chronic diarrhoea and intestinal pseudo-obstruction, leucodystrophy, lactic acidosis and ragged-red fibres. Simon *et al.* (1990) subsequently suggested the acronym POLIP (polyneuropathy, ophthalmoplegia, leucoencephalopathy and intestinal pseudo-obstruction) for their further four cases. Partial COX deficiency was found in muscle and liver of the original patient (Bardosi *et al.*, 1987) and in muscle biopsy specimens from two other patients (Blake *et al.*, 1990). Pedigree analysis suggests autosomal recessive inheritance, pointing to a defect in a nDNA-encoded subunit.

COMPLEX V DEFICIENCY

Complex V (ATP synthase) converts the transmembrane proton gradient generated in the respiratory chain into chemical energy by synthesizing ATP from adenosine diphosphate (ADP) and inorganic phosphorus (Pi). It is composed of 12 to 14 subunits, two of which (subunits 6 and 8) are encoded by mtDNA (Hatefi, 1985). Defects of ATPase were demonstrated indirectly by polarographic analysis of isolated muscle mitochondria in two patients with a different clinical phenotype. One was a 37-year-old woman with congenital, slowly progressive myopathy, ragged-red fibres, and paracrystalline inclusions in virtually all mitochondria (Schotland *et al.*, 1976), the other a 17-year-old boy with a multisystem disorder characterized by weakness, ataxia, retinopathy, dementia and peripheral neuropathy (Clark *et al.*, 1983) resembling the affected members of a family with a maternally inherited multisystem disorder and a mutation in subunit 6 of complex V (Holt *et al.*, 1990) (see below).

COMBINED DEFECTS

Combined defects of the respiratory chain have been reported in several patients with myopathy or, more often, encephalomyopathies. Because the mtDNA encodes subunits of four of the five complexes, combined defects can be explained by mutations of mtDNA affecting its overall function, such as deletions, point-mutations of tRNA genes, or depletion. In fact, most of the mtDNA-related diseases are characterized biochemically by combined defects of the respiratory chain (see below). Mutations of nDNA, however, may theoretically also cause defects of multiple respiratory chain complexes by a number of potential mechanisms, which include: 1) mutations of regulatory genes controlling more than one complex; 2) mutations of subunits shared by two or more complexes; 3) mutations affecting the milieu of the complexes, such as the phospholipid composition of the inner membrane; and 4) defects of mitochondrial protein import affecting subunits of multiple complexes. A combined defect of complexes I and IV affecting muscle, heart and liver but sparing brain and kidney was reported by Zheng *et al.* (1989) in an infant with a lethal disorder, characterized by growth retardation, diffuse weakness, progressive cardiomyo-

pathy, hepatic insufficiency, severe lactic acidosis and ragged-red fibres. They postulated a mutation in the mature isoform of a nDNA-encoded, tissue-specific and developmentally regulated subunit shared by complexes I and IV. Conversely, it was suggested that a mutation affecting the fetal isoform of the same subunit might explain the benign, spontaneously reversible myopathy described by Roodhooft *et al.* (1986) which also had a combined defect of complexes I and IV. A combined defect of complexes III and IV was reported by Takamiya *et al.* (1986) in an infant with diffuse weakness, lactic acidosis and cardiorespiratory insufficiency who died at 5 months. It was postulated that the primary defect may involve a nDNA-encoded protein controlling mtDNA translation or processing of the polycistronic mRNAs.

DEFECTS OF MITOCHONDRIAL PROTEIN TRANSPORT

Schapira *et al.* (1990) described a 14-year-old girl with congenital myopathy whose muscle biopsy showed increased lipid droplets, scattered COX-negative fibres, and complete lack of the SDH histochemical reaction, but no ragged-red fibres. Biochemical analysis showed combined defects of the respiratory chain, with a specific defect of both the 27.7 kD iron-sulphur protein of SDH and the Rieske protein of complex III. Because the Rieske protein was present both in muscle homogenate and in the cytosol, but not in isolated mitochondria, it was suggested that the primary defect in this patient involved mitochondrial protein import.

DISEASES CAUSED BY DEFECTS OF MITOCHONDRIAL DNA

The main mutations in mtDNA are deletions and point mutations and, much less commonly, duplications, which have the same effect as deletions.

DELETIONS AND DUPLICATIONS

The single deletion in mtDNA is identical in all tissues in any one patient, but the number of copies of the deleted genome varies from tissue to tissue because of heteroplasmy. From the clinical point of view, three major syndromes have been associated with deletions: Kearns–Sayre syndrome (KSS), sporadic progressive external ophthalmoplegia (PEO) with RRF, and Pearson marrow/pancreas syndrome. Although the underlying genetic defect and pathogenesis may be similar, the distribution of deletions among tissues determines these syndromes. Intermediate cases, such as patients with incomplete KSS, or evolving cases, such as patients with Pearson syndrome developing KSS, have been reported, but are not common.

KEARNS–SAYRE SYNDROME —————————

Kearns and Sayre first described this condition in 1958, way ahead of the molecular explosion, in a patient with retinitis pigmentosa, external ophthalmoplegia and complete heart block. Additional features were gradually added to the list. The dominant clinical features include progressive eye signs such as ptosis, restricted eye movements and pigmentary retinopathy. Neurological symptoms include incoordination, cerebellar involvement, mental retardation and episodic coma. Seizures are infrequent, and usually associated with concomitant hypoparathyroidism. Complete heart block may lead to sudden death. The cardiac abnormality begins with left anterior fascicular heart block, occasionally in combination with right bundle branch block. Insertion of a pacemaker may be life-saving. Short stature and sensorineural hearing loss are common in KSS, as in other mtDNA-associated conditions (see Table 5-1). Endocrine disturbances include diabetes mellitus, hypoparathyroidism, and isolated growth hormone deficiency.

Elevated lactate and pyruvate values are found in plasma and in CSF. Cranial computed tomography and magnetic resonance imaging demonstrated lesions in the cerebral white matter, corresponding to the spongy degeneration of brain that has been reported in all autopsied cases (Pavlakis *et al.*, 1988). Calcification of the basal ganglia is also a feature, particularly in patients with hypoparathyroidism.

Muscle biopsy shows ragged-red fibres and a variable number of COX-negative fibres. Prognosis is poor; even after provision of a pacemaker, the course is progressively downhill and most patients die in the third or fourth decade.

Molecular genetics

Kearns–Sayre syndrome is a sporadic, non-familial disorder. Recognition of mtDNA deletions as the genetic basis of KSS by Zeviani *et al.* (1988) has helped to validate the clinical syndrome. In numerous large series from different parts of the world (Moraes *et al.*, 1989; Holt *et al.*, 1989; Zeviani *et al.*, 1990a; Goto *et al.*, 1990b; Degoul *et al.*, 1991; Trounce *et al.*, 1991), almost all patients with the clinical features of KSS had mtDNA deletions, a few had normal mtDNA by Southern analysis and occasional cases had a duplication. It has also helped

to identify cases of KSS associated with unusual features such as renal tubular acidosis (Goto *et al.*, 1990c; Eviatar *et al.*, 1990) and stroke-like episodes similar to MELAS syndrome (Zupanc *et al.* 1991).

Absence of deletions in muscle mtDNA from mothers of KSS patients (Moraes *et al.*, 1989; Zeviani *et al.*, 1990a) suggests the deletions are new mutations, probably in the zygote and affecting somatic rather than germ-line cells. This would also account for the occasional KSS women who reproduce having clinically normal children. However, Poulton *et al.* (1991) documented by polymerase chain reaction (PCR) the same mtDNA deletion in a child with KSS and in his asymptomatic mother and maternal aunt, suggesting germ-line mutations. In addition Poulton *et al.* (1989) found duplications of mtDNA in two patients with KSS.

Some patients have PEO plus only a few but not all of the features of KSS. These cases of *incomplete KSS* (Moraes *et al.*, 1989) may develop the full syndrome later in life and the presence of mtDNA deletions in most of them underlines the identity with KSS.

SPORADIC PEO WITH RRF —————————

This clinically benign condition is characterized by ophthalmoplegia, ptosis and proximal limb weakness. Onset is usually in adolescence or early adult life, and the course is slowly progressive and compatible with a relatively normal life. Muscle biopsy shows ragged-red fibres and COX-negative fibres. About 50% of all patients with progressive external ophthalmoplegia have mtDNA deletions (Moraes *et al.*, 1989). There is no family history, and this helps in the differential diagnosis from other forms of PEO, such as late-onset autosomal dominant oculopharyngeal muscular dystrophy and autosomal dominant PEO with multiple mtDNA deletions. Women with PEO reproduce normally and have asymptomatic children, suggesting the mutation affects only somatic cells or, if it affects germ-line cells, must be selected against in the course of oogenesis.

PEARSON MARROW/PANCREAS SYNDROME —————————

This non-neurological disease of childhood is characterized by refractory sideroblastic anaemia, vacuolization of marrow precursors and exocrine pancreatic dysfunction, and is usually fatal in early childhood, from sepsis secondary to bone marrow failure (Pearson *et al.*, 1979; Rotig *et al.*, 1990). The overlap with Kearns-Sayre syndrome has been established in some exceptional patients with Pearson syndrome who survived into adolescence, only to develop symptoms and signs of KSS (Larsson *et al.*, 1990; McShane *et al.*, 1991). The clinical improvement of the blood dyscrasia in these patients is probably due to a gradual decrease of the number of mtDNA deletions in blood cells, whereas the muscle, in contrast, on repeated biopsies in a patient who developed KSS showed an increase in the proportion of deletions with time (Larsson *et al.*, 1990).

DELETIONS OF mtDNA: MOLECULAR BIOLOGY

The deletions of mtDNA range in size from approximately 2 to 8.5 kb and are largely confined to an 11 kb region of the mitochondrial genome. Regardless of clinical presentation, a number of separate studies have shown that some 30–40% of all deletions are identical (the *common deletion*) and span 4977 bp from the ATPase 8 gene to the ND5 gene (see Figure 5-17) (Moraes *et al.*, 1989; Holt *et al.*, 1989; Schon *et al.*, 1989; Johns *et al.*, 1989; Shoffner *et al.*, 1989; Tanaka *et al.*, 1989).

Analysis of mtDNA heteroplasmy has shown, by polymerase chain reaction, abundant deletions in most postmortem tissues from patients with Kearns–Sayre syndrome, as well as the presence of deleted mtDNAs in accessible non-muscle tissues from patients with progressive external ophthalmoplegia. These observations suggest that the clinical phenotype is determined by the distribution and relative abundance of mtDNA deletions in different tissues.

POINT MUTATIONS

Point mutations of mtDNA have been found in association with five maternally inherited diseases: MERRF (Shoffner *et al.*, 1990); MELAS (Goto *et al.*, 1990a; Kobayashi *et al.*, 1990); Leber hereditary optic neuroretinopathy (LHON) (Wallace *et al.*, 1988a); neuropathy, ataxia and retinitis pigmentosa (NARP) (ATPase 6 mutation syndrome) (Holt *et al.*, 1990); and a maternally inherited disorder with adult-onset myopathy and cardiomyopathy (MIMyCa) (Zeviani *et al.*, 1991b).

MERRF (MYOCLONUS EPILEPSY WITH RAGGED-RED FIBRES)

In 1980, Fukuhara *et al.* described two patients with myoclonus epilepsy and ragged-red fibres. A subsequent review of the literature by Pavlakis *et al.* (1988) identified 25 potential examples of MERRF. In its full clinical expression, MERRF is characterized by myoclonic seizures, mitochondrial myopathy, and cerebellar ataxia. Additional, less common signs include dementia, hearing loss, optic atrophy, peripheral neuropathy and spasticity (Table 5-1). Given the clinical heterogeneity characteristic of mtDNA mutations, the disease may be fully expressed only in very few members of a given family, whereas other maternal relatives may show only some symptoms and signs or be totally asymptomatic. In the absence of at least one typical patient, the diagnosis of MERRF can be missed, and the hereditary pattern can be overlooked.

Recognition of a highly specific, although not exclusive, point mutation at nt 8344 in the tRNA[Lys] gene of mtDNA by Shoffner *et al.* (1990) has made possible the identification of patients independently of the severity of their clinical phenotype and has become an indispensable tool in the classification of MERRF. This point mutation has been present in most patients with clinical diagnosis of MERRF, but was lacking in four patients with typical MERRF, suggesting genetic heterogeneity (Zeviani *et al.*, 1991a; Hammans *et al.*, 1991).

Clinical features

Onset of symptoms can be in childhood or in adult life, and the course can be slowly progressive or rapidly downhill. Wallace *et al.* (1988b) suggested that the vulnerability of different organs parallels their dependence on oxidation/phosphorylation, with the brain suffering first, followed by muscle and heart, but this may vary from patient to patient. Clinical heterogeneity is well illustrated by the original family in which Tsairis *et al.* (1973) first described the association of myoclonic epilepsy and RRF. The mother, at age 33, presented with a myopathy diagnosed as limb girdle muscular dystrophy, despite the presence of RRF, and died of a lymphoma 13 years later without developing any brain symptoms. Of her four children, one had ragged-red fibres in a muscle biopsy at age 22 but was still asymptomatic at 40; two girls died at 12 and 16 years of age after rapidly progressive encephalomyopathy compatible with MERRF; the fourth child, in whom the point mutation at nt 8344 was documented, also had typical MERRF with onset in childhood, but the course was relatively slow and he died at age 36 (DiMauro, 1993).

In a well-characterized pedigree (Figure 5.19) documented by Wallace and Lott (1993), the proband had uncontrolled myoclonic jerking, dementia, cardiomyopathy, nephropathy, neurosensory

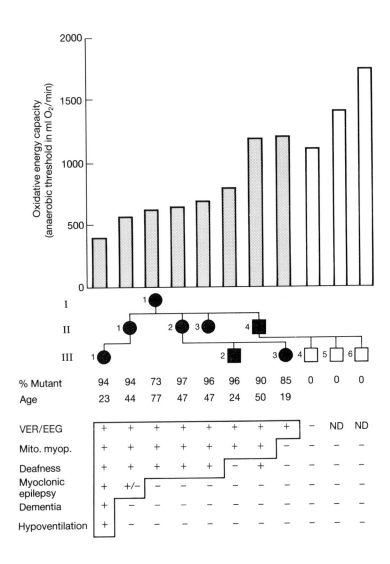

% Mutant	94	94	73	97	96	96	90	85	0	0	0
Age	23	44	77	47	47	24	50	19			
VER/EEG	+	+	+	+	+	+	+	+	−	ND	ND
Mito. myop.	+	+	+	+	+	+	+	−	−	−	−
Deafness	+	+	+	+	+	−	+	−	−	−	−
Myoclonic epilepsy	+	+/−	−	−	−	−	−	−	−	−	−
Dementia	+	−	−	−	−	−	−	−	−	−	−
Hypoventilation	+	−	−	−	−	−	−	−	−	−	−

Figure 5-19 The association between genotype, phenotype, and oxidative phosphorylation defect in myoclonus epilepsy and ragged-red fibres (MERRF) pedigree. Oxidative energy capacity (anaerobic threshold) was determined by an exercise stress test and the values are directly proportional to OXPHOS enzyme levels. The percentages of mutant mtDNA levels were determined by CviJI digestion of amplified patient mtDNA and together with age they determine the OXPHOS level and clinical phenotype. VER/EEG, visual evoked response/electroencephalography analysis; Mito.Myop., mitochondrial myopathy; ND, not determined. Reproduced with permission from Wallace and Lott, 1993.

hearing loss, mitochondrial myopathy, and aberrations in the visual evoked response and electroencephalographic tracings. Less severely affected family members had progressively fewer symptoms – the mother only an occasional myoclonic jerk plus hearing loss, mitochondrial myopathy and electrophysiological changes; two aunts hearing loss, mitochondrial myopathy and electrophysiological changes; and a maternal cousin, who was clinically normal, only mild electrophysiological aberrations.

Physiological analyses showed that the severity of these symptoms was directly proportional to the mitochondrial energy output as determined by exercise stress tests, muscle mitochondrial respiration rates and muscle mitochondrial oxidative phosphorylation (OXPHOS) enzyme activities. The severely affected proband had the lowest energy capacity, whereas the mildly affected cousin was in the normal range.

Although all of the maternal relatives of this

pedigree harboured varying proportions of the tRNA^{Lys} mutation (Figure 5-19), the percentage of mutant mtDNAs was not directly proportional with the severity of the OXPHOS defect or the symptoms. This discrepancy resulted from an additional variable, the progressive decline of OXPHOS with age. When members of the maternal lineage were stratified according to mtDNA genotype, the specific activities of all OXPHOS enzymes were observed to decline in parallel with age. Further, when the family members were stratified by age, the clinical phenotypes correlated well with genotype – the normal mtDNAs having a marked protective effect over mutant mtDNAs.

The marked phenotypic variability observed in heteroplasmic MERRF pedigrees is consistent with the concept that symptoms progressively accumulate as the mitochondrial energy generating capacity drops progressively below organ-specific expression thresholds. It also demonstrates the critical role that the age-related decline in OXPHOS plays in the appearance and progression of symptoms. Presumably, an individual born with over 90% mutant tRNA^{Lys} has sufficient residual OXPHOS capacity while young to function normally. As this individual grows older, however, OXPHOS declines further until organ thresholds are traversed, and symptoms appear in the young adult years (Figure 5-19).

Molecular genetics

The point mutation, an A to G transition in the TΨC loop of the tRNA^{Lys} gene, must be relatively mild because even small proportions of wild-type mtDNA have protective effects on the clinical phenotype (Shoffner *et al.*, 1990). The mutation was present in all tissues of a patient studied postmortem by Zeviani *et al.* (1991a,b). It was also detectable in blood cells of all five patients studied by Hammans *et al.* (1991), which should provide a useful way to confirm a suspected clinical diagnosis.

Muscle biopsy

The ragged-red fibres on muscle biopsy are an essential component of the syndrome, though an occasional, otherwise typical, case may not show them. Histochemistry shows numerous COX-negative fibres, and immunocytochemistry shows the presence of two populations of mitochondria in individual muscle fibres: a population with normal COX activity and immunoreactivity for subunit II and a population with decrease in COX activity and in COX-II immunoreactivity (Lombes *et al.*, 1989). Neuropathology has shown consistent central nervous system changes in all patients.

Biochemical studies

Biochemical studies of muscle have given divergent results, with defects of complex III; complexes II and IV; complexes I and IV; complexes I, III and IV; or complex IV alone. Combined partial defects of all complexes requiring mtDNA-encoded subunits probably occur and could explain these apparent discrepancies between patients.

MELAS (MITOCHONDRIAL ENCEPHALOMYOPATHY, LACTIC ACIDOSIS, AND STROKE-LIKE EPISODES)

The distinctive features of this clinical syndrome were first documented by Pavlakis *et al.* in 1984. There is a normal early development, followed by a devastating, progressive encephalomyopathy, punctuated by paroxysmal episodes resembling strokes.

Clinical features

Hirano *et al.* (1992) recently gave a progress report on the original case and reviewed some 70 additional cases from the literature. All patients became symptomatic before age 40 years; almost all had normal early development followed by the onset of exercise intolerance, stroke-like episodes, seizures and dementia. Almost all cases had evidence of lactic acidosis and had RRF in biopsied skeletal muscle. Recurrent migraine-like headaches preceded by nausea and vomiting were common in this patient population, as were hearing loss, short stature, learning difficulties, hemiparesis and hemianopia, and limb weakness. CSF protein value was normal in one-half of the patients and mildly elevated in the other 50%. One-third of patients had basal ganglia calcifications. The lateralizing cerebral abnormalities often immediately preceded seizures. Progressive external ophthalmoplegia was noted in approximately 10% of cases. One-quarter of cases had a positive family history consistent with maternal inheritance.

Muscle biopsy

Muscle biopsy usually shows ragged-red fibres, but these were lacking in three patients of Ciafaloni *et al.* (1992) and two of Hammans *et al.* (1991).

Biochemical studies

Biochemical studies of muscle have shown complex I deficiency in many patients (Kobayashi *et al.*, 1987; Nishizawa *et al.*, 1987; Ichiki *et al.*, 1988, 1989;

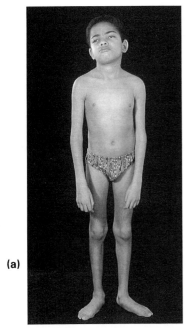

(a)

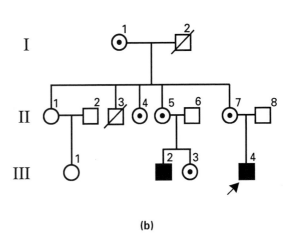

(b)

Figure 5-20 MELAS. The index patient (a,b; III,4) was referred to our muscle clinic for further investigation at the age of 7 years. He was born prematurely at 34 weeks and had delay in his motor milestones, sitting at 9 months, commando crawling at 15 months and walking at 18 months. At school he was noted by a physiotherapist to have poor coordination, and assessment showed poor muscle tone and generalized weakness, with inability to hop or jump. At 7 years he was referred to his local paediatrician because his eating was poor and he tired easily. His height and weight were below the 3rd centile, his muscle power and coordination below par, his CK elevated at 675 iu/litre. When referred to the Hammersmith Hospital his muscle power was MRC 4 in most groups, the muscle ultrasound normal and the blood lactate markedly elevated at 8.5 mmol/litre (n <1.8). Needle biopsy of the quadriceps showed a mitochondrial myopathy. At 8 years 11 months he was admitted for investigation of episodic blindness, occurring on several occasions in the preceding months when he awoke in the morning with marked loss of vision and only able to distinguish light and dark. No visual deficit could be demonstrated but a CT scan showed low attenuation areas in the occipital lobes involving predominantly the white matter. His blood lactate was 9.2 mmol/litre. A diagnosis of MELAS was made and he was treated with riboflavine and coenzyme Q without any clinically detectable effect. He subsequently had two transitory episodes of hemiplegia involving first the left and then the right side, associated with wedge-shaped infarcts on CT scanning, which also showed resolution of the previous occipital lesions. He was also admitted to hospital on several occasions with severe nausea and vomiting, and needed intravenous fluid replacement. He found it difficult coping at normal school and was being assessed for special school placement. His cousin (III,2) was also affected, but less severely and did not have any stroke-like episodes. His appetite was poor; he failed to thrive, and was noted at school to be lethargic and less active than his peers. He was investigated at another hospital at 6 years and found to have a normal CK, an elevated blood lactate (10.9 mmol/litre) and mitochondrial myopathy on biopsy. He subsequently had two grand mal convulsions but no stroke-like episodes. He was developmentally delayed and attending special school; he also had behaviour problems. DNA studies of the family (Dr Jo Poulton) revealed the classical bp 3243 point mutation in all members tested, including blood and muscle from the index patient, muscle only from his cousin and blood from the clinically normal females, II,4, 5 and 7 and III,3. The proportion of mutant DNA in the index patient was higher in muscle than in blood, and higher in his muscle than that of his cousin. The amount of mutant DNA was lower in the clinically unaffected individuals carrying the mutation. The mother of the index patient has some hearing loss and also migraine.

Koga *et al.*, 1988); whilst a combined defect of complexes I and IV was found by Byrne *et al.* (1988) in identical twins that had features of MERRF and MELAS. In their patients with MELAS, Ciafaloni *et al.* (1992) found multiple defects of the respiratory chain affecting complexes I, III and especially complex IV.

Molecular genetics

As MELAS is characterized by stroke-like episodes, in their absence it may be difficult to diagnose clinically. As with MERRF, the identification of a highly specific, although not exclusive, point mutation at nt 3243 in the tRNA$^{Leu(UUR)}$ gene of mtDNA has provided an indispensable diagnostic tool. The point mutation was found in 26 of 31 MELAS patients by Goto *et al.* (1990a) and in all six patients of Kobayashi *et al.* (1990). Hammans *et al.* (1991) reported the point mutation in 17 patients, eight of whom had stroke-like episodes, whilst the others had variable symptoms. Ciafaloni *et al.* (1992) found that 21 of 23 patients with MELAS had the mutation when they defined MELAS on the basis of 1) stroke-like episodes (with CT or MRI evidence of focal brain abnormalities); 2) lactic acidosis, RRF, or both; and 3) at least two of the following: focal or generalized seizures, dementia, recurrent headache and vomiting. They also found the mutation in all 11 oligosymptomatic and 12 of the 14 asymptomatic maternal relatives, a reminder that the MELAS mutation should be looked for in patients with non-specific symptoms and signs of mitochondrial encephalomyopathy and evidence of maternal inheritance. Onset was before age 15 in 62% of their MELAS patients, hemianopia or cortical blindness being the most common manifestation, and the first stroke-like episode occurred before age 40 in all but four. Seizures were present in all cases and lactic acidosis in all but one.

In two patients studied postmortem by Ciafaloni *et al.* (1991, 1992), the point mutation, an A to G transition at nt pair 3243, was found in all tissues, with a high proportion of the mutant mtDNA (93–96% of total). The percentages of mutant genomes, however, were lower in muscle from oligosymptomatic relatives (62–89%) and lowest in muscle from asymptomatic relatives (28–82%). Because the number of mutant genomes is lower in blood than in muscle, the mutation may not be detectable in blood cells from some patients in whom it would be detectable in muscle. Thus no mutations were found in blood from one asymptomatic relative who had 55% mutant mtDNAs in her muscle (Ciafaloni *et al.*, 1992), and Hammans *et al.* (1991) failed to find the mutation in the blood of one of their 11 patients with the MELAS mutation in muscle. Thus screening of blood cells for the MELAS mutation is useful, particularly if positive, but may give false negative results. Absence of the mutation at nt 3243 in occasional MELAS patients suggests genetic heterogeneity.

Prognosis in patients with the full syndrome is very poor, and there is currently no effective therapy (Figure 5-20).

ATPASE 6 MUTATION SYNDROME; NEUROPATHY, ATAXIA, RETINITIS PIGMENTOSA (NARP)

Holt *et al.* (1990) reported a new maternally-inherited, multisystem disorder, affecting four members in three generations of a family, with developmental delay, retinitis pigmentosa, dementia, seizures, ataxia, proximal weakness and sensory neuropathy. There were no ragged-red fibres in the muscle biopsy. They attributed the disease to a heteroplasmic point mutation at nt 8993 within the ATPase 6 gene. The different severity of the disease in different family members seemed to correlate with the relative abundance of mutant genomes in leucocytes. The acronym NARP has now become attached to this syndrome (neuropathy, ataxia, retinitis pigmentosa).

MATERNALLY INHERITED DISORDER WITH ADULT-ONSET MYOPATHY AND CARDIOMYOPATHY (MIMyCa)

Zeviani *et al.* (1991b) reported a large pedigree with several members affected by a maternally inherited condition involving skeletal and cardiac muscle. Serum lactate values were elevated and ragged-red fibres were present in biopsied skeletal muscle. The central nervous system was not involved.

A heteroplasmic point mutation was uncovered in the mtDNA gene for tRNA$^{Leu(UUR)}$. Although a different point mutation, the mtDNA gene was at the same site as the MELAS point mutation.

OTHER mtDNA POINT MUTATIONS

Many papers have appeared describing point mutations in tRNA genes, other than those involved in MERRF and MELAS, in individual patients with diverse clinical presentations, including fatal infantile cardiomyopathy (Tanaka *et al.*, 1990), fatal infantile myopathies or hepatopathies with lactic acidosis and respiratory chain defects (Yoon *et al.*, 1991), PEO, or MNGIE syndrome (Lauber *et al.*, 1991), but the pathogenetic role of these defects remains to be determined.

DISEASES CAUSED BY DEFECTS OF COMMUNICATION BETWEEN NUCLEAR AND MITOCHONDRIAL GENOME

MULTIPLE mtDNA DELETIONS

Zeviani *et al.* (1989) and Servidei *et al.* (1991) described an Italian family with autosomal dominant transmission of PEO, exercise intolerance, weakness of proximal limb and respiratory muscles, cataracts, hearing loss and early death. Southern analysis revealed multiple deletions of mtDNA associated with lactic acidosis and RRF. All affected family members had multiple deletions involving a large portion of mtDNA. In addition, the amount of deleted mtDNA increased with time and appeared to be roughly proportional to the clinical severity. Deletions also appeared to be tissue specific. The origin of all the deletions was in the displacement loop (D-loop) region of mtDNA (Figure 5-17), which is the site of interaction between the nuclear genome and the mitochondrial genome. The nuclear gene defect in these cases apparently alters the biological integrity of the mitochondrial genome and predisposes to multiple deletions that characterize this clinical syndrome.

Several other families have been described with autosomal dominantly inherited PEO (Zeviani *et al.*, 1990b; Cormier *et al.*, 1991), and multiple deletions of mtDNA have been documented in a family with PEO and RRF previously described by Iannaccone *et al.* in 1974 (DiMauro, 1993).

Associated symptoms and signs varied in different families but were suggestive of multisystem involvement: hearing loss, tremor, ataxia, peripheral neuropathy (Zeviani *et al.*, 1990b); ataxia, mental retardation, hypoparathyroidism and low-density areas in basal ganglia, centrum ovale and brain peduncle by CT scan (Cormier *et al.*, 1991); nystagmus and abnormal electroencephalogram (Iannaccone *et al.*, 1974). The French patient recorded by Cormier *et al.* (1991) presented in early childhood with recurrent attacks of incoordination, drowsiness, and coma associated with ketoacidosis. Ragged-red fibres were present in his muscle, and a defect in oxidative phosphorylation was found in muscle and lymphocytes. Various mtDNA deletions were detected in the proband as well as his healthy mother and maternal aunt, but not in the rest of the maternal progeny. Pigmentary retinopathy was absent in all of these cases.

Biochemical studies

Biochemical studies of muscle showed combined defects of the respiratory chain of varying severity in one family (Servidei *et al.*, 1991), and complex I deficiency in the patient of Cormier *et al.* (1991).

The clear autosomal dominant mode of transmission in most of these families suggests that the alteration of a nDNA-encoded trans-acting factor triggers the mtDNA deletions (Zeviani *et al.*, 1989), although the responsible factor remains elusive.

DEPLETION OF mtDNA ————————

This is the first hereditary human disorder characterized by a quantitative rather than qualitative abnormality of mtDNA (Moraes *et al.*, 1991). In 1983, Boustany *et al.* described a family in which two sisters had died in infancy of a myopathy, and a second cousin (related through the maternal grandfather) died in infancy of liver disease. Biochemical studies showed cytochrome oxidase, cytochrome *b*, and cytochrome aa_3 deficiencies in muscle of the sisters and in the liver of the cousin. Thinking that a skewed tissue distribution could explain the different clinical phenotypes in members of the same family, Moraes *et al.* (1991) studied muscle from one of the sisters and liver from the cousin by Southern blot. They found no evidence of a deletion but noted that mtDNA was barely detectable.

mtDNA depletion has been observed in other patients; a severe depletion in three unrelated infants and partial mtDNA depletion in four children (Tritschler *et al.*, 1992; Moraes *et al.*, 1991). Of the five infants with severe mtDNA depletion, four developed diffuse myopathy in the first weeks of life, requiring assisted ventilation. One had persistent external ophthalmoplegia (Boustany *et al.*, 1983). All had severe lactic acidosis and ragged-red fibres in the muscle biopsy. Two also had renal dysfunction with glycosuria, phosphaturia and generalized aminoaciduria (DeToni–Fanconi–Debre syndrome), making the differential diagnosis from the fatal infantile myopathy caused by cytochrome oxidase deficiency difficult on purely clinical grounds. The patient with liver disease died at 9 months of hepatic failure, and postmortem examination of the liver showed abnormal mitochondria. Family history suggested autosomal recessive inheritance in the cases of Boustany *et al.*; a brother of another patient had died at 6 hours of heart failure, and the mother had had three miscarriages. All parents were asymptomatic, and there was no evidence of maternal transmission. In each case, mtDNA depletion was observed only in affected tissues (muscle, liver, kidney) and not in unaffected tissues.

In the four patients with partial mtDNA depletion, the clinical picture was dominated by myopathy; onset was later, between 5 and 12 months, and the course was slower, but two children died at 11 months and 3 years, and one was tetraplegic and ventilator-dependent at 3½ years (Tritschler *et al.*, 1992). Blood lactates were normal. Muscle biopsies showed ragged-red fibres, but a biopsy obtained early in the course of the disease had shown only non-specific myopathic features. Two of the four patients were siblings, and all parents were asymptomatic.

Biochemical studies

Biochemical studies showed combined defects of respiratory chain complexes containing mtDNA-encoded subunits, such as complexes I, III, and IV, more marked in patients with severe than in those with partial mtDNA depletion. In patients with severe mtDNA depletion, there was a close correlation between degree of depletion and COX deficiency (Moraes *et al.*, 1991).

The decrease of mtDNA was documented by densitometry of Southern blots and confirmed by immunocytochemistry with anti-DNA antibodies and by *in situ* hybridization (Tritschler *et al.*, 1992; Moraes *et al.*, 1991; Andreetta *et al.*, 1991). The depletion of muscle mtDNA was almost complete (83–98%) in the more severely affected infants and varied between 66% and 92% in the less severely affected children. Considering that mitochondria are increased in number, it can be calculated that many organelles must be totally devoid of mtDNA in affected tissues.

As predicted by the scarcity of mtDNA and suggested by the biochemical results, immunocytochemistry using subunit-specific antibodies showed that mtDNA-encoded subunits, such as COX-II or ND1, were absent or markedly decreased, whereas nDNA-encoded subunits, such as COX-IV, were present.

GENETICS

The apparently mendelian inheritance of mtDNA depletion suggests that the genetic defect may involve a nuclear gene controlling mtDNA replication. On the other hand, the tissue-specific expression of the depletion would be more easily explained by uneven segregation to different tissues of a replication-deficient mtDNA population.

In a recent study of five patients with mitochondrial myopathy, Poulton *et al.* (1995) questioned whether mtDNA depletion was indeed a distinct clinical syndrome or possibly a relatively non-specific response of muscle to various pathological processes. They found a variation in the ratio of mtDNA to nDNA in samples from different muscles of the same individual and very low levels of mtDNA versus nDNA in fetal muscle and in ischaemic muscle from amputees. However, four patients with cytochrome oxidase deficiency had low levels of mtDNA, suggesting an association. Two of these cases had a benign course, in contrast to the uniformly severe course of those documented in the literature.

TREATMENT OF MITOCHONDRIAL DISEASE

The potential treatment of the various mitochondrial disorders has been reviewed by Przyrembel (1987) and more recently by Calvani *et al.* (1993). Many of the reports in the literature have been anecdotal case histories, either in isolated cases or in small trials over relatively short periods of time. Given the rarity of these disorders and the rationale for trying some of these compounds, it seems reasonable to attempt one-off therapeutic efforts in this way. The additional problem of trying to set up controlled clinical trials in these mitochondrial disorders is the remarkable variability of clinical phenotype, even within individual families.

The following is a summary of some of the approaches that have been tried:

DIETARY MEASURES; VITAMINS

Dietary manipulations can decrease endogenous production of toxic metabolites in relation to various specific disorders. A regimen of a high carbohydrate intake has been recommended to compensate for impaired gluconeogenesis and to decrease lipolysis; frequent meals with nocturnal feeding in patients suffering from hypoketotic hypoglycaemic dicarboxylic aciduria syndromes; additional fat restriction or a substitution of long- with medium-chain triglycerides for subjects affected by carnitine and carnitine-palmitoyl transferase deficiency.

Thiamine (vitamin B1), riboflavine (vitamin B2) and folates have been tried in several mitochondrial disorders without any apparent benefit.

Vitamin C together with vitamin K have been used to try and bypass some blocks in the electron transport chain and facilitate the transfer of electrons to cytochrome *c*, and especially defects of Complex III (CoQ-cytochrome *c*-reductase), with beneficial effects on energy metabolism in a single case (Eleff *et al.*, 1984). The same treatment, however, was ineffective in two other patients, an infant with encephalomyopathy (Przyrembel, 1987) and an adult with myopathy (Reichmann *et al.*, 1986). Vitamin C has been utilized alone in a patient with cytochrome *c* deficiency, and has been considered useful for the survival of the subject (over 5 years) (Przyrembel, 1987).

COENZYME Q_{10}

Coenzyme CoQ_{10} transfers electrons from Complexes I and II to Complex III, stabilizes respiratory complexes at the level of the inner mitochondrial membrane, and inhibits the effects of free radicals on mitochondrial membranes. In two sisters with encephalomyopathy and an apparently primary deficiency of CoQ_{10}, CoQ_{10} administration was effective (Ogasahara et al., 1989).

In a patient with Kearns–Sayre syndrome, Ogasahara et al. (1985) found a decreased concentration of CoQ_{10} both in serum and in skeletal muscle mitochondria. After treatment with CoQ_{10} (60–120 mg/day) for 3 months, serum levels of lactate and pyruvate normalized, and there was improvement of cardiac and ocular symptoms.

A subsequent clinical trial in seven cases of Kearns–Sayre syndrome showed after 1 year of CoQ_{10} treatment (120 mg/day) improvement in clinical features and lower serum lactate and pyruvate levels (Bresolin et al., 1988).

Some change in the biochemical abnormalities was documented in two case reports on MELAS syndrome (Yamamoto et al., 1987; Ihara et al., 1989). In a case of MELAS with partial cytochrome c oxidase deficiency in muscle, 1 year of CoQ_{10} administration (90 mg/day) did not improve CSF lactate but did decrease plasma lactate and may have ameliorated clinical weakness (Yamamoto et al., 1987). In another patient with MELAS, administration of 90 mg/day of idebenone in addition to 210 mg/day of CoQ_{10} for 3 months decreased CSF protein, lactate and pyruvate, whereas monoamines and their metabolites increased (Ihara et al., 1989).

On the other hand, Zierz et al. (1990) obtained no response to CoQ_{10} administration (50–100 mg/kg/day) in two patients with mitochondrial myopathy, and negative results were also obtained in a patient with mitochondrial encephalomyopathy and cytochrome c oxidase deficiency treated with CoQ_{10} (150 mg/day) for 2 years (Nishikawa et al., 1989); there was some improvement of the patient's 'fatiguability', but ophthalmoplegia and ptosis did not change.

A study investigating the efficacy of CoQ_{10} in association with menadione, ascorbic acid, thiamine, niacinamide and riboflavin in patients with progressive external ophthalmoplegia, myoclonus epilepsy and ragged-red fibres (MERRF) and pure myopathy found no improvement in objective measurements of oxidative metabolism (Ford et al., 1992).

CORTICOSTEROIDS

A positive response to corticosteroids has been claimed by some authors in patients with mitochondrial myopathy (Mastaglia et al., 1980; Patten et al., 1976). The mechanism of action may relate to membrane stabilization, enzyme induction, or inhibition of phospholipase activity.

Bachynski et al. (1986), however, showed that, in addition to the typical side-effects associated with steroid administration, there was further impairment of oxidative phosphorylation in a patient with Kearns–Sayre syndrome.

Corticosteroids, together with carnitine, have also been used to treat primary carnitine deficiency with some apparent benefit (Angelini et al., 1992). In patients with carnitine deficiency, there has been no clear correlation between dosage of corticosteroids and clinical improvement.

REFERENCES

Amendt, B.A., Green, C., Sweetman, L. et al. (1987) Short-chain acyl-coenzyme A dehydrogenase deficiency: clinical and biochemical studies in two patients. *Journal of Clinical Investigation* **79**: 1303–1309.

Amendt, B.A., Moon, A., Teel, L. et al. (1988) Long-chain acyl-coenzyme A dehydrogenase deficiency: biochemical studies in fibroblasts from three patients. *Pediatric Research* **23**: 603–605.

Anderson, S., Bankier, A.T., Barrell, B.G. et al. (1981) Sequence and organization of the human mitochondrial genome. *Nature* **290**: 457–465.

Andreetta, F., Tritschler, H-J, Schon, E.A. et al. (1991) Localization of mitochondrial DNA in normal and pathological muscle using immunological probes: A new approach to the study of mitochondrial myopathies. *Journal of the Neurological Sciences* **105**: 88–92.

Angelini, C., Martinuzzi, A. and Vergani, L. (1992) Treatment with L-carnitine of the infantile and adult for primary carnitine deficiency. In: Ferrari, R., DiMauro, S. and Sherwood, G. eds, *L-Carnitine and its Role in Medicine: From Function to Therapy*. London: Academic Press, pp. 139–153.

Argov, Z. and Bank, W.J. (1991) Phosphorus magnetic resonance spectroscopy (^{31}P MRS) in neuromuscular disorders. *Annals of Neurology* **30**: 90–97.

Bachynski, B.N., Flynn, J.T., Rodrigues, M.M. et al. (1986) Hyperglycemic acidotic coma and death in Kearns–Sayre syndrome. *Ophthalmology* **93**: 391–396.

Bardosi, A., Creutzfeldt, W., DiMauro, S. et al. (1987) Myo-, neuro-, gastrointestinal encephalopathy (MNGIE syndrome) due to partial deficiency of cytochrome c oxidase. *Acta Neuropathologica* **74**: 248–258.

Behbehani, A.W., Goebel, H., Osse, G. *et al.* (1984) Mitochondrial myopathy with lactic acidosis and deficient activity of muscle succinate-cytochrome *c* oxidoreductase. *European Journal of Pediatrics* **143**: 67–71.

Bet, L., Bresolin, N., Moggio, M. *et al.* (1990) A case of mitochondrial myopathy, lactic acidosis and complex I deficiency. *Journal of Neurology* **237**: 399–404.

Birch–Machin, M.A., Shepherd, I.M., Watmaugh, N.J. *et al.* (1989) Fatal lactic acidosis in infancy with a defect of complex III of the respiratory chain. *Pediatric Research* **25**: 553–559.

Blake, D., Lombes, A., Minetti, C. *et al.* (1990) MNGIE syndrome: Report of two new patients. *Neurology* **40** (Suppl 1): 294.

Blass, J.P., Avigan, J. and Uhlendorf, B.W. (1970) A defect in pyruvate decarboxylase in a child with an intermittent movement disorder. *Journal of Clinical Investigation* **49**: 423–432.

Bougnères, P-F., Saudubray, J-M., Marsac, C. *et al.* (1981) Fasting hypoglycaemia resulting from hepatic carnitine palmitoyltransferase deficiency. *Journal of Pediatrics* **98**: 742–746.

Boustany, R.N., Aprille, J.R., Halperin, J. *et al.* (1983) Mitochondrial cytochrome deficiency presenting as a myopathy with hypotonia, external ophthalmoplegia, and lactic acidosis in an infant and as fatal hepatopathy in a second cousin. *Annals of Neurology* **14**: 462–470.

Bresolin, N., Zeviani, M., Bonilla, E. *et al.* (1985) Fatal infantile cytochrome oxidase deficiency: decrease of immunologically detectable enzyme in muscle. *Neurology* **35**: 802–812.

Bresolin, N., Bet, L., Binda, A. *et al.* (1988) Clinical and biochemical correlations in mitochondrial myopathies treated with coenzyme Q10. *Neurology* **38**: 892–899.

Bressler, R. (1970) Carnitine and the twins. (Editorial). *New England Journal of Medicine* **282**: 745–746.

Byrne, E., Dennett, X., Trounce, I. *et al.* (1985) Partial cytochrome *c* oxidase deficiency in chronic progressive external ophthalmoplegia. *Journal of the Neurological Sciences* **71**: 257–271.

Byrne, E., Trounce, I., Dennett, X. *et al.* (1988) Progression from MERRF to MELAS phenotype in a patient with combined respiratory complex I and IV deficiencies. *Journal of the Neurological Sciences* **88**: 327–337.

Calvani, M., Koverech, A. and Caruso G. (1993) Treatment of mitochondrial diseases. In: DiMauro, S. and Wallace, D.C. eds, *Mitochondrial DNA in Human Pathology*. New York: Raven Press.

Ciafaloni, E., Ricci, E., Servidei, S. *et al.* (1991) Widespread tissue distribution of a tRNA$^{Leu(UUR)}$ mutation in the mitochondrial DNA of a patient with MELAS syndrome. *Neurology* **41**: 1663–1665.

Ciafaloni, E., Ricci, E., Shanske, S. *et al.* (1992) MELAS: clinical features, biochemistry, and molecular genetics. *Annals of Neurology* **31**: 391–398.

Clark, J.B., Hayes, D.J., Byrne, E. *et al.* (1983) Mitochondrial myopathies: defects in mitochondrial metabolism in human skeletal muscle. *Biochemical Society Transactions* **11**: 626–627.

Coates, P.M., Hale, D.E., Stanley, C.A. *et al.* (1985) Genetic deficiency of medium-chain acyl-coenzyme A dehydrogenase: studies in cultured skin fibroblasts and peripheral mononuclear leukocytes. *Pediatric Research* **19**: 671–676.

Coates, P.M., Hale, D.E., Finocchiaro, G. *et al.* (1988) Genetic deficiency of short-chain acyl-coenzyme A dehydrogenase in cultured fibroblasts from a patient with muscle carnitine deficiency and severe skeletal muscle weakness. *Journal of Clinical Investigation* **81**: 171–175.

Cormier, V., Rotig, A., Tardieu, M. *et al.* (1991) Autosomal dominant deletions of the mitochondrial genome in a case of progressive encephalomyopathy. *American Journal of Human Genetics* **48**: 643–648.

Cornelio, F., Di Donato, S., Peluchetti, P. *et al.* (1977) Fatal cases of lipid storage myopathy with carnitine deficiency. *Journal of Neurology, Neurosurgery and Psychiatry* **40**: 170–178.

Cruse, R.P., DiMauro, S., Towfighi, J. *et al.* (1984) Familial systemic carnitine deficiency. *Archives of Neurology (Chicago)* **41**: 301.

Darley-Usmar, V.M., Kennaway, N.G., Buist, N.R. *et al.* (1983) Deficiency in ubiquinone cytochrome *c* reductase in a patient with mitochondrial myopathy and lactic acidosis. *Proceedings of the National Academy of Sciences of the USA* **80**: 5103–5106.

Degoul, F., Nelson, I., Lestienne, P. *et al.* (1991) Deletions of mitochondrial DNA in Kearns-Sayre syndrome and ocular myopathies: Genetic, biochemical, and morphological studies. *Journal of the Neurological Sciences* **101**: 168–171.

Demaugre, F., Bonnefont, J-P., Colonna, M *et al.* (1991) Infantile form of carnitine palmitoyltransferase II deficiency with hepatomuscular symptoms and sudden death: Physiological approach to carnitine palmitoyltransferase II deficiencies. *Journal of Clinical Investigation* **87**: 859–864.

De Vivo, D.C. (1993) Mitochondrial DNA defects: Clinical features. In: DiMauro, S. Wallace, D.C. eds, *Mitochondrial DNA in Human Pathology*. New York: Raven Press.

Di Donato, S., Rimoldi, M., Cornelio, F. *et al.* (1982) Evidence for autosomal recessive inheritance in systemic carnitine deficiency. *Annals of Neurology* **11**: 190–192.

Di Donato, S., Pelucchetti, D., Rimoldi, M. *et al.* (1984) Systemic carnitine deficiency: clinical, biochemical, and morphological cure with L-carnitine. *Neurology* **34**: 157–162.

Di Donato, S., Gellera, C., Peluchetti, D. *et al.* (1989) Normalization of short-chain acyl-coenzyme A dehydrogenase after riboflavin treatment in a girl with multiple acylcoenzyme A dehydrogenase-deficient myopathy. *Annals of Neurology* **25**: 479–484.

DiMauro, S. (1993) Mitochondrial encephalomyopathies. In: Rosenberg, R.N., Prusiner, S.B., DiMauro, S. *et al.* eds, *The Molecular and Genetic Basis of*

Neurological Disease. Boston: Butterworth-Heinemann, pp. 665–694.

DiMauro, S. and DiMauro, P.M. (1973) Muscle carnitine palmityl-transferase deficiency and myoglobinuria. *Science* 182: 929–931.

DiMauro, S. and DeVivo, D.C. (1989) Diseases of carbohydrate fatty acid, and mitochondrial metabolism. In: Siegel, G.J. *et al.* eds, *Basic Neurochemistry: Molecular, Cellular and Medical Aspects* 4th edn. New York: Raven Press, p. 647.

DiMauro, S., Trevisan, C. and Hays, A. (1980) Disorders of lipid metabolism in muscle. *Muscle and Nerve* 3: 369–388.

DiMauro, S., Nicholson, J.F., Hays, A.P. *et al.* (1983) Benign infantile mitochondrial myopathy due to reversible cytochrome *c* oxidase deficiency. *Annals of Neurology* 14: 226–234.

DiMauro, S., Bonilla, E., Zeviani, M. *et al.* (1985) Mitochondrial myopathies. *Annals of Neurology* 17: 521–538.

DiMauro, S., Lombes, A., Nakase, H. *et al.* (1990) Cytochrome *c* oxidase deficiency. *Pediatric Research* 28: 536–541.

Duran, M., Hofkamp, M., Rhead, W.J. *et al.* (1986) Sudden child death and healthy affected family members with medium-chain acyl-coenzyme A dehydrogenase deficiency. *Pediatrics* 78: 1052–1057.

Egger, J., Lake, B.D. and Wilson, J. (1981) Mitochondrial cytopathy: a multisystem disorder with ragged red fibers on muscle biopsy. *Archives of Disease in Childhood* 56: 741–752.

Eleff, S., Kennaway, N.G., Buist, N.R.M. *et al.* (1984) 31-PNMR study of improvement in oxidative phosphorylation by vitamins K and C in a patient with a defect in electron transport at complex III in skeletal muscle. *Proceedings of the National Academy of Sciences of the USA* 81: 3529–3533.

Engel, A.G. and Angelini, C. (1973) Carnitine deficiency of human skeletal muscle with associated lipid storage myopathy: a new syndrome. *Science* 179: 899–902.

Engel, A.G., Rebouche, C.J., Wilson, D.M. *et al.* (1981) Primary systemic carnitine deficiency. II. Renal handling of carnitine. *Neurology* 31: 819–825.

Engel, W.K. and Cunningham, C.G. (1963) Rapid examination of muscle tissue: An improved trichrome stain method for fresh-frozen biopsy sections. *Neurology* 13: 919–923.

Engel, W.K., Vick, N.A., Glueck, C.J. *et al.* (1970) A skeletal muscle disorder associated with intermittent symptoms and a possible defect of lipid metabolism. *New England Journal of Medicine* 282: 697.

Eviatar, L., Shanske, S., Gauthier, B. *et al.* (1990) Kearns–Sayre syndrome presenting as renal tubular acidosis. *Neurology* 40: 1761–1763.

Ford, B., Mattheus, P.M., Karpati, G. *et al.* (1992) Coenzyme Q and vitamin therapy in mitochondrial disease (Abstract). *Neurology* 42 (Suppl 3): 418.

Fukuhara, N., Tokiguchi, S., Shirakawa, K. *et al.* (1980) Myoclonus epilepsy associated with ragged red fibers (mitochondrial abnormalities): disease entity or syndrome? *Journal of the Neurological Sciences* 47: 117–133.

Garavaglia, B., Antozzi, C., Girotti, F. *et al.* (1990) A mitochondrial myopathy with complex II deficiency. *Neurology* 40 (Suppl 1): 294.

Giles, R.E., Blanc, H., Cann, R.M. *et al.* (1980) Maternal inheritance of human mitochondrial DNA. *Proceedings of the National Academy of Sciences of the USA* 83: 9611–9615.

Goto, Y-I, Nonaka, I. and Horai, S. (1990a) A mutation in the tRNA[Leu(UUR)] gene associated with the MELAS subgroup of mitochondrial encephalomyopathies. *Nature* 348: 651–653.

Goto, Y, Koga, Y., Horai, S. *et al.* (1990b) Chronic progressive external ophthalmoplegia: A correlative study of mitochondrial DNA deletions and their phenotypic expression in muscle biopsies. *Journal of the Neurological Sciences* 101: 168–177.

Goto, Y., Itami, N., Kajii, N. *et al.* (1990c) Renal tubular involvement mimicking Bartter syndrome in a patient with Kearns–Sayre syndrome. *Journal of Pediatrics* 116: 904–910.

Hale, D.E., Barshaw, M.L., Coates, P.M. *et al.* (1985) Long-chain acyl-coenzyme A dehydrogenase deficiency: an inherited cause of nonketotic hypoglycaemia. *Pediatric Research* 19: 666–671.

Hale, D.E., Stanley, C.A. and Coates, P.M. (1990) The long-chain acyl-CoA dehydrogenase deficiency. In: Tanaka, K. and Coates, P.M. eds, *Fatty Acid Oxidation: Clinical, Biochemical and Molecular Aspects*. New York: Alan R. Liss, pp. 303–311.

Haller, R.G., Lewis, S.F., Eastabrook, R.W. *et al.* (1989) Exercise intolerance, lactic acidosis, and abnormal cardiopulmonary regulation in exercise associated with adult skeletal muscle cytochrome *c* oxidase deficiency. *Journal of Clinical Investigation* 84: 155–161.

Haller, R.G., Henriksson, K.G., Jorfeldt, L. *et al.* (1991) Deficiency of skeletal muscle succinate dehydrogenase and aconitase: pathophysiology of exercise in a novel human muscle oxidative defect. *Journal of Clinical Investigation* 88: 1197–1206.

Hammans, S.R., Sweeney, M.G., Brockington, M. *et al.* (1991) Mitochondrial encephalomyopathies: molecular genetic diagnosis from blood samples. *Lancet* 337: 1311–1313.

Hart, Z. and Chang, C.H. (1988) A newborn infant with respiratory distress and stridulous breathing. *Journal of Pediatrics* 113: 150–155.

Hatefi, Y. (1985) The mitochondrial electron transport and oxidative phosphorylation system. *Annual Review of Biochemistry* 54: 1015–1069.

Hayes, D.J., Lecky, B.R.F., Landon, D.N. *et al.* (1984) A new mitochondrial myopathy: Biochemical studies revealing a deficiency in the cytochrome *b-c$_1$* complex (complex III) of the respiratory chain. *Brain* 107: 1165–1177.

Hirano, M., Ricci, E., Koenigsberger, M.R. *et al.* (1992) MELAS: an original case and clinical criteria for diagnosis. *Neuromuscular Disorders* 2: 125–135.

Holt, I.J., Harding, A.E. and Morgan-Hughes, J.A. (1988) Deletions of muscle mitochondrial DNA in patients with mitochondrial myopathies. *Nature* 331: 717–719.

Holt, I.J., Harding, A.E., Cooper, J.M. *et al.* (1989) Mitochondrial myopathies: Clinical and biochemical features of 30 patients with major deletions of muscle mitochondrial DNA. *Annals of Neurology* **26**: 699–708.

Holt, I.J., Harding, A.E., Perry, R.K.H. *et al.* (1990) A new mitochondrial disease associated with mitochondrial DNA heteroplasmy. *American Journal of Human Genetics* **46**: 428–433.

Hoppell, C.L. and Tomec, R.J. (1972) Carnitine palmityl transferase: location of two enzymatic activities in rat liver mitochondria. *Journal of Biological Chemistry* **247**: 832–841.

Hoppell, C.L., Kerr, D.S., Dahms, B. *et al.* (1981) Deficiency of the reduced nicotinamide adenine dinucleotide dehydrogenase component of complex I of mitochondrial electron transport. *Journal of Clinical Investigation* **80**: 71–77.

Hug, G.., Bove, K.E. and Soukup, S. (1991) Lethal neonatal multi-organ deficiency of carnitine palmitoyltransferase II. *New England Journal of Medicine* **325**: 1862–1864.

Iannaccone, S.T., Griggs, R.C., Markesbery, W.R. *et al.* (1974) Familial progressive external ophthalmoplegia and ragged-red fibers. *Neurology* **24**: 1033–1038.

Ichiki, T., Tanaka, M., Nishikimi, M. *et al.* (1988) Deficiency of subunits of complex I and mitochondrial encephalomyopathy. *Annals of Neurology* **23**: 287–294.

Ichiki, T., Tanaka, M., Kobayashi, M. *et al.* (1989) Disproportionate deficiency of iron-sulfur clusters and subunits of complex I in mitochondrial encephalomyopathy. *Pediatric Research* **25**: 194–201.

Ihara, Y., Namba, R., Kuroda, S. *et al.* (1989) Mitochondrial encephalomyopathy (MELAS): pathological study and successful therapy with coenzyme Q10 idebenone. *Journal of the Neurological Sciences* **90**: 263–271.

Jackson, S. and Turnbull, D.M. (1993) Lipid disorders of muscle. In: Rosenberg, R.N., Prusiner, S.B., DiMauro, S. *et al.* eds, *The Molecular and Genetic Basis of Neurological Disease*. Boston: Butterworth-Heinemann, pp. 651–661.

Jackson, S., Bartlett, K., Land, J. *et al.* (1991) Long-chain 3-hydroxyacyl-CoA dehydrogenase deficiency. *Pediatric Research* **29**: 406–411.

Jerusalem, F., Angelini, C., Engel, A.G. *et al.* (1973) Mitochondria-lipid-glycogen (MLG) disease of muscle. *Archives of Neurology* **29**: 162–169.

Johns, D.R., Rutledge, S.L., Stine, O.C. *et al.* (1989) Directly repeated sequences associated with pathogenic mitochondrial DNA deletions. *Proceedings of the National Academy of Sciences of the USA* **86**: 8059–8062.

Johnson, M.A., Turnbull, D.M., Dick, D.J. *et al.* (1983) A partial defect of cytochrome *c* oxidase in chronic progressive external ophthalmoplegia. *Journal of the Neurological Sciences* **60**: 31–53.

Karpati, G., Carpenter, S., Engel, A.G. *et al.* (1975) The syndrome of systemic carnitine deficiency: Clinical, morphological, biochemical and pathophysiologic features. *Neurology* **25**: 16–24.

Kearns, T.P. and Sayre, G.P. (1958) Retinitis pigmentosa, external ophthalmoplegia, and complete heart block. *Ophthalmology* **60**: 280–289.

Kennaway, N.G. (1988) Defects in the cytochrome bc[1] complex in mitochondrial diseases. *Journal of Bioenergetics and Biomembranes* **20**: 325–352.

Kennaway, N.G., Buist, N.R., Darley-Usmar, V.M. *et al.* (1984) Lactic acidosis and mitochondrial myopathy associated with deficiency of several components of complex III of the respiratory chain. *Pediatric Research* **18**: 991–999.

Kobayashi, M., Morishita, H., Sugiyama, N. *et al.* (1987) Two cases of NADH-coenzyme Q reductase deficiency: Relationship to MELAS syndrome. *Journal of Pediatrics* **110**: 223–227.

Kobayashi, Y., Momo, M.Y., Tominaga, K. *et al.* (1990) A point mutation in the mitochondrial tRNA[Leu(UUR)] gene in MELAS. *Biochemical and Biophysical Research Communications* **173**: 816–822.

Koga, Y., Nonaka, I., Kobayashi, M. *et al.* (1988) Findings in muscle in complex I (NADH Coenzyme Q reductase) deficiency. *Annals of Neurology* **24**: 749–756.

Land, J.M., Mistry, S., Squier, M. *et al.* (1995) Neonatal carnitine palmitoyltransferase-2 deficiency: a case presenting with myopathy. *Neuromuscular Disorders* **5**: 129–138.

Larsson, N-G., Holme, E., Kristiansson, B. *et al.* (1990) Progressive increase of the mutated mitochondrial DNA fraction in Kearns–Sayre syndrome. *Pediatric Research* **28**: 131–136.

Lauber, J., Marsac, C., Kadenbach, B. *et al.* (1991) Mutations in mitochondrial tRNA genes: a frequent cause of neuromuscular diseases. *Nucleic Acid Research* **19**: 1391–1397.

Loehr, J.P., Goodman, W.I., Frerman, F.E. (1990) Glutaric acidemia type II: Heterogeneity of clinical and biochemical phenotypes. *Pediatric Research* **27**: 311–315.

Lombes, A., Mendell, J.R., Nakase, H. *et al.* (1989) Myoclonic epilepsy and ragged-red fibers with cytochrome *c* oxidase deficiency: neuropathology, biochemistry, and molecular genetics. *Annals of Neurology* **26**: 20–33.

Luft, R., Ikkos, D., Palmieri, G. *et al.* (1962) A case of severe hypermetabolism of nonthyroid origin with a defect in the maintenance of mitochondrial respiratory control: a correlated clinical, biochemical, and morphological study. *Journal of Clinical Investigation* **41**: 1776.

Mastaglia, F.L., Thompson, P.L. and Papadimitriou, J.M. (1980) Mitochondrial myopathy and cardiomyopathy, lactic acidosis and response to prednisone and thiamine. *Australia and New Zealand Journal of Medicine* **10**: 660–664.

McShane, M.A., Hammans, S.R., Sweeney, M. *et al.* (1991) Pearson syndrome and mitochondrial encephalopathy in a patient with a deletion of mtDNA. *American Journal of Human Genetics* **48**: 39–42.

Moraes, C.T., DiMauro, S., Zeviani, M. *et al.* (1989)

Mitochondrial DNA deletions in progressive external ophthalmoplegia and Kearns-Sayre syndrome. *New England Journal of Medicine* **320**: 1293–1299.

Moraes, C.T., Shanske, S., Tritschler, H-J. *et al.* (1991) MtDNA depletion with variable tissue expression: a novel genetic abnormality in mitochondrial diseases. *American Journal of Human Genetics* **48**: 492–501.

Moreadith, R.W., Batshaw, M.L., Ohnishi, T. *et al.* (1984) Deficiency of the iron-sulfur clusters of mitochondrial reduced nicotinamide-adenine dinucleotide-ubiquinone oxidoreductase (complex I) in an infant with congenital lactic acidosis. *Journal of Clinical Investigation* **74**: 685–697.

Morgan-Hughes, J.A. (1982) Mitochondrial myopathies. In: Mastaglia, F.L. and Walton, Sir John, eds, *Skeletal Muscle Pathology*. Edinburgh: Churchill Livingstone, p. 309.

Morgan-Hughes, J.A., Darveniza, P., Kahn, S.N. *et al.* (1977) A mitochondrial myopathy characterized by a deficiency in reducible cytochrome *b*. *Brain* **100**: 617–640.

Morgan-Hughes, J.A., Hayes, D.J., Cooper, M. *et al.* (1985) Mitochondrial myopathies: Deficiencies localized to complex I and complex III of the mitochondrial respiratory chain. *Biochemical Society Transactions* **13**: 648–650.

Morgan-Hughes, J.A., Schapira, A.H.V., Cooper, J.M. *et al.* (1988) Molecular defects of NADH-ubiquinone oxidoreductase (complex I) in mitochondrial diseases. *Journal of Bioenergetics and Biomembranes* **20**: 365–382.

Müller-Höcker, J., Pongratz, D. and Hubner, G. (1983) Focal deficiency of cytochrome oxidase in skeletal muscle of patients with progressive external ophthalmoplegia. *Virchows Archives* **402**: 61–71.

Nass, S. and Nass, M.M.K. (1963) Intramitochondrial fibers with DNA characteristics. *Journal of Cell Biology* **19**: 593–629.

Naylor, E.W., Mosovich, L.L., Guthrie, R. *et al.* (1980) Intermittent non-ketotic dicarboxylic aciduria in two siblings with hypoglycaemia: an apparent defect in β-oxidation of fatty acids. *Journal of Inherited Metabolic Diseases* **3**: 19–24.

Nishikawa, Y., Takahashi, M., Yorifuji, S. *et al.* (1989) Long term coenzyme Q_{10} therapy for a mitochondrial encephalomyopathy with cytochrome *c*-oxidase deficiency: a ^{31}P-NMR study. *Neurology* **39**: 399–403.

Nishizawa, M., Tanaka, K., Shinozawa, K. *et al.* (1987) A mitochondrial encephalomyopathy with cardiomyopathy: a case revealing a defect of complex I of the respiratory chain. *Journal of the Neurological Sciences* **78**: 189–201.

Nonaka, I., Koga, Y., Shikura, K. *et al.* (1988) Muscle pathology in cytochrome c oxidase deficiency. *Acta Neuropathologica* **77**: 152–160.

Ogasahara, S., Yorifuji, S., Nishikawa, Y. *et al.* (1985) Improvement of abnormal pyruvate metabolism and cardiac conduction defect with coenzyme Q_{10} in Kearns-Sayre syndrome. *Neurology* **35**: 372–377.

Ogasahara, S., Engel, A.G., Frens, D. *et al.* (1989) Muscle coenzyme Q deficiency in familial mitochondrial encephalomyopathy. *Proceedings of the National Academy of Sciences of the USA* **86**: 2379–2382.

Papadimitriou, A., Neustein, H.B., DiMauro, S. *et al.* (1984) Histiocytoid cardiomyopathy of infancy: deficiency of reducible cytochrome *b* in heart mitochondria. *Pediatric Research* **18**: 1023–1028.

Patten, B.M., Dodson, R.F., Hefferan, P. *et al.* (1976) Mitochondrial myopathy associated with abnormal lactate metabolism: response to prednisone in three patients. *Neurology* **26**: 370.

Pavlakis, S.G., Phillips, P.C., DiMauro, S. *et al.* (1984) Mitochondrial myopathy, encephalopathy, lactic acidosis, and stroke-like episodes: a distinctive clinical syndrome. *Annals of Neurology* **16**: 481–488.

Pavlakis, S.G., Rowland, L.P., De Vivo, D.C. *et al.* (1988) Mitochondrial myopathies and encephalomyopathies. In: Plum, F. ed., *Advances in Contemporary Neurology*. Philadelphia: F.A. Davis, pp. 95–133.

Pearson, H.A., Lobel, J.S., Kocoshis, S.A. *et al.* (1979) A new syndrome of refractory sideroblastic anemia with vacuolization of marrow precursors and exocrine pancreatic dysfunction. *Journal of Pediatrics* **95**: 976–984.

Petty, R.K.H., Harding, A.E. and Morgan-Hughes, J.A. (1986) The clinical features of mitochondrial myopathy. *Brain* **109**: 915–938.

Poulton, J., Deadman, M.E. and Gardiner, R.M. (1989) Duplications of mitochondrial DNA in mitochondrial myopathy. *Lancet* **i**: 236–240.

Poulton, J., Deadman, M.E., Ramacharan, S. *et al.* (1991) Germ-line deletions of mtDNA in mitochondrial myopathy. *American Journal of Human Genetics* **48**: 649–653.

Poulton, J., Sewry, C., Dubowitz, V. *et al.* (1995) Variation in mitochondrial DNA levels in normal controls: Is depletion of mtDNA in patients with mitochondrial myopathy a distinct clinical syndrome? *Journal of Inherited Metabolic Diseases* (in press).

Prick, M.J.J., Gabreels, F.J.M., Trijbels, J.M.F. *et al.* (1983) Progressive poliodystrophy (Alpers disease) with a defect in cytochrome aa_3 in muscle: A report of two unrelated patients. *Clinical Neurology and Neurosurgery* **85**: 57–70.

Przyrembel, H. (1987) Therapy of mitochondrial disorders. *Journal of Inherited Metabolic Diseases* **10**: 129–146.

Rebouche, C.J. and Engel, A.G. (1981) Primary systemic carnitine deficiency: I. Carnitine biosynthesis. *Neurology* **31**: 813–818.

Rebouche, C.J. and Engel, A.G. (1983) Carnitine metabolism and deficiency syndromes. *Mayo Clinic Proceedings* **58**: 533–540.

Reichmann, H., Rohkamm, R., Zeviani, M. *et al.* (1986) Mitochondrial myopathy due to complex III deficiency with normal reducible cytochrome *b* concentration. *Archives of Neurology* **43**: 957–961.

Riggs, J.E., Schochet, S.S., Fakadej, A.V. *et al.* (1984)

Mitochondrial encephalomyopathy with decreased succinate-cytochrome *c* reductase activity. *Neurology* **34**: 48–53.

Rocchiccioli, F., Wanders, R.J.A., Aubourg, P. *et al.* (1990) Deficiency of long-chain 3-hydroxyacyl-CoA dehydrogenase: A cause of lethal myopathy and cardiomyopathy in early childhood. *Pediatric Research* **28**: 657–662.

Roe, C.R. and Coates, P.M. (1989) Acyl-CoA dehydrogenase deficiencies. In: Scriver, C.R. *et al.* eds, *The Metabolic Basis of Inherited Disease*. New York: McGraw Hill, pp. 889–914.

Roodhooft, A.M., Van Acker, K.J., Martin, J.J. *et al.* (1986) Benign mitochondrial myopathy with deficiency of NADH-CoQ reductase and cytochrome *c* oxidase. *Neuropediatrics* **17**: 221–226.

Rotig, A., Cormier, V., Blanche, S. *et al.* (1990) Pearson's marrow-pancreas syndrome: A multisystem mitochondrial disorder in infancy. *Journal of Clinical Investigation* **86**: 1601–1608.

Rowland, L.P., Hays, A.P., DiMauro, S. *et al.* (1983) Diverse clinical disorders associated with morphological abnormalities of mitochondria. In Scarlato, G. and Cerri, C. eds, *Mitochondrial Pathology in Muscle Diseases*. Padova: Piccin, pp.141–158.

Sadeh, M. and Gutman, A. (1990) Carnitine palmitoyltransferase deficiency: a common cause of recurrent myoglobinuria. *Israel Journal of Medical Sciences* **26**: 510–515.

Schapira, A.H.V., Cooper, J.M., Morgan-Hughes, J.A. *et al.* (1990) Mitochondrial myopathy with a defect of mitochondrial protein transport. *New England Journal of Medicine* **323**: 37–42.

Schiffmann, R., Lahat, E. and Schechter, A. (1992) Severe periodic febrile myalgia in infancy due to carnitine palmitoyltransferase deficiency. *Neuromuscular Disorders* **2**: 285–288.

Schon, E.A., Rizzuto, R., Moraes, C.T. *et al.* (1989) A direct repeat is a hotspot for large-scale deletion of human mitochondrial DNA. *Science* **244**: 346–349.

Schotland, D.L., DiMauro, S., Bonilla, E. *et al.* (1976) Neuromuscular disorder associated with a defect in mitochondrial energy supply. *Archives of Neurology* **33**: 475–479.

Sengers, R.C.A., Fischer, J.C., Trijbels, J.M.F. *et al.* (1983) A mitochondrial myopathy with a defective respiratory chain and carnitine deficiency. *European Journal of Pediatrics* **240**: 332–337.

Servidei, S., Bertini, E., Dionisi-Vici, C. *et al.* (1988) Benign infantile mitochondrial myopathy due to reversible cytochrome *c* oxidase deficiency: A third case. *Clinical Neuropathology* **7**: 209–210.

Servidei, S., Zeviani, M., Manfredi, G. *et al.* (1991) Dominantly inherited mitochondrial myopathy with multiple deletions of mitochondrial DNA: clinical, morphologic, and biochemical studies. *Neurology* **41**: 1053–1059.

Shapira, Y., Harel, S. and Russell, A. (1977) Mitochondrial encephalomyopathies: A group of neuromuscular disorders with defects in oxidative metabolism. *Israel Journal of Medical Sciences* **13**: 161–164.

Shoffner, J.M., Lott, M.T., Voljavec, A.S. *et al.* (1989) Spontaneous Kearns-Sayre/chronic external ophthalmoplegia plus syndrome associated with mitochondrial DNA deletion: a slip-replication model and metabolic therapy. *Proceedings of the National Academy of Science, USA* **86**: 7952–7956.

Shoffner, J.M., Lott, M.T., Lezza, A.M.S. *et al.* (1990) Myoclonic epilepsy and ragged-red fibers (MERRF) is associated with a mitochondrial DNA tRNA^{Lys} mutation. *Cell* **61**: 931–937.

Shy, G.M. and Gonatas, N.K. (1964) Human myopathy with giant abnormal mitochondria. *Science* **145**: 493–496.

Shy, G.M., Gonatas, N.K. and Perez, M. (1966) Two childhood myopathies with abnormal mitochondria. I. Megaconial myopathy. II. Pleoconial myopathy. *Brain* **89**: 133.

Simon, L.T., Horoupian, D.S., Dorfman, L.J. *et al.* (1990) Polyneuropathy, ophthalmoplegia, leukoencephalopathy, and intestinal pseudo-obstruction: POLIP syndrome. *Annals of Neurology* **28**: 349–360.

Sperl, W., Ruitenbeek, W. and Trijbels, J.M.F. (1988) Mitochondrial myopathy with lactic acidemia, Fanconi-DeToni-Debre syndrome and a disturbed succinate:cytochrome *c* oxido-reductase activity. *European Journal of Pediatrics* **147**: 418–421.

Spiro, A.J., Moore, C.L., Prineas, J.W. *et al.* (1970) A cytochrome-related inherited disorder of the nervous system and muscle. *Archives of Neurology* **23**: 103–112.

Stanley, C.A., Hale, D.E., Coates, P.M. *et al.* (1983) Medium-chain acyl-CoA dehydrogenase deficiency in children with non-ketotic hypoglycemia and low carnitine levels. *Pediatric Research* **17**: 877–884.

Takamiya, S., Yanamura, W., Capaldi, R.A. *et al.* (1986) Mitochondrial myopathies involving the respiratory chain: a biochemical analysis. *Annals of the New York Academy of Sciences* **488**: 33–43.

Tanaka, M., Sato, W., Ohno, K. *et al.* (1989) Direct sequencing of deleted mitochondrial DNA in myopathic patients. *Biochemical and Biophysical Research Communications* **164**: 156–163.

Tanaka, M., Ino, H., Ohno, K. *et al.* (1990) Mitochondrial mutation in fatal infantile cardiomyopathy. *Lancet* **ii**: 1452.

Tein, I., De Vivo, D.C., Hale, D.E. *et al.* (1991) Short-chain L-3-hydroxyacyl-CoA dehydrogenase deficiency in muscle: a new cause for recurrent myoglobinuria and encephalopathy. *Annals of Neurology* **30**: 415–419.

Tritschler, H-J., Bonilla, E., Lombes, A. *et al.* (1991) Differential diagnosis of fatal and benign cytochrome *c* oxidase-deficient myopathies of infancy: an immunohistochemical approach. *Neurology* **41**: 300–305.

Tritschler, H-J., Andreetta, F., Moraes, C.T. *et al.* (1992) Mitochondrial myopathy of childhood associated with depletion of mitochondrial DNA. *Neurology* **42**: 209–217.

Trounce, I., Byrne, E., Marzuki, S. *et al.* (1991) Functional respiratory chain studies in subjects with chronic progressive external ophthalmoplegia and large heteroplasmic mitochondrial DNA deletions. *Journal of the Neurological Sciences* **102**: 92–99.

Tsairis, P., Engel, W.K. and Kark, P. (1973) Familial myoclonic epilepsy syndrome associated with skeletal muscle mitochondrial abnormalities. *Neurology* **24**: 408.

Turnbull, D.M., Bartlett, K., Stevens, D.L. *et al.* (1984) Short-chain acyl-CoA dehydrogenase deficiency associated with a lipid-storage myopathy and secondary carnitine deficiency. *New England Journal of Medicine* **311**: 1232–1236.

Turnbull, D.M., Shepherd, I.M., Ashworth, B. *et al.* (1988a) Lipid storage myopathy associated with low acyl-CoA dehydrogenase activities. *Brain* **111**: 815–828.

Turnbull, D.M., Bartlett, K., Eyre, J.A. *et al.* (1988b) Lipid storage myopathy due to glutaric aciduria type II: treatment of a potentially fatal myopathy. *Developmental Medicine and Child Neurology* **30**: 667–672.

Wallace, D.C. and Lott, M.T. (1993) Maternally inherited diseases. In: DiMauro, S. and Wallace, D.C. eds, *Mitochondrial DNA in Human Pathology*. New York: Raven Press, pp. 63–83.

Wallace, D.C., Singh, G., Lott, M.T. *et al.* (1988a) Mitochondrial DNA mutation associated with Leber's hereditary optic neuropathy. *Science* **242**: 1427–1430.

Wallace, D.C., Zheng, X., Lott, M.T. *et al.* (1988b) Familial mitochondrial encephalomyopathy (MERRF): Genetic, pathophysiological and biochemical characterization of a mitochondrial DNA disease. *Cell* **55**: 601–610.

Wanders, R.J.A., Ijlst, L., Van Gennip, A.H. *et al.* (1990) Long-chain 3-hydroxyacyl-CoA dehydrogenase deficiency: Identification of a new inborn error of mitochondrial fatty acid β-oxidation. *Journal of Inherited Metabolic Diseases* **13**: 311–314.

Willems, J.L., Monnens, L.A.H., Trijbels, J.M.F. *et al.* (1977) Leigh's encephalomyelopathy in a patient with cytochrome c oxidase deficiency in muscle tissue. *Pediatrics* **60**: 850–857.

Willner, J.H., DiMauro, S., Eastwood, A. *et al.* (1979) Muscle carnitine deficiency: genetic heterogeneity. *Journal of the Neurological Sciences* **41**: 235–246.

Wood, P.A., Amendt, B.A., Rhead, W.J. *et al.* (1989) Short-chain acyl-coenzyme A deficiency in mice. *Pediatric Research* **25**: 38–43.

Yamaguchi, S., Orii, T., Suzuki, Y. *et al.* (1991) Newly identified forms of electron transfer flavoprotein deficiency in two patients with glutaric aciduria type II. *Pediatric Research* **29**: 60–63.

Yamamoto, M., Sato, T., Anno, M. *et al.* (1987) Mitochondrial myopathy, encephalopathy, lactic acidosis, and stroke-like episodes with recurrent abdominal symptoms and coenzyme Q10 administration. *Journal of Neurology, Neurosurgery and Psychiatry* **50**: 1475–1481.

Yoon, K.L., Aprille, J.R. and Ernst, S.G. (1991) Mitochondrial tRNA[Thr] mutation in fatal infantile respiratory enzyme deficiency. *Biochemical and Biophysical Research Communications* **176**: 1112–1115.

Zeviani, M., Van Dyke, D.H., Servidei, S. *et al.* (1986) Myopathy and fatal cardiopathy due to cytochrome c oxidase deficiency. *Archives of Neurology* **43**: 1198–1202.

Zeviani, M., Peterson, P., Servidei, S. *et al.* (1987) Benign reversible muscle cytochrome c oxidase deficiency: A second case. *Neurology* **37**: 64–67.

Zeviani, M., Moraes, C.T., DiMauro, S. *et al.* (1988) Deletions of mitochondrial DNA in Kearns–Sayre syndrome. *Neurology* **38**: 1339–1346.

Zeviani, M., Servidei, S., Gellera, C. *et al.* (1989) An autosomal dominant disorder with multiple deletions of mitochondrial DNA starting at the D-loop region. *Nature* **339**: 309–311.

Zeviani, M., Gellera, C., Pannacci, M. *et al.* (1990a) Tissue distribution and transmission of mitochondrial DNA deletions in mitochondrial myopathies. *Annals of Neurology* **28**: 94–97.

Zeviani, M., Bresolin, N. Gellera, C. *et al.* (1990b) Nucleus-driven multiple large-scale deletions of the human mitochondrial genome: a new autosomal dominant disease. *American Journal of Human Genetics* **47**: 904–914.

Zeviani, M., Amati, P., Bresolin, N. *et al.* (1991a) Rapid detection of the A-to-G[(8344)] mutation of mtDNA in Italian families with myoclonus epilepsy and ragged-red fibers (MERRF). *American Journal of Human Genetics* **48**: 203–211.

Zeviani, M., Gellera, C., Antozzi, C. *et al.* (1991b) Maternally inherited myopathy and cardiomyopathy: association with mutation in mitochondrial DNA tRNA[Leu(UUR)]. *Lancet* **338**: 143–147.

Zheng, X., Shoffner, J.M., Lott, M.A. *et al.* (1989) Evidence in a lethal infantile mitochondrial disease for a nuclear mutation affecting respiratory complexes I and IV. *Neurology* **39**: 1203–1209.

Zierz, S., Von Wersebe, O., Bleistein, J. *et al.* (1990) Exogenous coenzyme Q fails to increase CoQ in the skeletal muscle of two patients with mitochondrial myopathies. *Journal of the Neurological Sciences* **95**: 283–290.

Zupanc, M.L., Moraes, C.T., Shanske, S. *et al.* (1991) Deletions of mitochondrial DNA in patients with combined features of Kearns–Sayre and MELAS syndromes. *Annals of Neurology* **29**: 680–683.

CHAPTER 6

Metabolic Myopathies III Ion Channel Disorders

INTRODUCTION

A series of spectacular advances in knowledge over the past few years has helped to bring together a number of somewhat diverse syndromes under a common umbrella of ion channel disorders (Table 6-1). The application of the new genetic techniques of linkage analysis, gene cloning and mutational analysis was helped by an already firmly established clinical and electrophysiological foundation, and in several instances has confirmed an existing hypothesis by going directly for a candidate gene. The syndromes involved are those with myotonia and periodic paralysis (Table 6-2), and the new techniques have also helped to clarify the overlap in clinical features between some of the traditional potential bed-fellows such as hyperkalaemic periodic paralysis and paramyotonia congenita (Table 6-3).

The commonest ion channel disorder is in fact cystic fibrosis, due to an abnormality in the non-voltage-dependent, chloride (Cl) channel (Riordan et al., 1989). As this protein is expressed in many tissues the resultant disease is a multi-system one. In contrast, abnormalities of the voltage-sensitive ion channels involve structures expressed only in muscle, and thus produce disorders confined predominantly to skeletal muscle.

PERIODIC PARALYSIS

This group of disorders is characterized by attacks of paralysis with associated flaccidity, and a tendency to remission and relapse. Different types have been recognized depending on whether the serum potassium (K) is low, high or normal in the attack.

HISTORICAL

One can trace the early descriptions of this muscle disorder to the German literature of the latter half of the last century (Westphal, 1885; Oppenheim, 1891). Although the apparent beneficial effects of potassium salts were already observed by Singer and Goodbody (1901) and Holzapple (1905), it was not until 1934 that Biemond and Daniels first documented the low serum potassium level. Aitken et al. (1937) subsequently found that the fall in serum potassium was not associated with an increased urinary output of potassium, suggesting that there may be a movement of the potassium from the serum into the muscle (Grob et al., 1957; Zierler and Andres, 1957).

In 1934 Schoenthal described a family with periodic paralysis starting in infancy and unresponsive to potassium. Subsequently Tyler et al. (1951) documented a similar family where the serum potassium did not fall during attacks and suggested this was a separate entity. Gamstorp (1956) made a detailed study of two large families with this condition and suggested the name adynamia episodica hereditaria. There was a clinical overlap between this hyperkalaemic form of periodic paralysis and paramyotonia congenita (Gamstorp, 1963).

Poskanzer and Kerr (1961) documented a third type of periodic paralysis, resembling the hyperkalaemic form but not associated with a rise in serum potassium during attacks. It has been questioned in recent times whether this is indeed a separate clinical entity and the recent major advances at a molecular genetic level have helped to resolve this.

266

Table 6-1 Disorders of ion channels and receptors and inherited dominant disorders (human and animal) in relation to current knowledge on channel or receptor involvement

Disease	Channel or receptor
Human	
Inherited	
Cystic fibrosis	Chloride channel (CFTR)[a]
Hyperkalaemic periodic paralysis	Sodium channel
Paramyotonia congenita	Sodium channel
Myotonia congenita (K-sensitive)	Sodium channel
Hypokalaemic periodic paralysis	Calcium channel (DHP receptor)[b]
Myotonia congenita Becker's generalized (recessive) Thomsen's (dominant)	Chloride channel (voltage-sensitive)
Malignant hyperthermia	Ryanodine receptor
Sporadic	
Myasthenia gravis	Acetylcholine receptor
Lambert–Eaton Myasthenic Syndrome	Calcium channel
Animal	
Hyperkalaemic periodic paralysis	Sodium channel
Myotonic goat	Chloride channel (voltage-sensitive)
Myotonic adr/adr mouse	Chloride channel
Dysgenic dys/dys mouse	Calcium channel (DHP receptor)[b]
Porcine malignant hyperthermia	Ryanodine receptor

[a] Cystic fibrosis transmembrane conductance regulator.
[b] Dihydropyridine receptor.

From Brown (1993).

HYPOKALAEMIC PERIODIC PARALYSIS

This familial disorder is inherited as an autosomal dominant trait, with full penetrance, although males appear to be more frequently and more severely affected than females. The attacks usually commence in the second decade and reach a peak frequency in early adult life (about 20–35 years), after which they tend to decline.

CLINICAL FEATURES

The classical picture is of a previously healthy young adult waking in the early hours of the morning finding himself unable to move but still able to breathe, swallow and speak. The weakness usually starts in the trunk and thighs, and gradually spreads to the rest of the legs, the upper limbs and the neck. The attack may last anything from a few hours to

Table 6-2 Classification of the syndromes with myotonia in relation to specific ion channel or other genetic abnormalities

Disease	Gene	Chromosome
Non-dystrophic		
Periodic paralysis		
Hyperkalaemic	Sodium channel	17
Hypokalaemic (rarely)	Calcium channel	1
Paramyotonic congenita	Sodium channel	17
Pure		
K-sensitive		
Myotonia congenita		
Autosomal dominant		
Typical (Thomsen's)	Chloride channel	7
K-sensitive	Sodium channel	17
Autosomal recessive	Chloride channel	7
(Becker's generalized)		
Schwartz–Jampel Syndrome	?	
Dystrophic		
Myotonic dystrophy	Protein kinase	19

From Brown (1993).

2 or 3 days or even longer and then fairly rapidly subsides. Death is rare in an attack. The external ocular and respiratory muscles are usually unaffected, possibly because of the normal continuous activity of these muscles. Patients at times note that if an attack starts during the day or they are awake at the onset at night it can be aborted by exercising the weak muscles. Attacks vary in severity from almost total paralysis to much milder and more focal weakness.

Predisposing factors appear to be a period of prolonged rest after vigorous exercise, a heavy carbohydrate meal a few hours before, cold, and anxiety. Clinically an attack may be provoked by frequent ingestion of glucose or by glucose plus insulin.

Smooth muscle is not affected but there may be evidence of cardiac involvement, with bradycardia and electrocardiographic changes with prolonged PR, QRS and QT intervals and flattened T waves, which probably reflect the low plasma potassium.

Between attacks patients are usually completely normal but occasionally there may be some permanent residual muscle weakness. The long-term outlook in most patients is good, with a tendency to gradual regression of the attacks which may subside completely, especially in females.

BIOCHEMICAL CHANGES

The plasma potassium falls coincident with the onset of paralysis, which may begin at a level of 3–3.5 mmol/litre and is usually marked at 2–2.5 mmol/litre. Some patients become severely paralysed at only slightly lowered potassium levels, which would not cause weakness in a normal individual, suggesting some additional factors. The plasma potassium remains low during the period of weakness and rises again with recovery.

ELECTROPHYSIOLOGICAL STUDIES

The muscle weakness is associated with complete inexcitability of the muscle to either faradic or galvanic stimulus. There is also a failure of propagation of the action potentials from the endplates along the muscle fibres (Grob *et al.*, 1957).

HISTOLOGY

Between attacks the muscle may be completely normal but during attacks there may be a vacuolar myopathy, already noted by Goldflam in 1890 and confirmed by recent authors. Electron microscopy shows marked dilatation of the sarcoplasmic reticulum (Shy *et al.*, 1961; Howes *et al.*, 1966) and t-system tubules (Engel, 1970).

TREATMENT

In the acute attack potassium chloride (KCl) can be given orally (up to 10g) and repeated within 1–2 hours if necessary. In severe cases K^+ may exceptionally have to be given intravenously. The continued use of KCl prophylactically has not been of much value but a combination of a slowly-released K^+ preparation (Slow-K^+) together with a low carbohydrate diet may be more beneficial. Griggs *et al.* (1970) reported good results with acetazolamide and McArdle (1974) with chlorothiazide in combination with Slow-K^+.

THYROTOXIC PERIODIC PARALYSIS

A form of periodic paralysis identical to the idiopathic hypokalaemic variety occurs in association with thyrotoxicosis. It seems to occur particularly in oriental races (Okinaka *et al.*, 1957; McFadzean and Yeung, 1967; Cheah *et al.*, 1975) and, like thyrotoxicosis and hypokalaemic periodic paralysis, is essentially a disorder of adults and seems predominantly to affect males. Treatment of the thyrotoxicosis cures the periodic paralysis and prevents attacks being provoked (Resnick *et al.*, 1969).

HYPERKALAEMIC PERIODIC PARALYSIS

This form of periodic paralysis is more likely to be seen in infancy and childhood. Like the hypokalaemic form, it is also inherited as an autosomal dominant trait. It was originally delineated because of the lack of response, or even aggravation of symptoms, with administration of potassium during attacks of periodic paralysis and the asssociated elevation rather than reduction in plasma potassium level during the attack (Tyler *et al.*, 1951; Gamstorp, 1956).

CLINICAL FEATURES

Attacks of weakness usually occur during a period of rest after exercise. Exercise seems to be the most important predisposing factor, but attacks may also be provoked by cold or by missing a meal. The weakness tends to start in the legs and then to progress to the arms. Swallowing may be affected but respiratory function is rarely involved. There may be involvement of ocular muscles, which may reflect myotonia rather than weakness of these muscles.

Attacks are usually short-lived and may reach a peak within 30 minutes and subside within 2–3 hours. Occasionally weakness may persist for several hours or even days. The attacks usually occur by day and active movement of the affected limbs may abort an incipient attack or hasten the recovery, but the weakness may recur as soon as the patient rests again.

The frequency of attacks may vary considerably from only occasional ones to daily severe attacks where the patient is hardly free of some residual weakness. There is also considerable variation in the extent and severity of weakness even in the same patient. In some it is fairly mild and relatively focal, whereas in others it may progress to a complete flaccid quadriplegia. Respiratory involvement is not a usual feature of the attacks and death in an attack has not been recorded.

Myotonia has been an associated feature in many cases (Gamstorp, 1956). Percussion myotonia is most readily demonstrable in the tongue and less frequently demonstrable peripherally; myotonic lid lag may also be elicited. This led to the suggestion that hyperkalaemic periodic paralysis and paramyotonia congenita might be the same disease (Drager *et al.*, 1958; Layzer *et al.*, 1967).

It has been suggested that three clinically different subtypes can be recognized: hyperkalaemic periodic paralysis (hyperPP) with myotonia, without myotonia, and with paramyotonia. In *myotonic hyperPP*, lid-lag and percussion myotonia can usually be elicited at any time, and virtually all affected members of a family show bursts of fibrillation potentials in the EMG. In *non-myotonic hyperPP*, both clinical and electrical myotonia are absent. In both types weakness, but not stiffness, is induced by cooling. Rewarming of the muscles quickly re-establishes full force. *Paramyotonic hyperPP*, is characterized by attacks of generalized weakness triggered by potassium intake or a workload with subsequent rest and by the induction of stiffness and weakness on cooling (Ricker *et al.*, 1986).

From a clinical point of view, however, the predominant feature of hyperkalaemic periodic paralysis is the muscle weakness with the myotonia being an incidental and relatively minor component, whereas in paramyotonia congenita the main clinical feature is the myotonia which is precipitated by cold, and the associated weakness, while marked in some cases, may be absent in others. It is of interest that myotonic lid lag has on rare occasions also been documented in hypokalaemic periodic paralysis (Resnik and Engel, 1967).

BIOCHEMICAL FEATURES ────────────

The cardinal feature is the elevation of the plasma K^+ during the attacks. However the elevation may at times be minimal, and mild weakness may even be associated with levels of under 5 mmol/litre. Severe paralysis is likely to develop at levels of 7 mmol/litre, which would not cause symptoms in normal subjects. The urinary K^+ is increased during attacks suggesting that the increased plasma K^+ is due to leakage from the muscles (McArdle, 1962).

ELECTROPHYSIOLOGICAL STUDIES ────

Creutzfeldt *et al.* (1963) found a low resting membrane potential between attacks with a further drop during paralysis. Since change in K^+ could not adequately explain this they postulated an increased membrane permeability to sodium $(Na)^+$.

Routine electromyography during an attack shows a reduced interference pattern and myotonic discharges.

HISTOLOGY ────────────────────

Vacuoles similar to those in hypokalaemic periodic paralysis have been observed (Olivarius and Cristensen, 1965). These have corresponded to dilatation of the sarcoplasmic reticulum on electron microscopy and in addition non-specific tubular abnormalities have been documented (MacDonald *et al.*, 1968; Bradley, 1969). Engel (1966, 1970) studied the evolution of the vacuoles and defined four stages: evolving, intermediate-stage, mature and remodelling vacuoles. He also showed the involvement of the sarcoplasmic reticulum, the T system and varying cytoplasmic degradation products in the evolution of the vacuole. In subsequent studies, Engel (1977) demonstrated the similarity in the changes in different types of periodic paralysis and that the morphological changes in the muscle were reactive, representing a delayed consequence of the physiological abnormalities.

TREATMENT ───────────────────

Many of the attacks may be short lived and not require treatment. In more severe and persistent attacks intravenous calcium gluconate and glucose infusion, with or without insulin, have been used, with variable response.

Diuretics such as acetazolamide or hydrochlorothiazide have proved beneficial in the long-term prevention of attacks.

Wang and Clausen (1976) showed that salbutamol by inhalation in patients with hyperkalaemic periodic paralysis can prevent the rise in serum potassium and the associated paralysis provoked by either ingestion of potassium or by exercise. They also found the drug to be effective in the long-term prevention of attacks in these patients by inhalation at the first sign of an attack starting.

Patients should be encouraged to take regular exercise and to avoid vigorous exertion. They usually learn to adapt their activities to prevent severe attacks. The long-term prognosis is good and attacks tend to become less severe and less frequent as the child reaches adulthood.

NORMOKALAEMIC PERIODIC PARALYSIS

The periodic paralysis described by Poskanzer and Kerr (1961) also had a dominant inheritance and resembled hyperkalaemic periodic paralysis but the attacks were more severe and persistent, lasting for several days or even weeks. The serum K^+ was not raised, even in severe attacks. Paralysis was, however, induced or made worse by administration of potassium and improved by NaCl. Treatment with acetazolamide and 9-α-fluorohydrocortisone prevented attacks being provoked by potassium. The family described by Meyers *et al.* (1972) had shorter attacks which were not provoked by potassium and were not improved by acetazolamide.

MYOTONIC SYNDROMES

The clinical feature common to all the myotonic disorders is myotonia, which is a state of delayed relaxation, or sustained contraction, of skeletal muscle. It may manifest after a voluntary muscle contraction, so-called active myotonia. The patient may be aware of difficulty in relaxing the grip after grasping something. This is best demonstrated by the delayed extension of the fingers following tight closure of the hand. With repetition of the same movement, the myotonia gradually becomes less and

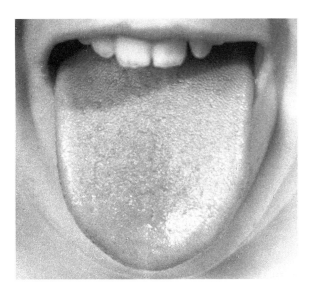
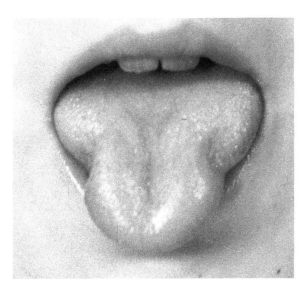

Figure 6-1 Percussion myotonia of the tongue in a case of myotonia congenita (see Figure 6-3).

then disappears. The term paradoxical myotonia has been applied to cases where the myotonia, instead of improving with activity, becomes worse with successive movements.

In infants the first manifestation of myotonia may occasionally be observed as a delayed opening of the eyes after their closure with crying. In some patients the myotonia may be fairly localized to only some muscle groups; in others there may be a more general 'stiffness' during the bouts of myotonia.

Myotonia may also be elicited by percussion of a muscle, so-called percussion mytonia. This can usually be demonstrated clinically by percussion with a finger. Suitable sites include the tongue (midline tap with finger), which often gives a bilateral contraction notch and slow relaxation (Figure 6-1), the thenar eminence giving an adduction and flexion of the thumb with slow return, or various other sites such as the deltoid, the brachioradialis or the gluteal muscles which give a local contraction dimple. Percussion myotonia also becomes less marked with repetitive tapping of the same muscle.

The clinical myotonia can be confirmed on electromyography which shows a characteristic pattern. With the use of the concentric needle, there is increased insertional activity and irritability of the muscle as the needle is inserted and spontaneous myotonic bursts may be produced. The myotonic bursts can also be elicited if the muscle is tapped with a finger in the vicinity of the needle, or when the patient voluntarily contracts the muscle.

These myotonic bursts consist of a prolonged series of rhythmical activity, initially of high frequency (around 20–80 Hz) and high amplitude, and then gradually waning in amplitude and also slowing down (Figure 6-2). The burst may continue for several seconds and an acoustic amplification gives a characteristic sound, likened to a dive-bomber (in the pre-jet age) or a motor cyclist taking off at speed and disappearing into the distance. The individual elements of the myotonic discharge usually resemble either positive sharp waves or fibrillation potentials, and represent action potentials from single muscle fibres.

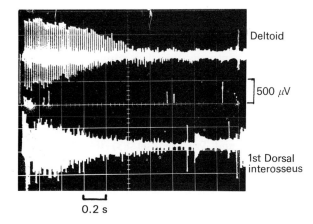

Figure 6-2 EMG showing spontaneous myotonic burst of approximately 60 discharges per second with steady waning of amplitude.

Table 6-3 Comparison of clinical features of hypokalaemic and hyperkalaemic periodic paralysis, myotonia congenita and paramyotonia congenita

| | Periodic paralyses | | Paramyotonia congenita | Myotonia congenita |
	Hypokalaemic	Hyperkalaemic		
Recurrent weakness:	Yes	Yes	Rarely	No
Onset:	Puberty	Infancy	Infancy	Infancy
Attack duration:	Hours to days	Minutes to days	Minutes to days	Minutes to days
Interictal interval:	Hours to days	Minutes to days	Minutes to days	Minutes to days
Myotonia:	No	Yes	Yes	Yes
Triggered by:	Cold	Cold	Cold	Cold
	Rest after exercise	Rest after exercise	Rest after exercise	Rest after exercise
	Carbohydrates	Fasting	Fasting	Fasting
Ameliorated by:	Potassium	Carbohydrates	Warming	
	Exercise	Exercise	Exercise	Exercise
Therapy:	Acetazolamide	Acetazolamide mexiletine	Acetazolamide mexiletine	Acetazolamide mexiletine

From Brown (1993).

'Pseudomyotonia' is sometimes noted on EMG in other neuromuscular disorders such as type II glycogenosis. The bursts are usually shorter and less striking than true myotonia and do not show the characteristic decrement. One cannot elicit clinical myotonia in these patients.

MYOTONIA IN ANIMALS

Extensive experimental studies have been done on hereditary myotonia occurring in goats in some of the Southern States of the USA. The myotonia in these animals is brought on by sudden exertion or following a sudden surprise such as a loud noise. Legend has it that they would freeze rigid in their tracks and keel over at the sound of the whistle of an oncoming train. The condition has many similarities to human myotonia congenita. An hereditary condition affecting horses, known as springhalt, has some resemblances to human paramyotonia congenita.

CHEMICALLY INDUCED MYOTONIA

Myotonia has also been produced by monocarboxylic aromatic acids (Brody, 1973) and a cholesterol-lowering agent, diazocholesterol (Somers and Winer, 1966).

MYOTONIA CONGENITA (THOMSEN'S DISEASE)

HISTORICAL

The classical treatise on myotonia congenita by the Danish physician Thomsen (1876) was based on his personal experience of the condition, which had already affected four generations of his family and could be traced back to his great grandmother, whose family had emigrated to Denmark from North Germany in the eighteenth century. What prompted Thomsen to document the disease, at the age of 61 years, was apparently the refusal of the Prussian army medical officers to accept his medical certificate that his affected son, who had been conscripted into the Prussian army, was unfit for military service. Thomsen described the disease as 'tonic cramps' and also highlighted the 'psychotic disposition', which also ran in his family and which he considered an integral part of the condition. Strümpell (1881) suggested the term 'myotonia congenita' and Westphal (1883) the designation 'Thomsen's disease'. In 1886 Wilhelm Erb incorporated both these suggestions in the exhaustive monograph on 'Die Thomsen'sche Krankheit (myotonia congenita)' he wrote to commemorate the 500th Anniversary of Heidelberg University. He described for the first time the production of myotonia by electrical stimulus, and also gave a description of the histological features of the muscle.

In 1923 Thomsen's grandnephew, Nissen, updated the Thomsen family tree with an additional two generations and pointed out that the hereditary psychosis affecting the family was independent of the myotonia congenita. In his monograph on myotonia, Thomasen (1948) (no relation) documented further details about branches of the Thomsen family still living in Denmark.

CLINICAL FEATURES

The condition is inherited as an autosomal dominant trait and, as the name implies, symptoms may be present from birth, but usually come on later. The essential manifestation is the myotonia, which may vary considerably in severity and may at times be fairly mild and localized. The diagnosis, in the absence of a positive family history, is largely dependent on an accurate history and, once suspected, the diagnosis may readily be confirmed by the demonstration of myotonia (Figures 6-1, 6-2).

Patients often first become aware of active myotonia either in the arms or the legs. In the arms this usually manifests as difficulty in releasing an object after grasping it firmly. In the legs there may be difficulty with walking or other activities such as climbing stairs, brought on particularly after a period of prolonged rest or inactivity. It is thus often worse on waking in the morning and can often be 'worked off' with repeated movement, a characteristic feature of myotonia. At times other muscles are affected and the mother may have noted prolonged closure of an infant's eyes following crying.

Myotonia may be aggravated by cold, by mood and by fatigue. Some patients may develop a marked generalized myotonia or stiffness in response to a sudden fright or sudden diffuse muscular tension.

Clinically the active myotonia may be demonstrated following sustained contraction of a muscle group such as clenching the hand. Where the myotonia affects other isolated muscle groups unusual features may be demonstrable, such as lid lag following upward gaze or squint and diplopia following sustained conjugate movement of the eyes in one direction.

The other common feature of myotonia congenita is muscle hypertrophy. This is usually generalized and affects males as well as females.

GENETICS

Becker (1971) reviewed several large pedigrees of myotonia congenita in West Germany and concluded that there were two separate entities with a different genetic basis. The one is the classical Thomsen's disease, inherited as a autosomal dominant trait, and the number of affected to unaffected individuals in the pedigree studies was the anticipated 50%. There was full penetrance of the gene, with no apparent skipping of generations. The other form is an autosomal recessive variety in which siblings were affected but the parents were found to be normal. The incidence of affected to unaffected members in siblings approached the 25% region expected for an autosomal recessive inheritance. There was also a high incidence of consanguinous marriages among the parents.

MYOTONIA CONGENITA (BECKER)

Becker noted some clinical differences between the dominant and recessive forms. Usually, the myotonia in the recessive form was later in onset and more generalized and more marked than in the dominant. The onset was gradual and tended to affect the legs before the arms or face. His cases also tended to have more striking hypertrophy of their muscles (Figures 6-3–6-5). Associated weakness of muscles was also a more common feature in the recessive than in the dominant variety. The dominant form, however, seemed more prone to aggravation of the myotonia by cold. The incidence of the recessive form was higher and it also seemed likely that this was an underestimate since many of the persons suffering from myotonia were found to conceal their disability as they tended to be looked upon as malingerers.

INVESTIGATIONS

The diagnosis is essentially a clinical one and can readily be confirmed by the classical EMG pattern.

Muscle biopsy shows an essentially normal histological picture apart from the presence of true hypertrophy of fibres in some cases, the occurrence of isolated atrophic fibres and the presence of internal nuclei. On histochemical study there is an interesting absence of type 2B fibres (Dubowitz and Brooke, 1973; Crews *et al.*, 1976).

TREATMENT

Many patients learn to cope with the disability, which may tend to be relatively mild. Repetitive muscle activity may overcome the myotonia so that by avoiding postures of continuous rest the myotonia can be prevented. Thus one of my patients with dominantly inherited myotonia always sat on an aisle seat in the cinema or theatre, in order to 'keep his legs going' so that he was not stiff or immobile at

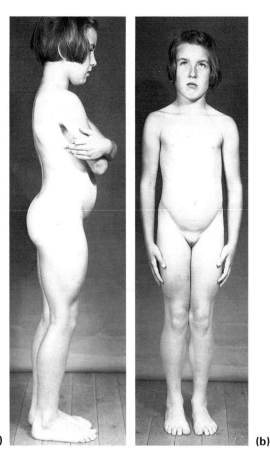

(a)   **(b)**

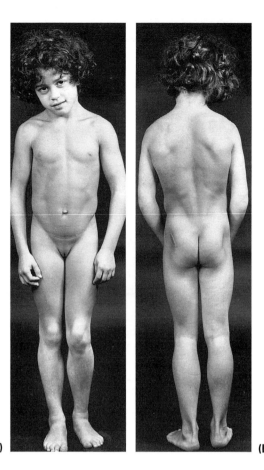

(a)   **(b)**

Figure 6-3a,b Recessive congenital myotonia in an 8-year-old girl. Her mother had consulted many physicians since first becoming concerned about the child's gait at about 2 years of age. No abnormality was found and initially the mother and subsequently the daughter were labelled as neurotic. The daughter's history was classical for myotonia congenita. In the mornings she was so stiff on waking she could scarcely get out of bed and practically stumbled down stairs to prepare tea for her parents. By the time she took the tea upstairs her gait was normal. She was also fond of competitive running at school but was often left behind, stuck to the starting line – although once away she gradually caught up. She showed generalized hypertrophy and percussion myotonia of the tongue (see Figure 6-1) and of various skeletal muscles. The parents were normal.

Figure 6-4a,b Recessive congenital myotonia in a 9-year-old girl in whom myotonia congenita was diagnosed on a characteristic history from her father: 'When we travel by tube [underground] train from Neasden to Wembley, which is only one stop, she is unable to get off the train but stumbles and has to be helped. Within a few minutes she is walking normally again.' She showed generalized muscle hypertrophy (a,b) and percussion myotonia could be elicited in the tongue and thenar muscles. There was a delayed opening of the eyes after closure. The parents were normal.

the end of the show. Each patient thus has to be assessed on his own merits and the benefits of treatment weighed against the degree of disability and the possible side-effects of therapy.

The mainstay in the treatment of myotonia is the type I class of cardiac anti-arrhythmic agents. These drugs act on the voltage-dependent Na channel to reduce the rate of channel activation, thereby prolonging the effective channel refractory period. In essence, these drugs reduce the ease with which an

action potential can be triggered by a preceding potential with a given interpotential latency. In the context of repetitive action potential generation in myotonia, the result is a reduction in the frequency of repetitive spikes and in the duration of spiking activity.

The type I anti-arrhythmic agents available in clinical practice include phenytoin, procainamide, quinine, mexiletine and tocainide. Some of these agents, such as phenytoin and quinine, are relatively

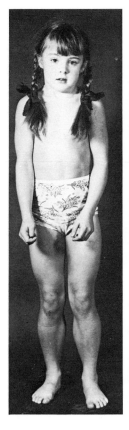
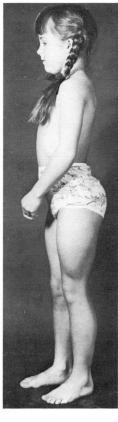

(a)   **(b)**

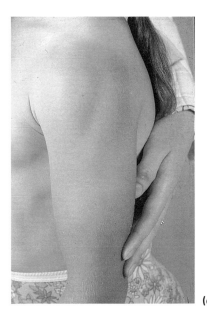

(c)

Figure 6-5a-c Recessive congenital myotonia in an 8-year-old girl presenting with stiffness of muscles after rest. Note the marked muscle hypertrophy (a,b) and percussion myotonia of deltoid (c). The parents were normal. There was no clinical weakness.

innocuous, while others, such as tocainide, have been associated with serious side-effects. There is a serious question as to whether it is justifiable to expose a patient to the risk of a potentially fatal complication of drug therapy to treat a non-lethal complication of a chronic disease. In some cases, however, the effects of severe myotonia can be so disabling that therapy might be considered if other less risky alternatives are exhausted. In these cases, initial therapy with phenytoin (Munsat, 1967) or quinine (Wolf, 1936) is often chosen.

In patients where phenytoin is not effective, a trial of procainamide may be tried. In resistant cases, mexiletine is often found useful. This drug does not appear to carry the risk of fatal haematological complications seen with tocainide. Myotonia associated with paramyotonia congenita or with hyperkalaemic periodic paralysis may be particularly sensitive to tocainide (Streib *et al.*, 1983; Streib, 1987; Ricker *et al.*, 1980; 1983) and its use in selected cases may be indicated.

PARAMYOTONIA CONGENITA (EULENBURG'S DISEASE)

HISTORICAL

Paramyotonia congenita was originally described by Eulenburg (1886, 1916) in 26 members from six generations of a family in East Germany, and is characterized by myotonia which is brought on or aggravated by cold. Many reports have appeared since and it has been reviewed in detail by Becker (1970). It is possible that most cases can be traced back to the same mutant gene occurring in the second half of the seventeenth century. Another classical description was that of an American physician, Dr Ezra Clark Rich (1894), who documented the dominantly inherited, cold-sensitive, myopathy in his own family. Because the myotonia of myotonia congenita may also be aggravated by cold, the question has been raised from time to time as to whether paramyotonia is indeed a distinct nosological entity.

CLINICAL FEATURES

The symptoms of the disease are usually mild and more of a nuisance than a handicap. The condition particularly affects the muscles of the face and hands and will usually respond rapidly to warming (Figures 6-6 and 6-7). As in myotonia congenita there is a tendency to hypertrophy of the musculature. The stiffness of the muscles may be followed by transitory weakness but the episodes usually subside within a matter of hours.

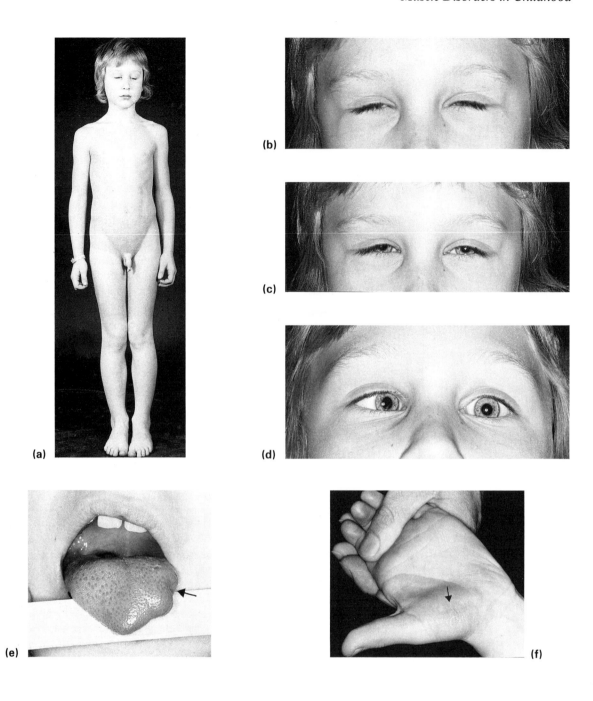

Figure 6-6a-f Congenital paramyotonia in an 8-year-old boy (a) whose mother was also affected. Myotonia of the face was first noticed by the mother when he was sneezing when a few months old, and also episodes of coughing and choking with feeds were noticed. Motor milestones, and power, were normal. He tended to experience stiffness when running. There was striking exacerbation with a visit to his estranged father, due to increased physical activity. There was marked myotonia of eyelids (b,c,d) when he tried to open them after tight closure. Myotonia was also present in external ocular muscles after a gaze in one direction. Rubbing of the eyelids to release myotonia seemed to work. Percussion myotonia elicited in tongue (e) and thenar eminence (note furrow and flexion of finger) (f) and various other muscles. There was no muscle hypertrophy.

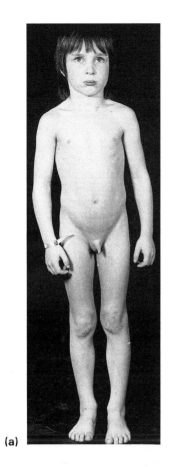

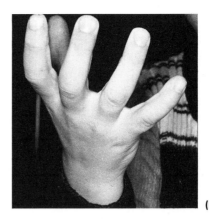

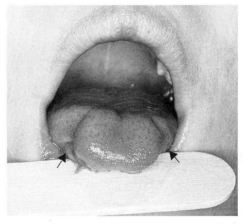

Figure 6-7a-c The 6-year-old brother (a) of child in Figure 6-6 with similar features. Diagnosis was by the mother within first 2 months of life on the basis of choking spasms when breast feeding. The motor milestones were normal. Myotonia was more severe than in the brother; this child was also very cold sensitive. There was a marked delay in opening hand (b) and eyes, as in the brother. Myotonia of the eyelids was relieved by rubbing. Myotonia of the external ocular muscles was also present. There was percussion myotonia of the tongue (c) and various other muscles. There was no hypertrophy. Their mother was similarly affected, as was her mother and maternal grandmother. She experienced marked myotonia on exposure to cold, and at times general stiffness precipitated by fright. She also had episodes of weakness, aggravated by continued activity. She had striking myotonia of the eyelids and also external ocular muscles which 'get all knotted up' after she fixated in one direction and tried to look in another direction. In spite of her myotonia she used to work as a dancer in a circus and it was only the extra pressures of marriage which made it difficult for her to cope. The myotonia became much worse in her first pregnancy. (Seen by courtesy of Dr Christopher Pallis.)

Becker (1970) delineated as a separate category a group of patients with paramyotonia congenita who, in addition to the paramyotonia, also had longer periods of weakness independent of exposure to cold.

An overlap has been observed between paramyotonia congenita, and also myotonia congenita, and hyperkalaemic periodic paralysis (adynamia episodica hereditaria) by several authors and also on rare occasions in cases with hypokalaemic periodic paralysis. It is also of interest that myotonic lid lag has been observed in association with paramyotonia congenita in several of the reported cases and also in association with hyperkalaemic and hypokalaemic periodic paralysis. These astute clinical observations anticipated the recent advances in the molecular genetics of this group of disorders.

CHONDRODYSTROPHIC MYOTONIA; SCHWARTZ–JAMPEL SYNDROME

A syndrome of myotonia, dwarfism, diffuse bone disease and unusual ocular and facial abnormalities delineated by Aberfeld *et al.* (1965) is probably similar to the syndrome of congenital blepharophimosis with myopathy described by Schwartz and Jampel (1962), whose names are now associated with the syndrome. Two further cases were reported by Aberfeld *et al.* (1970) under the title of 'chondrodystrophic myotonia'. The condition is readily suspected in children who show the striking blepharospasm and unusual facial appearance in addition to their myotonia, muscle weakness and stunted growth (Figure 6-8).

In most patients, symptoms are obvious at birth, and the diagnosis is typically made in the first year of life. Affected infants have narrow palpebral fissures, blepharospasm, micrognathia, and flattened facies (Farrell *et al.*, 1987). They may also have a harsh cry with laryngeal stridor. They almost invariably have limitation of joint movement. Skeletal abnormalities include short neck, kyphosis and pectus carinatum. The muscles are typically hypertrophic and clinically

stiff. The symptoms are not progressive. About 20% of reported cases also had mild mental retardation (Huttenlocher *et al.*, 1969; Ferrannini *et al.*, 1982).

Electrophysiologically, there is nearly continuous electrical activity and electrical silence is difficult to obtain. The characteristic muscle stiffness arises from sustained muscle membrane electrical activity (Spaans *et al.*, 1990). Discharges differ from those of myotonia congenita and recessive generalized myotonia in that there is relatively little waxing and waning in either amplitude or frequency. The electrical activity in chondrodysplastic myotonia does not disappear with sleep, and is not affected by curarization (Cao *et al.*, 1978; Spaans *et al.*, 1990). Benzodiazepines and other drugs that modify spinal cord synaptic activity also have no effect on the muscle electrical activity. Some therapeutic benefit has been reported with procainamide (Huttenlocher *et al.*, 1969; Spaans *et al.*, 1991) and recently with carbamazepine (Topaloglu *et al.*, 1993).

Muscle biopsy in chondrodystrophic myotonia exhibits mostly non-specific changes (Fowler *et al.*, 1974; Spaans *et al.*, 1990), including vacuoles between myofibrils, interpreted to be dilated elements of the T-tubular system, focal disarrangement and discontinuities in myofibrils, and Z-line streaming.

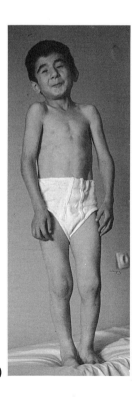 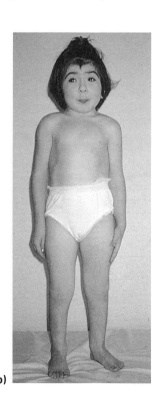 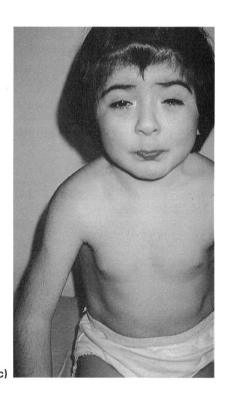

(a) (b) (c)

Figure 6-8a-c Schwartz–Jampel syndrome (chondrodystrophic myotonia). (a,b) Two unrelated children with typical dwarfism, postural abnormality and myotonia. Note blepharosparm after eye closure (c). (Courtesy Dr Haluk Topaloglu.)

The disorder is inherited as an autosomal recessive trait. However, some cases with possible autosomal dominant inheritance have been reported (Ferrannini *et al.*, 1982).

Electrophysiological studies by Lehmann-Horn *et al.* (1990) at the single channel level showed abnormal sodium channel kinetics in the sarcolemma of muscle, obtained at biopsy from patients with the Schwartz–Jampel syndrome. Bursts of single channel opening were obtained with patch clamp in response to depolarization. Genetic analysis, however, still awaits resolution.

PATHOPHYSIOLOGY

The electrophysiological basis of the myotonias has been extensively studied and has helped elucidate the defects in membrane excitability and to suggest possible candidate genes, which in turn helped to short-circuit the resolution of the molecular basis of some of these disorders.

In normal nerve and muscle in the resting state, the intracellular compartment is electrically hyperpolarized with respect to the extracellular milieu. At least three factors contribute to this resting potential: (1) a gradient of ions across the semi-permeable cell membrane, with potassium and chloride ions concentrated extracellularly, while sodium ions are concentrated intracellularly; (2) the presence of impermeable, negatively-charged proteins within the cytoplasm; and (3) an electrogenic Na-K exchange pump in the membrane which extrudes three Na ions in exchange for two K. For each individual ion, movement across the membrane is dictated by membrane permeability, the ion's concentration gradient and the electrical membrane profile across the membrane. For each permeant ion, an equilibrium condition exists at which there is no net ion movement (the so-called Nernst or reversal potential).

At equilibrium the membrane potential is the weighted average of the reversal potentials for each ion species, where the weighting factors are the conductances for the ion. At rest, the conductances for K and Cl are much greater than that of Na. When the membrane is depolarized to the threshold for all-or-nothing excitation, the conductance for sodium increases rapidly so that it becomes much greater than that for K plus Cl. Repolarization occurs for two reasons. The abrupt rise in the Na conductance is self-terminating and the depolarized Na channel rapidly closes or inactivates. Slightly thereafter, an outward K current is activated. Thus, the Na conductance falls and K conductance rises. Both factors will drive membrane potential back toward reversal potential of K and Cl.

Two hypotheses evolved relevant to myotonia and the periodic paralyses. The first, 'depolarization hypothesis', is that myotonia could theoretically arise from any conductance change which slightly depolarizes the membrane potential, rendering it closer to the firing threshold. An increase in Na conductance or a decrease in either K or Cl conductance could act to depolarize the cell and trigger myotonic bursts of repetitive firing.

In the second hypothesis, the Nernstian hypothesis for periodic paralysis, based on the Nernst potential for K, predicted that during paralytic episodes in hypokalaemic periodic paralysis the membrane would be hyperpolarized, while in hyperkalaemic paralysis it would be depolarized.

HYPERKALAEMIC PERIODIC PARALYSIS AND PARAMYOTONIA CONGENITA

Some 30 years ago, Creutzfeld *et al.* (1963) studied the membrane potential of normal and periodic paralysis muscle *in situ* in patients, either under normal conditions or during attacks of paralysis with corresponding abnormalities in serum potassium. They noted that in both hyperkalaemic and hypokalaemic paralysis there was depolarization of the patient's muscle, and that in the hyperkalaemic patients the degree of depolarization exceeded that predicted by the Nernst equation for the change in K. They concluded that hyperkalaemic paralysis arises from excessive depolarization because of a defect in Na conductance.

This hypothesis was subsequently supported by the extensive studies of Lehmann-Horn and colleagues (1983). In their *in vitro* studies with muscle biopsies from hyperkalaemic periodic paralysis, they documented that increasing K levels in the medium bathing the muscle increased inward current and simultaneously depolarized the membrane potential (Lehmann-Horn *et al.*, 1983; Lehmann-Horn and Rüdel, 1987), and that the extent of depolarization exceeded the predictions of the Nernst equation. They further showed that both the increment in background current and the depolarization induced by elevated bath potassium could be reversed by addition of a sodium channel blocking agent, tetrodotoxin.

Cannon *et al.* (1991) extended these observations by analysing the function of single muscle sodium channels, using patch clamping of muscle grown in culture from biopsies of a hyperkalaemic paralysis patient. At normal potassium concentrations, the behaviour of the channels was normal. However, at

7 mM potassium, the sodium channels in hyperkalaemic paralysis muscles behaved distinctly abnormally: opening time became dramatically longer and, during a single depolarization, abnormal repetitive openings were seen. In effect, the mutant channels showed imperfect inactivation.

The few clinical and experimental investigations that have been made to elucidate the pathophysiology of paramyotonia congenita indicated that the defect lies in the muscle fibre membrane, probably also in the sodium channel (Lehmann-Horn et al., 1981, 1987). *In vitro* investigations of membrane resting potential and conductance showed that at 37°C, these parameters are normal but that on cooling to 27°C, a pathological depolarization on the membrane sets in. During the depolarization process, long-lasting series of low-frequency action potentials occur that resemble those in the EMG *in vivo*. When the depolarization reaches a steady state at −40 mV, the fibres are inexcitable, causing the paramyotonic weakness. This depolarization is prevented *in vitro* by tetrodotoxin. Anti-arrhythmic drugs that block the sodium channel with a pronounced use dependence are effective in preventing cold-induced stiffness and weakness in the patients. The long-lasting persistence of the weakness, even after rewarming, could have its origin in the fact that in paramyotonia the muscle fibres depolarize much more than in the other periodic paralyses. During such long-lasting strong depolarization, the fibres take up potassium chloride, and this slows the repolarization process. There is no indication that a channel alteration persists beyond the period of cooling, for when repolarization was forced with the voltage clamp, the channels were normal.

These studies convincingly incriminated a defect in sodium conductance in the pathogenesis of both hyperkalaemic paralysis and possibly paramyotonia congenita. Both the conventional physiological studies and the patch clamp data suggested that both factors which trigger the clinical symptoms, elevated potassium and reduced temperature, act to augment sodium conductance. These findings were in striking accord with the simple 'depolarization hypothesis' that the abnormal excitability in these disorders arises because membrane potential is depolarized by an increased sodium conductance, and pointed to the skeletal muscle sodium channel as an excellent candidate gene in these two disorders.

MYOTONIA CONGENITA

The early literature also provided convincing evidence that the 'depolarization hypothesis' pertained to myotonia congenita muscle as well; in this instance because of a reduced chloride conductance

rather than an increased sodium conductance. In normal skeletal muscle Bryant and Morales-Aguilera (1971) observed that reduction of chloride conductance produces a tendency toward easily triggered, sustained, repetitive membrane firing, whilst Lipicky et al. (1971) documented that membrane chloride conductance is reduced in muscle of patients with myotonia congenita (Thomsen's disease), which was subsequently confirmed by Rüdel et al. (1988) and Franke et al. (1991).

ANIMAL MODELS

The role of an abnormal chloride conductance in myotonia was further supported by animal studies. Adrian and Bryant (1974) demonstrated that sustained, repetitive myotonic bursting requires both a reduced chloride conductance and an intact t-tubule system, and Bryant (1979) showed that congenital myotonia in the goat arises from a reduction in skeletal muscle chloride permeability.

Several studies have documented that, like the myotonic goat, the *adr/adr* mouse has an abnormally low skeletal muscle chloride conductance. (*adr* = arrested development of righting response: if the animal is dropped on a table it becomes stiff and cannot right itself.) Steinmeyer and colleagues (1991a) cloned a mammalian, voltage-dependent, developmentally regulated, chloride channel, 'ClC-1', and demonstrated that this was disrupted in the *adr/adr* mouse by the presence of a transposon within the gene for ClC-1 (Steinmeyer et al., 1991b). Thus, like the Na channel in hyperkalaemic paralysis and paramyotonia congenita, the chloride channel ClC-1 provided an excellent candidate gene for human myotonia congenita.

MOLECULAR GENETICS

HYPERKALAEMIC PERIODIC PARALYSIS AND PARAMYOTONIA CONGENITA

To determine whether the skeletal muscle sodium channel is genetically linked to hyperkalaemic periodic paralysis, Fontaine et al. (1990) used a partial cDNA for the α-subunit of this protein to perform genetic linkage analysis. In a single family, a lod score of 4.0 was obtained; with multi-point analysis testing for co-inheritance of the disease with both the test allele of the sodium channel and a tightly linked marker (the gene for human growth hormone), Fontaine obtained a lod score of just over 7. These scores pointed to a high probability that

Table 6-4 Mutations recognized to date in sodium channel α-subunit in relation to hyperkalaemic periodic paralysis (HYPERPP), paramyotonia congenita (PMC) and myotonia congenita (MC)

	Mutation	Position	Domain	Disease	Reference
1.	Met → Val	1592	IV, S6	HYPERRPP	Rojas *et al.* (1991)
2.	Thr → Met	704	II, S5	HYPERPP	Ptacek *et al.* (1991c)
3.	Ala → Thr	1156	III, S4-5	HYPERPP-PMC	McClatchey *et al.* (1992c)
4.	Gly → Val	1306	III-IV loop	PMC	McClatchey *et al.* (1992b)
5.	Thr → Met	1313	III-IV loop	PMC	McClatchey *et al.* (1992b)
6.	Arg → His	1448	IV, S4	PMC	Ptacek *et al.* (1992a)
7.	Arg → Cys	1448	IV, S4	PMC	Ptacek *et al.* (1992a)
8.	Ser → Phe	804	II, S6	PMC/MC	McClatchey *et al.* (1992c)
9.	Leu → Arg	1433	IV, S3	PMC	Ptacek *et al.* (1992b)
10.	Phe → Leu	1421	IV, S3	HYPERPP[a]	Rudolph *et al.* (1992)

(For reference list on nomenclature of amino acids see Chapter 15)
[a] equine
From Brown (1993).

defects within the sodium channel gene cause hyperkalaemic paralysis. Several further studies confirmed the close linkage of hyperkalaemic periodic paralysis to the sodium channel gene on chromosome 17q (Ptacek *et al.*, 1991a; Koch *et al.*, 1991a) and also that paramyotonia congenita is linked to the same locus (Ebers *et al.*, 1991; Koch *et al.*, 1991b; Ptacek *et al.*, 1991b; McClatchey *et al.*, 1992a) so that the two conditions are allelic.

Further progress followed rapidly, and several groups identified missense mutations in nine different human hyperkalaemic paralysis pedigrees (Ptacek *et al.*, 1991c, 1992a,b; Rojas *et al.*, 1991; McClatchey *et al.*, 1992b,c). A similar mutation has also been found in a pedigree of quarter horses, which had been selectively bred for their muscle bulk (Rudolph *et al.*, 1992). As seen in Table 6-4 and Figure 6-9 these mutations produce relatively minor amino acid changes. It remains highly likely that the number of mutations will grow considerably.

Feero *et al.* (1993) recently studied point mutations of the human adult, voltage-gated, skeletal muscle sodium channel gene in 12 families with hyperkalaemic periodic paralysis, from diverse ethnic backgrounds. Three of the 12 families showed the *Met*1592*Val* mutation, the remaining six had the *Thr*704*Met* mutation; in three families the mutation was not identified. In one of these latter three families, the disease was not linked to the human adult voltage-gated sodium channel gene, suggesting the existence of a clinically similar but molecularly distinct form of hyperkalaemic periodic paralysis. Genotype/phenotype correlations showed the variable and subjective nature of the illness, although the clinical distinctions between hyperkalaemic periodic paralysis and paramyotonia congenita were reinforced by the molecular data.

To date, 23 hyperkalaemic periodic paralysis families have shown linkage to the sodium-channel gene locus, with no recombinants (LOD = 50.01), and 23 paramyotonia congenita families have shown similar results (LOD = 32.96) (Wang *et al.*, 1993). All mutations are single base changes resulting in an amino acid substitution of a highly conserved residue in the sodium-channel protein.

SODIUM-CHANNEL MYOTONIA ———

A dominantly inherited myotonia congenita, resembling Thomsen's disease, has recently been shown to be due to a mutation in the Na channel (Iaizzo *et al.*, 1991a; Lerche *et al.*, 1993; Heine *et al.*, 1993). It is characterized by aggravation of the myotonia by potassium intake and the fact that, unlike periodic paralysis and paramyotonia congenita, muscle weakness is not a significant feature.

ANDERSEN'S SYNDROME ———

This syndrome comprises a triad of autosomal dominant hyperkalaemic periodic paralysis together with ventricular arrhythmia and a mildly dysmorphic facies. It is not linked to the Na channel (Tawill *et al.*, 1994).

HYPOKALAEMIC PERIODIC PARALYSIS ———

It has been shown that hypokalaemic paralysis is not linked to the skeletal muscle sodium channel locus (Fontaine *et al.*, 1992). The defect in hypokalaemic periodic paralysis is currently still not known, but one possibility is a reduction in potassium conductance, in view of the reduced excitability in hypokalaemic periodic paralysis and the observation that

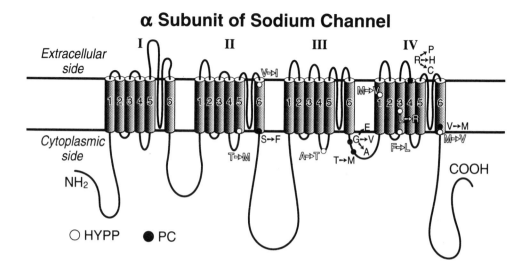

Figure 6-9 Schematic diagram of the 270 kD α-subunit of the adult skeletal muscle voltage-sensitive sodium channel, indicating the individual amino acid changes causing either hyperkalaemic periodic paralysis (HYPP) or paramyotonia congenita (PC). The protein is organized into four domains (I, II, III, IV), each of which has multiple transmembrane segments. All the indicated amino acid changes are only seen in human patients affected with either hyperkalaemic periodic paralysis or paramyotonia congenita, with the exception of the F→L change in domain IV which causes hyperkalaemic periodic paralysis in quarter horses. C, cysteine; F, phenylalanine; L, leucine; G, guanine; H, histidine; M, methionine; P, proline; R, arginine; V, valine; NH_2 and COOH, amino- and carboxyl-termini of proteins, respectively. (Courtesy Dr Eric Hoffman; Hoffman and Wang, 1993.)

cromakilin, a substance that increases potassium conductance, is able to repolarize hypokalaemic periodic paralysis fibres *in vitro* so that they regain their strength (Grafe *et al.*, 1990).

The gene for hypokalaemic periodic paralysis has just been localized to chromosome 1q31-32 (Fontaine *et al.*, 1994). The gene encoding the α1-subunit of the muscle dihydropyridine-sensitive calcium channel is localized in the same region (Gregg *et al.*, 1993), so that it is a potential candidate gene. It is also of special interest that the hereditary mouse disorder, muscular dysgenesis (Pai, 1965a,b), in which there is a failure of excitation–contraction coupling, with death from respiratory failure soon after birth, is due to the same gene and has an absence of the α_1-subunit of the skeletal DHP-sensitive Ca^{2+} channel (Knudson *et al.*, 1989; Adams and Beam, 1990).

MYOTONIA CONGENITA

It is now clear that mutations in the gene for the chloride channel, ClC-1, underly at least two types of myotonia congenita. Linkage of the dominant form, Thomsen's disease, to chromosome 7q was established by Abdalla *et al.* in 1991 (a,b), and in 1992 Koch *et al.* reported that Becker's autosomal recessive myotonia congenita is also linked to the ClC-1 locus on human chromosome 7q. By examin-

ing co-inheritance of the generalized myotonia trait with haplotypes for ClC-1 and a closely linked marker (TCRB), Koch's group obtained a lod score of 5.79 in a single family. Sequence analysis documented the presence of a T to G substitution within an exon of the gene, predicted to produce a substitution of cysteine for phenylalanine. Koch *et al.* also examined four families with autosomal dominant myotonia congenita for linkage to the ClC-1 locus and obtained a maximum lod score of 4.58, strongly implicating a mutation in ClC-1 in this disease as well.

CHANNEL BIOPHYSICS

The sodium channel is believed to be composed of a large α-subunit and at least two, relatively small, β-subunits (Catterall, 1988). The α-subunit consists of about 2000 amino acids. There are four domains (I-IV), each consisting of six membrane spanning α-helices (S1-S6) (see Figure 6-9). In each domain, the fourth helix (S4) bears several positive charges. This general organization is highly conserved, both across several different sodium channel isoforms in skeletal muscle and brain, and also across different species. There is also a high degree of homology with voltage-sensitive calcium channels, and each specific sodium channel domain is highly homologous to single, voltage-sensitive, potassium channels.

Several lines of basic investigation over the years have suggested that specific domains of the channel are associated with specific functions.

The mutations to date in hyperkalaemic paralysis families fall loosely into three groups. Three mutations causing well-defined hyperkalaemic paralysis are located within the membrane, more toward the cytoplasmic end of the respective α-helices (Ptacek, 1991c; Rojas *et al.*, 1991). Five mutations producing the phenotype of paramyotonia congenita are located either in the III-IV cytoplasmic loop or toward the extracellular ends of S3 and S4 in domain IV (McClatchey *et al.*, 1992b; Ptacek *et al.*, 1992a,b). The remaining two mutations were associated with somewhat variable phenotypes (McClatchey *et al.*, 1992c).

Little is currently known about the domains of the voltage-sensitive chloride channel, so that one cannot relate the single myotonia congenita mutation reported by Koch *et al.* (1992) to the observed reduction in conductance in ClC-1. Recently, George *et al.* (1993) used single-strand conformational polymorphism analysis to screen DNA from members of four unrelated pedigrees with autosomal dominant myotonia congenita (Thomsen's disease) for mutations in the human skeletal muscle chloride channel gene (HUMCLC) on chromosome 7q35. Abnormal bands were detected in all affected, but no unaffected, individuals in three of the families. Directed sequencing revealed a G to A transition that results in the substitution of a glutamic acid for a glycine residue, located between the third and fourth predicted membrane spacing segments. This glycine residue is conserved in all known members of this class of chloride channel proteins. These results establish HUMCLC as the gene for Thomsen's disease.

THERAPEUTIC IMPLICATIONS ———————

The beneficial effect of mexiletine on myotonia almost certainly is a consequence of the sodium channel blocking effects of this lidocaine analogue. Indeed, it is precisely an actively-dependent sodium channel blocking agent which one would expect to be beneficial in a disorder characterized by incomplete sodium channel inactivation.

The mechanism of action of acetazolamide in preventing attacks of both hypokalaemic and hyperkalaemic periodic paralysis is unclear. Ricker *et al.* (1989) suggested that the acidosis produced by this carbonic anhydrase inhibitor may be central to its effect. They noted that, like normal individuals, patients with hyperkalaemic paralysis develop hyperkalaemia during extensive exercise. However, the patients do not develop weakness while exer-

cising; rather, only after rest and partial recovery from the exercise-induced hyperkalaemia. Evidently something occurs concurrently with intense exercise to mitigate the paralysis, despite significant hyperkalaemia, and one possibility is systemic acidosis.

MYOTONIC DYSTROPHY; STEINERT'S DISEASE

This condition, inherited as an autosomal dominant trait, is the most common muscular dystrophy of adult life, with a prevalence of about 5 per 100 000 (Harper, 1989). Whilst affecting predominantly adults, it also occurs in childhood and infancy. It is characterized by myotonia in association with muscle weakness and wasting plus a whole syndrome complex with additional features such as frontal balding (in males), cataracts, cardiomyopathy with conduction defects, gonadal atrophy and possible infertility, and low intelligence or dementia.

CLASSIFICATION ———————

Whilst myotonic dystrophy is loosely linked to the other myotonic syndromes by its associated myotonia, it is not primarily a channel disorder and the myotonia is often a relatively insignificant component in relation to the other features of the syndrome. Similarly, the muscle dystrophic element is but one component of the syndrome, so that it does not sit very comfortably either amidst the muscular dystrophies.

The basic molecular abnormality has now been shown to be an unstable expansion of DNA with a variable number of triplet repeats, associated with the gene for a protein kinase. From a molecular point of view it now joins a growing family of somewhat disparate and clinically divergent disorders associated with an unstable expansion of triplet repeats, which currently includes the fragile-X syndrome, Huntington's chorea, X-linked spinobulbar muscular atrophy, and spinocerebellar ataxia.

For the present I have thus decided to leave myotonic dystrophy in its current locus with the other myotonic syndromes.

HISTORICAL ———————

Looking back in the literature it is perhaps surprising how long it took for this striking symptom complex to be recognized as a distinct entity. After Erb's

(1886) classical monograph on Thomsen's disease, there were numerous papers on atypical Thomsen's disease with associated wasting and weakness. It was not until 1909, however, that Batten and Gibb in England and Steinert in Germany clearly delineated the condition as separate from myotonia congenita and drew attention to the consistent selective and symmetrical involvement of the facial, sternomastoid and forearm muscles in these patients. Batten and Gibb also stressed the hereditary nature of the condition and the fact that the myotonia might precede the muscle wasting and weakness. Steinert noted in addition the presence of ptosis and of bulbar paralysis, with disturbances of speech and swallowing, and also documented some of the non-muscle features such as frontal baldness, testicular atrophy, vasomotor disturbances and mental disturbances.

Comprehensive monographs on myotonic dystrophy ('dystrophia myotonica') have been written by Thomasen (1948), de Jong (1955), Caughey and Myrianthopoulos (1963), and in more recent times by Harper (1989).

CLINICAL FEATURES

The disorder is usually looked upon as a disease of adult life and the classical form usually has its onset in adolescence or adulthood.

The fullblown picture is readily recognizable (Figure 6-10) and the muscle weakness commonly includes ptosis and facial weakness as well as wasting of the sternomastoids and involvement of distal rather than proximal limb muscles. There may be associated swallowing difficulties and dysarthria and some cases have an external ophthalmoplegia. Myotonia may be an early symptom and often affects the hands, with inability to release a grasp. The patient illustrated in Figure 6-10 first became aware of the condition when he was unable to release his suitcase on Waterloo station on the day he was demobilized from the army in 1945. In the course of the disease, however, the muscle weakness soon becomes the predominant problem, to be followed by respiratory or cardiac problems. Cataracts are common in the late stages of the disease but may be detected in earlier cases on slit lamp examination. In the real world, however, most patients do not present with the classical, full-blown picture. Many may present with relatively minor symptoms or may in fact be subclinical and may only be recognized for the first time after family appraisal following the diagnosis of the index case, which may be a neonate with the severe congenital myotonic syndrome.

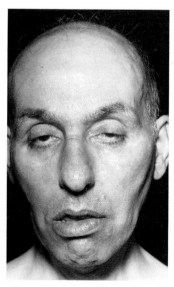 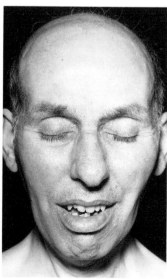

Figure 6-10   Adult patient (aged 51) with classical myotonic dystrophy showing characteristic facies, frontal balding and inability to close eyes or to show teeth. The patient looked older than his years.

Childhood forms

The condition also presents in childhood and may take various forms. The classical adult type may be recognized in childhood in affected families (Figure 6-11). These children are often symptom-free at this stage but myotonia may be demonstrated either clinically or on EMG and they also usually show a myopathic facies. Mild degrees of facial muscle weakness can often be demonstrated by the inability to screw the eyes up tightly and completely bury the eyelashes. The children subsequently follow the classical course of the disease with progression of weakness and also myotonia. As in other dominantly inherited conditions, there is marked variability in clinical severity within a family and careful family studies will often reveal subclinical cases.

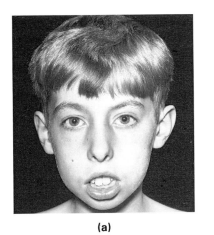
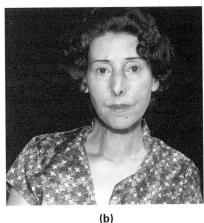
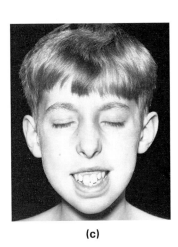

(a)	**(b)**	**(c)**

Figure 6-11a-c Myotonic dystrophy. Childhood onset. (a) The 10-year-old symptom-free son of a woman (b) with myotonic dystrophy. Note myopathic facies and inability to bury eyelashes (c).

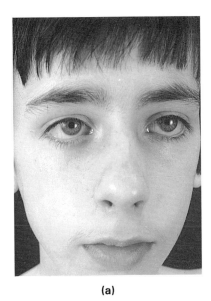
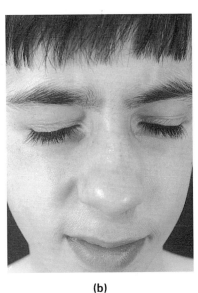
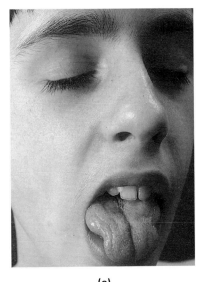

(a)	**(b)**	**(c)**

Figure 6-12a-c A 13-year-old boy with myotonic dystrophy diagnosed during routine admission for dental extractions. Note the facial weakness (a) with inability to close the eyes tightly (b) and percussion myotonia of the tongue (c). His mother was found to be similarly affected, although apparently symptom-free. Extreme caution must be exercised when administering anaesthesia to patients with myotonic dystrophy, in view of their sensitivity to relaxants as well as analgesics.

The condition may also be discovered fortuitously in children with facial weakness, or with delayed intellectual development, or with constipation (Figures 6-12 to 6-14). Some cases may present with orthopaedic problems such as talipes or scoliosis (Figures 6-15 and 6-16). It is important for these previously undiagnosed cases of myotonic dystrophy to be recognized when referred for surgery in view of the danger of anaesthesia (see below).

Smooth muscle involvement

There have been numerous reports on dysphagia and involvement of the swallowing mechanism in myotonic dystrophy. This may of course largely reflect involvement of striated muscle in the pharynx and upper oesophagus. Smooth muscle elsewhere has also been implicated. Harvey *et al.* (1965) undertook a comprehensive study of possible smooth muscle involvement in 16 adult cases of myotonic dystrophy. Of the 12 patients in whom oesophageal function was studied, all showed evidence of involvement of the striated muscle in the pharynx and upper oeophagus and 11 had a reduction in the amplitude of peristaltic contraction of 50% or more.

In addition, six patients showed a diminution of amplitude of contraction by more than 50% in the lower third of the oesophagus. Of nine patients subjected to cholangiographic study, six showed a prompt contraction of the gallbladder after cholecystokinin, two showed no response and one had a slow response. Studies of intestinal absorption in nine patients showed delay in reaching a peak with both lysine and glucose. Intestinal biopsy was normal. Manometric studies of the anal sphincter reflex in response to transient distension by a balloon in the rectum showed prompt and prolonged contraction and slow relaxation in both the internal (involuntary) and external (voluntary) components of the anal sphincter in seven of the eight cases studied. On digital examination all eight patients appeared to have very relaxed anal sphincters, but were not incontinent of faeces. Further studies on the functional deficit of the anal sphincter in adults with myotonic dystrophy have been documented by Hamel-Roy *et al.* (1984) and Eckardt and Nix (1991), whilst Reardon *et al.* (1992) drew attention to laxity of the anal sphincter in childhood cases of myotonic dystrophy and its possible confusion with childhood sex abuse.

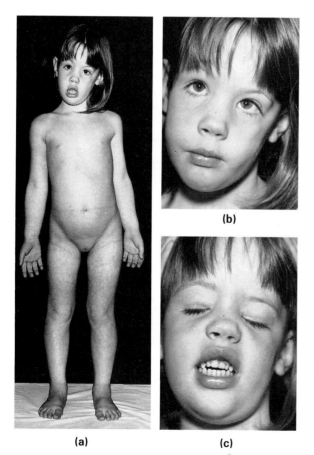

(a) (b) (c)

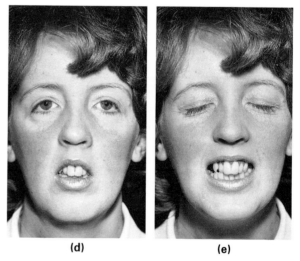

(d) (e)

Figure 6-13a-e Myotonic dystrophy. A 5-year-old girl (a) referred to general outpatient clinic for investigation of chronic constipation was noted to have (b) a somewhat droopy face and (c) inability to bury eyelashes. The mother (d, e) also had 'myopathic' facies and inability to bury eyelashes, and showed clinical myotonia of hands after clenching her fist. She was not aware of any stiffness, but had been receiving treatment for 'ulcerative colitis'. No clinical myotonia was present in the daughter, but myotonia was demonstrated in both of them on EMG.

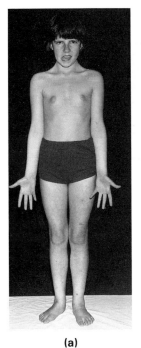

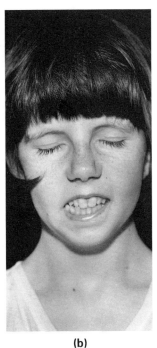

(a)　　　　　　　　　　(b)

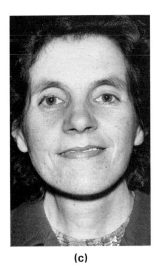

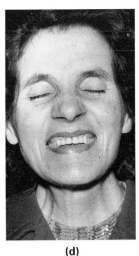

(c)　　　　　　　　　　(d)

Figure 6-14a-d Myotonic dystrophy in an 8-year-old girl (a) with chronic constipation seen at same clinic as the patient in Figure 6-13. She was also noted to have a slightly droopy face and inability to bury the eyelashes (b). Her mother (c) had a reasonably normal-looking face with good general movements but (d) inability to screw up the eyes and bury the eyelashes. No clinical myotonia was seen in either mother or daughter. There were no bowel symptoms in the mother. Diagnosis in both of them was confirmed by demonstration of myotonic bursts on EMG.

Constipation

Although swallowing difficulty is a well recognized feature of myotonic dystrophy, the condition is not usually included in the differential diagnosis of constipation. I had the unusual experience of seeing two patients with constipation at the same general outpatient clinic, in both of whom a myopathic facies suggested a possible myotonic dystrophy and was supported by a similar observation in both mothers (Figures 6-13 and 6-14). I have not seen another such case since. The association with constipation is probably a rare one, but worth bearing in mind. It may reflect involvement of the smooth muscle, or possibly the inability of the anal sphincter to relax normally. The constipation in my two patients showed no improvement on procainamide or quinine.

Cardiac involvement

Cardiac muscle is frequently affected in myotonic dystrophy. In a review of 98 cases from the literature de Wind and Jones (1950) found 61 cases (65%) with abnormal electrocardiograms, and a similar study by Fisch (1951) revealed 68% of abnormal tracings in a review of 85 cases. In a study of the ECG in 19 patients, Caughey and Myrianthopoulos (1963) found abnormalities of conduction or rhythm in 15. These patients are usually free of cardiac symptoms but some may present with Stokes–Adams syncope attacks (Wolintz *et al.*, 1966).

In a further extensive review of published cases, Church (1967) found ECG abnormalities in 202 of 236 patients, whilst only 16% had any cardiac symptoms, with about half attributed to arrhythmias. Subsequent prospective studies have shown a similar high prevalence of electrocardiographic abnormality in symptom-free patients, with mainly impairment of conduction and arrhythmias (Perloff *et al.*, 1984; Olofsson *et al.*, 1988; Hawley *et al.*, 1991), whilst intracardiac electrophysiological studies and histological studies showed abnormalities in all areas of the conducting system, and most frequently in the His–Purkinje system (Perloff *et al.*, 1984; Motta *et al.*, 1979; Nguyen *et al.*, 1988). Of 10 patients investigated by Hartwig *et al.* (1983) with radionuclide angiography, nine had abnormality of the ventricular wall motion during exercise. Mitral valve prolapse has been found in about 30% of patients (Streib *et al.*, 1985).

Cardiac failure is rare in myotonic dystrophy but sudden death is well recognized and one report suggested that as many as 30% of patients might die in this way (Hiromasa *et al.*, 1988). Whilst conduction block may be a possible mechanism, it has also been reported in patients with pacemakers, so that ventricular arrhythmia seems more likely a cause.

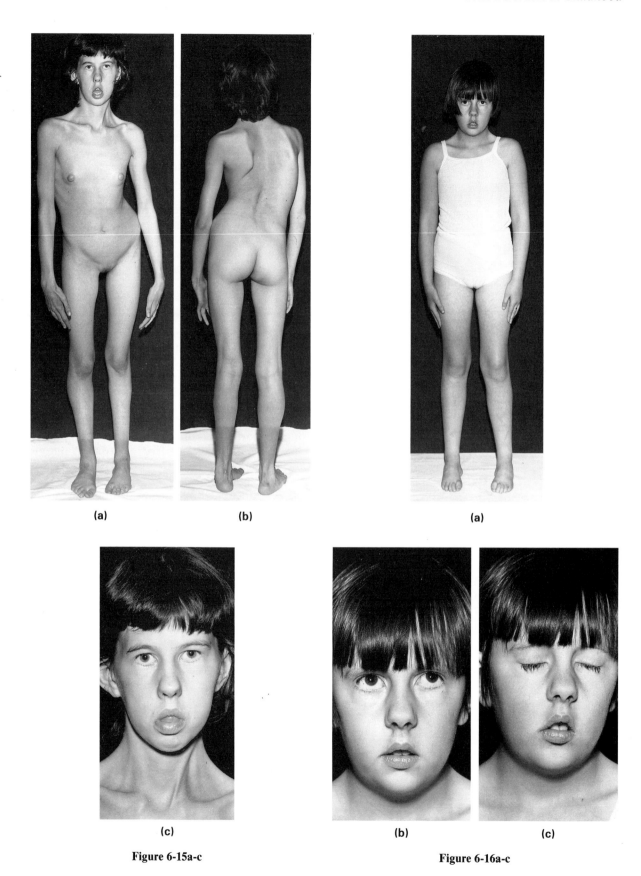

(a)   (b)   (a)

(c)   (b)   (c)

Figure 6-15a-c   **Figure 6-16a-c**

In view of the high frequency of electrocardiographic abnormality and the potential risk of sudden death, it is probably advisable to monitor these patients with routine ECG on an annual basis and, in those with evidence of significant abnormality or with clinical symptoms, to consider further assessment such as 24-hour monitoring with a view to possible intracardiac electrophysiological studies and insertion of a pacemaker.

Anaesthetic risk

A number of authors have drawn attention to the particular risks these patients have with anaesthesia, especially with thiopentone, which can result in sudden death (Dundee, 1952; Bourke and Zuck, 1957; Gillam *et al.*, 1964). They are particularly sensitive to relaxants and also to sedation and analgesia in general and need very close monitoring in the postoperative period until they have fully regained consciousness. The risk is independent of the clinical severity of the myotonic dystrophy and catastrophies can also occur in subclinical cases. This may be compounded by the cardiac involvement, and in addition these patients often have severe pulmonary insufficiency as a result of involvement of the intercostal muscles and diaphragm.

CONGENITAL MYOTONIC DYSTROPHY

In recent years attention has been focused on the congenital form of myotonic dystrophy, which may be one of the common modes of presentation of this condition. Vanier (1960) first drew attention to it and numerous subsequent reports highlighted the fairly consistent clinical features. Harper and Dyken (1972) and Dyken and Harper (1973) reviewed a series of cases in the USA, and subsequently Harper (1975a,b) undertook a detailed study of all available

cases in Great Britain, comprising 70 patients from five sibships. Hageman *et al.* (1993) recently documented the clinical data in 13 cases and the neuropathological findings in five, which did not show any specific features in the muscle or brain.

CLINICAL FEATURES

The main presenting features in the newborn period are general hypotonia and difficulty with sucking and swallowing, usually to the degree of necessitating tube feeding. Some patients may in addition have severe respiratory difficulties (which can be fatal) or associated deformities such as talipes equinovarus. A history of hydramnios during pregnancy is also a common feature and is presumably due to the inability of the fetus to swallow amniotic fluid *in utero* (Dunn and Dierker, 1973; Moosa, 1974). The mother may also have noted diminished fetal movements. Premature delivery is also a common problem, possibly precipitated by the hydramnios. It provides an additional compounding factor in relation to the respiratory deficit and may be an important factor in prognosis, both for survival and for associated intellectual retardation.

On clinical examination these infants have a striking facial diplegia, usually associated with an open, triangular-shaped, 'tented' mouth and inability to close the eyes fully (Figures 6-17 to 6-21). Myotonia is not a feature of the condition at this stage and is also not detectable on EMG. Skeletal deformities are common, particularly talipes.

The diagnosis is confirmed by examination of the mother who will almost invariably show subclinical or overt features of myotonic dystrophy, although she is often symptom-free. The two most consistent signs are mild facial weakness with inability to screw the eyes closed and bury the eyelashes and clinical myotonia after clenching the fist. Percussion myotonia can often be demonstrated in the tongue. The myotonia can be confirmed in the mother on EMG. Muscle biopsy in the infant is not helpful and may in fact be confusing and lead to misdiagnosis of other pathologies (Dubowitz, 1992).

Figure 6-15a-c (*left, facing page*) Myotonic dystrophy in a 13-year-old girl, with (a,b) scoliosis and left pes cavus, referred by an orthopaedic surgeon for possible underlying myopathy prior to operative treatment of her scoliosis. Note (c) myopathic facies and wasting of sternomastoids. A clinical diagnosis of myotonic dystrophy was confirmed on EMG.

Figure 6-16a-c (*right, facing page*) Myotonic dystrophy in the 10-year-old, symptom-free, sister of girl in Figure 6-15, noted to have (a) bilateral pes cavus and (b,c) a somewhat expressionless face and inability to bury the eyelashes. Diagnosis was confirmed on EMG. The mother was also found to have subclinical myotonic dystrophy.

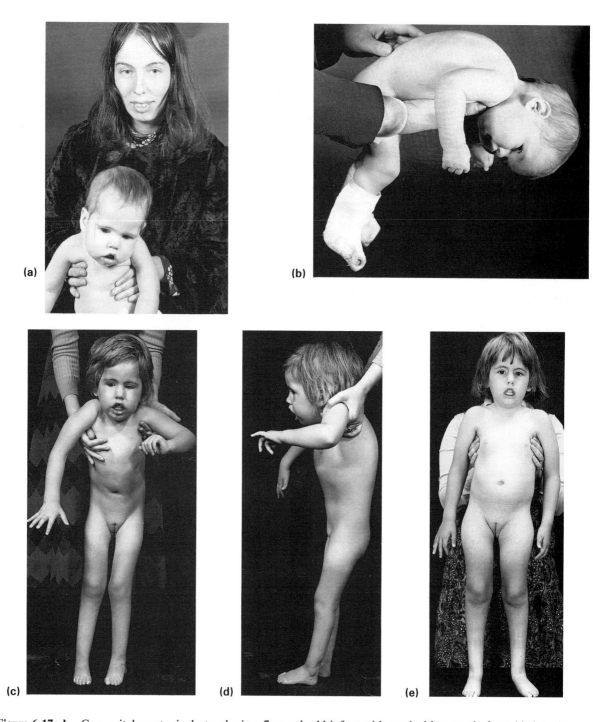

Figure 6-17a-h Congenital myotonic dystrophy in a 7-month-old infant with marked hypotonia from birth and transitory feeding difficulty in the neonatal period (a,b). Note the myopathic facies, and tent-shaped mouth. She also had a fixed equinovarus deformity of both feet, treated with plaster casts to maintain the posture, and a moderate kyphosis. Her mother, who was symptom-free, had a myopathic facies, was unable to screw her eyes tightly and bury her eyelashes, and showed mild myotonia on closure of her hands. EMG showed no abnormality in the infant but striking myotonic bursts in the mother. The hypotonia and motor function gradually improved and she was able to support her weight after the age of 3 years (c,d), at which time she had surgical correction of her foot deformities. Note the kyphosis. She walked with support at 5 years (e) and unsupported about 6 months later. Note the persistence of the myopathic facies and tent-shaped mouth. She continued independent ambulation (f, aged 9½ years) and managed at a normal school. The facial weakness persisted (g,h) but her facial expression improved and she was able to voluntarily close her mouth and purse her lips.

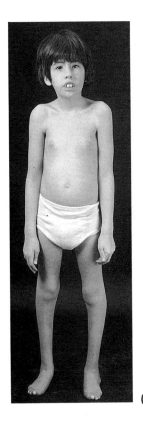

(f)

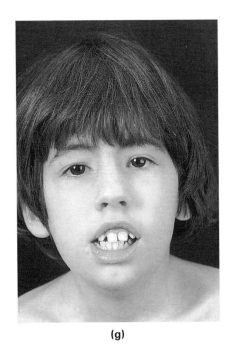

(g)

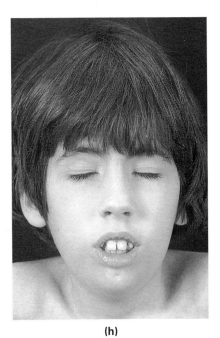

(h)

Figure 6-17f-h   (*for caption see facing page*)

There is a high incidence of death from respiratory failure in these cases, many of which may go undiagnosed. Harper (1975a) observed an unusually high neonatal mortality in siblings of his patients and many of these had been associated with hydramnios as well as talipes, and in retrospect were presumptive cases of myotonic dystrophy. There have also been autopsy reports of hypoplasia of the diaphragm, which may be suspected on an X-ray showing diaphragmatic elevation. The presence of thin ribs on chest X-ray is also a common feature, pinpointing an antenatal origin, and may help in the retrospective diagnosis in previous siblings who may have died of respiratory distress in the newborn period (Fried *et al.*, 1975).

There is usually no clinical evidence of cardiomyopathy but the ECG may show abnormality in some of these cases.

Lenard *et al.* (1977) demonstrated an associated involvement of smooth muscle, manifesting as megacolon and associated bowel symptoms, in two brothers with congenital myotonic dystrophy.

Mental retardation is a common feature of the congenital form of myotonic dystrophy. Some cases do fall within the normal range but in general there is a marked shift to the left, as in the case of Duchenne dystrophy, but probably even more marked. The mental retardation is not progressive. Many of these infants also have evidence of intraventricular haemorrhage and ventricular dilatation, even if born near term; this seems to be more frequent and extensive than could be accounted for by the associated prematurity alone (Regev *et al.*, 1987).

CLINICAL COURSE

Patients with congenital myotonic dystrophy show a gradual improvement in the hypotonia and will eventually walk, although this may be considerably delayed. They subsequently show clinical myotonia and EMG evidence of myotonia, usually after the age of 2–3 years, and later show progressive deterioration as in the adult form of the disease. Once they get past the neonatal period there is also a tendency to improvement in those with respiratory distress. The sucking and swallowing difficulties usually resolve in about 8–12 weeks in full-term infants, but may of course take longer in those born prematurely.

Harper (1975b) suggested that the most likely explanation for the congenital form of myotonic dystrophy, with its transient hypotonia and neonatal

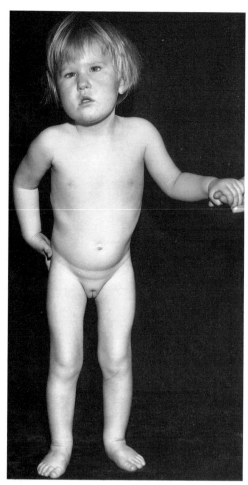

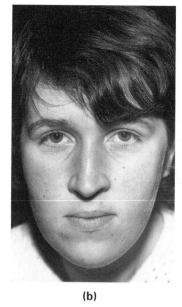

(b)

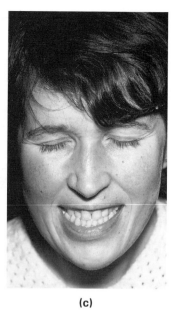

(c)

(a)

Figure 6-18a-c Congenital myotonic dystrophy in 4-year-old girl with hypotonia since birth, who had just managed to walk unaided. Note (a) expressionless face and triangular mouth. Her symptom-free mother (b) had a rather expressionless face and (c) was unable to bury her eyelashes. She had no clinical myotonia; EMG showed myotonic bursts in both the child and her mother.

problems, was an additional maternal intrauterine factor, affecting those individuals who already have the dominant gene for myotonic dystrophy. Another recent hypothesis has been imprinting with some additional influence from the maternal 19 chromosome. In spite of the major recent advances in the molecular genetics of myotonic dystrophy (see below), the pathogenesis of this unusual congenital floppy infant syndrome is still not fully understood.

INVESTIGATIONS OF MYOTONIC DYSTROPHY

Serum enzymes

These are usually non-contributory. The creatine kinase may be elevated in some of the adult cases but in others it is within normal limits. In the congenital form and in their minimally affected mothers the CK is usually normal.

Electromyography

The EMG in the adult patients as well as in the minimally affected mothers of infants with the congenital form will usually show the pathognomonic spontaneous myotonic bursts of activity with gradual decrement, giving the typical 'dive bomber' or 'departing motor cycle' sound on acoustic amplification (Figure 6-2). Where myotonia is not apparent in a proximal muscle, attempts should also be made to elicit it from a distal muscle, such as the first dorsal interosseous of the hand. Tapping the muscle with a finger may help to set off the myotonic bursts, but usually this is apparent on insertion of the concentric needle. In the congenital form the myotonia is usually not present but will appear later, usually after the age of 2 or 3 years. In addition to the myotonia, patients with associated weakness will show evidence of myopathy, with small amplitude, short duration, polyphasic potentials, as in other myopathies.

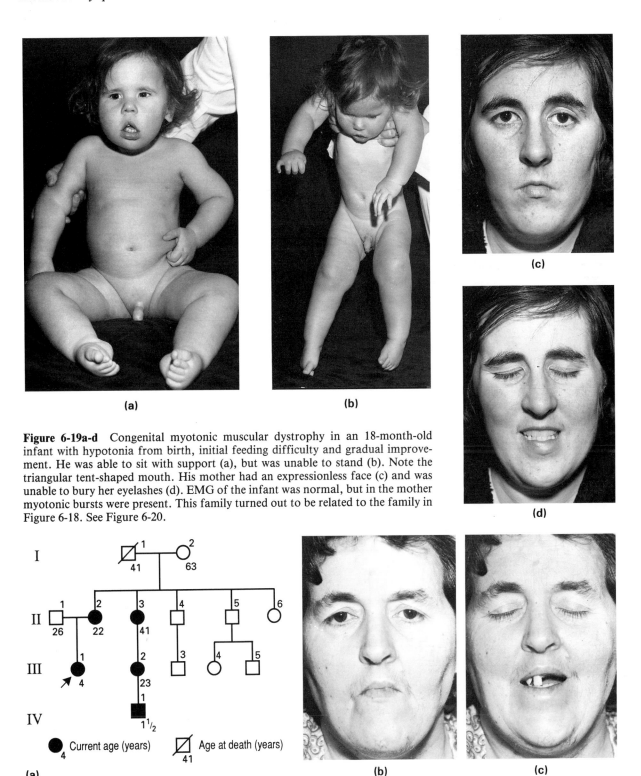

Figure 6-19a-d Congenital myotonic muscular dystrophy in an 18-month-old infant with hypotonia from birth, initial feeding difficulty and gradual improvement. He was able to sit with support (a), but was unable to stand (b). Note the triangular tent-shaped mouth. His mother had an expressionless face (c) and was unable to bury her eyelashes (d). EMG of the infant was normal, but in the mother myotonic bursts were present. This family turned out to be related to the family in Figure 6-18. See Figure 6-20.

Figure 6-20a-c (a) Pedigree chart of families in Figures 6-18 (III,1 and II,2) and 6-19 (IV,1 and III,2). Although said to be symptom-free, the grandmother of the second infant (II,3) was eventually examined and found to have an expressionless face with limited facial mobility and the inability to bury her eyelashes (b,c). EMG showed myotonia. This family demonstrates the classical dominant pattern of inheritance of myotonic dystrophy and also the subclinical involvement of the mothers of the two severely hypotonic affected infants. These two mothers themselves had a normal neonatal period.

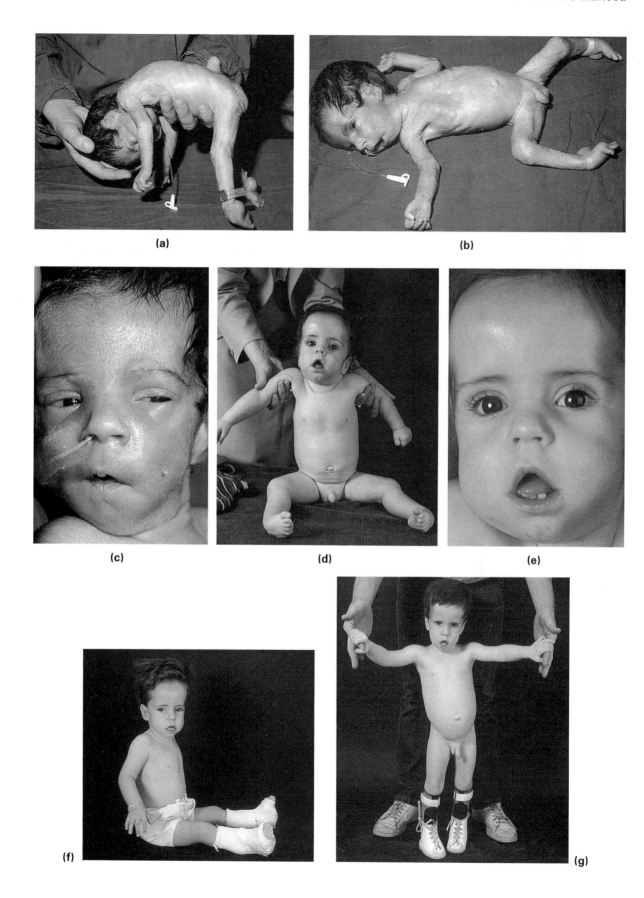

(a)

(b)

(c)

(d)

(e)

(f)

(g)

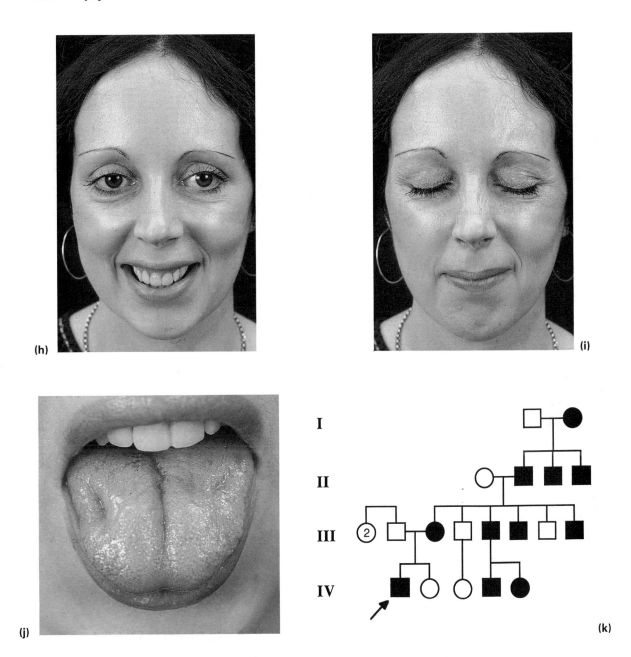

Figure 6-21a-k Congenital myotonic dystrophy. This 3-week-old infant was born prematurely at 34 weeks gestation. Marked hypotonia was present with poor head control and associated swallowing difficulty and transitory respiratory distress (a-c). Note the marked equinovarus deformity of the feet (b). He also had facial weakness and a prominent looking head with evidence of ventricular dilation on cranial ultrasound. He later showed steady improvement, although remaining retarded in developmental milestones. Correction of the foot deformities was deferred until he was able to bear weight on his legs to prevent recurrence or the need for prolonged immobilization. Regular passive stretching of the feet was done by the parents under the supervision of physiotherapists. At 9 months he was sitting with support but still had facial weakness, a tent-shaped mouth and deformity of the feet (d,e). At 18 months he was sitting unsupported, took weight on his legs and surgical correction of the foot deformities was recommended (f). By 2 years he stood well and walked with support (g) and at 3 years was showing still further improvement and walking well unsupported. His mother was also affected, but had previously been unaware of any problem. She had facial weakness with inability to close the eyes tightly and bury the eyelashes (h, i), myotonia of the hands and percussion myotonia of the tongue (j). On further assessment of the family, two of her brothers were found to be affected and also two children of one brother (k). A younger brother (III,9) had experienced a reaction following anaesthesia for a hernia operation and had later remained in a coma after tooth extractions under general anaesthesia and died after several months of ventilator support.

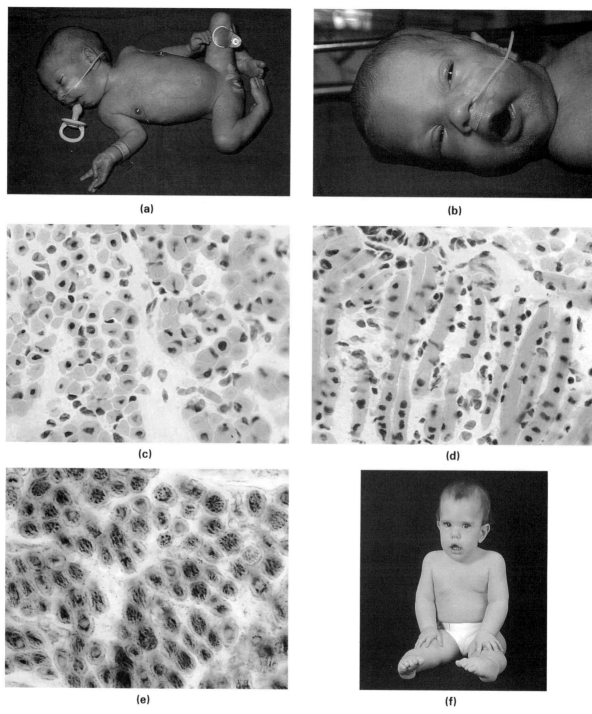

Figure 6-22a-f Congenital myotonic dystrophy. This 4-week-old infant presented with marked hypotonia from birth and associated equinovarus deformity of the feet and had difficulty in swallowing. Some facial weakness was also present (a,b). There was reasonable respiratory function. Facial weakness and myotonia were demonstrated in the mother who had been symptom-free. Needle biopsy of the infant's quadriceps showed a strikingly abnormal picture with prominent central nuclei and aggregation of oxidative enzyme activity, reminiscent of myotubular myopathy (c-e). The muscle was undifferentiated into fibre types and immunocytochemical techniques showed prescence of only slow myosin. When reviewed at 6 months she was showing good progress; at 11 months she was sitting without support (f). Muscle biopsy in congenital muscular dystrophy usually shows only non-specific changes, such as type 1 fibre atrophy, and is unhelpful or, at times, such as in this case, even misleading and may lead to an erroneous diagnosis.

Muscle biopsy

The classical adult type cases usually show extensive pathological change in the muscle with variation in fibre size, a remarkable proliferation of internal nuclei, ring fibres, sarcoplasmic masses at the periphery of the fibre and varying degrees of degeneration of fibres and connective tissue and adipose tissue proliferation.

The congenital patients do not show such change and may appear remarkably normal apart from a selective atrophy of type 1 fibres, which may also show internal nuclei. Occasionally the histological and histochemical picture may be indistinguishable from congenital (X-linked) myotubular myopathy (Dubowitz, 1989, 1992) (Figure 6-22).

Electron microscopic studies may show some evidence of maturational delay in the muscle, but this is non-specific and not helpful diagnostically. In general, muscle biopsy in the congenital cases is more likely to be confusing rather than helpful and diagnosis is best made on clinical and electrophysiological assessment of the mother.

MANAGEMENT

In the adult form the muscle weakness is usually the major problem and treatment of the myotonia is unlikely to produce much functional improvement. It is important for these patients to be encouraged to remain mobile and ambulant in order to retain their independence as long as they can. The condition is usually a chronic and slowly progressive one.

All cases of 'idiopathic' scoliosis and talipes coming to the attention of orthopaedic surgeons should be screened for underlying myotonic dystrophy, which may be apparent on careful clinical assessment and confirmed by EMG.

In the congenital form of the disease, attention to the early respiratory problems is important since there is subsequently a tendency to gradual improvement and if the infant can be tided over the first few weeks he will usually be able to cope after that. One is often faced with a therapeutic and ethical dilemma in severely affected neonates, who also are born prematurely and are making no effort at all at spontaneous respiration. The prognosis in some of these may be very poor and withdrawal of ventilator support may be indicated after full appraisal and review.

The associated deformities should be actively treated and can often be managed with a non-surgical approach. Any surgical intervention for deformities such as talipes should be deferred until much later, when the child reaches the stage of taking some weight on his legs and can then maintain the corrected posture. Early surgery often leads to recurrence of the deformity and any attempts at prolonged immobilization, postoperative or otherwise, may in fact aggravate the fixed deformities. Regular passive stretching can be very helpful in improving the range of mobility in the interim. Much of this can be done by the parents themselves with intermittent supervision by a physiotherapist.

The swallowing difficulty is usually self-limiting and the majority will achieve the ability to suck and swallow by about 2 months of age. Prior to this, tube feeding is usually necessary and may be followed by feeding from a spoon rather than bottle and teat.

Once the neonatal problems of hypotonia and respiratory and swallowing difficulties have resolved, the infant then has to face the later onset and gradual progression of the underlying disease itself. The problems are likely to be multiple, with the physical as well as the intellectual disability to contend with.

DRUG THERAPY

Various drugs have been shown to be effective in the treatment of myotonia. These include quinine, steroids, phenytoin and cardiac anti-arrhythmia drugs such as procainamide and mexiletine.

The question of therapy for the myotonia has to be individually assessed in every patient and depends on the amount of disability produced by the myotonia. In most cases of myotonic dystrophy the muscle weakness is the major problem and the myotonia of little significance.

GENETIC COUNSELLING

Myotonic dystrophy (DM) was the first autosomal dominant disease in humans to be linked. Mohr reported in 1954 a linkage to the Lutheran (LU) blood group and the ABH secretor locus (FUT2). The DM-FUT2-LU linkage group was not localized to a chromosome until it was linked to the third component of complement (C3), which in turn was localized to chromosome 19, using somatic cell hybrid techniques. Over a relatively short period of time, several DNA genetic markers were found to be informative and tightly linked to the DM locus on the proximal long arm of chromosome 19 (19q13.3) (Shaw *et al.*, 1985; Pericak-Vance *et al.*, 1986; Brunner *et al.*, 1989; Yamaoka *et al.*, 1990), and this provided a more accurate means for genetic counselling in informative families (Meredity *et al.*, 1986; Speer *et al.*, 1990). Linkage studies in large pedigrees provided additional information concerning carriers of the DM gene, who could not be reliably recognized or diagnosed by detailed physical examination and clinical laboratory studies. However, it took another decade before the genomic region containing the gene itself was cloned, following chromosome walking between flanking genetic markers and the use of cosmid contigs and yeast artificial chromosomes.

MOLECULAR ADVANCES ————————

Within the region of DNA that was defined by linkage techniques, a variable trinucleotide repeat insert consisting of 50 to several thousand CTG repeats has been discovered (Aslandis *et al.*, 1992; Buxton *et al.*, 1992; Harley *et al.*, 1992a). The inheritance of the inserted element, designated p(CTG)n repeat, was found to be a dynamic mutation and did not remain of constant size in individuals within a pedigree. Normal individuals have CTG repeats varying in length up to approximately 38 repeats. The normal inheritance of different alleles is stable. In myotonic dystrophy one of the alleles is enlarged over the range of 50 to several thousand CTG repeats. The length of the CTG repeat usually increases in subsequent generations, and the measurement in blood DNA correlates roughly with the general severity of the disease. Thus a genetic basis for the long-recognized phenomenon of anticipation has now been related to the size of the CTG repeat (Harper *et al.*, 1992). However, the size of the CTG repeat varies between tissues of the same individual and may be related directly to the characteristic variable expressivity that is exhibited in myotonic dystrophy. Thus in some individuals the length of the CTG repeat decreases in blood DNA, but the patient may have more severe clinical expression in muscle or other tissues. The variability of the CTG repeat is therefore an early mitotic event and probably occurs at an early stage of embryogenesis. From a clinical point of view, measurement of the CTG repeat is an accurate diagnostic test, but blood or chorionic villus DNA *cannot predict* the severity of the disease in an individual with absolute accuracy (Roses, 1993).

The site of the dynamic mutation interrupts the 3′ untranslated region of a protein kinase gene that has been named myotonin protein kinase (Brook *et al.*, 1992; Mahadevan *et al.*, 1992; Fu *et al.*, 1992). This is a completely novel type of genetic mutation and a similar dynamic mutation has also been found in fragile X syndrome, Huntington's chorea and in X-linked spinobulbar muscular atrophy (Kennedy syndrome).

It is still unclear how the interruption of the myotonin protein kinase is related to the pathogenesis of the disease, although abnormalities of endogenous membrane protein kinase were reported almost two decades ago (Roses and Appel, 1974, 1975; Wong and Roses, 1977). Interferences with transcription of a small region surrounding the CTG repeat may lead to diminished expression of a gene in that region that is critical for function.

Expression of the myotonic dystrophy protein kinase (DMPK) in RNAs has been studied in various tissues and shown to be highly expressed in skeletal muscle, heart and smooth muscle, and at a much lower level in brain. There is currently still controversy on the expression of DMPK mRNA in myotonic dystrophy tissues; some reports say it is up (Sabouri *et al.*, 1993), some say it is down (Fu *et al.*, 1993) and some say it is neither up nor down!

Currently, experimental studies with knockout genes in mice, and with transgenic mice with the trinucleotide expansion, are also being pursued in order to try and resolve the pathogenesis of the clinical phenotype in relation to the DNA expansion.

Clinical application

Harley *et al.* (1992b) recently reviewed the potential clinical impact of this new genetic breakthrough. A study of the DNA in 127 patients and 73 normal controls (mainly unaffected spouses) showed that the increase in length of the CTG repeats correlated broadly with disease severity and that there was expansion of the sequence in successive generations in the same family. This provides a possible molecular explanation for the well-documented 'anticipation' in myotonic dystrophy, with apparently earlier onset and increasing severity in successive generations.

They suggest that the technique could also be helpful in confirming the diagnosis of congenital myotonic dystrophy in a newborn floppy infant. They quote one subject who had been diagnosed initially on clinical grounds as congenital myotonic dystrophy, but the diagnosis had been revised on muscle biopsy to fibre type disproportion. [I would consider this an obvious misinterpretation because fibre type disproportion is a pathological, not a clinical, diagnosis and should not be made in the context of cases that have a specific clinical diagnosis.] They were subsequently able to show that the patient, at 11 years of age, had obvious clinical myotonia, as also did the mother, and the DNA analysis now revealed an expansion of 3–4 kilobases with a smaller expansion (0.5 kilobases) in the mother. The authors conclude that, 'availability of this specific molecular test at the initial assessment would have prevented subsequent misdiagnosis and an inappropriate assessment, prognosis and genetic risks, which was not corrected for 10 years'. One might add that if they had not done a biopsy on the infant and had instead followed the recommended practice of confirming the diagnosis of myotonic dystrophy in the mother, by clinical examination and EMG, they might have avoided the initial misdiagnosis.

They also quote another case where a child was wrongly diagnosed as having myotonic dystrophy, despite normal clinical findings and EMG, and they were now able to dispel the continued concern of the parents by showing a normal gene with no evidence of expansion in the child, although expansions were found in the affected mother and both affected sisters. This erroneous diagnosis was apparently based on a pathology report of 'typical features of congenital myotonic dystrophy'. As there are no typical histological changes of congenital myotonic dystrophy, one has to view such reports with caution, and should still pursue the more logical and reliable course of confirming the diagnosis in the mother, once the condition is suspected on clinical grounds in the infant. There would be no indication for a muscle biopsy in a clinically normal infant, and EMG would also be unhelpful as it usually shows no myotonia in infants affected with myotonic dystrophy.

In clinical practice one has to be cautious that advances in technology do not replace good clinical practice or common sense.

The variable sequence may help in accurate diagnosis in individuals with mild or minimal symptoms and signs suggestive of myotonic dystrophy. This includes older cases where cataract may be the only abnormality.

Prenatal diagnosis

With the advent of chorionic villus sampling, it is now possible accurately to diagnose affected fetuses, using the CTG repeat, early in pregnancy. However, as mentioned above, one cannot prognosticate on the severity of the clinical condition in relation to the size of the repeat.

MUSCLE STIFFNESS ON EXERCISE (Ca^{2+}-ATPase DEFICIENCY IN SARCOPLASMIC RETICULUM) (BRODY'S DISEASE)

In 1969 Brody reported an unusual disorder of muscle function, present since childhood in a 26-year-old male, characterized by painless contractures occurring with exercise, particularly vigorous exercise or sudden rapid movement. Muscle contraction was normal but the relaxation phase became increasingly slow during exercise. Myotonia was ruled out by the absence of muscle action potentials during the slow relaxation. Biochemically, there was a marked decrease in the ability of the sarcoplasmic reticulum to accumulate calcium ions. Muscle phosphorylase was normal but the proportion of the active form was exceptionally high and there was a high venous lactate during rest. Brody postulated that the slow relaxation might be due to decreased uptake of calcium by the sarcoplasmic reticulum, and that the persistently high level of free calcium expected as a result might explain the persistent activation of muscle phosphorylase and hence the high resting lactate. He attributed the disease to a selective defect of relaxing factor in the sarcoplasmic reticulum.

Karpati et al. (1986) documented similar features in four adult males from two families and demonstrated in addition a very low ATP-dependent calcium transport rate and a marked reduction in the 100-kD phosphoprotein corresponding to Ca^{2+}-ATPase of sarcoplasmic reticulum. Immunocytochemical studies suggested these changes were confined to the histochemical type 2 fibres. In view of consanguinity in the parents of the two affected siblings in family 1, they suggested an autosomal recessive inheritance, but since all four affected were males an X-linked inheritance was also possible.

Danon et al. (1988) subsequently documented a family in which four members in two generations (a mother, her son, and two daughters) suffered from impaired muscle relaxation aggravated by exercise, associated with marked reduction in sarcoplasmic reticulum ATPase protein, confined to histochemical type 2 fibres. Inheritance in this family appeared to be autosomal dominant.

MALIGNANT HYPERPYREXIA

This dramatic and often fatal condition was first described in 1960 by Denborough and Lovell in an Australian family in which there had been 10 deaths after anaesthesia. Since then several hundred cases have been reported. It is characterized by a rapid and sustained rise in temperature during general anaesthesia (often as rapid as 1°C every 5 minutes and going up to 43°C or higher), accompanied by generalized muscle rigidity, tachycardia, tachypnoea and cyanosis. There is also a severe respiratory and metabolic acidosis. Extensive muscle necrosis follows, with subsequent myoglobinuria and renal shutdown (Heffron, 1988). The serum creatine kinase (CK) is grossly elevated (up to 50 000 iu/litre or more), as is the serum potassium.

The attack can be precipitated by almost any anaesthetic agent, but halogenated hydrocarbons, such as halothane, and succinylcholine are the ones most frequently involved. Patients with the genetic trait do not necessarily react to each exposure with an episode of malignant hyperthermia, and nearly half of the patients have been previously exposed to triggering agents without incident. Additionally, episodes of malignant hyperthermia vary widely among different individuals as well as at different times in the same individual. In addition to anaesthetics, other chemical substances as well as environmental stress have also been implicated as triggers (Gronert, 1980; Nelson and Flewellen, 1983; Tomarken and Britt, 1987).

The condition is inherited as an autosomal dominant trait and the most valuable warning sign for the patient at risk is thus a family history of a catastrophe during anaesthesia. Those patients who survive anaesthesia may show evidence of myopathy during remission and some clinically normal relatives who are at risk have also been shown to have a subclinical myopathy with moderately raised serum CK levels (Isaacs and Barlow, 1970; Denborough et al., 1970) as well as electromyographic or structural abnormality in the muscle (Denborough et al., 1970; Steers et al., 1970; King et al., 1972; Denborough et al., 1973; Ellis et al., 1973; Isaacs and Barlow, 1973). Unfortunately not all cases at risk have a raised CK or an abnormal EMG so that care should be exercised when giving anaesthesia to any relative of a known case of malignant hyperpyrexia.

The histological changes in the muscle, both at light and electron microscopic level, are non-specific and the only reliable method of diagnosis is the demonstration of abnormal sensitivity of the muscle in vitro to halothane, succinylcholine or caffeine (Moulds and Denborough, 1972; Ellis et al., 1978; European Malignant Hyperpyrexia Group, 1984; Fletcher and Rosenberg, 1985; Larach, 1989; Allen et al., 1990). This is a sophisticated technique requiring specialized laboratory facilities. The standardized European in vitro contracture test provides for three possible diagnoses: malignant hyperthermia susceptible (MHS), malignant hyperthermia normal (MHN) and malignant hyperthermia equivocal (MHE).

Harriman (1982) reviewed the histological changes in a series of 200 patients investigated for malignant hyperthermia, both by in vitro testing of muscle strips as well as by light and electron microscopy of motor point biopsies. The biopsies were subdivided into those from 'susceptible' patients (80) with a positive in vitro test, and the remainder (120) looked upon as 'controls', where the in vitro test was negative. In the biopsies from 35 of the 80 malignant hyperthermia-susceptible group

there were myopathic changes; the remainder were considered normal. Histological changes were also found in 61 of the 120 'control' biopsies. Fourteen of these control patients had themselves actually suffered a malignant hyperpyrexia episode under anaesthesia, whereas the remainder were from at-risk families. So much for the reliability and consistency of the in vitro testing.

The presence of myopathic changes in the biopsies from malignant hyperpyrexia-susceptible patients does not necessarily relate to a previous episode of malignant hyperpyrexia following anaesthesia, and, conversely, patients who have previously had a reaction to anaesthesia can still have a normal biopsy.

Denborough et al. (1973) drew attention to a possible link between malignant hyperpyrexia and central core disease after discovering the presence of cores in more than 50% of the type 1 fibres of a patient with malignant hyperpyrexia. There was, however, no type 1 predominance in the biopsy, a feature usually present in central core disease. It was not clear whether the presence of cores in the fibres merely reflected one of the various relatively non-specific changes found in the muscle in malignant hyperpyrexia, or whether patients with the dominantly inherited central core disease (usually presenting with a mild non-progressive weakness from early childhood) are more susceptible to malignant hyperpyrexia. A child subsequently documented by Eng et al. (1978) seemed to have had a genuine association of both disorders, and this has been substantiated in subsequent publications (Frank et al., 1980) and has now been reinforced by the recent molecular genetic revelations (see below and also Chapter 3).

MOLECULAR GENETICS

Although autosomal dominant inheritance with reduced penetrance and variable expression of the gene seems well established, multiple alleles or several different genes may be involved (Kalow et al., 1979; Tomarken, 1987). Recent linkage studies have mapped at least one locus for the disease to chromosome 19q12-13.2 (McCarthy et al., 1990; MacLennan et al., 1990).

In the corresponding malignant hyperthermia in pigs, an association has also been established with the ryanodine receptor at that site, and subsequently also in the human disease (Fujii et al., 1991; Gillard et al., 1991; 1992; MacLennan and Phillips, 1992).

DNA polymorphisms flanking the malignant hyperthermia locus can identify those at risk in large families with malignant hyperthermia mapping to 19q with a high degree of accuracy, and should replace more invasive investigations such as the *in vitro* contracture test requiring muscle biopsy. Mutations in the ryanodine receptor gene have recently been identified in families with malignant hyperthermia or central core disease (Gillard *et al.*, 1991, 1992; Zhang *et al.*, 1993; Quane *et al.*, 1993). One of these mutations occurred in both disorders (Quane *et al.*, 1993).

Evidence for genetic heterogeneity was provided by Levitt *et al.* (1991) in a study of three unrelated families with malignant hyperthermia susceptibility (MHS) who were unlinked to markers at the 19q13.1 locus. Levitt *et al.* (1992) subsequently extended this study in an assessment of 16 MHS families. Four showed linkage to the 19q12-q13.2 region, five families were unlinked to the 19q locus but found to be closely linked to an anonymous marker (NME1) on chromosome 17q11.2-q24, two families were clearly unlinked to either of these two loci, and the five additional families gave insufficient data to establish linkage. They concluded that there were probably at least three separate genetic loci for malignant hyperthermia susceptibility and that the 17q gene locus (MHS2) might well have a gene frequency equal to that of the MHS1 locus on 19q. The additional gene locus on 17q has subsequently been confirmed in further families (Deufel *et al.*, 1992; Fagerlund *et al.*, 1992). Further studies by Levitt and his colleagues (Olckers *et al.*, 1992) have suggested a sodium channel α-subunit (SCN4A), which localizes to the same 17q region, as a candidate gene for MHS2.

PATHOPHYSIOLOGY

Although the precise molecular defect has not yet been elucidated, it is apparently at the level of excitation-contraction coupling, where altered sarcoplasmic calcium transport has been demonstrated. At rest, patients with susceptibility to episodes of malignant hyperthermia have elevated levels of free sarcoplasmic calcium ions (Lopez *et al.*, 1985). Further increases in free sarcoplasmic calcium ion concentration, by release from the sarcoplasmic reticulum induced by the triggering anaesthetics or succinylcholine, produce maximal fibre contraction. The inability of normal homeostatic pump mechanisms to sequester all these free calcium ions does not allow fibre relaxation and depletes muscle fibre energy reserves. Mitochondrial uptake of large quantities of free calcium ions uncouples oxidation and phosphorylation (Wrogemann and Pena, 1976). Energy production becomes relatively ineffective, and increased metabolic activity, attempting to restore ATP levels in muscle fibres throughout the body, generates heat that is clinically evident as hyperthermia. The lactic acid generated by the increased metabolic activity is released into the circulation producing acidosis. The contracture from depletion of muscle fibre ATP and phosphocreatine is followed by rhabdomyolysis.

TREATMENT

Treatment involves the administration of dantrolene before the stage of contracture develops (Kolb *et al.*, 1982; Tomarken and Britt, 1987). Dantrolene reduces the resting elevation of free sarcoplasmic calcium ions and also impedes calcium release from the sarcoplasmic reticulum (Lopez *et al.*, 1985, 1987). Thus, intravenous administration of dantrolene can abort the development of an episode of malignant hyperthermia. Dantrolene can also be used prophylactically in susceptible patients by slow intravenous infusion prior to induction of anaesthesia. Once the stage of rhabdomyolysis and hyperthermia has developed, supportive treatment (including cooling) is also required.

DIAGNOSIS

Because of potential mortality with episodes of malignant hyperthermia, considerable attention has been focused on tests to identify susceptible individuals. Although many susceptible individuals have slight elevations of serum CK, most blood studies have proven unreliable in detecting susceptibility to malignant hyperthermia (Ørding, 1988). Unless an individual has survived a previous episode of malignant hyperthermia or has a close relative who experienced an episode of malignant hyperthermia, however, no method is available to identify susceptible or potentially susceptible individuals without properly studying muscle biopsy specimens.

Muscle biopsies taken immediately after an episode of malignant hyperthermia show the expected changes of rhabdomyolysis (fibre destruction and regeneration), whereas biopsies taken before or some months following an episode show only minor non-specific changes, such as scattered smaller fibres and fibres with central nuclei. Thus, the routine muscle biopsy is of no value in diagnosing the disorder or in predicting the potential susceptibility to development of the syndrome in the individual patient.

Investigations of patients (and an animal model in pigs) have indicated that the most reliable diagnostic test consists of an *in vitro* study of contraction-related events on exposure of an unfixed muscle biopsy specimen to halothane or caffeine or both, along with histological study, since a lack of type 1 fibres in the biopsy could potentially produce false negative results (Ørding, 1988; Larach, 1989; Iaizzo and Lehmann-Horn, 1989; Iaizzo *et al.*, 1991b). In this contracture test, biopsies from individuals susceptible to malignant hyperthermia show a lower threshold for developing contracture than do specimens from normal individuals. Attempts have been made to standardize these *in vitro* tests (European Malignant Hyperpyrexia Group, 1984).

DISEASES WHICH APPEAR TO BE ASSOCIATED WITH MALIGNANT HYPERTHERMIA

In addition to the clear-cut relationship between malignant hyperthermia (MH) and central core disease, there have been a small number of further close associations, and a large number of loosely associated muscle disorders.

THE KING–DENBOROUGH SYNDROME (KDS)

Described in 1973, this syndrome was characterized by the association of a slowly progressive myopathy in young boys with short stature, pectus carinatum, cryptorchidism, kyphoscoliosis and distinctive facial features, with known susceptibility to malignant hyperpyrexia (King and Denborough, 1973 a,b) (Figures 6-23, 6-24). Subsequently, the syndrome was described in a female patient who died of an apparent fulminant MH episode (McPherson and Taylor, 1981). Heiman-Patterson *et al.* (1986) described abnormal contracture testing, indicating susceptibility to MH, in an affected male child and his mother, suggesting an autosomal dominant pattern of inheritance, although the mother had no dysmorphic features. Elevation of serum CK has been noted in a large proportion of patients with King–Denborough syndrome, though this finding is not invariable. It is still unclear whether the association of malignant hyperthermia with the King–

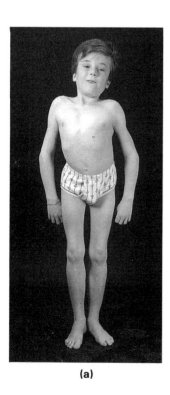 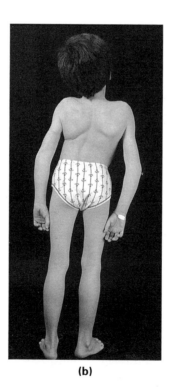 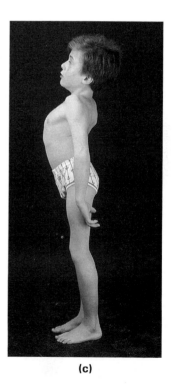

(a)   (b)   (c)

Figure 6-23a-c King–Denborough syndrome. This 9-year-old boy was originally referred at 2 years for investigation of scoliosis. He had no associated weakness but a persistently elevated CK of around 300–400 iu/litre. Radiography of the spine showed a bony abnormality (diastematomyelia) and he was referred for myelography. During anaesthesia for this he had a full-blown malignant hyperthermia reaction, which responded to dantrolene. This established a diagnosis of malignant hyperthermia and also of King–Denborough syndrome in view of his associated short stature, pectus carinatum and facial features. The family history was negative. He subsequently continued well, but had bouts of rigidity in association with febrile illness, resembling a malignant hyperthermia episode, which responded to dantrolene. He died suddenly at the age of 11 years during one of these febrile illnesses.

Denborough syndrome is coincidental or is part of a multiple congenital anomalies syndrome characterized by a primary myopathy with secondary deformities. The syndrome appears to be sporadic rather than familial, though variability of associated clinical findings may result in underdiagnosis of the syndrome. In any case, all patients with known King–Denborough syndrome should be treated as MH susceptible, and evaluation of other family members is recommended to determine whether MH susceptibility is present.

DUCHENNE AND BECKER DYSTROPHY

Sudden cardiac arrest and post-anaesthetic skeletal muscle breakdown have been reported in Duchenne dystrophy following volatile anaesthetics or succinylcholine, as well as clinical episodes which may represent MH (Miller *et al.*, 1978; Boltshauser *et al.*, 1980; Linter *et al.*, 1982; Oka *et al.*, 1982; Brownell *et al.*, 1983; Kelfer *et al.*, 1983; Henderson, 1984; Sethna and Rockoff, 1986; Solares *et al.*, 1986; Marks *et al.*, 1987; Chalkiadis and Branch, 1990).

Contracture testing in some, though not all, patients with Duchenne muscular dystrophy indicates MH susceptibility (Heiman-Patterson *et al.*, 1988; Lehmann-Horn and Iaizzo, 1989). It is difficult to determine whether this association is independent or genetically associated as evaluations of large pedigrees are not available.

Published reports of MH-like episodes in patients with Duchenne muscular dystrophy may overemphasize the risk of this association, as rhabdomyolysis and cardiac abnormalities could be ascribed to the underlying muscle disorder rather than a hypermetabolic response. However, it would be prudent to treat all patients with Duchenne muscular dystrophy as possibly MH susceptible and to avoid triggering anaesthetics (Rosenberg and Heiman-Patterson, 1983).

Bush and Dubowitz (1991) recently documented a case of cardiac arrest during anaesthesia in a 7-year-old boy with a mild Becker muscular dystrophy and a deletion of exons 3-7 in the gene. They reviewed the differences between the delayed onset of bradycardia and cardiac arrest, usually without hyperthermia, occurring in these Duchenne/Becker cases, and the classical MH reaction.

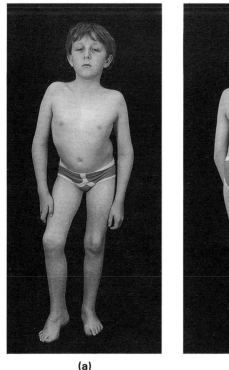
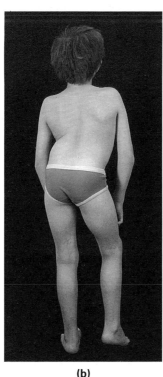
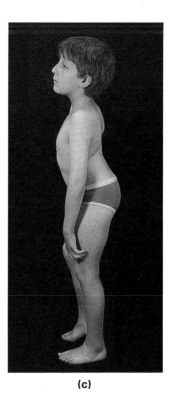

(a)   (b)   (c)

Figure 6-24a-c King–Denborough syndrome. This 13-year-old boy was referred after a malignant hyperthermia reaction during anaesthesia. Note the striking similarity in his facial appearance, stature, posture, and deformities to the boy in Figure 6-23. The family history was negative.

DISEASES WHICH APPEAR TO BE ASSOCIATED WITH MALIGNANT HYPERTHERMIA BUT WHICH ARE UNLIKELY TO BE ————————————

There have been a large number of reports in the literature suggesting the association of other neuromuscular diseases with MH-like clinical findings or positive *in vitro* contracture testing (reviewed by Wedel, 1992).

The list of these diseases includes myoadenylate deaminase deficiency, the Schwartz–Jampel syndrome, the Fukuyama type of congenital muscular dystrophy, limb girdle dystrophy, facioscapulohumeral dystrophy, periodic paralysis, myotonia congenita, mitochondrial myopathy, and minimal change myopathy. It is difficult to know whether the occurrence is mere chance or whether in some disorders there is an inter-relationship.

Some cases of so-called 'hyperCKemia' with unexplained high serum CK on screening, who do not turn out to be Becker muscular dystrophy or other forms of muscular dystrophy, may possibly be latent cases of malignant hyperthermia (Wedel, 1992).

Many of the signs and symptoms of heatstroke are similar to those seen in MH, including muscle damage which can result in rhabdomyolysis. Case reports of heat- and exercise-induced hyperthermia and muscle breakdown often bear striking resemblance to intraoperative fulminant MH episodes (Denborough *et al.*, 1984). Investigators have also described heat- and exercise-induced, mild MH-like episodes in individuals who are known to be MH susceptible, the symptoms of which respond to oral doses of dantrolene (Gronert *et al.*, 1980).

Denborough *et al.* (1982) reported a higher than expected incidence of muscle biopsy proven MH susceptibility in parents of infants who succumbed to sudden infant death syndrome (SIDS), but Ellis and Heffron (1985) were not able to show a higher incidence of SIDS in MH affected families than in the general population (2–8 episodes per 1000 live births).

In the absence of a simple, inexpensive screening test for MH, its true incidence in a given population will remain unknown. It is apparent that this trait is highly heterogeneous in humans, making a diagnosis on clinical symptoms alone highly inaccurate. Contracture testing is a sensitive indicator of MH susceptibility, but this technique is invasive and expensive, and evaluation can only be recommended for those individuals who are identified by clinical or family history. Evaluation of large pedigrees will help clarify the questions regarding associated diseases and enable the molecular geneticists to contribute more effectively to diagnosis in individual cases in the future.

Patients with neuromuscular diseases, laboratory evidence of muscle membrane abnormalities, or diagnoses of other suggested associated disorders need not be treated as MH susceptible, except for those patients with a diagnosis of central core disease, which is clearly associated with this trait. However, succinylcholine should be avoided in any patient with significant neuromuscular disease, and all patients should be carefully monitored for evidence of MH episodes (Wedel, 1992).

MYOGLOBINURIA/RHABDOMYOLYSIS

The appearance of myoglobin in the urine reflects an acute necrosis of muscle, with severe damage and loss of permeability of the muscle fibre membrane. Being a relatively small protein molecule (molecular mass 17 000 daltons), myoglobin has a low renal threshold and is readily cleared by the kidney. Renal shutdown can occur in severe cases. There is often a history of preceding muscle cramps and the muscles involved are frequently contracted and painful as well as firm and tender to palpation. There may also be localized oedema. Myoglobinuria will usually occur within 24 hours of the acute episode. Large quantities of myoglobin produce a mahogany-coloured urine, resembling vinegar or Coca-Cola.

There is an associated leak of enzymes from the damaged muscle with grossly elevated serum creatine kinase levels. Other constituents such as glycogen, potassium and creatine will also be released. The associated hyperkalaemia may produce life-threatening cardiac arrhythmia.

NOMENCLATURE ————————————

Bowden *et al.* (1956) suggested the term rhabdomyolysis to highlight the fact that the fundamental problem in myoglobinuria is in the muscle and not related to either myoglobin or renal failure. No case with abnormality of the myoglobin molecule, comparable with the haemoglobinopathies, has yet been described. The term myoglobinuria is, however, firmly entrenched in the medical literature.

AETIOLOGY

In some cases the underlying cause may be apparent, whereas others occur in isolation. Myoglobinuria is merely a symptom and the causes can be conveniently classified as follows:

1. Metabolic
2. Toxic
3. Inflammatory
4. Traumatic and ischaemic
5. Paroxysmal myoglobinuria
6. Idiopathic rhabdomyolysis

1. Metabolic

As noted in earlier chapters, myoglobinuria is a recognized feature of some of the glycogenoses associated with impaired glycolysis, such as types V and VII, and is also a feature of abnormal lipid metabolism due to carnitine palmitoyl transferase deficiency. Myoglobinuria also occurs in malignant hyperpyrexia in which the basic biochemical abnormality probably predisposes the muscle to acute necrosis when exposed to anaesthetic agents. Muscle cramps and myoglobinuria on exertion may occasionally be a presenting feature of a mild Becker or limb girdle muscle dystrophy, with no recognizable metabolic abnormality in the muscle (see case history, Figures 2-43 and 2-44). Most of these are cases of Becker muscular dystrophy and can now be confirmed with the new molecular genetic techniques. The CK usually remains elevated after the attack has subsided and the muscle biopsy looks dystrophic.

Tonin *et al.* (1990) reviewed the possible metabolic causes in 77 consecutive patients with myoglobinuria (documented in 44, suspected in 33). Enzyme defects were found in 36 patients: carnitine palmitoyl transferase deficiency in 17, phosphorylase kinase in four, myoadenylate deaminase in three, phosphoglycerate kinase in one, and a combined defect of carnitine palmitoyl transferase and myoadenylate deaminase in one. Exercise was the main precipitating factor, both in patients with and in those without detectable enzymopathies, including 14 with phosphorylase deficiency, nine with myoadenylate deaminase, three with phosphorylase kinase, three with phosphofructokinase and one with phosphoglycerate mutase deficiency. Systematic biochemical evaluation of muscle biopsy specimens revealed specific enzymopathies in about half of the patients with idiopathic myoglobinuria. The rest may have had blocks of metabolic pathways not yet studied routinely, such as beta oxidation, or genetic defects of the sarcolemma, such as Becker muscular dystrophy.

2. Toxic

Myoglobinuria has been recorded in association with a whole host of toxic causes, ranging from alcohol and barbiturates (Fahlgren *et al.*, 1957), heroin (Richter *et al.*, 1971), carbon monoxide (Loughbridge *et al.*, 1958), amphotericin B (Drutz *et al.*, 1970) and liquorice (Tourtellotte and Hirst, 1970) to Malayan sea snake bite (Reid, 1961) and hornet venom (Shilkin *et al.*, 1972), and the interesting Haff disease, in which lakeside communities in Eastern Europe get myoglobinuria after ingestion of fish and eels caught in inlets ('haff') thought to be contaminated by factory waste products (Berlin, 1948).

3. Inflammatory

Myoglobinuria may be a rare associated feature in severe cases of acute dermatomyositis in childhood and may even be severe enough to be associated with renal shutdown. Myoglobinuria may also occur in association with acute infections involving muscle, either as a result of viral infections such as Coxsackie, or acute bacterial infections such as staphylococcal or clostridial.

4. Traumatic and ischaemic

The association of myoglobinuria with trauma was first noted in severe crush injuries of the limbs during air raids in the second world war (Bywaters, 1944) and it may be followed by renal failure. Myoglobinuria may also occur with muscle necrosis in association with arterial occlusion (Bywaters and Stead, 1945; Haimovici, 1960) or occasionally with the more local ischaemic effects of the anterior tibial compartment syndrome (Hughes, 1948).

5. Paroxysmal myoglobinuria

This is characterized by attacks of muscle cramps and tenderness associated with weakness and followed by myoglobinuria. It usually resolves within a few days but severe cases may go on to renal damage, anuria and death. Korein *et al.* (1959) defined two types; type I related to exertion and occurring predominantly in males, and type II usually following an infection and more common in childhood. Some of these cases tend to be familial. It is quite likely some of these earlier cases of paroxysmal exertional myoglobinuria (march myoglobinuria) are in fact examples of McArdle's disease and other metabolic myopathies. In time all exertional myoglobinuria will presumably be found to have some metabolic basis.

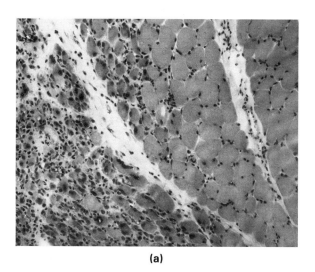

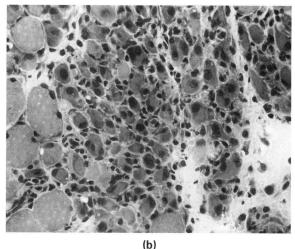

(a)   (b)

Figure 6-25a,b   Acute rhabdomyolysis. This 8-year-old girl developed acute rhabdomyolysis and associated severe hypotonia and some respiratory distress after a sore throat, treated with penicillin. CK was over 50 000 iu/litre; glutamate oxalacetic transaminase 3000 units. She did not develop any renal problems (blood urea 32 mg/100 ml) and the condition gradually resolved. Overt myoglobinuria was not present, but myoglobin was detected on analysis of the urine. Muscle biopsy of the quadriceps during the second week of her illness, when she was already recovering, showed extensive regenerative activity in the areas of previous necrosis (a, H & E × 95; b, H & E × 225). She had never had a previous attack and did not have another during 3 years follow-up.

6. Idiopathic rhabdomyolysis

This condition overlaps with type II paroxysmal myoglobinuria. It is a rare condition but may occur in childhood and may follow an upper respiratory infection (Figure 6.25). Savage *et al.* (1971) reported two female siblings aged 3½ years and 14 months who died within 2 days and 14 days respectively of the onset, and a third unrelated 7-year-old male patient with a milder form which resolved within 3 weeks. They also reviewed in detail the literature on paediatric cases of type II myoglobinuria.

REFERENCES

Abdalla, J.A., Casey, W.L., Cousin, H.K. *et al.* (1991a) Linkage of Thomsen disease to the T-cell receptor beta (TCRB) locus on chromosome 7q35. *American Journal of Human Genetics* **51**: 579–584.

Abdalla, J.A., Casey, W.L., Hudson, A.J. *et al.* (1991b) Linkage analysis of candidate loci in autosomal dominant myotonia congenita. *Neurology* **42**: 1561–1564.

Aberfeld, D.C., Hinterbuchner, L.P. and Schneider, M. (1965) Myotonia, dwarfism, diffuse bone disease and unusual ocular and facial abnormalities (a new syndrome). *Brain* **88**: 313.

Aberfeld, D.C., Namba, T., Vye, M.V. and Grob, D. (1970) Chondrodystrophic myotonia: report of two cases. *Archives of Neurology* **22**: 455–462.

Adams, B.A. and Beam, K.G. (1990) Muscular dysgenesis in mice: a model system for studying excitation-contractions coupling. *FASEB Journal* **4**: 2809-2816.

Adrian, R.H. and Bryant, S.H. (1974) On the repetitive discharge in myotonic muscle fibers. *Journal of Physiology* **240**: 505–515.

Aitken, R.S., Allott, E.N., Castleden, L.I.M. and Walker, M. (1937) Observations on a case of familial periodic paralysis. *Clinical Science* **3**: 47–57.

Allen, G.C., Fletcher, J.E., Huggins, F.J. *et al.* (1990) Caffeine and halothane contracture testing in swine using the recommendations of the North American Malignant Hyperthermia Group. *Anesthesiology* **72**: 71–76.

Aslandis, C., Jansen, G., Amemiya, C. *et al.* (1992) Cloning of the essential myotonic dystrophy region and mapping of the putative defect. *Nature* **355**: 548–551.

Barchi, R.L. (1988) The myotonic syndromes. *Neurology Clinics* **6**: 473–483.

Batten, F.E. and Gibb, H.P. (1909) Myotonia atrophica. *Brain* **32**: 187–205.

Becker, P.E. (1970) Paramyotonia congenita (Eulenburg). In: Becker, P.E., Lenz, W., Vogel, F. and Wendt, G.G. eds, *Advances in Human Genetics* Vol. 3. Stuttgart: Thieme, pp. 1–134.

Becker, P.E. (1971) Genetic approaches to the nosology of muscle disease: myotonias and similar diseases. In: *The Second Conference on the Clinical Delineation of Birth Defects*. Part VII. *Muscle*. Birth Defects: Original Article Series, Vol. VII, No. 2. Baltimore: Williams and Wilkins, pp. 52–62.

Berlin, R. (1948) Haff disease in Sweden. *Acta Medica Scandinavica* **129**: 560.

Biemond, A. and Daniels, A.P. (1934) Familial periodic paralysis and its transition into spinal muscular atrophy. *Brain* **57**: 91–108.

Bolthauser, E., Steinmann, B., Meyer, A. *et al.* (1980) Anaesthesia-induced rhabdomyolysis in Duchenne muscular dystrophy. *British Journal of Anaesthesia* **52**: 559.

Bourke, T.D. and Zuck, D. (1957) Thiopentone in dystrophia myotonica. *British Journal of Anaesthesia* **29**: 35.

Bowden, D.H., Fraser, D., Jackson, S.H. and Ford Walker, N. (1956) Acute recurrent rhabdomyolysis (paroxysmal myohaemoglobinuria). *Medicine* **35**: 335–353.

Bradley, W.G. (1969) Ultrastructural changes in adynamia episodica hereditaria and normokalaemic periodic paralysis. *Brain* **92**: 379.

Brody, I.A. (1969) Muscle contracture induced by exercise: a syndrome attributable to decreased relaxing factor. *New England Journal of Medicine* **281**: 187–192.

Brody, I.A. (1973) Myotonia induced by monocarboxylic aromatic acids: a possible mechanism. *Archives of Neurology* **28**: 243.

Brook, J.D., McCurrach, M.E., Harley, H.G. *et al.* (1992) Molecular basis of myotonic dystrophy: expansion of a trinucleotide (CTG) repeat at the 3′ end of a transcript encoding a protein kinase family member. *Cell* **68**: 799–808.

Brown, R.H. Jr. (1993) Inherited disorders of ion channels in neurology: the molecular basis of myotonia and hyperkalemic period paralysis. New York AAN Meeting, Course No 341.

Brownell, A.K.W., Paasuke, R.T., Elash, A. *et al.* (1983) Malignant hyperthermia in Duchenne muscular dystrophy. *Anesthesiology* **58**: 1880–182.

Brunner, H.G., Korneluk, R.G., Coerwinkel-Driessen, M. *et al.* (1989) Myotonic dystrophy is closely linked to the gene for muscle-type creatine kinase (CKMM). *Human Genetics* **81**: 308–310.

Bryant, S.H. (1979) Myotonia in the goat. *Annals of the New York Academy of Sciences* **317**: 314–325.

Bryant, S.H. and Morales-Aguilera, A. (1971) Chloride conductance in normal and myotonic muscle fibres and the action of monocarboxylic aromatic acids. *Journal of Physiology* **219**: 367–383.

Bush, A. and Dubowitz, V. (1991) Fatal rhabdomyolysis complicating general anaesthesia in a child with Becker muscular dystrophy. *Neuromuscular Disorders* **1**: 201–204.

Buxton, J., Shelbourne, P., Davies, J. *et al.* (1992) Detection of an unstable fragment of DNA specific to individuals with myotonic dystrophy. *Nature* **355**: 547–548.

Bywaters, E.G.L. (1994) Ischemic muscle necrosis: crushing injury, traumatic edema, the crush syndrome: a type of injury seen in air raid casualties following burial beneath debris. *Journal of the American Medical Association* **124**: 1103–1109.

Bywaters, E.G.L. and Stead, J.K. (1945) Thrombosis of femoral artery with myohaemoglobinuria and low serum potassium concentration. *Clinical Science* **5**: 195.

Cannon, S.C., Brown, R.H. Jr. and Corey, D.P. (1991) A sodium channel defect in hyperkalemic periodic paralysis: potassium induced failure of inactivation. *Neuron* **6**: 619–626.

Cao, A., Cianchetti, C., Calisti, L. *et al.* (1978) Schwartz-Jampel syndrome: Clinical, electrophysiological and histopathological study of a severe variant. *Journal of the Neurological Sciences* **36**: 175–187.

Catterall, W. (1988) Structure and function of voltage-sensitive ion channels. *Science* **242**: 50–61.

Caughey, J.E. and Myrianthopoulos, N.C. (1963) *Dystrophia Myotonica and Related Disorders*. Springfield, Illinois: Charles C. Thomas.

Chalkiadis, G.A. and Branch, K.G. (1990) Cardiac arrest after isoflurane anaesthesia in a patient with Duchenne's muscular dystrophy. *Anaesthesia* **45**: 22–25.

Cheah, J.S., Tock, E.P.C. and Kan, S.P. (1975) The light and electron microscopic changes in the skeletal muscles during paralysis in thyrotoxic periodic paralysis. *American Journal of the Medical Sciences* **269**: 365.

Church, S.C. (1967) The heart in myotonia atrophica. *Archives of Internal Medicine* **119**: 176–181.

Creutzfeldt, O.D., Abbott, B.C., Fowler, W.M. and Pearson, C.M. (1963) Muscle membrane potentials in episodic adynamia. *Electroencephalography and Clinical Neurophysiology* **15**: 508–515.

Crews, J., Kaiser, K.K. and Brooke, M.H. (1976) Muscle pathology of myotonia congenita. *Journal of the Neurological Sciences* **28**: 449–457.

Danon, M.J., Karpati, G., Charuk, J. *et al.* (1988) Sarcoplasmic reticulum adenosine triphosphatase deficiency with probable autosomal dominant inheritance. *Neurology* **38**: 812–815.

de Jong, J.G.Y. (1955) *Dystrophia Myotonica, Paramyotonia and Myotonia Congenita*. Utrecht: van Gorcum.

Denborough, M.A. and Lovell, R.R.H. (1960) Anaesthetic deaths in a family. *Lancet* **ii**: 45 (letter).

Denborough, M.A., Ebeling, P., King, J.O. and Zapf, P. (1970) Myopathy and malignant hyperpyrexia. *Lancet* **i**: 1138.

Denborough, M.A. Dennett, X. and Anderson, R.McD. (1973) Central-core disease and malignant hyperpyrexia. *British Medical Journal* **i**: 272.

Denborough, M.A., Galloway, G.J. and Hopkinson, K.C. (1982) Malignant hyperpyrexia and sudden infant death. *Lancet* **2**: 1068–1069.

Denborough, M.A., Collins, S.P. and Hopkinson, K.C. (1984) Rhabdomyolysis and malignant hyperpyrexia. *British Medical Journal* **288**: 1878.

Deufel, T., Golla, A., Iles, D. *et al.* (1992) Evidence for genetic heterogeneity of malignant hyperthermia susceptibility. *American Journal of Human Genetics* **50**: 1151–1161.

de Wind, L.T. and Jones, R.J. (1950) Cardiovascular observations in dystrophia myotonica. *Journal of the American Medical Association* **144**: 299–303.

Drager, G.A., Hammill, J.F. and Shy, G.M. (1958) Paramyotonia congenita. *Archives of Neurology and Psychiatry (Chicago)* **80**: 1.

Drutz, D.J., Fan, J.H., Tai, T.Y., Cheng, J.T. and Hsieh, W.C. (1970) Hypokalemic rhabdomyolysis and myoglobinuria following amphotericin B therapy. *Journal of the American Medical Association* **211**: 824–826.

Dubowitz, V. (1989) *A Colour Atlas of Muscle Disorders in Childhood.* London: Wolfe Medical.

Dubowitz, V. (1992) Lesson for the month: Genetic counselling. *Neuromuscular Disorders* **2**: 85–86.

Dubowitz, V. and Brooke, M.H. (1973) *Muscle Biopsy: A Modern Approach.* London and Philadelphia: W.B. Saunders.

Dundee, J.W. (1954) Thiopentone in dystrophia myotonica. *Current Researches in Anesthesia and Analgesia* **31**: 257.

Dunn, L.J. and Dierker, L.J. (1973) Recurrent hydramnios in association with myotonia dystrophica. *Obstetrics and Gynecology* **42**: 104.

Dyken, P.R. and Harper, P.S. (1973) Congenital dystrophia myotonica. *Neurology* **23**: 465.

Ebers, G.C., George, A.L., Barchi, R.L. *et al.* (1991) Paramyotonia congenita and hyperkalemic periodic paralysis are linked to the adult muscle sodium channel gene. *Annals of Neurology* **30**: 810–816.

Eckardt, V.F. and Nix, W. (1991) The anal sphincter in patients with myotonic muscular dystrophy. *Gastroenterology* **100**: 424–430.

Ellis, F.R. and Heffron, J.J.A. (1985) Clinical and biochemical aspects of malignant hyperpyrexia. In: Atkinson, R.S. and Adams, A.P. eds, *Recent Advances in Anaesthesia and Analgesia.* Edinburgh: Churchill Livingstone, pp. 173–207.

Ellis, F.R., Keaney, N.P. and Harriman, D.G.F. (1973) Histopathological and neuropharmacological aspects of malignant hyperpyrexia. *Proceedings of the Royal Society of Medicine* **66**: 66.

Ellis, F.R., Harriman, D.G.F., Currie, S. *et al.* (1978) Screening for malignant hyperthermia in susceptible patients. In: Aldrete, J.A. and Britt, B.A. eds, *Second International Symposium on Malignant Hyperthermia.* New York: Grune & Stratton, p. 273.

Eng, G.D., Epstein, B.S., Engel, W.K. *et al.* (1978) Malignant hyperthermia and central core disease in a child with congenital dislocating hips. *Archives of Neurology (Chicago)* **35**: 189–197.

Engel, A.G. (1966) Electron microscopic observations in primary hypokalemic and thyrotoxic periodic paralyses. *Mayo Clinic Proceedings* **41**: 797.

Engel, A.G. (1970) Evolution and content of vacuoles in primary hypokalemic periodic paralysis. *Mayo Clinic Proceedings* **45**: 774–814.

Engel, A.G. (1977) Hypokalemic and hyperkalemic periodic paralysis. In: Goldensohn, E.C. and Appel, S.H. eds, *Scientific Approach to Clinical Neurology.* Philadelphia: Lea & Febiger, pp. 1742–1765.

Engel, A.G. (1986) The periodic paralyses. In: Engel, A.G. and Banker, B.W. eds, *Myology.* McGraw Hill, pp. 1843–1870.

Erb, W. (1886) *Die Thomsen'sche Krankheit (myotonia congenita).* Leipzig, 128 pp.

Eulenburg, A., von (1886) Ueber eine familiäre, durch 6 Generationen verfolgbare Form congenitaler Paramyotonie. *Neurologisches Zentralblatt* **5**: 265, 1886.

Eulenburg, A. von (1916) Ueber Paramyotonia congenita. *Medizinische Klinik,* **12**: 505–507.

European Malignant Hyperpyrexia Group (1984) A protocol for the investigation of malignant hyperpyrexia (MH) susceptibility. *British Journal of Anaesthesia* **56**: 1267–1271.

Fagerlund, T., Islander, G., Ranklev, E. *et al.* (1992) Genetic recombination between malignant hyperthermia and calcium release channel in skeletal muscle. *Clinical Genetics* **41**: 270–272.

Fahlgren, H., Hed, R. and Lundmark, C. (1957) Myonecrosis and myoglobinuria in alcohol and barbiturate intoxication. *Acta Medica Scandinavica* **158**: 405–412.

Farrell, S.A., Davidson, R.G. and Thorp, P. (1987) Neonatal manifestations of Schwartz-Jampel syndrome. *American Journal of Medical Genetics* **27**: 799–805.

Feero, W.G., Wang, J., Barany, F. *et al.* (1993) Hyperkalemic periodic paralysis: rapid molecular diagnosis and relationship of genotype to phenotype in 12 families. *Neurology* **43**: 668–673.

Ferrannini, E., Perniola, T., Krajewska, G. *et al.* (1982) Schwartz–Jampel syndrome with autosomal dominant inheritance. *European Neurology* **21**: 137–146.

Fisch, C.: The heart in dystrophia myotonica. *American Heart Journal* **41**: 525.

Fletcher, J.E. and Rosenberg, H. (1985) *In vitro* interaction between halothane and succinylcholine in human skeletal muscle: Implications for malignant hyperthermia and masseter muscle rigidity. *Anesthesiology* **63**: 190–194.

Fontaine, B., Khurana, T., Hoffman, E. *et al.* (1990) Hyperkalemic periodic paralysis and the adult muscle sodium channel alpha-subunit gene. *Science* **250**: 1000–1002.

Fontaine, B., Toffater, J., Rouleau, G.A. *et al.* (1992) Different gene loci for hyperkalemic and hypokalemic periodic paralysis. *Neuromuscular Disorders* **1**: 235–238.

Fontaine, B., Vale-Santos, J., Jurkat-Rott, K. *et al.* (1994) Mapping of the hypokalaemic periodic paralysis (HypoPP) locus to chromosome 1q31-q32 in three European families. *Nature Genetics* **6**: 267–272.

Fowler, W.M. Jr., Layzer, R.B., Taylor, T.D. *et al.* (1974) The Schwartz–Jampel syndrome: its clinical, physiological and histological expressions. *Journal of the Neurological Sciences* 22: 127–146.

Frank, J.P., Harati, Y., Butler, I.J. *et al.* (1980) Central core disease and malignant hyperthermia syndrome. *Annals of Neurology* 7: 11–17.

Franke, C., Iaizzo, P.A., Hatt, H. *et al.* (1991) Altered Na+ channel activity and reduced Cl-conductance cause hyperexcitability in recessive generalized myotonia (Becker). *Muscle and Nerve* 14: 762–770.

Fried, K., Pajewski, M., Mundel, G., Caspi, E. and Spira, R. (1975) Thin ribs in neonatal myotonic dystrophy. *Clinical Genetics* 7: 417–420.

Fu, Y-H., Pizzuti, A., Fenwick, R.G. Jr. *et al.* (1992) An unstable triplet repeat in a gene related to myotonic muscular dystrophy. *Science* 255: 1256–1258.

Fu, Y-H., Friedman, D.L., Richards, S. *et al.* (1993) Decreased expression of myotonin-protein kinase messenger RNA and protein in adult form of myotonic dystrophy. *Science* 260: 235–238.

Fujii, J., Otsu, K., Zorato, F. *et al.* (1991) Identification of a mutation in porcine ryanodine receptor associated with malignant hyperthermia. *Science* 253: 448–451.

Gamstorp, I. (1956) Adynamia episodica hereditaria. *Acta Paediatrica* (Suppl.) 108: 1–126.

Gamstorp, I. (1964) Adynamia episodica hereditaria and myotonia. *Acta Neurologica Scandinavica* 39: 41–58.

George, A.L. Jr, Crackower, M.A., Abdallah, J.A. *et al.* (1993) Molecular basis of Thomsen's disease (autosomal dominant myotonia congenita). *Nature Genetics* 3: 305–309.

Gillam, P.M.S., Heaf, P.J.D., Kaufman, L. and Lucas, B.G.B. (1964) Respiration in dystrophia myotonica. *Thorax* 19: 112.

Gillard, E., Otsu, K., Fujii, J. *et al.* (1991) A substitution of cysteine for arginine in the ryanodine receptor is potentially causative of human malignant hyperthermia. *Genomics* 11: 751–755.

Gillard, E., Otsu, K., Fujii, J. *et al.* (1992) Polymorphisms and deduced amino acid substitutions in the coding sequence of the ryanodine receptor (RYR1) gene in individuals with malignant hyperthermia. *Genomics* 13: 1247–1254.

Goldflam, S. (1980) Ueber eine eigenthumliche Form von periodischer, familiarer, wahrscheinlich autointoxicationischer Paralyse. *Wiener Medizinische Presse* 31: 1418.

Grafe, P., Quasthoff, S., Strupp, M. *et al.* (1990) Enhancement of K+ conductance improves in vitro the contraction force of skeletal muscle in hypokalemic periodic paralysis. *Muscle and Nerve* 13: 451–457.

Gregg, R.G., Couch, F., Hogan, K. *et al.* (1993) Assignment of the human gene for the α_1 subunit of the skeletal muscle DHP-sensitive Ca^{2+} channel (CACNL1A3) to chromosome 1q31-q32. *Genomics* 15: 107–112.

Griggs, R.G., Engel, W.K. and Resnick, J.S. (1970) Acetazolamide treatment of periodic paralysis. Prevention of attacks and improvement of persistent weakness. *Annals of Internal Medicine* 73: 39.

Grob, D., Liljestrand, A. and Johns, R.J. (1957) Potassium movement in patients with familial periodic paralysis: relationship of the defect in muscle function. *American Journal of Medicine* 23: 356–375.

Gronert, G.A. (1980) Malignant hyperthermia. *Anesthesiology* 53: 395–423.

Gronert, G.A., Thompson, R.L. and Onofrio, B.M. (1980) Human malignant hyperthermia: awake episodes and correction by dantrolene. *Anesthesia and Analgesia* 59: 277–278.

Hageman, A.T., Gabreels, F.J., Liem, K.D. *et al.* (1993) Congenital myotonic dystrophy: a report on thirteen cases and a review of the literature. *Journal of the Neurological Sciences* 115: 95–101.

Haimovici, H. (1960) Arterial embolism with acute massive ischaemic myopathy and myoglobinuria: evaluation of hitherto unreported syndrome with report of two cases. *Surgery* 47: 739.

Hamel-Roy, J., Devroede, G., Arhan, P. *et al.* (1984) Functional abnormalities of the anal sphincters in patients with myotonic dystrophy. *Gastroenterology* 86: 1469–1474.

Harley, H.G., Brook, J.D., Rundle, S.A. *et al.* (1992a) Expansion of an unstable DNA region and phenotypic variation in myotonic dystrophy. *Nature* 355: 545–546.

Harley, H.G., Rundle, S.A., Reardon, W. *et al.* (1992b) Unstable DNA sequence in myotonic dystrophy. *Lancet* 339: 1125–1128.

Harper, P.S. (1975a) Congenital myotonic dystrophy in Britain. I. Clinical aspects. *Archives of Disease in Childhood* 50: 505.

Harper, P.S. (1975b) Congenital myotonic dystrophy in Britain II. Genetic basis. *Archives of Disease in Childhood* 50: 514.

Harper, P.S. (1989) *Myotonic Dystrophy* 2nd edn. London: W.B. Saunders.

Harper, P.S. and Dyken, P.R. (1972) Early-onset dystrophia myotonica. Evidence supporting a maternal environment factor. *Lancet* ii: 53.

Harper, P.S., Harley, H.G., Reardon, W. *et al.* (1992) Anticipation in myotonic dystrophy: new light on an old problem. *American Journal of Human Genetics* 51: 10–16.

Harriman, D.G.F. (1982) The pathology of malignant hyperpyrexia. In: Mastaglia, F.L. and Walton, J. eds, *Skeletal Muscle Pathology*. Edinburgh: Churchill Livingstone, pp. 575–591.

Hartwig, G.B., Rao, K.R., Radoff, F.M. *et al.* (1983) Radionuclide angiocardiographic analysis of myocardial function in myotonic muscular dystrophy. *Neurology* 33: 657–660.

Harvey, J.C., Sherbourne, D.H. and Siegel, C.I. (1965) Smooth muscle involvement in myotonic dystrophy. *American Journal of Medicine* 39: 81–90.

Hawley, R.J., Milner, M.R., Gottdiener, J.S. *et al.* (1991) Myotonic heart disease: a clinical follow-up. *Neurology* 41: 259–262.

Heffron, J.J.A. (1988) Malignant hyperthermia: biochemical aspects of the acute episode. *British Journal of Anaesthesia* 60: 274–278.

Heiman-Patterson, T.D., Rosenberg, H.R., Binning, C.P.S. *et al.* (1986) King-Denborough syndrome: contracture testing and literature review. *Pediatric Neurology* **2**: 175–177.

Heiman-Patterson, T.D., Rosenberg, H., Fletcher, J.E. *et al.* (1988) Halothane-caffeine contracture testing in neuromuscular diseases. *Muscle and Nerve* **11**: 453–457.

Heine, R., Pika, U., Lehmann-Horn, F. (1993) A novel SCN4A mutation causing myotonia aggravated by cold and potassium. *Human Molecular Genetics* **2**: 1349–1353.

Henderson, W.A.V. (1984) Succinylcholine induced cardiac arrest in unsuspected Duchenne muscular dystrophy. *Canadian Anaesthesiology Society Journal* **31**: 444–446.

Hiromasa, S., Ikeda, T., Kubota, K. *et al.* (1988) Ventricular tachycardia and sudden death in myotonic dystrophy. *American Heart Journal* **115**: 914–915.

Hoffman, E.P. and Wang, J.Z. (1993) Duchenne/Becker muscular dystrophy and the non-dystrophic myotonias: paradigms for loss-of-function and change-of-function gene products. *Archives of Neurology* **50**: 1227–1237.

Holzapple, G.E. (1905) Periodic paralysis. *Journal of the American Medical Association* **45**: 1224–1231.

Howes, E.L. Jr, Price, H.M. and Blumberg, J.M. (1966) Hypokalemic periodic paralysis: electron microscopic changes in the sarcoplasm. *Neurology (Minneapolis)*, **16**: 242.

Hughes, J.R. (1948) Ischaemic necrosis of anterior tibial muscle due to fatigue. *Journal of Bone and Joint Surgery* **30B**: 581.

Huttenlocher, R.P., Landwirth, J., Hanson, V., Gallagher, B.B. and Bensch, K. (1969) Osteochondro-muscular dystrophy: a disorder manifested by multiple skeletal deformities, myotonia, and dystrophic changes in muscle. *Pediatrics* **44**: 945–958.

Iaizzo, P.A. and Lehmann-Horn, F. (1989) The *in vitro* determination of susceptibility to malignant hyperthermia. *Muscle and Nerve* **12**: 184–190.

Iaizzo, P.A., Franke, C., Hatt, N. *et al.* (1991a) Altered sodium channel behaviour causes myotonia in dominantly inherited myotonia congenita. *Neuromuscular Disorders* **I**: 47–53.

Iaizzo, P.A., Wedel, D.J. and Gallagher, W.J. (1991b) *In vitro* contracture testing for determination of susceptibility to malignant hyperthermia: a methodologic update. *Mayo Clinic Proceedings* **66**: 998–1004, 1991b.

Isaacs, H. and Barlow, M.B. (1970) Malignant hyperpyrexia during anaesthesia; possible association with subclinical myopathy. *British Medical Journal* **i**: 275.

Isaacs, H. and Barlow, M.B. (1973) Malignant hyperpyrexia. *Journal of Neurology, Neurosurgery and Psychiatry* **36**: 228.

Kalow, W., Britt, B.A. and Chan, F.Y. (1979) Epidemiology and inheritance of malignant hyperthermia. *International Anesthesiology Clinics* **17**: 119–139.

Karpati, G., Charuk, J., Carpenter, S. *et al.* (1986) Myopathy caused by a deficiency of Ca^{2+}-adenosine triphosphatase in sarcoplasmic reticulum (Brody's disease). *Annals of Neurology* **20**: 38–49.

Kelfer, H.M., Singer, W.D. and Reynolds, R.N. (1983): Malignant hyperthermia in a child with Duchenne muscular dystrophy. *Pediatrics* **71**: 118–119.

King, J.O. and Denborough, M.A. (1973a) Malignant hyperpyrexia in Australia and New Zealand. *Medical Journal of Australia* **1**: 525–528.

King, J.O. and Denborough, M.A. (1973b) Anesthetic induced malignant hyperpyrexia in children. *Journal of Pediatrics* **83**: 37–40.

King, J.O., Denborough, M.A. and Zapf, P.W. (1972) Inheritance of malignant hyperpyrexia. *Lancet* **i**: 365.

Knudson, C.M., Chaudhari, N., Sharp, A.H. *et al.* (1989) Specific absence of the α_1 subunit of the dihydropyridine receptor in mice with muscular dysgenesis. *Journal of Biological Chemistry* **264**: 1345–1348.

Koch, M.C., Ricker, K., Otto, M. *et al.* (1991a) Confirmation of linkage of hyperkalemic periodic paralysis to chromosome 17. *Journal of Medical Genetics* **28**: 583–586.

Koch, M.C., Ricker, K., Otto, M. *et al.* (1991b) Linkage data suggesting allelic heterogeneity in paramyotonia congenita and hyperkalemic periodic paralysis on chromosome 17. *Human Genetics* **88**: 71–74.

Koch, M.C., Steinmeyer, K., Lorenz, C. *et al.* (1992) The skeletal muscle chloride channel in dominant and recessive myotonia. *Science* **257**: 797–800.

Kolb, M.E., Horne, M.L. and Martz, R. (1982) Dantrolene in human malignant hyperthermia: a multicenter study. *Anesthesiology* **56**: 254–262.

Korein, J., Coddon, D.R. and Mowrey, F.H. (1959) The clinical syndrome of paroxysmal paralytic myoglobinuria. *Neurology (Minneapolis)* **9**: 767–785.

Larach, M.G. (1989) Standardization of the caffeine halothane muscle contracture test. North American Malignant Hyperthermia Group. *Anesthesia and Analgesia* **69**: 511–515.

Layzer, R.B., Lovelace, R.E. and Rowland, L.P. (1967) Hyperkalemic periodic paralysis. *Archives of Neurology (Chicago)* **16**: 455.

Lehmann-Horn, F. and Iaizzo, P.A. (1989) Neuromuscular diseases and their relationship to malignant hyperthermia. In: Serratrice, G., Pellissier, J.S., Desnuelle, C. *et al.* eds, *Advances in Neuromuscular Diseases*. Expansion Scientifique, Francaise, pp. 260–266.

Lehmann-Horn, F. and Rüdel, R. (1987) Membrane defect in paramyotonia congenita (Eulenberg). *Muscle and Nerve* **10**: 633–641.

Lehmann-Horn, F., Rüdel, R., Dengler, R. *et al.* (1981) Membrane defects in paramyotonia congenita with and without myotonia in a warm environment. *Muscle and Nerve* **4**: 396–406.

Lehmann-Horn, F., Rüdel, R., Ricker, K. *et al.* (1983) Two cases of adynamia episodica hereditaria: *in vitro* investigations of muscle cell membrane contraction parameters. *Muscle and Nerve* **6**: 113–121.

Lehmann-Horn, F., Küther, G., Ricker, K. *et al.* (1987) Adynamia episodica hereditaria with myotonia: A non-activating sodium current and the effect of extracellular pH. *Muscle and Nerve* **10**: 363–374.

Lehmann-Horn, F., Iaizzo, P.A., Franke, C. *et al.* (1990) Schwartz–Jampel syndrome: II. Na channel defect causes myotonia. *Muscle and Nerve* **13**: 528–535.

Lenard, H.G., Goebel, H.H. and Weigel, W. (1977) Smooth muscle involvement in congenital myotonic dystrophy. *Neuropädiatrie* **8**: 48–52.

Lerche, H., Heine, R., Pika, U. *et al.* (1993) Sodium channel myotonia: slowed channel inactivation due to substitutions within the III/IV linker. *Journal of Physiology* **470**: 13–22.

Levitt, R.C., Nouri, N., Jedlicka, A.E. (1991) Evidence for genetic heterogeneity in malignant hyperthermia susceptibility. *Genomics* **11**: 543–547.

Levitt, R.C., Olckers, A., Meyers, S. *et al.* (1992) Evidence for the localization of a malignant hyperthermia susceptibility locus (MHS2) to human chromosome 17q. *Genomics* **14**: 562–566.

Linter, S.P.K., Thomas, P.R., Withington, P.S. *et al.* (1982) Suxamethonium associated hypertonicity and cardiac arrest in unsuspected pseudohypertrophic muscular dystrophy. *British Journal of Anaesthesia* **54**: 1331–1332.

Lipicky, R.J., Bryant, S.H. and Salmon, J.H. (1971) Cable parameters, sodium, potassium and chloride and water content and potassium efflux in isolated external intercostal muscle of normal volunteers and patients with myotonia congenita. *Journal of Clinical Investigation* **50**: 2091–2103.

Lopez, J.R., Alamo, L., Caputo, C. *et al.* (1985) Intracellular ionized calcium concentration in muscles from humans with malignant hyperthermia. *Muscle and Nerve* **8**: 355–358.

Lopez, J.R., Medina, P. and Alamo, L. (1987) Dantrolene sodium is able to reduce the resting ionic [Ca^{2+}] in muscle from humans with malignant hyperthermia. *Muscle and Nerve* **10**: 77–79.

Loughbridge, L.W., Leader, L.P. and Bowen, D.A.L. (1958) Acute renal failure due to muscle necrosis in carbon-monoxide poisoning. *Lancet* **ii**: 349.

MacDonald, R.D., Rewcastle, N.B. and Humphrey, J.G. (1968) Myopathy of hyperkalemic periodic paralysis. An electron microscopic study. *Archives of Neurology (Chicago)* **19**: 274.

MacLennan, D.H. and Phillips, M.S. (1992) Malignant hyperthermia. *Science* **256**: 789–794.

Mahadevan, M., Tsilfidis, C., Sabourin, L. *et al.* (1992) Myotonic dystrophy mutation: an unstable CTG repeat in the 3′ untranslated region of the gene. *Science* **255**: 1253–1255.

Marks, W.A., Bodensteiner, J.B. and Reitz, R.D. (1987) Cardiac arrest during anesthetic induction in a child with Becker type muscular dystrophy. *Journal of Child Neurology* **2**: 160–161.

McArdle, B. (1962) Adynamia episodica hereditaria and its treatment. *Brain* **85**: 121.

McArdle, B. (1974) Metabolic and endocrine myopathies.

In: Walton, J.N ed, *Disorders of Voluntary Muscle* 3rd edn. Edinburgh, London: Churchill Livingstone, p. 729.

McCarthy, T.V., Healy, J.M.S., Heffron, J.J.A. *et al.* (1990) Localization of the malignant hyperthermia susceptibility locus to human chromosome 19q12–13. *Nature* **343**: 562–564.

McClatchey, A.I., Troffater, J., McKenna-Yasek, D. *et al.* (1992a) Dinucleotide repeat polymorphisms at the SCN4A locus suggest allelic heterogeneity of hyperkalemic periodic paralysis and paramyotonia congenita. *American Journal of Human Genetics* **50**: 896–901.

McClatchey, A.I., Van den Bergh, P., Pericak-Vance, M.P. *et al.* (1992b) Temperature-sensitive mutations in the III-IV cytoplasmic loop region of the skeletal muscle sodiumchannel gene in paramyotonia congenita. *Cell* **68**: 769–774.

McClatchey, A.I., McKenna-Yasek, D., Cros, D. *et al.* (1992c) Novel mutations in families with unusual and variable disorders of the skeletal muscle sodium channel. *Nature Genetics* **2**: 148–152.

McFadzean, A.J.S. and Yeung, R. (1967) Periodic paralysis complicating thyrotoxicosis in Chinese. *British Medical Journal* **i**: 451.

MacLennan, D.H., Duff, C., Zorzato, F. *et al.* (1990) Ryanodine receptor gene is a candidate for predisposition to malignant hyperthermia. *Nature* **343**: 559–561.

McPherson, E.W. and Taylor, C.S. Jr. (1981) The King syndrome: malignant hyperthermia, myopathy and multiple anomalies. *American Journal of Medical Genetics* **8**: 159–165.

Meredity, A.L., Huson, S.M., Lunt, P.W. *et al.* (1986) Application of a closely-linked polymorphism of restriction fragment length to counselling and prenatal testing in families with myotonic dystrophy. *British Medical Journal* **293**: 1353–1357.

Meyers, K.R., Gilden, D.H., Rinaldi, F.J. and Hansen, J.L. (1972) Periodic muscle weakness, normakalemia and tubular aggregates. *Neurology (Minneapolis)* **22**: 269.

Miller, E.D. Jr., Sanders, D.B., Rowlingson, J.C. *et al.* (1978) Anaesthesia-induced rhabdomyolysis in a patient with Duchenne's muscular dystrophy. *Anesthesiology* **48**: 146–148.

Mohr, J. (1954) *A Study of Linkage in Man*. Vol. 33. Opera ex domo biologiae hereditariae humanae universitatis hafniensis. Copenhagen: Munksgaard.

Moosa, A. (1974) The feeding difficulty in infantile myotonic dystrophy. *Developmental Medicine and Child Neurology* **16**: 824–825.

Motta, J., Guilleminault, C., Billingham, M. *et al.* (1979) Cardiac abnormalities in myotonic dystrophy: electrophysiologic and histopathologic studies. *American Journal of Medicine* **67**: 467–473.

Moulds, R.F.W. and Denborough, M.A. (1972) Procaine in malignant hyperpyrexia. *British Medical Journal* **iv**: 526–528.

Munsat, T.L. (1967) Therapy of myotonia. A double-blind evaluation of diphenylhydantoin, procainamide and placebo. *Neurology (Minneapolis)* **17**: 359.

Nelson, T.E. and Flewellen, E.H. (1983) The malignant hyperthermia syndrome. *New England Journal of Medicine* 309: 416–418.

Nguyen, H.H., Wolfe, J.T., Holmes, D.R. Jr. *et al.* (1988) Pathology of the cardiac conduction system in myotonic dystrophy: a study of 12 cases. *Journal of the American College of Cardiologists* 11: 662–671.

Nissen, L. (1923) Beiträge zur Kenntnis der Thomsen'schen Krankheit (Myotonia congenita) mit besonderer Berücksichtigung des heriditären Momentes und seinen Beziehungen zu den Mendelschen Vererbungsregeln. *Zeitschift für klinische Medizin* 97: 58–93.

Novelli, G., Gennarelli, M., Menegazzo, E. *et al.* (1993) (CTG)n triplet mutation and phenotype manifestations in myotonic dystrophy patients. *Biochemical Medicine and Metabolic Biology* 50: 85–92.

Oka, S., Igarashi, Y., Takagi, A. *et al.* (1982) Malignant hyperpyrexia and Duchenne muscular dystrophy: a case report. *Canadian Anaesthesiology Society Journal* 29: 627–629.

Okinaka, S., Shizume, J. and Watanabe, A. (1957) The association of periodic paralysis and hyperthyroidism in Japan. *Journal of Clinical Endocrinology* 17: 1454.

Olivarius, B. de F. and Cristensen, E. (1965) Histopathological muscular changes in familial periodic paralysis. *Acta Neurologica Scandinavica* 41: 1.

Olckers, A., Meyers, D.A., Meyers, S. *et al.* (1992) Adult muscle sodium channel α-subunit is a gene candidate for malignant hyperthermia susceptibility. *Genomics* 14: 829–831.

Olofsson, B-O., Forsberg, H., Andersson, S. *et al.* (1988) Electrocardiographic findings in myotonic dystrophy. *British Heart Journal* 59: 47–52.

Oppenheim, H. (1891) Neue Mittheilungen über den von Professor Westphal beschriebende Fall von periodischer Lahmung aller vier Extremitaten. *Charité-Annalen* 16: 350–372.

Ørding, H. (1988) Diagnosis of susceptibility to malignant hyperthermia in man. *British Journal of Anaesthesia* 60: 287–302.

Pai, A.C. (1965a) Developmental genetics of a lethal mutation, muscular dysgenesis (*mdg*) in the mouse. I. Genetic analysis and gross morphology. *Developmental Biology* 11: 82–92.

Pai, A.C. (1965b) Developmental genetics of a lethal mutation, *muscular dysgenesis (mdg)* in the mouse. II. Developmental analysis. *Developmental Biology* 11: 93–109.

Pericak-Vance, M.A., Yamaoka, L.H., Assinder, R.I.F. *et al.* (1986) Tight linkage of apilipoprotein C2 (ApoC2) to myotonic dystrophy (DM) on chromosome 19. *Neurology* 36: 1418–1423.

Perloff, J.K., Stevenson, W.G., Roberts, N.K. *et al.* (1984) Cardiac involvement in myotonic muscular dystrophy (Steinert's disease): a prospective study of 25 patients. *American Journal of Cardiology* 54: 1074–1081.

Poskanzer, D.C. and Kerr, D.N.S. (1961) A third type of periodic paralysis, with normokalemia and favorable response to sodium chloride. *American Journal of Medicine* 31: 328.

Ptacek, L.J., Tyler, F. and Timmer, J.S. (1991a) Analysis in a large hyperkalemic periodic paralysis pedigree supports tight linkage to a sodium channel locus. *American Journal of Human Genetics* 49: 378–382.

Ptacek, L.J., Trimmer, J.S., Agnew, W.S. *et al.* (1991b) Paramyotonia congenita and hyperkalemic periodic paralysis map to the same sodium channel gene locus. *American Journal of Human Genetics* 49: 851–854.

Ptacek, L.J., George, A.L., Griggs, R.C. *et al.* (1991c) Identification of a mutation in the gene causing hyperkalemic periodic paralysis. *Cell* 67: 1021–1027.

Ptacek, L.J., George, A.L. Jr., Barchi, R.L. *et al.* (1992a) Mutations in an S4 segment of the adult skeletal muscle sodium channel cause paramyotonia congenita. *Neuron* 8: 891–897.

Ptacek, L.J., McMannis, P., Kwiecinski, H. *et al.* (1992b) Genetic heterogeneity in patients with the temperature-sensitive paramyotonia congenita phenotype. *Annals of Neurology* 32: 250(A).

Quane, K.A., Healy, J.M.S., Keating, K.E. *et al.* (1993) Mutations in the ryanodine receptor gene in central core disease and malignant hyperthermia. *Nature Genetics* 5: 51–55.

Reardon, W., Hughes, H.E., Green, S.H. *et al.* (1992) Anal abnormalities in childhood myotonic dystrophy — a possible source of confusion in child sexual abuse. *Archives of Disease in Childhood* 67: 527–528.

Regev, R., De Vries, L.S., Heckmatt, J.Z. *et al.* (1987) Cerebral ventricular dilatation in congenital myotonic dystrophy. *Journal of Pediatrics* 111: 372–376.

Reid, H.A. (1961) Myoglobinuria and sea-snakebite poisoning. *British Medical Journal* i: 1284–1289.

Resnick, J.S. and Engel, W.K. (1967) Myotonic lid lag in hypokalemic periodic paralysis. *Journal of Neurology, Neurosurgery and Psychiatry* 30: 47.

Resnick, J.S., Dorman, J.D. and Engel, W.K. (1969) Thyrotoxic periodic paralysis. *American Journal of Medicine* 47: 831.

Rich, E.C. (1894) A unique form of motor paralysis due to cold. *Medical News* 65: 210–213.

Richter, R.W., Challenor, Y.B., Pearson, J., Kagan, L.J., Hamilton, L.L. and Ramsey, W.H. (1971) Acute myoglobinuria associated with heroin addiction. *Journal of the American Medical Association* 216: 1172–1176.

Ricker, K., Böhlen, R., Haass, A. *et al.* (1980) Successful treatment of paramyotonia congenital (Eulenberg): muscle stiffness and weakness prevented by tocainide. *Journal of Neurology, Neurosurgery and Psychiatry* 43: 268–271.

Ricker, K., Böhlen, R. and Rohkamm, R. (1983) Different effectiveness of tocainide and hydrochlorothiazide in paramyotonia congenita with hyperkalemic episodic paralysis. *Neurology* 33: 1615–1618.

Ricker, K., Rohkamm, R. and Böhlen, R. (1986) Adynamia episodica and paralysis periodica paramyotonica. *Neurology* 36: 682–686.

Ricker, K., Camacho, I.M., Grafe, P. *et al.* (1989)

Adynamia episodica hereditaria: what causes the weakness? *Muscle and Nerve* 12: 883–891.

Riordan, J.R., Rommens, J.M., Keremn, B. *et al.* (1989) Identification of the cystic fibrosis gene: cloning and characterization of a complementary cDNA. *Science* 245: 1066–1073.

Rojas, C.V., Wang, J., Schwartz, L.S. *et al.* (1991) A methionine to valine mutation in the skeletal muscle sodium channel alpha-subunit in human hyperkalemic periodic paralysis. *Nature* 354: 387–389.

Rosenberg, H. and Heimann-Patterson, T. (1983) Duchenne's muscular dystrophy and malignant hyperthermia: another warning. *Anesthesiology* 59: 362.

Roses, A.D. (1993) Myotonic Dystrophy. In: Rosenberg, R.N., Prusiner, S.B., DiMauro, S. *et al.* eds, *The Molecular and Genetic Basis of Neurological Disease*. Boston: Butterworth-Heinemann, pp. 633–646.

Roses, A.D. and Appel, S.H. (1974) Muscle membrane protein kinase in myotonic muscular dystrophy. *Nature* 250: 245–247.

Roses, A.D. and Appel, S.H. (1975) Phosphorylation of component 'a' of the human erythrocyte membrane in myotonic dystrophy. *Journal of Membrane Biology* 20: 51–58.

Roses, A.D., Pericak-Vance, M.A., Ross, D.A. *et al.* (1986) RFLPs at the D19S19 locus of human chromosome 19 linked to myotonic dystrophy. *Nucleic Acids Research* 14: 55–69.

Rüdel, R. (1986) The pathophysiological basis of the myotonias and the periodic paralyses. In: Engel, A.G. and Banker, B.Q. eds, *Myology*. McGraw Hill, pp. 1297–1311.

Rüdel, R. and Lehmann-Horn, F. (1985) Membrane changes in cells from myotonia patients. *Phys Rev* 65: 310–356.

Rüdel, R., Ricker, K. and Lehmann-Horn, F. (1988) Transient weakness and altered membrane characteristic in recessive generalized myotonia (Becker). *Muscle and Nerve* 11: 202–211.

Rudolph, J.A., Spier, S.J., Byrns, G. *et al.* (1992) Periodic paralysis in quarter horses: a sodium channel mutation disseminated by selective breeding. *Nature Genetics* 2: 144–147.

Sabouri, L.A., Mahadevan, M.S., Narang, M. *et al.* (1993) Effect of the myotonic dystrophy (DM) mutation on mRNA levels of the DM gene. *Nature Genetics* 4: 233–238.

Savage, D.C.L., Forbes, M. and Pearce, G.W. (1971) Idiopathic rhabdomyolysis. *Archives of Disease in Childhood* 46: 594.

Schoenthal, L. (1934) Family periodic paralysis, with review of literature. *American Journal of Diseases of Children* 48: 799–813.

Schwartz, O. and Jampel, R.S. (1962) Congenital blepharophimosis associated with an unique generalized myopathy. *Archives of Ophthalmology* 68: 52.

Sethna, N.F. and Rockoff, M.A. (1986) Cardiac arrest following inhalation induction of anaesthesia in a child with Duchenne's muscular dystrophy.

Canadian Anaesthesiology Society Journal 33: 799–802.

Shaw, D.J. and Harper, P.S. (1992) Myotonic dystrophy: advances in molecular genetics. *Neuromuscular Disorders* 2: 241–243.

Shaw, D.J., Meredity, A.L., Sarfarazi, M. *et al.* (1985) The apolipoprotein CII gene: subchromosomal localization and linkage to the myotonic dystrophy locus. *Human Genetics* 70: 271–273.

Shilkin, K.B., Chen, B.T.M. and Khoo, O.T. (1972) Rhabdomyolysis caused by hornet venom. *British Medical Journal* i: 156.

Shy, G.M., Wanko, T., Rowley, P.T. and Engel, A.G. (1961) Studies in familial periodic paralysis. *Experimental Neurology* 3: 53.

Singer, H.D. and Goodbody, F.W. (1901) A case of family periodic paralysis with a critical digest of the literature. *Brain* 24: 257–285.

Solares, G., Herranz, J.L. and Sanz, M.D. (1986) Suxamethonium-induced cardiac arrest as an initial manifestation of Duchenne muscular dystrophy. *British Journal of Anaesthesia* 58: 576.

Somers, J.E. and Winer, N. (1966) Reversible myopathy and myotonia following administration of a hypocholesterolemic agent. *Neurology* 16: 761.

Spaans, F., Theunissen, P., Reekers, A.D. *et al.* (1990) Schwartz–Jampel syndrome: I. Clinical, electromyographic and histologic studies. *Muscle and Nerve* 13: 516–527.

Spaans, F., Wagenmakers, A., Saris, W. *et al.* (1991) Procainamide therapy, physical performance and energy expenditure in the Schwartz–Jampel syndrome. *Neuromuscular Disorders* 1: 371–374.

Speer, M.C., Pericak-Vance, M.A., Yamaoka, L. *et al.* (1990) Presymptomatic and prenatal diagnosis in myotonic dystrophy by genetic linkage studies. *Neurology* 40: 671–676.

Steers, A.J.W., Tallack, J.A. and Thompson, D.E.A. (1992) Fulminating hyperyrexia during anaesthesia in a member of a myopathic family. *British Medical Journal* ii: 341.

Steinert, H. (1909) Myopathologische beiträge. I. Über das klinische und anatomische Bild des Muskelschwunds der Myotoniker. *Deutsche Zeitschrift für Nervenheilkunde* 37: 58.

Steinmeyer, K., Ortland, C. and Jentsch, T.J. (1991a) Primary structure and functional expression of a developmentally regulated skeletal muscle chloride channel. *Nature* 354: 301–304.

Steinmeyer, K., Klocke, R., Ortland, C. *et al.* (1991b) Inactivation of muscle chloride channel by transposon insertion in myotonic mice. *Nature* 354: 304–308.

Streib, E.W. (1987) Paramyotonia congenita: successful treatment with tocainide. Clinical and electrophysiologic findings in seven patients. *Muscle and Nerve* 10: 155–162.

Streib, E.W., Sun, S.F. and Hanson, M. (1983) Paramyotonia congenita: clinical and electrophysiologic studies. *Electromyography and Clinical Neurophysiology* 23: 315–325.

Streib, E.W., Meyers, D.G. and Sun, S.F. (1985) Mitral

valve prolapse in myotonic dystrophy. *Muscle and Nerve* **8**: 650–653.

Strümpell, A. (1881): Tonische Krämpfe in willkürlich bewegten Muskeln (myotonia congenita). *Berliner klinische Wochenschrift* **18**: 119.

Tawil, R., Ptacek, L.J., Pavlakis, S.G. *et al.* (1994) Andersen's syndrome: potassium-sensitive periodic paralysis, ventricular ectopy and dysmorphic features. *Annals of Neurology* **35**: 326–330.

Thomasen, E. (1948) *Myotonia: Thomsen's Disease (Myotonia Congenita), Paramyotonia and Dystrophia Myotonica.* Universitetsforlaget i Aarhus, Denmark.

Thomsen, J. (1876) Tonische Krämpfe in willkürlich beweglichen Muskeln in Folge von ererbter psychischer Disposition (Ataxia muscularis?). *Archiv für Psychiatrie und Nervenkrankheiten* **6**: 702.

Tomarken, J.L. and Britt, B.A. (1987) Malignant hyperthermia. *Annals of Emergency Medicine* **16**: 1253–1265.

Tonin, P., Lewis, P., Servidei, S. *et al.* (1990) Metabolic causes of myoglobinuria. *Annals of Neurology* **27**: 181–185.

Topaloglu, H., Serdaroglu, A., Okan, M. *et al.* (1993) Improvement of myotonia with carbamazepine in three cases with the Schwartz–Jampel syndrome. *Neuropediatrics* **24**: 232–234.

Tourtellotte, C.R. and Hirst, A.E. (1970) Hypokalemia, muscle weakness, and myoglobinuria due to licorice ingestion. *California Medicine* **113**: 51–53.

Tyler, F.H., Stephens, F.E., Gunn, F.D. and Perkoff, G.T. (1951) Studies in disorders of muscle. VII. Clinical manifestations and inheritance of a type of periodic paralysis without hypopotassemia. *Journal of Clinical Investigation* **30**: 492–502.

Vanier, T.M. (1960) Dystrophia myotonica in childhood. *British Medical Journal* **ii**: 1284.

Wang, P. and Clausen, T. (1976) Treatment of attacks in hyperkalaemic familial periodic paralysis by inhalation of salbutamol. *Lancet* **i**: 221–223.

Wang, J., Zhou, J., Todorovic, S.M. *et al.* (1993)

Molecular genetic and genetic correlations in sodium channelopathies: lack of founder effect and evidence for a second gene. *American Journal of Human Genetics* **52**: 1074–1084.

Wedel, D.J. (1992) Malignant hyperthermia and neuromuscular disease. *Neuromuscular Disorders* **2**: 157–164.

Westphal, C. (1883) Demonstration zweier Fälle von Thomsen'scher Krankheit. *Berliner klinische Wochenchrift* **20**: 153.

Westphal, C. (1885) Ueber einen merkwurdigen Fall van periodischer Lahmung aller vier Extremitaten mit gleichzeitigen Erloschen der elektrischen Erregbarkeit wahrend der Lähmung. *Berliner klinische Wochenschrift* **22**: 489–491.

Wolf, A. (1936) Quinine: an effective form of treatment for myotonia. Preliminary report of four cases. *Archives of Neurology and Psychiatry* **36**: 382.

Wolintz, A.H., Sonnenblick, E.H. and Engel, W.K. (1966) Stoke–Adams syndrome and atrial arrythmias as the presenting symptoms of myotonic dystrophy, with response to electrocardioversion. *Annals of Internal Medicine* **65**, 1260.

Wong, P. and Roses, A.D. (1977) Altered component 'a' phosphorylation in erythrocyte membrane in myotonic muscular dystrophy. *Journal of Membrane Biology* **45**: 145–166.

Wrogemann, K. and Pena, S.D.J. (1976) Mitochondrial calcium overload: a general mechanism for cell-necrosis in muscle disease. *Lancet* **1**: 672–673.

Yamaoka, L.H., Pericak-Vance, M.A., Speer, M.C. *et al.* (1990) Tight linkage of creatine kinase (CKMM) to myotonic dystrophy on chromosome 19. *Neurology* **40**: 222–226.

Zhang, Y., Chen, H.S., Khanna, V.K. *et al.* (1993) A mutation in the human ryanodine receptor gene associated with central core disease. *Nature Genetics* **5**: 46–50.

Zierler, K.L. and Andres, R. (1957) Movement of potassium into skeletal muscle during spontaneous attack in family periodic paralysis. *Journal of Clinical Investigation* **36**: 730–737.

CHAPTER 7

Endocrine Myopathies

Myopathies have been described in association with a wide range of endocrine disorders. In most instances the muscle involvement is an incidental feature, and may even be subclinical and only identified because of special investigations such as serum enzymes, electromyography or muscle biopsy. In other instances muscle weakness may be a presenting feature and lead to the diagnosis of the underlying disorder.

The vast majority of these disorders occur in adults and, with a few exceptions, one is unlikely to meet these conditions in children.

This is a potentially fruitful area for basic research into the reasons why different hormones may influence muscle function, which in turn may throw light on some of the aspects of normal muscle function.

The molecular genetic revolution does not seem to have had any appreciable impact yet on this group of disorders.

THYROID DISORDERS

THYROTOXICOSIS

There are four different syndromes of muscle disorder associated with hyperthyroidism.

Thyrotoxic myopathy

This usually presents as a chronic disorder with generalized or mainly proximal muscle weakness and may precede overt thyrotoxicosis. Moreover, in cases of thyrotoxicosis without clinical muscle weakness there is a high incidence of abnormality on electromyography or muscle biopsy (Havard *et al.*, 1963).

Acute thyrotoxic myopathy with associated bulbar and ocular involvement is less common and may well be myasthenic rather than myopathic in origin.

Myasthenia

The association of myasthenia and thyrotoxicosis is well documented. The incidence of hyperthyroidism in the course of myasthenia is about 5%, which is considerably higher than the general prevalence of thyrotoxicosis of about 0.4–1%, whereas the occurrence of myasthenia in thyrotoxicosis is much lower, and probably under 0.5% (Simpson, 1968; Kissel *et al.*, 1970). This is about 30 times greater than the prevalence of myasthenia in the general population. There may be a genetic predisposition for the autoimmune origin of both myasthenia gravis and thyrotoxicosis. In individual patients one has to treat both disorders to achieve therapeutic resolution.

Periodic paralysis

Thyrotoxic periodic paralysis is very similar to hypokalaemic periodic paralysis. It occurs almost exclusively in oriental races and predominantly in adult males. About 75% of reported cases have been of Japanese or Chinese descent. It is possible that susceptibility to thyrotoxic periodic paralysis may be inherited as an autosomal dominant trait (Kufs *et al.*, 1989). The clinical manifestations are similar to hypokalaemic periodic paralysis and attacks usually respond to oral potassium. Treatment of the thyrotoxicosis usually prevents further attacks.

Exophthalmic ophthalmoplegia

Although usually looked upon as a complication of thyrotoxicosis, many cases do not have associated hyperthyroidism at the time of its development. Overproduction of thyroid-stimulating hormone, long-acting thyroid stimulator, or a specific exophthalmos-producing factor have been invoked but the mechanism still remains unknown (Havard, 1972).

HYPOTHYROIDISM ———————————

Muscle symptoms are common in hypothyroid patients (Figure 7-1) and may take the form of weakness, or of cramps, pain or stiffness, which may be precipitated by cold. A number of traditional eponymous syndromes have been described in association with hypothyroidism.

Kocher–Debré–Semelaigne syndrome

The rare syndrome of 'hypertrophia musculorum vera' in children was first described by Kocher in 1892 and the term popularized by Debré and Semelaigne (1935) who stressed the relation with hypothyroidism. This syndrome has been described in congenital hypothyroidism and in children of all ages with hypothyroidism and also following surgical or radioactive ablation of the thyroid. The hypertrophy is completely reversible by treatment of the hypothyroidism (Hesser, 1940).

Hoffmann's syndrome

Another form of hypothyroid myopathy with 'myotonoid' features but no muscle hypertrophy was described by Hoffmann (1897) in a patient following thyroidectomy. The patient had a myotonia congenita-like syndrome which was reversible on thyroid medication. It has been suggested that Hoffmann's syndrome is probably not a distinct entity but overlaps with the Kocher–Debré–Semelaigne syndrome (Salick *et al.*, 1968).

In hypothyroidism there is usually a slowness of movements as well as fatiguability and 'myotonic' tendon reflexes with delayed return. This is normally obvious with the Achilles tendon or triceps jerks. Lambert *et al.* (1951) showed that both the contraction and relaxation phases were delayed without any associated delay in nerve conduction or transmission. They suggested that the 'myotonic' reflex represents an abnormality of the contractile mechanism of the muscle, presumably due to an alteration in the muscle metabolism.

These patients do not show percussion myotonia but may instead produce a mound of 'myoedema' on percussion of the muscle which is electrically silent (Salick *et al.*, 1968). At times EMG does reveal increased insertional activity of the muscle and long bursts of repetitive discharge without the typical decrement of myotonia.

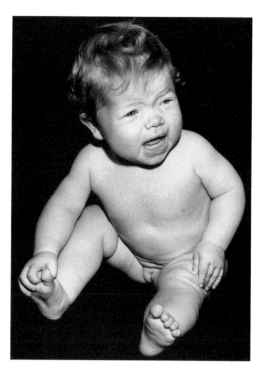

Figure 7-1 Hypothyroidism in a 16-month-old child presenting with delay in motor and intellectual milestones and associated hypotonia.

Cretins have a consistent elevation of serum creatine kinase (CK) even in the absence of any overt muscle weakness. In addition there is delayed myelination of the peripheral nerves, with slow nerve conduction velocity, which becomes normal after treatment (Moosa and Dubowitz, 1971). If hypothyroidism is acquired after the age of about 3–4 years, when the peripheral nerves are fully myelinated and the conduction velocity has reached adult levels, this slowing of conduction velocity will not be present.

Histology. In the few reports in the literature the muscle has usually been normal or shown only minimal change. These changes are relatively nonspecific, such as type 2 fibre atrophy and on electron microscopy Z-line streaming or mitochondrial changes.

Most of the *physiological* changes in hypothyroidism have been attributed to reduced myosin ATPase (Ianuzzo *et al.*, 1977; Wiles *et al.*, 1979; Nwoye *et al.*, 1982) and decreased calcium (Ca) uptake by the sarcoplasmic reticulum (Peter *et al.*, 1970).

The weakness of hypothyroidism has been attributed to a complex series of biochemical effects of thyroid hormone deficiency on skeletal muscle structure and function. There is a shift towards the physiological characteristics of slow muscle (Salviati *et al.*, 1985) and a decreased energy requirement for contraction (Wiles *et al.*, 1979; Leijendekker *et al.*, 1983). Decreased activities have been found in mitochondrial enzyme activities in human hypothyroid muscle (Khaleeli *et al.*, 1983 a,b,c) and this has been supported by recent studies with magnetic resonance spectroscopy (Argov *et al.*, 1988). Taylor *et al.* (1992), in a study of seven hypothyroid subjects ranging in age from 16 to 79 years, found that glycogen breakdown in skeletal muscle was delayed, thereby limiting the substrate supply for both glycolytic and oxidative production of ATP at the beginning of exercise.

Treatment. The underlying myopathy usually resolves completely with treatment of the hypothyroidism, as do the elevated CK and the slow reflexes.

DISORDERS OF THE PARATHYROIDS AND OSTEOMALACIA

Vicale (1949) gave a detailed clinical description of a myopathy in two cases of hyperpathyroidism and one of renal tubular acidosis and associated osteomalacia. The main clinical features are easy fatiguability, a waddling gait with symmetrical proximal weakness of the limb muscles, hypotonia, brisk tendon reflexes and discomfort on effort and sometimes spontaneous muscle cramps. Further cases were reviewed by Henson (1966), Smith and Stern (1967, 1969) and Lafferty (1981). Mental symptoms, particularly depression, are common and probably related to the hypercalcaemia. Diagnosis is easily missed due to the variable presentation, but readily confirmed by serum calcium and alkaline phosphatase studies and bone X-rays. The myo-

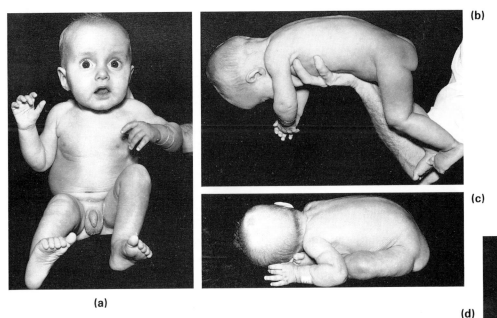

(b)

(c)

(e)

(a)

(d)

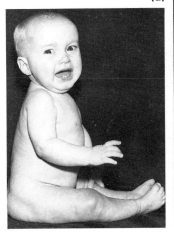

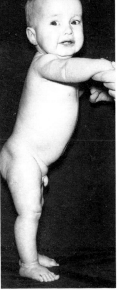

Figure 7-2a-e Renal tubular acidosis. This infant was referred at 9 months with a history of failure to thrive from 6 weeks. He had marked hypotonia and delay in motor and intellectual milestones (a,b,c) with head control at approximately a 6-week level. A diagnosis of renal tubular acidosis was established on the basis of a standard serum bicarbonate of 14 meq/litre and a persistently alkaline urine. There was an associated hypokalaemia (range 1.8–3.4 meq/litre) but other electrolytes were normal. Within a week of therapy with potassium citrate and potassium lactate there was marked improvement in his clinical condition, as well as the hypotonia and motor and intellectual functions. The biochemical changes reverted to normal. At 1 year he was sitting unsupported and standing well with support, had good head control, and tone in the limbs was normal (d,e).

pathy of osteomalacia usually responds to vitamin D, while the hyperparathyroidism requires surgical removal of adenoma, which can result in complete resolution of symptoms (Frame *et al.*, 1968; Patten *et al.*, 1974).

This is essentially a disorder of adult life but counterparts in infancy are provided by the hypotonia which is a component of idiopathic hypercalcaemia, renal tubular acidosis (Figure 7-2) and also nutritional rickets (see below) (Glorieux, 1991). The neuromuscular components of these metabolic and nutritional disorders usually resolve with treatment of the underlying disorder.

RENAL RICKETS

Patients with rickets secondary to renal disease may also present with neuromuscular symptoms; these may include muscle weakness, hypotonia, and also associated bone pain. The renal rickets in turn may be a manifestation of a rare underlying disorder such as Lowe's syndrome, and this was in fact the presentation of a female infant with hypotonia, weakness and delayed motor milestones who was found to have renal rickets and in addition ocular and cerebral manifestations. Following my comment that if only she were a male we would have diagnosed the X-linked Lowe's syndrome, chromosome studies were done which showed an X:3 translocation, with the breakpoint at Xq25 (Hodgson *et al.*, 1986), which in turn helped to locate the gene for Lowe's syndrome (Reilly *et al.*, 1990; Okabe *et al.*, 1992) (Figure 7-3).

Figure 7-3a-f (*facing page*)   Lowe's (oculo-cerebro-renal) syndrome; X:3 translocation. This girl, the second child of healthy unrelated parents, presented at 2 years with hypotonia and inability to stand (a). She had appeared to have weakness of the arms and legs, was generally irritable, and resented being touched. She was born at term and the neonatal period was uneventful. At 2 months abnormal eye movements were noted and she was found to have bilateral cataracts. Operation on the cataracts resulted in a progressive staphyloma of the right eye, with raised intra-ocular pressure, and subsequently needed enucleation. She smiled at 7 weeks, reached for large objects at 4½ months and sat at 9 months. When assessed at 2 years she sat steadily but was unable to take weight on her legs and her bones seemed to be tender to touch, and there was prominence of the epiphyses. Radiography showed marked rickets (b). Her height and weight were around the 3rd centile, but her head circumference around the 90th. Blood chemical studies showed a metabolic acidosis, an elevated chloride level with a base excess of -8, and a pH of 7.37. The urine pH was 6 and there was persistent aminoaciduria. The creatinine clearance and renal concentrating ability were normal. There was no excess loss of calcium or phosphate in a 24-hour urine collection. She had normal levels of parathyroid hormone and vitamin D metabolites. The serum alkaline phosphatase was elevated. There was no nephrocalcinosis on a plain abdominal X-ray film. A diagnosis was made of Fanconi syndrome, with proximal type II renal tubular acidosis due to bicarbonate wasting, rickets and generalized aminoaciduria. Treatment with oral phosphate, vitamin D, calcium and alkali supplements led to a marked improvement in her general well-being, the rickets healed (b) and her motor ability improved. She was able to take weight on her legs and to stand with callipers. She subsequently became ambulant with below-knee callipers (d, 5½ years; e, 7 years) and later without orthotic support. Following treatment she also showed a marked improvement in intellectual function and by 3½ years she had about 50 intelligible words and was making short sentences. At 15 years she currently continues fully ambulant and is coping well at a school for the blind. Following my comment that if she had been a boy we would have diagnosed a Lowe's syndrome to explain her combination of renal and ocular involvement with developmental delay, a chromosome analysis showed a *de novo* balanced translocation between chromosome 3 and the X-chromosome, with the breakpoint in the X-chromosome at Xq25. This provided a clue to the locus for the Lowe's syndrome gene.

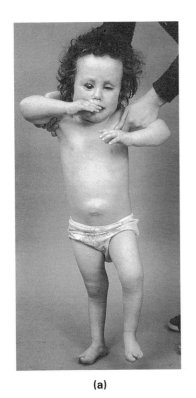

(a)

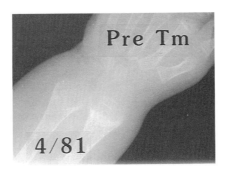

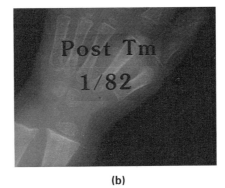

(b)

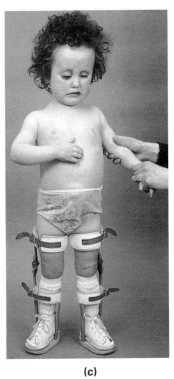

(c)

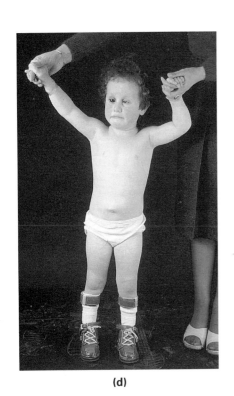

(d)

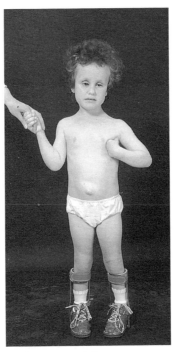

(e)

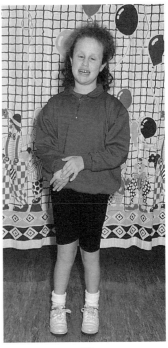

(f)

DISORDERS OF THE PITUITARY AND ADRENALS

HYPERPITUITARISM

In acromegaly there is a general hypertrophy and increased strength of the muscles but later this may be followed by muscle weakness (Lundberg *et al.*, 1970; Mastaglia *et al.*, 1970). Muscle biopsy has shown relatively minor changes, but a case studied by Cheah *et al.* (1975) showed mitochondrial abnormalities, which improved after hypophysectomy.

Two cases of pituitary gigantism documented by Lewis (1972) had an associated peripheral neuropathy, but the muscle biopsy in one showed some 'myopathic' features.

HYPOPITUITARISM

In children with hypopituitarism the muscle tends to be underdeveloped, in parallel with body growth generally, but there is no documented evidence of any associated myopathy.

CUSHING'S SYNDROME

Proximal weakness, especially of the lower limbs, is a well recognized complication of Cushing's syndrome (Müller and Kugelberg, 1959), and Pleasure *et al.* (1970) demonstrated a selective type 2 fibre atrophy and diminution of potassium in the muscle.

STEROID MYOPATHY

Myopathy as a result of steroid therapy was first documented in the same year as the Cushing's myopathy (Harman, 1959; Perkoff *et al.*, 1959; Williams, 1959) and many reports have followed, especially since the introduction of the 9-α-fluoro steroids. There also seems to be a possibility of a superadded steroid myopathy in apparently unresponsive cases of dermatomyositis on long-term high dosage steroid therapy (Dubowitz, 1976).

Steroid myopathy can be difficult to diagnose in the face of a disease under treatment, such as dermatomyositis, which in itself causes muscle weakness. Circumstantial evidence includes other side-effects of steroids, especially if given in high dosage and for a prolonged period. The CK may not be influenced and even the biopsy changes of a type 2 fibre atrophy are not necessarily specific.

The pathogenesis of steroid-induced myopathy has been extensively studied in experimental animals (Shoji, 1989) and in the occasional human subject (Pacy and Halliday, 1989) and suggests an increase

in protein catabolism with high-dosage steroids in addition to the decreased protein synthesis.

Catabolic effects of steroids also seem to be more pronounced in less active muscles. It is of interest in this context that exercise may lessen the effects of steroids on muscle (Horber *et al.*, 1985, 1987) and that in immobilized muscle the number of glucocorticoid receptors increases (Dubois and Almon, 1980).

Treatment of steroid myopathy requires reduction in the dosage, and this has to be done gradually and with close monitoring of the patient to avoid relapse of the underlying primary disorder under treatment. As steroid myopathy is largely an iatrogenic disorder and usually related to excessive and unnecessary high dosages of steroids, it can be prevented by cautious usage (see Chapter 11).

ADDISON'S DISEASE

Generalized muscle weakness and fatigue are an integral part of Addison's disease and probably related to the water and electrolyte changes in the plasma and muscle rather than any structural myopathy.

A sense of fatigue, subjective weakness and myalgia are also a feature of withdrawal from corticosteroid therapy, particularly if the dosage has been high, the duration of treatment prolonged and the rate of reduction too rapid. This can often be resolved by temporarily raising the steroid dose again and then tapering very slowly.

HYPERALDOSTERONISM

When Conn (1955) first described primary aldosteronism, he drew attention to the associated periodic attacks of weakness, presumably due to the hypokalaemia. In a subsequent review of 145 cases (Conn *et al.*, 1964) muscle weakness was one of the most common presenting features. The condition somewhat resembles hypokalaemic periodic paralysis but the low K+ persists between attacks and there is associated hypertension, alkalosis and hypernatraemia (Gallai, 1977; Atsumi *et al.*, 1979). The weakness may be unresponsive to KCl and surgery may be required for removal of an adrenal tumour.

NUTRITIONAL MYOPATHIES

PROTEIN–CALORIE MALNUTRITION

A high incidence of neurological involvement occurs in kwashiorkor, with mental changes as well as hypotonia and hyporeflexia (Udani, 1960). In addition, Sachdev *et al.* (1971) have also demon-

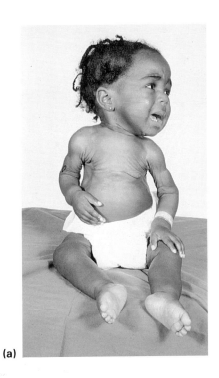

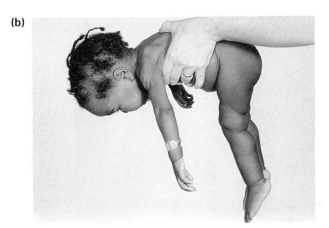

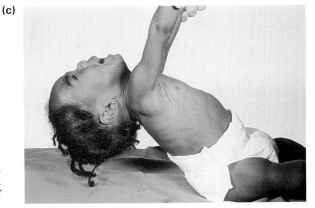

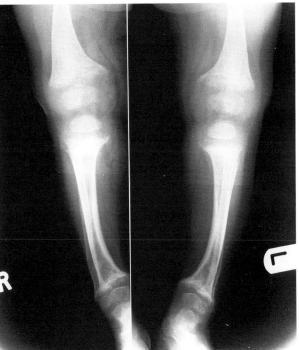

Figure 7-4a-c Rickets; malnutrition. A 14-month-old child presenting with marked hypotonia, associated with severe rickets and malnutrition. Note the prominence of the right wrist (a). (Courtesy of Professor Alex Mowat.)

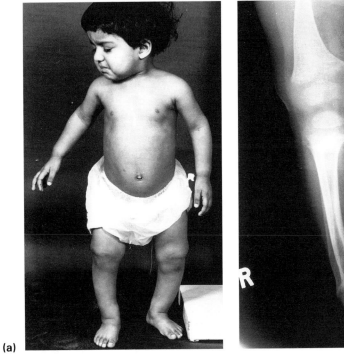

Figure 7-5a,b Rickets in a 2-year-old child presenting with bowing of legs, abnormal gait and associated hypotonia. Note prominence of wrists and lower femoral epiphyses (a); X-ray of legs showed typical epiphysial changes (b).

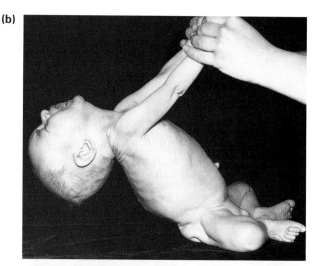

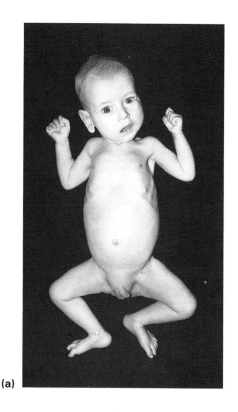

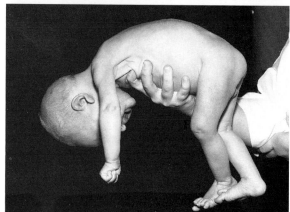

Figure 7-6a-c Coeliac disease in a 21-week-old child with failure to thrive from age 16 weeks and marked hypotonia, with poor head control but good muscle power. Note prominent abdomen and wasted buttocks.

strated slowing of motor nerve conduction and abnormalities on electromyography.

The symptoms usually resolve with correction of the malnutrition.

OTHER NUTRITIONAL DISORDERS

Hypotonia is an almost constant feature of rickets and usually responds to therapy with vitamin D (Figures 7-4, 7-5). In some cases of severe rickets the hypotonia and apparent associated weakness may be so profound, together with indrawing of the rib cage with respiration, as to suggest a clinical diagnosis of Werdnig–Hoffmann disease.

Children with coeliac disease often have associated hypotonia, which at times may be the most striking and presenting feature (Figure 7-6). It usually resolves as the child responds to a gluten-free diet.

REFERENCES

Argov, Z., Renshaw, P.F., Boden, B. *et al.* (1988) Effects of thyroid hormones on skeletal muscle bioenergetics. *Journal of Clinical Investigation* **18**: 1695–1701.

Atsumi, T., Ishikawa, S., Miyatake, T. *et al.* (1979) Myopathy and primary aldosteronism: electromicroscopic study. *Neurology* **29**: 1348–1353.

Cheah, J.S., Chua, S.P. and Ho, C.L. (1975) Ultrastructure of the skeletal muscles in acromegaly – before and after hypophysectomy. *American Journal of the Medical Sciences* **269**: 183.

Conn, J.W. (1955) Primary aldosteronism, a new clinical syndrome. *Journal of Laboratory and Clinical Medicine* **45**: 661.

Conn, J.W., Knopf, R.F. and Nesbit, R.M. (1964) Clinical characteristics of primary aldosteronism from an analysis of 145 cases. *American Journal of Surgery* **107**: 159.

Debré, R. and Semelaigne, G. (1935) Syndrome of diffuse muscular hypertrophy in infants causing athletic appearance: its connection with congenital myxedema. *American Journal of Diseases of Children* **50**: 1351–1361.

Dubois, D.C. and Almon, R.R. (1980) Disuse atrophy of skeletal muscle is associated with an increase in number of glucocorticoid receptors. *Endocrinology* **107**: 1649–1651.

Dubowitz, V. (1976) Treatment of dermatomyositis in childhood. *Archives of Disease in Childhood* **51**: 494–500.

Frame, B., Heinze, E.G., Block, M.A. *et al.* (1968) Myopathy in primary hyperparathyroidism: observations in three patients. *Annals of Internal Medicine* **68**: 1022–1027.

Gallai, M. (1977) Myopathy with hyperaldosteronism. *Journal of the Neurological Sciences* **32**: 337–345.

Glorieux, F.H. (1991) Rickets, the continuing challenge. *New England Journal of Medicine* **325**: 1875–1877.

Harman, J.B. (1959) Muscular wasting and corticosteroid therapy. *Lancet* **i**: 887.

Havard, C.W.H. (1972) Clinical endocrinology: endocrine exophthalmos. *British Medical Journal* **i**: 360.

Havard, C.W.H., Campbell, E.D.R., Ross, H.B. and Spence, A.W. (1963) Electromyographic and histological findings in the muscles of patients with thyrotoxicosis. *Quarterly Journal of Medicine* **32**: 145.

Henson, R.A. (1966) The neurological aspects of hypercalcaemia with special reference to primary hyperparathyroidism. *Journal of the Royal College of Physicians of London* **1**: 41.

Hesser, F.H. (1940) Hypertrophia musculorum vera (dystrophia musculorum hyperplastica) associated with hypothyroidism: a case study. *Bulletin of the Johns Hopkins Hospital* **66**: 353–377.

Hodgson, S.V., Heckmatt, J.Z., Hughes, E. *et al.* (1986) A balanced *de novo* X/autosome translocation in a girl with manifestations of Lowe syndrome. *American Journal of Medical Genetics* **23**: 837–847.

Hoffmann, J. (1897) Weiterer Beitrag zur Lehre von der Tetanie. *Deutsche Zeitschrift für Nervenheilkunde* **9**: 278–290.

Horber, F.F., Scheidegger, J.R., Grunig, B.E. *et al.* (1985) Evidence that prednisone-induced myopathy is reversed by physical training. *Journal of Clinical Endocrinology and Metabolism* **61**: 83–88.

Horber, F.F., Hoopeler, H., Scheidegger, J.R. *et al.* (1987) Impact of physical training on the ultrastructure of midthigh muscle in normal subjects and in patients treated with glucocorticoids. *Journal of Clinical Investigation* **79**: 1181–1190.

Ianuzzo, D., Patel, P., Chen, V. *et al.* (1977) Thyroidal trophic influence on skeletal muscle myosin. *Nature* **270**: 74–76.

Khaleeli, A.A., Griffith, D.G. and Edwards, R.H.T. (1983a) The clinical presentation of hypothyroid myopathy and its relationship to abnormalities in structure and function of skeletal muscle. *Clinical Endocrinology* **19**: 365–376.

Khaleeli, A.A., Gohil, K., McPhail, G. *et al.* (1983b) Muscle morphology and metabolism in hypothyroid myopathy: effects of treatment. *Journal of Clinical Pathology* **36**: 519–526.

Khaleeli, A.A., Edwards, R.H.T., Gohil, K. *et al.* (1983c) Corticosteroid myopathy: a clinical and pathological study. *Clinical Endocrinology* **18**: 155–156.

Kissel, P., Schmitt, J., Duc, M. and Duc, M.L. (1970) Myasthenia and thyrotoxicosis. In: Walton, J.N., Canal, N. and Scarlato, G. eds, *Muscle Diseases*. Amsterdam: Excerpta Medica, I.C.S. No. 199, p. 464.

Kocher (1892). (Quoted by Debré and Semelaigne, 1935.)

Kufs, W.M., McBiles, M. and Jurney, T. (1989) Familial thyrotoxic periodic paralysis. *Western Journal of Medicine* **150**: 461–463.

Lafferty, F.W. (1981) Primary hyperparathyroidism: changing clinical spectrum, prevalence of hypertension, and discriminant analysis of laboratory tests. *Archives of Internal Medicine* **141**: 1761–1766.

Lambert, E.H., Underdahl, L.O., Beckett, S. and Mederos, L.O. (1951) A study of the ankle jerk in myxedema. *Journal of Clinical Endocrinology* **11**: 1186.

Leijendekker, W.J., van Hardeveld, C. and Kassenaar, A.H. (1983) The influence of the hypothyroid state on energy turnover during tetanic stimulation in the fast-twitch (mixed type) muscle of rats. *Metabolism* **32**: 615–621.

Lewis, P.D. (1972) Neuromuscular involvement in pituitary gigantism. *British Medical Journal* **i**: 499.

Lundberg, P.O., Osterman, P.O. and Stålberg, E. (1970) Neuromuscular signs and symptoms in acromegaly. In: Walton, J.N., Canal, N. and Scarlato, G. eds, *Muscle Diseases*. Amsterdam: Excerpta Medica, I.C.S. No. 199, p. 531.

Mastaglia, F.L., Barwick, D.D. and Hall, R. (1970) Myopathy in acromegaly. *Lancet* **ii**: 907.

Moosa, A. and Dubowitz, V. (1971) Slow nerve conduction velocity in cretins. *Archives of Disease in Childhood* **46**: 852–854.

Müller, R. and Kugelberg, E. (1959) Myopathy in Cushing's syndrome. *Journal of Neurology, Neurosurgery and Psychiatry* **22**: 314.

Nwoye, L., Mommaerts, W.F.H.M., Simpson, D.R. *et al.* (1982) Evidence for a direct action of thyroid hormone in specifying muscle properties. *American Journal of Physiology* **242**: R401–R408.

Okabe, I., Attree, O., Bailey, L.C. *et al.* (1992) Isolation of cDNA sequences around the chromosomal breakpoint in a female with Lowe syndrome by direct screening of cDNA libraries with yeast artificial chromosomes. *Journal of Inherited Metabolic Diseases* **15**: 526–531.

Pacy, P.J. and Halliday, D. (1989) Muscle protein synthesis in steroid-induced proximal myopathy: a case report. *Muscle and Nerve* **12**: 378–381.

Patten, B.M., Bilezikian, J.P., Mallette, L.E. *et al.* (1974) Neuromuscular disease in primary hyperparathyroidism. *Annals of Internal Medicine* **80**: 182–193.

Perkoff, G.T., Silber, R., Tyler, F.H., Cartwright, G.E. and Wintrobe, M.M. (1959) Studies in disorders of muscle. XII. Myopathy due to the administration of therapeutic amounts of 17-hydroxycortico-steroids. *American Journal of Medicine* **26**: 891.

Peter, J.B., Verhaag, D.A. and Worsfold, M. (1970) Studies of steroid myopathy: examination of the possible effect of triamcinolone on mitochondria and sarcotubular vesicles of rat skeletal muscle. *Biochemical Pharmacology* **19**: 1627–1636.

Pleasure, D.E., Walsh, G.O. and Engel, W.K. (1970) Atrophy of skeletal muscle in patients with Cushing's syndrome. *Archives of Neurology* **22**: 118.

Reilly, D.S., Lewis, R.A. and Nussbaum, R.L. (1990) Genetic and physical mapping of Xq24-q26 markers flanking the Lowe oculocerebrorenal syndrome. *Genomics* **8**: 62–70.

Sachdev, K.K., Taori, G.M. and Pereira, S.M. (1971) Neuromuscular status in protein-calorie malnutrition. *Neurology (India)* **21**: 801.

Salick, A.I., Colachis, S.C. Jr and Pearson, C.M. (1968) Myxedema myopathy: clinical, electrodiagnostic, and pathologic findings in advanced case. *Archives of Physical Medicine and Rehabilitation* **49**: 230–237.

Salviati, G., Zeviani, M., Betto, R. *et al.* (1985) Effects of thyroid hormones on the biochemical specialization of human muscle fibres. *Muscle and Nerve* **8**: 363–371.

Shoji, S. (1989) Myofibrillar protein catabolism in rat steroid myopathy measured by 3-methylhistidine excretion in the urine. *Journal of the Neurological Sciences* **93**: 333–340.

Simpson, J.A. (1968) The correlations between myasthenia gravis and disorders of the thyroid gland. In: Research Committee of the Muscular Dystrophy Group of Great Britain: *Research in Muscular Dystrophy.* Proceedings of the Fourth Symposium. London: Pitman Medical. p. 31.

Smith, R. and Stern, G. (1967) Myopathy, osteomalacia and hyperparathyroidism. *Brain* **90**: 593.

Smith, R. and Stern, G. (1969) Muscular weakness in osteomalacia and hyperparathyroidism. *Journal of the Neurological Sciences* **8**: 511–520.

Taylor, D.J., Rajagopalan, B. and Radda, G.K. (1992) Cellular energetics in hypothyroid muscle. *European Journal of Clinical Investigation* **22**: 358–365.

Udani, P.M. (1960) Neurological manifestations in kwashiorkor. *Indian Journal of Child Health* **9**: 103.

Vicale, C.T. (1949) The diagnostic features of a muscular syndrome resulting from hyperparathyroidism, osteomalacia owing to renal tubular acidosis, and perhaps to related disorders of calcium metabolism. *Transactions of the American Neurological Association* **74**: 143.

Wiles, C.M., Young, A., Jones, D.A. *et al.* (1979) Muscle relaxation rate, fibre-type composition and energy turnover in hyper- and hypothyroid patients. *Clinical Science* **57**: 375–384.

Williams, R.S. (1959) Triamcinolone myopathy. *Lancet* **i**: 698.

CHAPTER 8

Disorders of the Lower Motor Neurone
The Spinal Muscular Atrophies

A vast number of clinical disorders, both acute and chronic, hereditary and acquired, affect the lower motor neurone (Dyck *et al.*, 1992). The lesion may be in the anterior horn cell or more distally along the course of the peripheral nerve. Some disorders affect only motor nerves, others the sensory as well. In some, the peripheral neuropathy occurs in isolation, in others it is associated with involvement of the spinal tracts or other parts of the central nervous system.

A full review of all of them is patently beyond the scope of this book. I shall concentrate on those disorders, mainly hereditary, which predominantly affect the motor nerves and are thus likely to overlap with other disorders of muscle. Emphasis will be placed on those disorders more likely to occur in childhood.

provide a fully up-to-date review of the various clinical syndromes in the light of the advances at the molecular level.

One can subdivide the disorders of the lower motor neurone into two broad categories — those affecting the anterior horn cells of the spinal cord, the spinal muscular atrophies, and those affecting the nerve itself, the motor neuropathies, involving either the axon (axonal) or the myelin sheath (demyelinating). The spinal muscular atrophies will be reviewed in this chapter, the motor neuropathies in Chapter 9.

NOMENCLATURE AND CLASSIFICATION

As in the case of the muscular dystrophies, clinical classification of the hereditary neuropathies has been based mainly on the location of the primary pathology, the distribution of muscle weakness, the severity and progression of the disease, genetic factors, associated features and, where known, any specific aetiological factors. Recent advances in molecular genetics have now added a completely new dimension. The gene location has been found for several of the syndromes and in some the DNA mutation identified and the protein abnormality established. The coming years will undoubtedly see a remarkable further resolution in many of these disorders, and this may well provide a more rational approach to classification. Meanwhile I have tried to

THE SPINAL MUSCULAR ATROPHIES

I have reserved the term spinal muscular atrophy (SMA) for the group of hereditary proximal symmetrical muscular atrophies associated with degeneration of the anterior horn cells of the cord and also, in the more severe forms, of the bulbar motor nuclei. This is one of the most common forms of neuromuscular disorder in childhood.

From a clinical point of view one can readily recognize the severe infantile spinal muscular atrophy (Werdnig–Hoffmann disease) and the mild 'pseudomyopathic' spinal muscular atrophy (Kugelberg–Welander disease), which resembles limb girdle muscular dystrophy and was confused with it in the past. Between these two syndromes is a group of cases of spinal muscular atrophy with a range of disability extending through all gradations from the severe infantile muscular atrophy at the one extreme to the mild ambulant form at the other (Dubowitz, 1967).

HISTORICAL SURVEY

In a series of detailed and well-documented papers Werdnig (1891, 1894) of the Institute of Pathology of the University of Graz in Austria, and Hoffmann (1893, 1897, 1900a,b), attached to Erb's clinic in Heidelberg, described the disease which bears their names.

The two brothers described by Werdnig had progressive weakness from the age of 10 months, starting in the legs and subsequently affecting the back and arm muscles. The first child also had an associated hydrocephalus and died of pertussis at 3 years of age. Autopsy revealed atrophy of the anterior horns, especially in the cervical and lumbar enlargements, and degeneration of the anterior roots. The gastrocnemius, the only muscle examined, showed 'simple atrophy'. The second boy had choreiform movements and fibrillary tremors of the muscles in addition to his weakness and he survived until 6 years of age. The cord showed atrophy of the cells in the anterior horns, especially in the cervical and lumbar regions, and also some degeneration in the V and VII nerve nuclei. The anterior roots as well as the peripheral nerves showed considerable degeneration. The cerebral cortex, pyramidal tracts, the cells of Clarke's column and the lateral horns all appeared normal. Most of the muscles showed mainly simple atrophy but large round fibres were present in some areas, suggesting a 'mixed' process.

Hoffmann described seven cases from four different families. They were also normal at birth and did not develop weakness until the latter part of the first year of life. Survival ranged from 14 months to 5 years of age. Autopsy in a number of cases revealed degeneration of the anterior horn cells of the spinal cord and extensive atrophy of muscle.

Although both Werdnig and Hoffmann stressed the late onset of the weakness, Beevor in 1902 recognized a familial case of congenital infantile spinal muscular atrophy, with weakness already present at birth.

In the first study of a large series of cases Brandt (1950) reviewed 112 patients coming from 69 families in Denmark. He drew attention to the variability in the clinical picture. As regards the onset of first clinical manifestation, 97 of the 112 (87%) were under 1 year of age. Of these 73 (65%) were less than 6 months of age, and in 41 (36%) weakness was already present at birth. In nine children the onset began after the age of 1 year and in the remaining six no information was available.

The overall prognosis was very poor, but again showed considerable variation. Fifty-three children (56%) died by the age of 1 year, 76 (80%) by the age of 4 years, eight cases between 4 and 10 years, and ten between 10 and 20 years. Of the 17 patients still alive at the time of the study, seven were under 6 years old, eight were between 6 and 15 years, one was 18 and one 20 years of age. All were severely disabled. Brandt made no attempt to categorize them into groups on the basis of severity.

Wohlfart *et al.* (1955) and Kugelberg and Welander (1956) subsequently described a much milder form of spinal muscular atrophy with proximal symmetrical weakness affecting predominantly the lower limbs. In Kugelberg and Welander's patients, onset was between 2 and 17 years of age and survival was into adult life, with continued ability to walk. Seven of their 12 cases were able to walk 20 years or more after the onset of their disease.

In a review of 52 cases of infantile muscular atrophy, Byers and Banker (1961) subdivided them 'for descriptive purposes' into three groups, according to age of onset. In the first group, onset of weakness was *in utero* or within the first 2 months of life; these children had severe generalized weakness and early death. In the second group onset was from age 2 to 12 months; weakness was more localized and survival longer. In the third group, with onset in the second year of life, weakness was very localized and survival was in terms of years rather than months.

In 1964 I reviewed a series of 12 cases of infantile muscular atrophy with prolonged survival (Dubowitz, 1964a). One child achieved the ability to walk; the others, including the brother of the ambulant child, could sit but were unable to stand (see Figures 8-5 to 8-10). Onset of symptoms, based on the history of the parents, was usually between 9 and 16 months. This reflects the period between the child's achieving the ability to sit, but subsequently failing to progress with standing or walking. All had survived into their teens. In one family with two affected sisters, a brother with a more severe spinal muscular atrophy, who had not been able to sit up, had died of pneumonia at 23 months and the diagnosis was confirmed at autopsy (see Figure 8-9).

Whilst this group of cases seemed to comprise a clearly defined clinical entity, with ability to sit but not to walk, I subsequently highlighted the difficulty of drawing any clearcut dividing line between the most severe cases, the cases of intermediate severity and the milder Kugelberg–Welander syndrome, in view of cases bridging the demarcation lines between the three groups, and suggested that there might be a continuum of cases of spinal muscular atrophy between the most severe infantile form at one end and the most mild juvenile or adult forms at the other (Dubowitz, 1964b, 1967).

NUMBER OF SYNDROMES

Clinicians traditionally fall into two groups, the lumpers and the splitters. This is well illustrated

Table 8-1   Spinal muscular atrophy: clinical classification

Type	Onset	Course	Age at death
1 (severe)	Birth to 6 months	Never sit	Usually <2 years
2 (intermediate)	<18 months	Never stand	>2 years
3 (mild)	>18 months	Stand alone	Adult

From: International Consortium on SMA (Munsat, 1991).

again in the case of infantile spinal muscular atrophy. While some have strongly supported the unitary hypothesis of a single genetic condition with variation in clinical severity (Byers and Banker, 1961; Dubowitz, 1964b, 1967, 1969a; Dunne and Chutorian, 1966; Hausmanowa-Petrusewicz *et al.*, 1966; Gardner-Medwin *et al.*, 1967; Munsat *et al.*, 1969) there have been equally determined efforts to define individual syndromes (Hausmanowa-Petrusewicz, 1970; Emery, 1971; Fried and Emery, 1971). Zellweger (1971) stressed the genetic heterogeneity of the spinal muscular atrophies and Becker (1966) suggested the possibility of three separate allelomorphic genes to account for the varying clinical phenotypes (which are discussed in the section on genetics). Fried and Emery (1971) suggested that there were at least three clinically and genetically distinct forms of spinal muscular atrophy of childhood: type 1 (Werdnig–Hoffmann disease) with onset at birth or within the first few months of life and death before the age of 2 years; type 2 (intermediate form) with onset between 3 and 15 months of age and survival beyond 4 years; and type 3 (Kugelberg–Welander disease) with onset after 24 months and a more benign course. The main problem with such a classification is that from a clinical point of view the age of onset is a very indistinct point to define in a condition which often has an insidious onset, especially in the milder forms. Moreover, some cases with onset of symptoms before 15 months seem to follow a course similar to the Kugelberg–Welander syndrome, which can certainly have typical cases with onset before 24 months of life. The definition of specific subtypes is of some value to the geneticist trying to define how many genes are involved.

In a genetic study of spinal muscular atrophy, using sib–sib correlation analysis in familial cases, Pearn *et al.* (1973) were able to identify, with a high concordance among sibs, an 'acute Werdnig–Hoffmann disease', which was fatal before the third birthday, caused delayed motor milestones 'certainly by 6 months and almost certainly by 3 months', and always resulted in the child being taken

to a doctor before 6 months. All the remaining cases they classified as chronic.

With the recent impact of molecular genetics there was an active search in several laboratories for the gene location of childhood spinal muscular atrophies. As it was not certain at the outset whether we would be dealing with one allelic gene for all the different grades of severity or whether there might prove to be more than one gene locus, accurate clinical diagnosis was essential in order to ensure a homogeneous cohort of patients for study (Dubowitz, 1991). An international consortium was established of clinicians and molecular geneticists involved in this SMA research programme and a consensus was obtained for a clinical classification of the childhood spinal muscular atrophies, together with clinical inclusion and exclusion criteria for patients enrolled into the study (Munsat, 1991; Munsat and Davis, 1992) (Table 8-1).

CLINICAL PICTURE ————————————

As has already been suggested, there is an infinitely variable picture of clinical severity. Some of the original cases described by Werdnig and Hoffmann would now be looked upon as of intermediate severity and not conforming to the most severe form, which has an even earlier onset than Werdnig and Hoffmann's cases and does not usually survive beyond the first year. In general, the age of onset is an unreliable criterion for classification, although there is an overall broad correlation between the age of onset and severity – the earlier the onset the more severe the phenotype. However, some cases of intermediate severity may have a very early onset (even at birth) and some of the most severe cases may not manifest until 4 or 5 months of age and yet be as severely affected as those with very early onset and still die before 1 year of age. The only practical guide to prognosis is the actual clinical severity of the disease itself, irrespective of the age of onset, and in particular the extent of respiratory muscle involvement and respiratory deficit. From a descriptive point of view one can readily define the most severe and the least severe forms and the cases who fall midway between. One can then also recognize those cases which bridge the gap between the three defined categories.

In clinical practice I have found it most practical to subdivide these cases of spinal muscular atrophy of severe, intermediate or mild form on the basis of the child's ability to sit unaided and to stand and walk unaided, as follows:

1. Severe. Unable to sit unsupported.
2. Intermediate. Able to sit unsupported. Unable to stand or walk unaided.
3. Mild. Able to stand and walk.

Note that this subdivision into three groups is arbitrary and there is variability within each group and an overall continuum of severity.

SEVERE SPINAL MUSCULAR ATROPHY (WERDNIG–HOFFMANN DISEASE) (TYPE 1)

The onset is early, either *in utero* or within the first 2–3 months of life. The onset may appear acute and a previously active infant may suddenly lose the ability to move his limbs. There does appear to be a period of complete normality before the onset of the disease in some of these infants. In one family where previously an infant had died at 8 months from spinal muscular atrophy, I had the opportunity of assessing a subsequent infant on the first day of life and throughout the first week. He was completely normal in all his motor activities, tendon reflexes and other neonatal responses. When he returned to clinic at 5 weeks he had the typical weakness of severe spinal muscular atrophy, which had come on 1 week before, and he also subsequently died at 8 months. Occasionally the mother may notice a cessation of previously active movements *in utero* and the infant may be born floppy.

The infant shows generalized hypotonia and there is practically generalized paralysis of the limbs and trunk (Figure 8-1). The lower limbs are more severely affected than the upper, and the proximal muscles

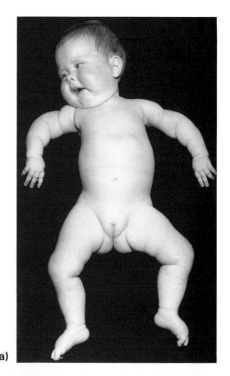

(a)

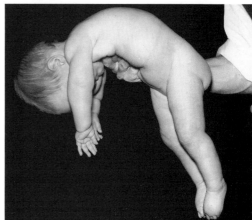

(b)

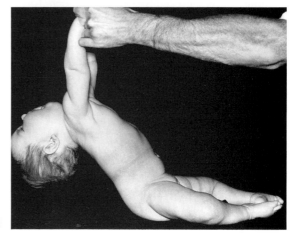

(c)

Figure 8-1a-c   Severe infantile spinal muscular atrophy in a 6-week-old infant with weakness and hypotonia from birth, showing (a) frog-like posture in supine position, (b) marked flaccid weakness of limbs and trunk in ventral suspension and (c) head lag in supine position. Note the normal facial expression (a).

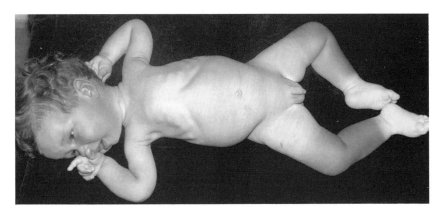

Figure 8-2 Severe spinal muscular atrophy in a 1-year-old infant showing intercostal recession and diaphragmatic breathing. Note frog posture of legs, ability to flex elbows and move hands and normal facial expression.

more than distal. Any residual spontaneous movement is usually confined to the ankles and toes, and in the upper limbs the child may be able to flex and extend the elbows, in addition to moving the hands and fingers, but is not able to move the shoulders or raise the arms against gravity.

There is marked weakness of all the axial muscles and the child has poor head control in both a prone and in the supine position (Figure 8-1). These infants are never able to raise their heads or to roll over and cannot raise their legs against gravity. The face is spared, and the child's expression appears normal (Figures 8-1 to 8-4). However, bulbar weakness is often present, with difficulty in sucking and swallowing and an associated accumulation of mucus in the pharynx. Fasciculation and atrophy of the tongue are not a striking feature. Fasciculation is probably present in many of them but difficult to identify and to distinguish from tongue tremor in a small infant.

The intercostal muscles are severely affected and breathing is almost entirely diaphragmatic. This gives the chest a bell-shaped appearance with associated distension of the abdomen with inspiration and costal recession (Figures 8-2, 8-3). This is a very characteristic feature of infantile spinal muscular atrophy and helps to distinguish it from other neuromuscular disorders presenting in early infancy, which do not give this selective respiratory muscle involvement and frequently have evidence of diaphragmatic weakness. The cry is weak and ineffectual, as is any effort at coughing.

The tendon reflexes are always absent. Contractures of any severity are not a feature of severe SMA, but mild contractures frequently occur. Involvement of the internal rotators of the shoulders gives the arms an internally rotated, 'jug-handle' position by the side of the body, with the hands facing outwards (Figure 8-4). This is a remarkably frequent and

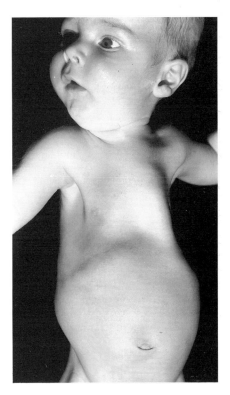

Figure 8-3 Severe infantile spinal muscular atrophy in a 3-month-old infant showing marked respiratory deficit with intercostal paralysis and reduction in chest size, and marked costal recession, with normal diaphragmatic function. (Note alert, expressive face.)

consistent feature and may suggest a 'spot' diagnosis on initial assessment of the infant. There may be some limitation of abduction of the hips (Figure 8-4) or of full extension of the knees or elbows. This is of minor degree and any more extensive contractures or

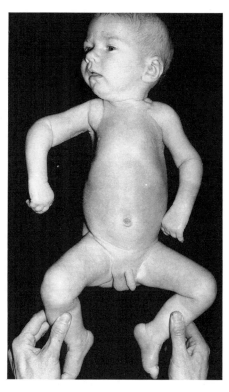

Figure 8-4 Severe spinal muscular atrophy with contractures of internal rotators of shoulders giving 'jug-handle' posture of arms, and of hip adductors giving limitation of hip adduction. Note normal facial expression.

arthrogryposis should raise the suspicion of an alternative diagnosis. Range of movement in the hands and feet is usually full, but occasionally the finger flexors are affected.

These infants are prone to recurrent respiratory infections and as a result rarely survive beyond the first two years of life. Cardiac muscle is not affected.

INTERMEDIATE SEVERITY SPINAL MUSCULAR ATROPHY (TYPE 2)

The typical history is of a child progressing quite normally in the first 6 months or so of life and usually achieving the ability to sit unaided. The child is then unable to take any weight on the legs and never achieves the ability to stand independently or walk. As in the severe form, the weakness is symmetrical, the proximal muscles are more affected than the distal, and the lower limbs more than the upper. The power in the arms may be reasonably good with ability to abduct the shoulders against gravity but some degree of weakness is usually present in them

from early on (Figure 8-5). The tendon reflexes are usually depressed or absent. The intercostal muscles are affected, but usually not severely, and as a rule there is no evidence of respiratory difficulty, although this may develop later, particularly after respiratory infections. As in the severe form, the diaphragm tends to be spared, so that the breathing is predominantly diaphragmatic.

There are no bulbar symptoms, but fasciculation and atrophy of the tongue are a common feature (Figure 8-6). Fasciculation of skeletal muscle is usually not apparent. An additional clinical feature common in these cases is a tremor of the hands, which may be marked enough for the parents to observe (Moosa and Dubowitz, 1973).

These cases usually have a benign course and patients survive into adolescence or adulthood. The muscle power in general tends to remain fairly static (Figures 8-7 to 8-10). Some may even show an apparent improvement in muscle power, presumably from reinnervation of atrophic muscle by surviving neurons. A few patients, however, do show definite deterioration in power, which may be gradual or may occur in episodes.

The single most important factor in determining prognosis is respiratory function. Those cases with equal weakness of the skeletal muscles but more striking intercostal involvement have a correspondingly poor outlook. As in any chairbound patient, these children are prone to develop contractures and deformities related to their consistent posture. This takes the form of flexion contractures of the hips and knees and equinus deformity of the feet, but the most disastrous complication is the development of scoliosis, which can be very rapidly progressive and have a marked effect on the respiratory function, as well as the comfort, of the child (see Figure 8-5). They are often hypotonic and may have an increased range of movement of joints – often striking in the hands. The metacarpophalangeal joints can often be extended to 90° and the outstretched fingers have a swan-neck like hyperextended posture. This joint hypermobility may also be an aggravating factor in the scoliosis, which often remains remarkably mobile even when pretty extensive.

Cardiac involvement is not a feature of spinal muscular atrophy and the ECG is usually normal. However, the ECG may be 'diagnostic' of SMA since the baseline consistently shows an irregular tremulous pattern, particularly in the limb leads, probably reflecting the fasciculation of the skeletal muscle (Figure 8-11).

These children also have a normal intellect, or possibly as a group even an above-average intellect. They often speak at an early age and may be able to make long sentences by the age of 2 years, well in advance of the norm for that age.

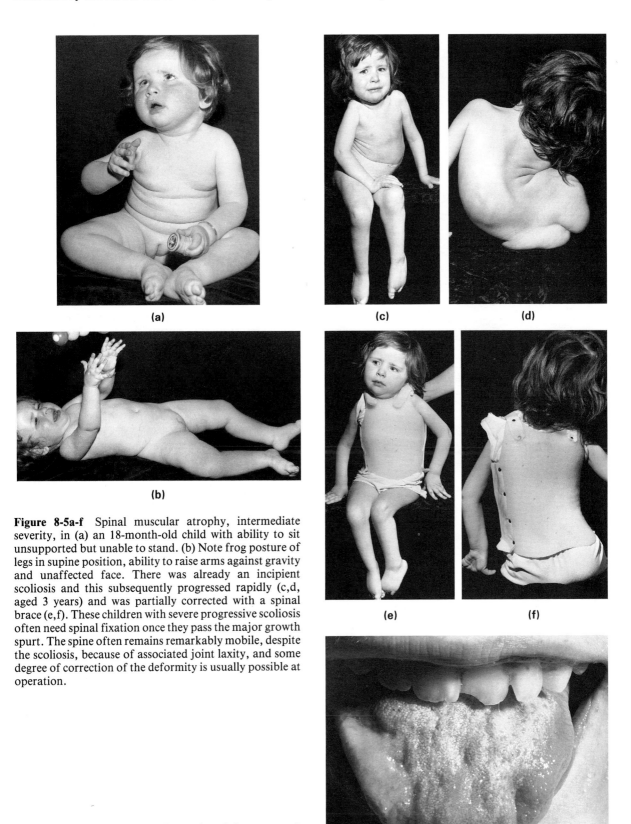

Figure 8-5a-f Spinal muscular atrophy, intermediate severity, in (a) an 18-month-old child with ability to sit unsupported but unable to stand. (b) Note frog posture of legs in supine position, ability to raise arms against gravity and unaffected face. There was already an incipient scoliosis and this subsequently progressed rapidly (c,d, aged 3 years) and was partially corrected with a spinal brace (e,f). These children with severe progressive scoliosis often need spinal fixation once they pass the major growth spurt. The spine often remains remarkably mobile, despite the scoliosis, because of associated joint laxity, and some degree of correction of the deformity is usually possible at operation.

Figure 8-6 Fasciculation and atrophy of the tongue. A common feature in intermediate severity spinal muscular atrophy.

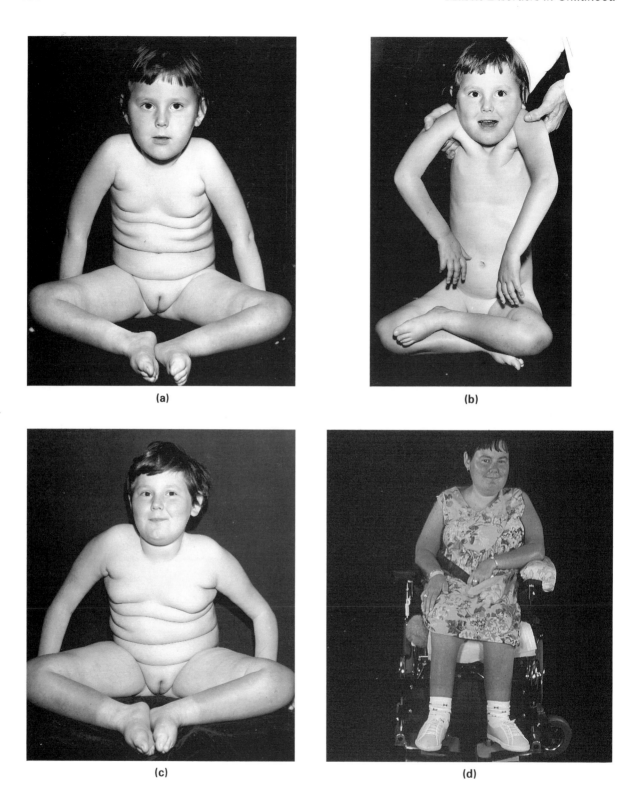

(a)

(b)

(c)

(d)

Figure 8-7a-d   Intermediate severity spinal muscular atrophy in a 5-year-old girl (a) who sat unsupported at 7 months, but was never able to stand or walk. Note associated hypotonia and joint hypermobility (b). Same child at 10 years (c) showed no apparent deterioration. Note straight back. There was no subsequent change at regular follow-up over a 6-year period, and a recent review some 20 years later, at the age of 34 years, has shown a remarkably stable condition (d).

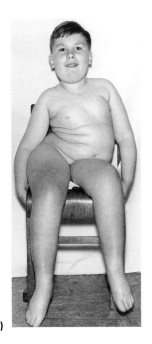
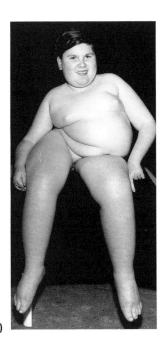
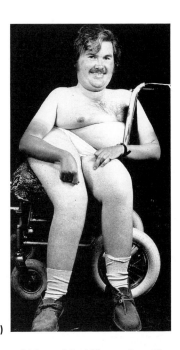

(a) (b) (c)

Figure 8-8a-c   Intermediate spinal muscular atrophy, static course, in (a) a 9-year-old boy with ability to sit at 12 months but never able to stand or walk. There was early onset of scoliosis. During a 15-year follow-up there was little apparent deterioration (b, aged 14 years; c, aged 24 years). Note normal facies.

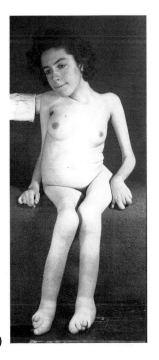
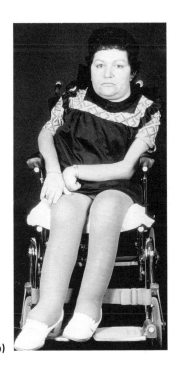
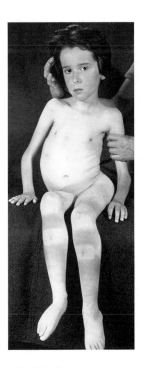

(a) (b) (c)

Figure 8-9a-c   Intermediate spinal muscular atrophy, static course, in (a) a 17-year-old girl who sat unsupported at 7 months but was never able to stand or walk. Onset of scoliosis was at 4 years of age. (b) At follow-up 17 years on, the patient, aged 34 years, showed no apparent deterioration over the years and was leading an independent and comparatively active life. During the ensuing 10 years she has continued to be fairly stable in muscle function but has had several severe chest infections. (c) Her 8-year-old sister with a similar degree of disability died 2 years later of pneumonia. A brother had severe spinal muscular atrophy. He developed generalized weakness at 6 months, was never able to sit and died of pneumonia at 23 months. Autopsy confirmed the diagnosis of Werdnig–Hoffmann disease.

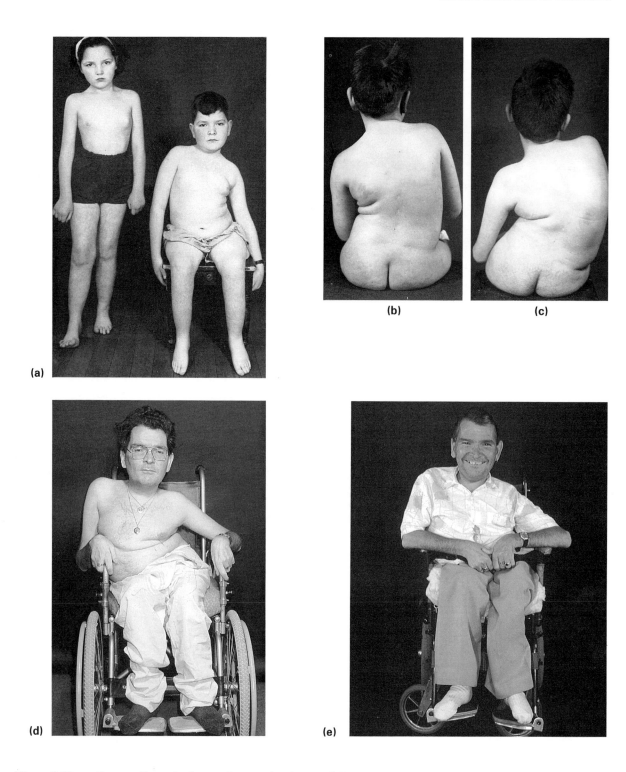

Figure 8-10a-e   Intermediate spinal muscular atrophy; 34-year follow-up. This 11-year-old boy (a) sat unsupported at 7 months but was never able to stand independently or to walk. He developed a scoliosis at an early age and this showed some progression over the years (b, 11 years; c, 15 years). His condition subsequently remained remarkably stable and he was still managing well, apart from recurrent bouts of pneumonia and some deterioration in respiratory function, when reviewed at 36 years (d) and recently at 45 years of age (e). His younger sister (a) was also affected and reluctant to stand in infancy, but following encouragement by her parents achieved independent ambulation and remained static throughout childhood. She subsequently lost ambulation in her early 20s during pregnancy.

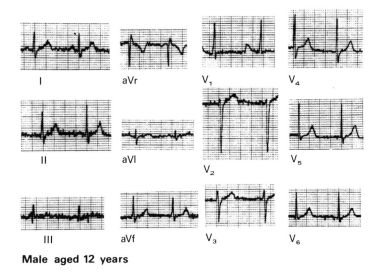

Male aged 12 years

Figure 8-11 Normal electrocardiogram of a 12-year-old boy with spinal muscular atrophy, showing the characteristic tremor of the baseline. (Compare ECG in muscular dystrophy, Figure 2-14.)

MILD SPINAL MUSCULAR ATROPHY (KUGELBERG–WELANDER DISEASE) (TYPE 3)

Into this category fall those patients who usually have normal milestones in the first year of life and subsequently achieve the ability to walk, either at a normal age or somewhat late, but then show evidence of mild weakness (Figure 8-12). Clinically they present in a similar fashion to a muscular dystrophy, with a waddling gait, difficulty in climbing steps, and getting up from the floor by the Gowers' manoeuvre (Figures 8-12, 8-13). Many subjects, however, get up from the floor with a different manoeuvre, not seen in Duchenne dystrophy, by going from a supine into a squatting position and rising straight from that position. They often walk 'flat-footed' with a tendency to eversion of the feet, in contrast to the tendency to toe-walking and equinovarus posture in Duchenne dystrophy. Weakness is mainly confined at that stage to the muscles of the pelvic girdle but the arms may be involved as well and a tremor of the hands is also a common feature. The reflexes may be normal or depressed.

The prognosis is good and these patients usually maintain ambulation over many years and may show little or no decline. In some cases, subjects show definite improvement in function, presumably as a result of compensatory reinnervation of the muscle. Active encouragement and physiotherapy may also have a beneficial effect on motor function in both the intermediate and mild groups. There is usually no associated respiratory deficit. These patients conform to the Kugelberg–Welander syndrome. Some who have remained relatively stable over several years may show an unexpected deterioration, with increasing difficulty in ambulation. This is in fact not due to any loss of muscle power but usually relates to a growth spurt, often between about 8 and 10 years of age. Loss of ambulation may also be precipitated by an incidental problem such as an injury, and even a fractured arm may at times tip the delicate balance from a stable and ambulant child to a non-ambulant one. Active supportive help is important under such circumstances to maintain ambulation. An increase in weight may also be a contributory factor in tipping the scales, with loss of ambulation.

PROGNOSIS/CLINICAL TYPES/ CLINICAL COMMON SENSE

There have been several reports in recent times of long-term survival into late childhood, adolescence or even early adult life of type 1 SMA (based on the international classification, with inability to sit unsupported). This has caused confusion and controversy and also introduced an element of false optimism for clinicians giving a prognosis in clinically severe cases. Some even went as far as to start telling parents that one could not predict whether the infant might survive 1 year or 20.

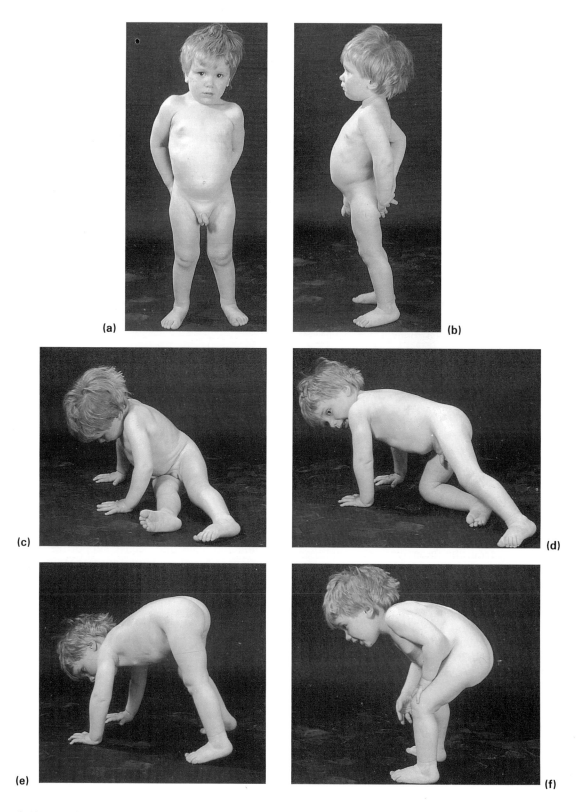

Figure 8-12a-f   Mild spinal muscular atrophy in (a,b) a 2-year-old boy with normal motor milestones and independent ambulation at 16 months. He had difficulty running and going up steps. Note lordotic posture (b), and Gowers' manoeuvre to get up from floor (c-f).

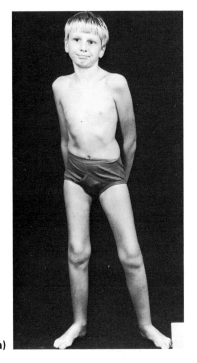 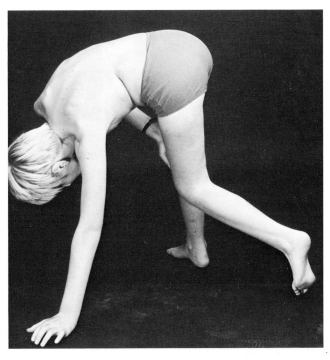

(a) **(b)**

Figure 8-13a,b Mild spinal muscular atrophy (Kugelberg–Welander) in (a) an 11-year-old boy with normal motor milestones and a history of walking at 18 months. There was proximal weakness of the pelvic girdle. He got up from the floor by Gowers' manoeuvre (b).

BORDERLINE CASES

Although it is usually easy to compartmentalize most cases of infantile spinal muscular atrophy into one of the above three categories, there are some cases which are borderline between severe and intermediate or between intermediate and mild. It is important to recognize these cases and to give a prognosis that is tailored to the functional status of the individual case, and not to a preconceived idea for the 'type' as a whole.

Some subjects may be overtly less severely affected than the typical severe form and may acquire some degree of head control and be able to raise the arms against gravity. However, they do not quite attain the intermediate category as they remain unable to sit unsupported (Figures 8-14, 8-15). Although they are prone to respiratory infections, they may yet survive beyond the first few years of life.

Similar severe cases with early onset and surviving 'against the odds' are illustrated in Figure 8-16. Much of the severe scoliosis deformity noted in such cases in the past should be preventable by adequate early spinal bracing, although it is difficult to completely stop the progression of the scoliosis.

As the enthusiasm for numerical classifications (types 1, 2, 3, etc.) rather than on descriptive clinical severity (severe, intermediate, mild) (which I personally prefer) seems well entrenched in many quarters of the medical fraternity, and has introduced an element of rigidity which does not readily reflect the variability within each type, I thought that one way around this might be to provide a concept of variability within each type by giving it a mathematical subdivision into first decimal (and strictly not beyond that) subdivisions, thus type 1.1 to 1.9, type 2.1 to 2.9, and type 3.1 to 3.9, with 4.0 representing normality (Table 8-2) (Dubowitz, 1995).

Table 8-2

Type 1:	Severe (variable):	Type 1.1 to 1.9
Type 2:	Intermediate (variable):	Type 2.1 to 2.9
Type 3:	Mild (variable):	Type 3.1 to 3.9
	(continuum)	
	Type 4.0 = Normal	

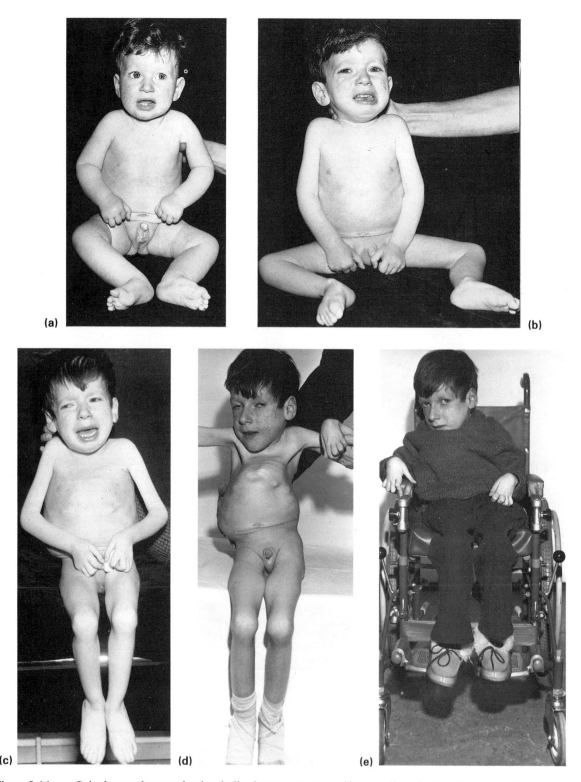

Figure 8-14a-e Spinal muscular atrophy, borderline between severe and intermediate, in (a) a 10-month-old boy who was unable to sit without support. His general power at 10 months when first seen was much better than the severe spinal muscular atrophy group. He seems to have just fallen short of the intermediate group. Subsequently muscle power remained fairly static (b, 2 years; c, 5 years; d, e, 10 years). He had severe respiratory deficit with many bouts of pneumonia from which he persistently recovered, but subsequently died of pneumonia at 12 years.

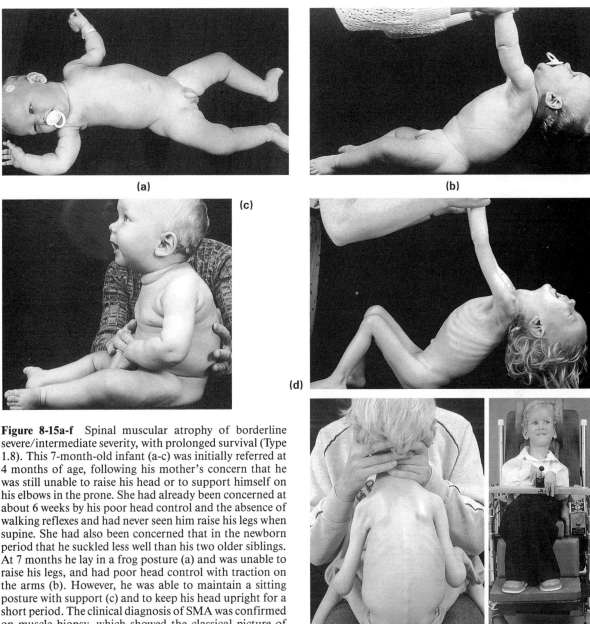

Figure 8-15a-f Spinal muscular atrophy of borderline severe/intermediate severity, with prolonged survival (Type 1.8). This 7-month-old infant (a-c) was initially referred at 4 months of age, following his mother's concern that he was still unable to raise his head or to support himself on his elbows in the prone. She had already been concerned at about 6 weeks by his poor head control and the absence of walking reflexes and had never seen him raise his legs when supine. She had also been concerned that in the newborn period that he suckled less well than his two older siblings. At 7 months he lay in a frog posture (a) and was unable to raise his legs, and had poor head control with traction on the arms (b). However, he was able to maintain a sitting posture with support (c) and to keep his head upright for a short period. The clinical diagnosis of SMA was confirmed on muscle biopsy, which showed the classical picture of large group atrophy. He had severe pneumonia at 10 months, needing a week's treatment in hospital and at 15 months had measles, followed by another bout of pneumonia and was critically ill. He was successfully treated without ventilator support on both occasions. After the second illness he lost a considerable amount of weight which he never regained, and also lost some muscle power, particularly in his head control (d). The muscle function subsequently remained fairly stable. Breathing was predominantly diaphragmatic. He had recurrent bouts of pneumonia, necessitating hospital treatment, every few weeks and had a number of respiratory arrests, from which his mother resuscitated him, and also two episodes of cardiac arrest. At 2 years he also had a spontaneous pneumothorax with collapse of the right lung, which never fully re-expanded again. He was provided with a plastizote jacket to support his back but could not tolerate this owing to constraints on his breathing. His head control and trunk support remained poor (d,e, aged 2 years) but with careful posturing his back remained remarkably straight. He had remarkable intellect, with early and advanced speech and at 6 years was fully confident with a computer and was assimilating some of the mathematical and other lessons of his older sisters. He was provided with an electrical wheelchair, with supportive inserts to maintain his sitting posture and a specially adapted and sensitized central controlling knob (f). He was subsequently able to operate a turbo chair. He died at 6 years 3 months, and a few days earlier had a remarkable premonition and told his mother he was going to die and wanted to be taken to the hospital, despite his chest being clear at the time.

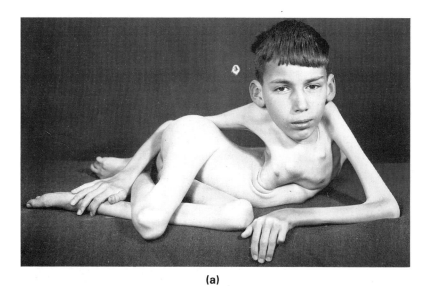

(a)

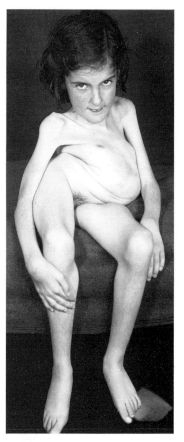

(b)

Figure 8-16a,b Two further cases (seen in the 1950s) of borderline severe/intermediate spinal muscular atrophy in patients who survived till 8 and 10 years respectively. Note the normal facies and the disastrously progressive scoliosis, resulting partly from no active intervention to try and prevent it at an early stage.

One can thus visualize that type 1.1 or 1.2 represents the severe end of the spectrum *within* the severe type 1 group, usually with early onset of severe weakness and hypotonia, plus severe intercostal muscle weakness and also bulbar involvement. The prognosis in this subgroup will be proportionately worse and many subjects may die within the first year of life, and indeed even within the first months. At the other end of the type 1 group are the type 1.8 and 1.9 patients, who are almost within the type 2 group but not quite, because they are unable to sit unsupported, although almost there, and certainly have better head control and respiratory function than the type 1.1 to 1.3 subjects. These are the cases that I have previously classed as straddling the arbitrary demarcation line between type 1 and type 2, and are accordingly the type 1 subjects with a predictably better outlook and longer survival (Figures 8-14, 8-15).

Similarly with group 2, there are the type 2.1 and 2.2 subjects, who are just able to sit unsupported but are very floppy and may have poor head control and marked weakness of the legs and not able to take any weight, whereas at the other end of the scale are the type 2.8 and 2.9 subjects who can take good weight on their legs and stand with support but are not quite able to stand independently (Figures 8-17, 8-18). Likewise, within the mild group are those subjects (type 3.1, 3.2) who have just made it into this group with ability to stand independently, but only just, and who can walk independently but are very limited (Figure 8-19). These are the ones who are likely to

lose ambulation very readily with any additional compromising factor, such as a growth spurt, a gain in weight or a minor injury. At the other end of this group the type 3.9 subjects are practically normal and present with good ambulation and only a modest disability, such as difficulty with running or going up steps, and are thus likely to have a much more active life. The degree of respiratory muscle weakness within these groups is also variable, particularly within the type 2, and may not necessarily correlate directly with the extent of skeletal muscle weakness.

In contrast to the general tendency of the disease to remain relatively static, in all grades of severity, a few cases do show a definite progression of disability. Many of these may relate to a change in other factors such as body dimensions, length and weight, associated with a growth spurt, rather than any change in muscle power as such. Thus children who are ambulant, either independently (type 3) or with orthoses (types 2.7 to 2.9 say) may lose their ambulation as a result of such extraneous factors (Figures 8-20, 8-21). Occasional cases, in contrast, may show an actual deterioration in power and a corresponding loss of function (Figure 8-22), but this seems to be the exception rather than the rule.

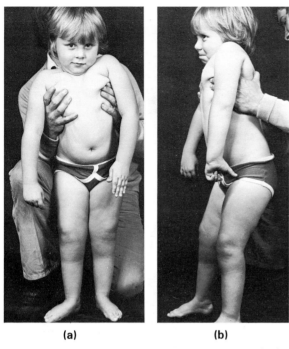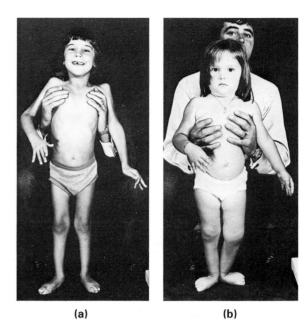

(a) **(b)**

Figure 8-17a,b Intermediate spinal muscular atrophy in a 5-year-old boy who was almost, but not quite able to stand without support (type 2.9).

(a) **(b)**

Figure 8-18a,b Intermediate spinal muscular atrophy in a 6-year-old boy (a) taking good weight on his legs (type 2.9), whereas his sister (b), aged 3 years, had much more difficulty (type 2.7).

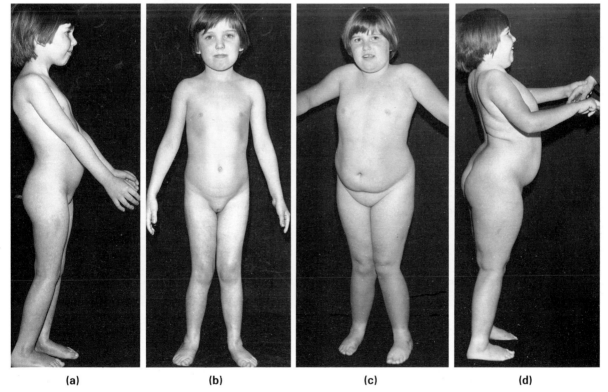

(a) **(b)** **(c)** **(d)**

Figure 8-19a-d Mild spinal muscular atrophy in a 6-year-old girl with good ambulation (a,b). The same child aged 9 years (c,d) showed marked obesity and difficulty standing without support.

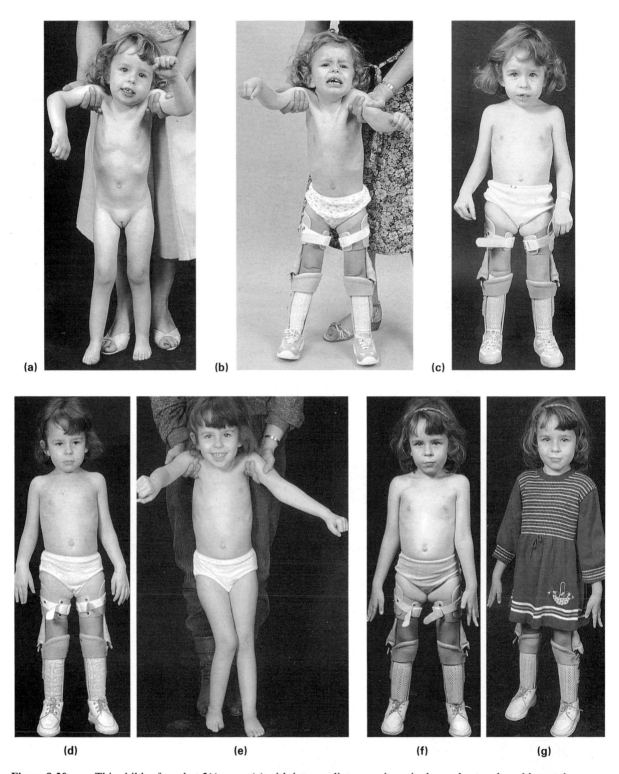

Figure 8-20a-n   This child referred at 2½ years (a) with intermediate severity spinal muscle atrophy, able to take some weight on the legs but unable to stand independently or with support (type 2.7). She was stabilized in knee–ankle–foot orthoses (b) and achieved independent ambulation, which she maintained through the ensuing years, although still unable to stand without callipers (c, 3½ years; d,e, 4½ years; f,g, 5 years; h, 6 years). At 8 years she had a growth spurt and had increasing difficulties, put on weight, and became chairbound (i,j,k,l) and also developed an incipient scoliosis (k). This was subsequently treated at 13 years with Luque spinal fixation (m,n).

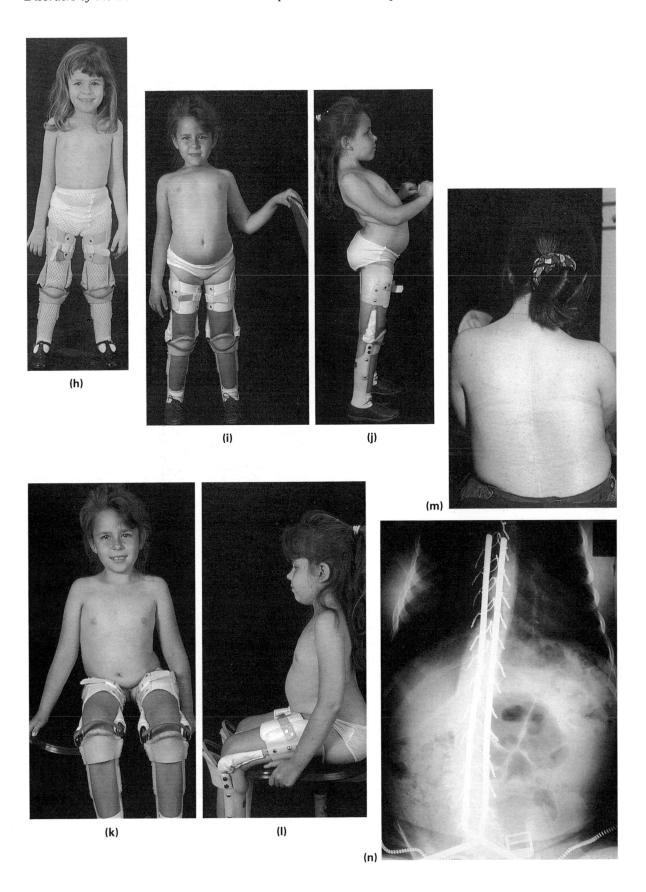

(h)

(i)　　　　(j)

(m)

(k)　　　　(l)

(n)

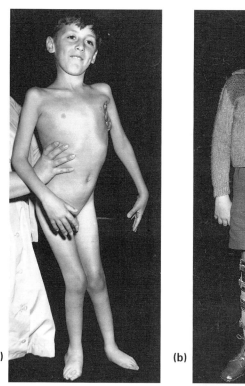
(a)

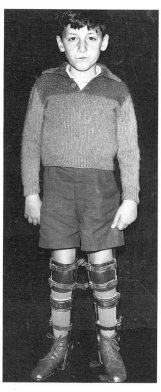
(b)

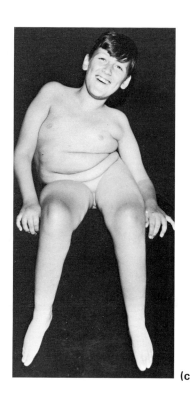
(c)

(d)

Figure 8-21a-d Intermediate spinal muscular atrophy in an 8-year-old boy (a) unable to stand without support, who achieved independent ambulation with traditional heavy-weight callipers (b). He subsequently became reluctant to wear his callipers, lost the ability to walk at 11 years and (c) developed a rapidly progressive scoliosis. It is difficult to assess whether the reluctance to walk was volitional or due to a genuine fall-off in muscle function, perhaps related to his growth spurt, as he was not seen at the time. A recent review (d), at age 26 years showed that he had been remarkably stable in muscle power, had recently married and had been free of respiratory problems.

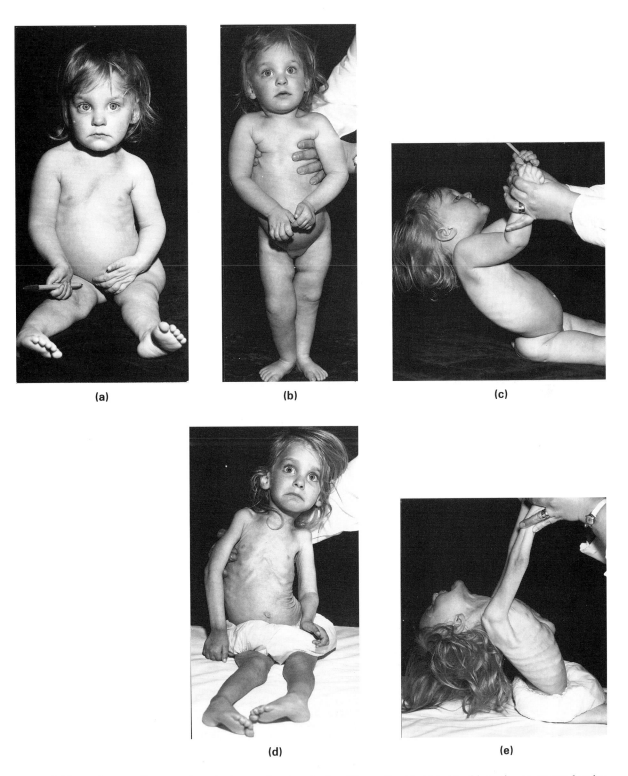

Figure 8-22a-e   Intermediate severity spinal muscular atrophy in a 20-month-old girl (a,b), able to sit unsupported and to stand with support. Note early scoliosis (a) and reasonable head control (c). In the course of the next year she had recurrent respiratory infections and showed a marked decline in her general health. At 2 years 10 months (d,e) she was no longer able to sit unsupported and had much poorer head control. This is a most unusual and exceptional degree of deterioration for an intermediate spinal muscular atrophy. Possibly the recurrent infections and the ensuing nutritional effects may have been important in the loss of muscle function, rather than any primary change in the disease process itself.

SPECIAL INVESTIGATIONS

Serum enzymes

Creatine kinase (CK) is invariably normal in the severe infantile spinal muscular atrophy. However, it is occasionally elevated in the milder forms with intermediate severity and more frequently shows some elevation in the Kugelberg–Welander syndrome. This elevation is usually slight or moderate but at times may be quite marked (up to tenfold or more). A normal CK in a mild case thus supports the evidence for a spinal muscular atrophy, against a limb girdle dystrophy, but a mildly or moderately raised CK does not exclude the disease. Higher levels are more suggestive of dystrophy.

Ultrasound imaging

This is a very useful screening tool and in our clinic has now largely replaced electromyography. In spinal muscular atrophy there is a characteristic picture of increased echo in the muscle, together with loss of muscle bulk, so that the diameter of the muscle is less than half the distance from the skin to the bone (see Figure 8-23).

Electromyography

This is a very useful diagnostic tool and in experi-

enced hands can usually provide evidence of a neurogenic atrophy associated with anterior horn cell degeneration to support the clinical diagnosis (Figures 8-24 and 8-25). In the case of small infants where voluntary co-operation cannot be expected, experience with handling infants is helpful in obtaining satisfactory results.

Motor nerve conduction is usually said to be normal in spinal muscular atrophy (Munsat *et al.*, 1969; Hausmanowa-Petrusewicz, 1970). In an extensive study of motor nerve conduction velocity in the ulnar and posterior tibial nerves Moosa and Dubowitz (1976) observed that the velocity is frequently slow in the most severe cases but tends to be normal in the milder forms. One technical problem is that the motor response in some cases, especially the severe ones, may be so small that it is difficult to make any measurement at all. These results would imply a selective loss of the fastest motor units in the severe form of the disease.

Muscle biopsy

Although the diagnosis may be reasonably certain on clinical, ultrasound or electromyographic grounds, it is always worth performing a biopsy for additional confirmation, since a number of conditions can closely mimic spinal muscular atrophy and may even show a denervation picture on EMG.

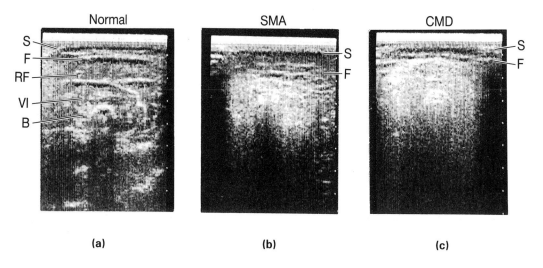

Figure 8-23a-c Ultrasound imaging, showing a transverse scan of the thigh in a normal child (a), a 2-year-old child with intermediate spinal muscular atrophy (b), and a 2-year-old with congenital muscular dystrophy (c). Note the relatively echo-free rectus femoris (RF) and vastus intermedius (VI) muscles in the normal and the marked increase in echo in both the spinal atrophy and congenital muscular dystrophy, with loss of distinction between the muscle, and also loss of the bone echo from the femur (B). In addition, there is atrophy of the muscle in spinal muscular atrophy, with increase in the distance between the skin (S) and fascia (F), in comparison with the normal or congenital muscular dystrophy muscle.

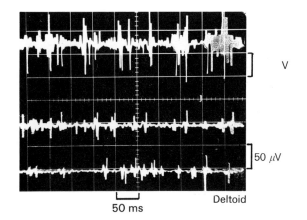

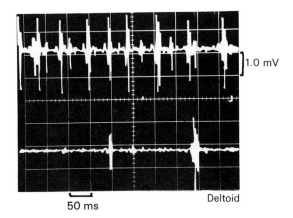

Figure 8-24 Concentric needle EMG of 7-month-old infant with severe spinal muscular atrophy. Top trace shows reduced interference pattern on activity. Motor units of normal amplitude. Lower trace shows small spontaneous fibrillation potentials at rest, usually at a frequency of 5–15 per second. This is characteristic of severe spinal muscular atrophy.

Figure 8-25 Concentric needle EMG of 5-year-old child with mild spinal muscular atrophy. Upper trace shows reduced interference pattern with discrete large polyphasic potentials. Lower trace shows spontaneous large polyphasic potentials at rest, characteristic of chronic anterior horn cell disease.

The muscle should be adequately processed for a full range of histological and histochemical techniques (Dubowitz and Brooke, 1973; Dubowitz, 1985) (see Chapter 1). The basic histological pattern is very similar in the severe and intermediate forms of spinal muscular atrophy and it is, indeed, quite impossible to make any judgement on the severity of the condition or the prognosis from the biopsy picture (Figures 8-26 to 8-36).

Atrophic fibres are a consistent feature of all biopsies in spinal muscular atrophy, and involve both type 1 and type 2 muscle fibres. Unlike other neurogenic atrophies, such as peripheral neuropathies, the atrophic fibres in SMA tend to be rounded in outline, are usually clustered in large groups, often whole bundles, and are interspersed with fascicles containing clusters of markedly hypertrophied fibres which may be three to four times the normal size for the patient's age (Figures 8-26 to 8-28). Whereas the atrophic fibres are usually a mixture histochemically of type 1 and type 2 fibres, as in the normal, the hypertrophic fibres tend to show complete uniformity of type 1 fibres, suggesting they are reinnervated fibres rather than unaffected normal fibres which would presumably have a mixed chequerboard of light- and dark-staining fibres (Figures 8-26 to 8-31). As these clusters of large type 1 fibres suggest a compensatory reinnervation process, it follows that extensive areas of such fibres might suggest a better outlook, but once again the degree of pathological change does not correlate accurately with clinical severity. One may see the identical pattern of large group atrophy with small

clusters of large type 1 fibres in cases both of severe SMA and intermediate SMA. Moreover, different areas of the same muscle may show different proportions of the large fibres.

The nuclei are usually in their normal peripheral location in the large fibres as well as in the atrophic ones. When the fibres become very markedly atrophic their nuclei may cluster together into pyknotic nuclear clumps.

Degenerative changes in the fibres are not a feature of severe spinal muscular atrophy, but the milder, more chronic forms may show so-called myopathic changes in the fibres (Figure 8-35). Core or target fibres are also found in the chronic denervations. Muscle spindles are often a striking feature of these biopsies; they may possibly appear conspicuous owing to the atrophy of the extrafusal fibres, but they do at times also seem increased in number and as many as ten or more may be seen in a single transverse section.

In a number of cases of severe spinal muscular atrophy that we biopsied within a few weeks of onset of weakness, the muscle has not shown the classical picture but a universal atrophy of all fibres, with a tendency for type 1 fibres to be more atrophic than the type 2 (see Figure 8-32). This 'pre-pathological' picture is probably the result of universal atrophy from severe denervation, but can be difficult to distinguish from hypoplasia of the muscle from other causes and may possibly be confused with congenital fibre type disproportion (see Chapter 3). Later biopsy or autopsy in such infants shows a classical picture in the muscle (see Figure 8-32e).

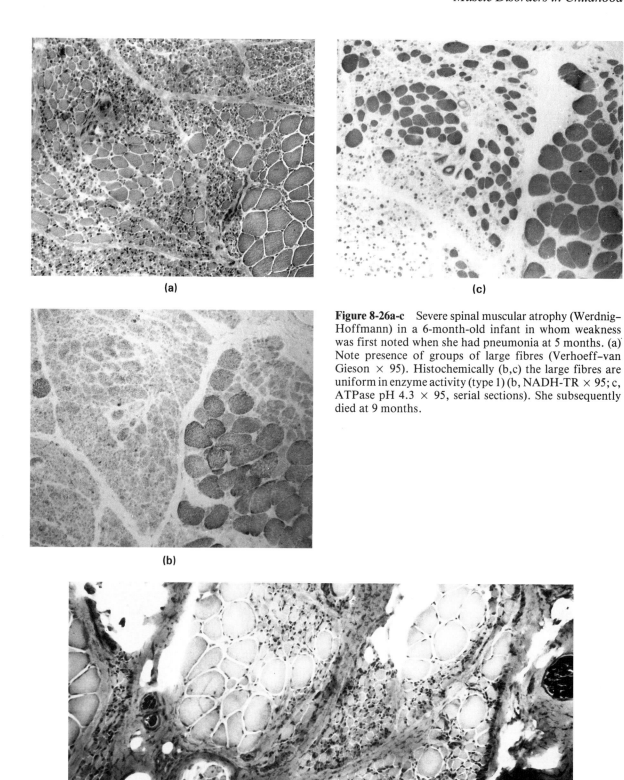

(a)

(c)

(b)

Figure 8-26a-c   Severe spinal muscular atrophy (Werdnig–Hoffmann) in a 6-month-old infant in whom weakness was first noted when she had pneumonia at 5 months. (a) Note presence of groups of large fibres (Verhoeff–van Gieson × 95). Histochemically (b,c) the large fibres are uniform in enzyme activity (type 1) (b, NADH-TR × 95; c, ATPase pH 4.3 × 95, serial sections). She subsequently died at 9 months.

Figure 8-27   Spinal muscular atrophy of intermediate severity, in a 2-year-old infant, showing large group atrophy and an unusual degree of connective tissue (dark area) and adipose tissue (clear area) proliferation (Verhoeff–van Gieson × 120).

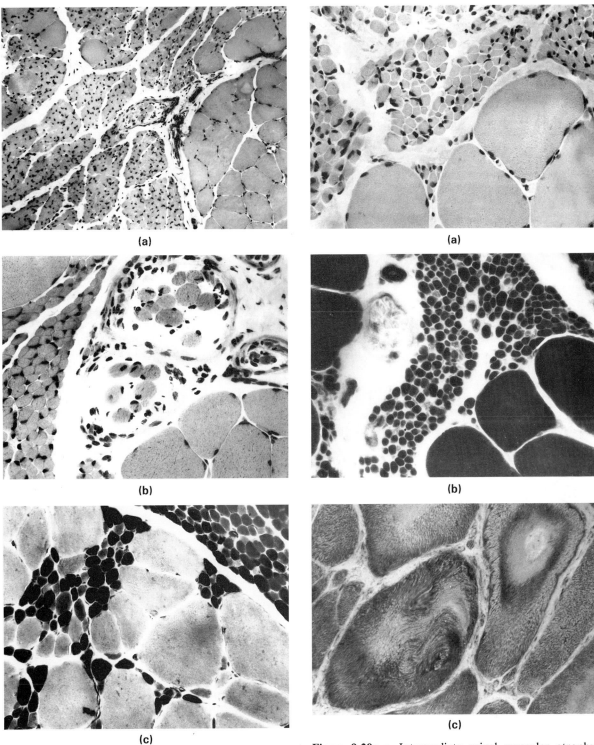

Figure 8-28a-c Spinal muscular atrophy of intermediate severity, in a 20-month-old infant. (a) Note the uniform atrophy of whole bundles of fibres (H & E × 90). (b) Atrophic fibres are smaller than intrafusal fibres of muscle spindles (H & E × 240). (c) Histochemically the large fibres show uniform activity compatible with type 1 fibres (ATPase pH 9.4 × 240).

Figure 8.29a-c Intermediate spinal muscular atrophy (almost mild), in a 2-year-old infant. Biopsy shows (a) large group atrophy comparable with severe cases (H & E × 190). (b) Large fibres uniform in enzyme type (ATPase pH 9.4 × 190). (c) Some of the large fibres show bizarre architectural changes such as whorling and cores (targets) (NADH-TR × 190). Subsequently the patient was able to walk with callipers.

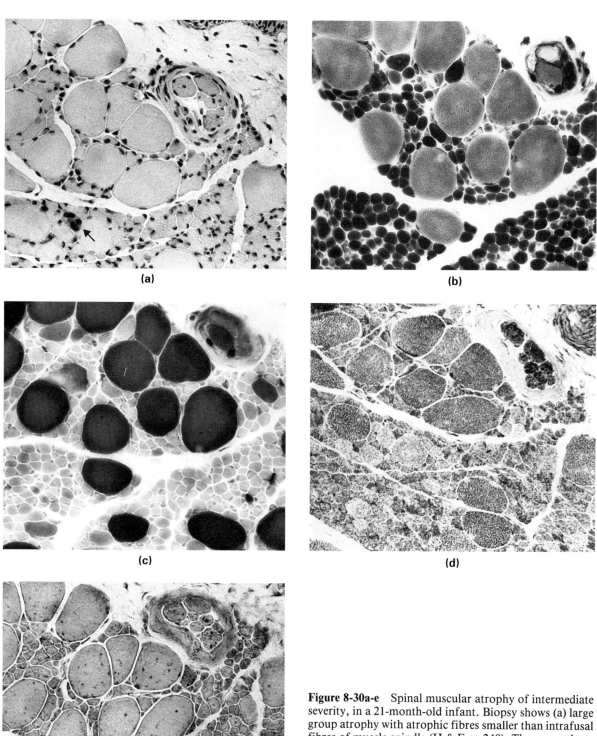

(a)

(b)

(c)

(d)

(e)

Figure 8-30a-e Spinal muscular atrophy of intermediate severity, in a 21-month-old infant. Biopsy shows (a) large group atrophy with atrophic fibres smaller than intrafusal fibres of muscle spindle (H & E × 240). There was also a number of unusual multinucleate fibres with very large nuclei in the section. See (a), arrow. Histochemically (b,c,d) the large fibres were of one type, conforming to type 1, but showing some variation of oxidative activity (serial sections) (b, ATPase pH 9.4 × 240; c, ATPase 4.3 × 240; d, NADH-TR × 240). (e) The atrophic fibres show high acid phosphatase activity, as do the muscle spindle fibres (acid phosphatase × 240).

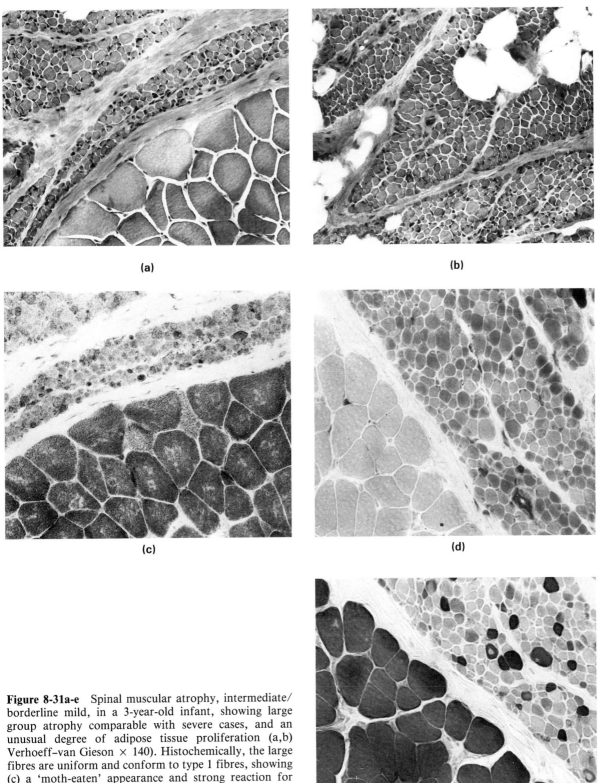

Figure 8-31a-e Spinal muscular atrophy, intermediate/borderline mild, in a 3-year-old infant, showing large group atrophy comparable with severe cases, and an unusual degree of adipose tissue proliferation (a,b) Verhoeff–van Gieson × 140). Histochemically, the large fibres are uniform and conform to type 1 fibres, showing (c) a 'moth-eaten' appearance and strong reaction for oxidative enzymes (NADH-TR × 140), (d) a weak activity for standard ATPase (ATPase pH 9.4 × 225) and (e) a strong activity for ATPase at pH 4.3 (ATPase 4.3 × 225), serial section to (d).

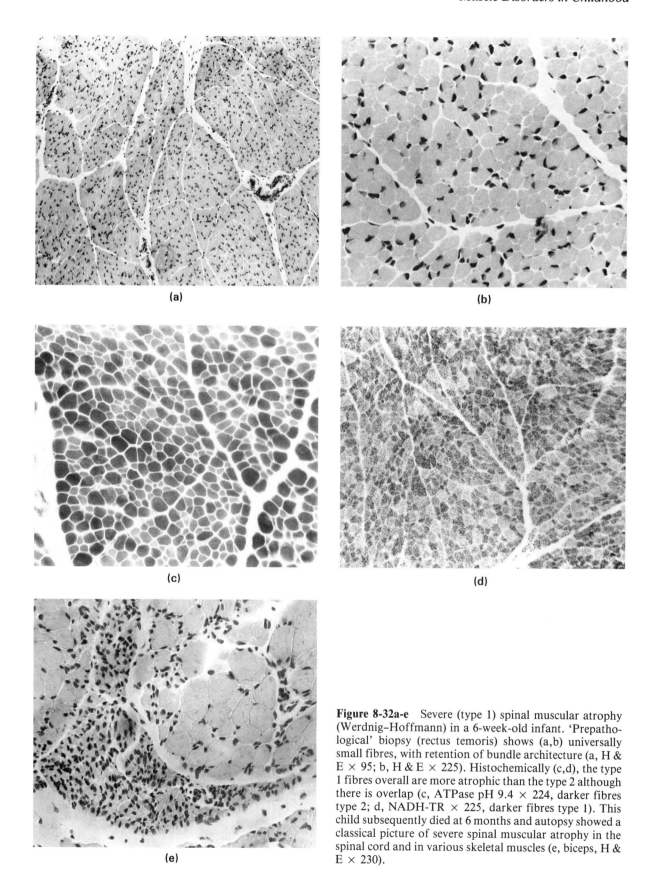

(a)

(b)

(c)

(d)

(e)

Figure 8-32a-e Severe (type 1) spinal muscular atrophy (Werdnig–Hoffmann) in a 6-week-old infant. 'Prepathological' biopsy (rectus temoris) shows (a,b) universally small fibres, with retention of bundle architecture (a, H & E × 95; b, H & E × 225). Histochemically (c,d), the type 1 fibres overall are more atrophic than the type 2 although there is overlap (c, ATPase pH 9.4 × 224, darker fibres type 2; d, NADH-TR × 225, darker fibres type 1). This child subsequently died at 6 months and autopsy showed a classical picture of severe spinal muscular atrophy in the spinal cord and in various skeletal muscles (e, biceps, H & E × 230).

The milder (Kugelberg–Welander) variety shows a number of slight differences in histological pattern. Group atrophy is still a consistent feature but takes the form of small groups rather than large groups (see Figures 8-33, 8-34). The non-atrophic large fibres frequently show fibre type grouping, and type 2 fibre predominance is also a common feature. Architectural changes within the fibres are common and take the form of central cores, target fibres and moth-eaten, whorled fibres or coil fibres. Fibres with internal nuclei and isolated fibres undergoing splitting or degeneration may also occur (see Figure 8-35). A number of early authors highlighted these 'myopathic' changes in the muscle in chronic spinal atrophy and caused much confusion in the classification of clinical cases and led some authors to dismiss entirely the existence of limb girdle muscular dystrophy or to erroneously diagnose spinal muscular atrophy in the face of dystrophic disorders such as Becker dystrophy or facioscapulohumeral dystrophy, purely on the basis of focal clusters of atrophic fibres in the presence of an otherwise dystrophic muscle – a patent example of missing the wood for the trees. In general there is no difficulty in categorizing a biopsy in one or other of these two categories (Dubowitz and Brooke, 1973; Dubowitz, 1985), and in the few cases that are difficult the distinction will probably be possible in future on the basis of the molecular genetic mutations or specific protein changes at tissue level in relation to either a muscular dystrophy or a spinal muscular atrophy, and adults with a longstanding, relatively benign, chronic weakness.

Neuropathology

The essential changes are in the anterior horn cells at all levels of the spinal cord and in the motor nuclei of the V–XIIth cranial nerves. There is striking loss of the large anterior horn cells and many of the remaining cells show varying degrees of degenerative change, with alteration in shape, eccentric nucleus and chromatolysis (see Figure 8-36). Some cells are ballooned out whereas others are pyknotic and shrunken. There is associated neurophagia and gliosis. Although there have been reports from time to time of changes in other parts of the nervous system, Byers and Banker (1961), in their careful study of a number of autopsy cases, ascribed the changes present in the cerebrum and cerebellum to terminal anoxia and found no abnormality in the long tracts of the cord or the cells of the intermediolateral column, Clarke's column or the posterior column. Other cases of mixed central nervous system involvement have usually been atypical cases and presumably separate disorders (see below).

While there are many documentations of cases of severe infantile muscular atrophy, the reports on the central nervous system in Kugelberg–Welander disease have been relatively few, owing to the good prognosis, but have shown the typical degenerative changes in the anterior horn cells (Kohn, 1968; Kennedy et al., 1968).

GENETICS

All the forms of spinal muscular atrophy have an hereditary basis. In the severe form, as well as the milder forms, the pattern of inheritance has usually been autosomal recessive, with the characteristic appearance of multiple cases in a sibship, a previously negative family history and a high incidence of consanguinity (Brandt, 1950). Within a family, concordance has been the rule and there have also been reports of similarly affected identical twins (Brandt, 1950; Zellweger et al., 1969). However, one of the unusual features has been the occasional occurrence of cases of varying severity within an affected sibship so that individual cases would fall into different clinical categories (Dubowitz, 1964a; Amick et al., 1966; Dunne and Chutorian, 1966; Hausmanowa-Petrusewicz et al., 1966; Gamstorp, 1967; Rowland et al., 1967; Munsat et al., 1969; Hausmanowa-Petrusewicz, 1970; Zellweger, 1971) (see Figures 8-9 and 8-10). This has been one of the supportive arguments in favour of a single genetic basis for the various clinical subtypes of spinal muscular atrophy, but could also be explained on the basis of multiple alleles.

The heterozygotes do not show any clinical manifestation of the disease, and no abnormality has been found on EMG or muscle biopsy to help in detecting the heterozygote carriers.

Apart from the usual autosomal recessive mechanism that appears to operate in most cases there were a number of reports in the 1960s of spinal muscular atrophy with dominant inheritance. These have usually been a milder disease, resembling the Kugelberg–Welander syndrome, with late onset and ability to walk. A number had atypical features such as more distal or diffuse weakness, or associated bulbar involvement, and may well be examples of hereditary motor neuropathy (see Chapter 9).

From a genetic counselling point of view one can, with the exception of the isolated mild dominant cases, give advice appropriate to an autosomal recessive inheritance with a 1:4 risk of recurrence. As a rule there is concordance of severity within a family but, on occasion, a family may show a severe case with early death, as well as a mild case with survival into adolescence (see Figure 8-9).

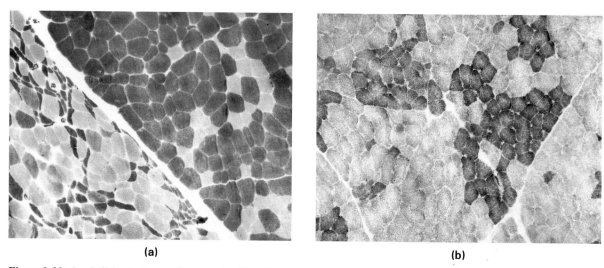

(a)　　　　　　　　　　　　　　　　　　　**(b)**

Figure 8-33a,b　Mild spinal muscular atrophy (Kugelberg–Welander) in an 8½-year-old child. The biopsy was reasonably normal looking with routine stains but showed some focal atrophy and also fibre type grouping of the normal looking fibres, indicative of a denervation/reinnervation process (a, ATPase pH 9.4 × 85; b, NADH-TR × 85).

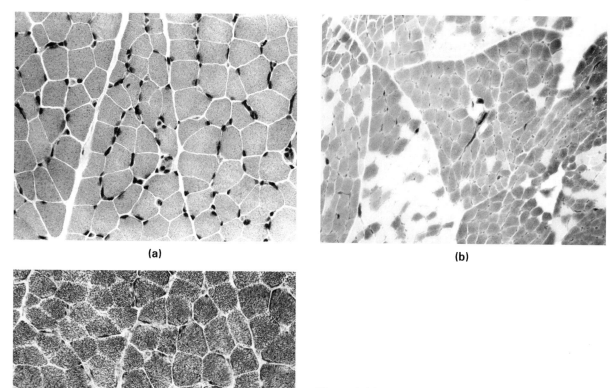

(a)　　　　　　　　　　　　　　　　　　　**(b)**

(c)

Figure 8-34a-c　Spinal muscular atrophy, mild/border-line intermediate in a 5-year-old child, who was ambulant but who later required callipers after elongation procedures for flexion contractures of hip and knees and shortening of tendo Achillis. Biopsy of rectus femoris shows (a) normal looking muscle apart from isolated atrophic fibres (H & E × 240). Histochemically (b,c), there is fibre type grouping, with large clusters of fibres of uniform fibre type (b, ATPase pH 4.3 × 90; c, NADH-TR × 225).

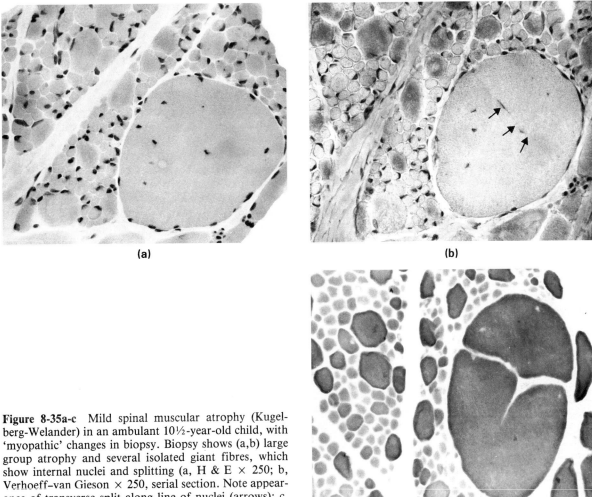

(a)

(b)

(c)

Figure 8-35a-c Mild spinal muscular atrophy (Kugelberg-Welander) in an ambulant 10½-year-old child, with 'myopathic' changes in biopsy. Biopsy shows (a,b) large group atrophy and several isolated giant fibres, which show internal nuclei and splitting (a, H & E × 250; b, Verhoeff–van Gieson × 250, serial section. Note appearance of transverse split along line of nuclei (arrows); c, ATPase pH 4.6 × 250 showing cleavage of fibre along line of splits).

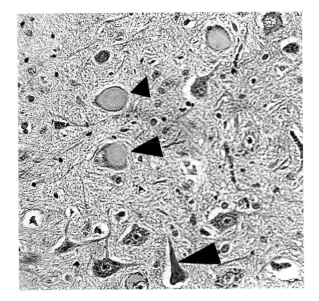

Figure 8-36 Severe spinal muscular atrophy showing degenerative changes in the nerve cells of the hypoglossal nucleus (H & E stain). Some nerve cells are ballooned and amorphous, others pyknotic and shrunken (arrows).

MOLECULAR GENETICS ————————

Another of the major contributions of the new genetics has been the location of the gene for the childhood spinal muscular atrophies and the demonstration that there is a single gene responsible for all the different phenotypes of varying severity, which are thus allelic, comparable with the Duchenne/Becker gene. This vindicates the views of the 'lumpers'.

The initial search for the gene for the SMAs of infancy and childhood was clouded by two major problems. In the severe infantile form the prognosis was so poor that cases rarely survived beyond the first year or two of life so it was difficult to find families with two living children, the minimum required for mapping a recessive disorder. In the milder clinical phenotypes, families were certainly available with multiple affected children, but the clinical picture was much more heterogeneous and, as there was still conflict of opinion as to whether

one was dealing with a single genetic disorder, there was the added problem of possible genetic heterogeneity. In the event, the gene location was established on the basis of seven large families with the mild or intermediate phenotype, each with three or four affected children (Brzustowicz *et al.*, 1990). With the use of eight DNA markers, spanning about 30 centimorgan, they were able to establish a gene locus at 5q11.2-13.3. The available data in this collaborative Anglo-American study suggested that the severe form of SMA was probably also at the 5q location, on the basis of DNA from five families with two affected siblings and one family with three, but the Lod score did not reach significance on this limited material. Confirmation of this came soon after from an application of the technique of homozygosity mapping in four consanguineous families with severe SMA (Gilliam *et al.*, 1990), including one large inbred family that we had documented through five generations and personally examined all the affected siblings as well as an affected cousin who had previously died (Figure 8-37).

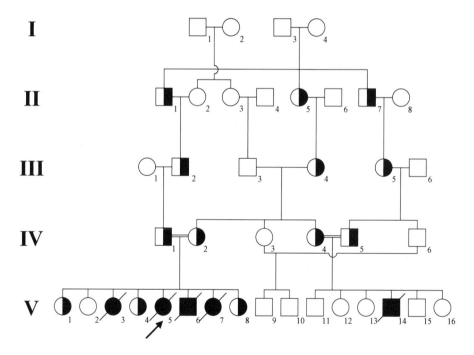

Figure 8-37 Pedigree chart of consanguineous family with severe spinal muscular atrophy. The index case (V,5) as well as 2 subsequently affected siblings (V,6,7) were personally examined, as was a previously affected cousin seen some years earlier (V,14). All had classical severe (type 1) spinal muscular atrophy and died during their second year, as did a previously affected sibling (V,3). Note the two consanguinity loops in this family affecting the couples IV, 1 and 2, and IV, 4 and 5. The mutant gene can be traced back through five generations of this family to one or other of the individuals I,3 or I,4. An additional female infant (V,8) was recently born at term and caused some anxiety because of respiratory distress and associated hypotonia. I had the opportunity of examining her within 24 hours of birth and thought she was probably unaffected because of antigravity power in the legs. I had never seen an infant with severe spinal muscular atrophy and respiratory deficit in the absence of limb weakness. Her respiratory symptoms subsided within a week and DNA linkage studies showed that she had a different haplotype to her previously affected siblings.

In an independent study by a French group, the gene location on 5q was confirmed, with close linkage to a single DNA marker D5S39, in 16 multiplex families with type 2 SMA and eight with type 3, each family having two affected siblings (Melki *et al.*, 1990a). Melki's group were subsequently able to show linkage to the same marker in a study of 25 families with type 1 SMA, all but one family having only a single affected case available plus normal siblings (Melki *et al.*, 1990b). They concluded that the three forms of SMA, separated clinically on the basis of age of onset and clinical course, were probably due to different mutations at a single locus on chromosome 5.

In a subsequent study of four sibships in which there was occurrence of both type 2 and type 3 SMA, Muller *et al.* (1992) found no evidence for multiple alleles to account for the differences in phenotype and concluded that the variation in severity might be due to other factors, genetic or environmental. This seemed to lay to rest Becker's somewhat complex, multi-allelic hypothesis.

Current research in a number of key laboratories of the international consortium is closing in on the gene itself, which should be isolated and cloned before long, given the power of current molecular genetic techniques (Munsat and Davies, 1992).

These laboratories have focussed on further refining the exact locus of SMA in relation to the nearest linked probes, and to identifying recombinants in informative families. Deletions have recently been identified in this region that may involve the SMA gene (Lefebvre *et al.*, 1995; Roy *et al.*, 1995).

Antenatal diagnosis

Closely-linked DNA markers can already be used for prenatal diagnosis. In families where the index case may no longer be alive and blood for DNA analysis had not been stored, the test could be done on Guthrie blood spots that might have been retained, or on other tissues such as muscle biopsy or even fixed autopsy material.

The closely linked probes will also continue to provide further data on possible families not conforming to a 5q location. It currently looks as if all classical cases, using strict diagnostic criteria, do conform to a 5q locus and in our own pooled molecular data on personal cases and a comparable cohort from Finland there have been no cases supporting genetic heterogeneity. However, Gilliam's group (Brzustowicz *et al.*, 1993) have still found some evidence for genetic heterogeneity in their review of 38 families, and only time will tell, once the gene is fully characterized, whether these families represent an alternative locus for a classical SMA or clinical misdiagnosis of a different neurogenic syndrome.

These probes can also be used to exclude 5q linkage in cases with other disorders associated with anterior horn cell disease (see below).

AETIOLOGY AND PATHOGENESIS ————

Apart from the genetic basis, the underlying cause and pathogenesis of the disease remain obscure. Whatever the mechanism, one has to explain the unusual nature of the disease in which a previously completely normal and active infant becomes severely paralysed over a relatively short period of time, and then remains fairly static. Either the process is a slowly developing one since embryonic life and reaches a point where a critical individual mass of nerve cells is unable to function adequately, or there is a process where some event, either prenatally determined or due to an additional environmental factor, suddenly becomes manifest. The picture is not unlike those inborn errors of metabolism with a complete deficiency of an enzyme which may not manifest until after a variable latent period, e.g. type 2 glycogenosis with acid maltase deficiency.

A number of authors have commented on the apparent onset of symptoms following fairly acutely after some episode such as smallpox vaccination (Dubowitz, 1964a), diphtheria-pertussis immunization (Gardner-Medwin *et al.*, 1967; Meadows *et al.*, 1969), or miscellaneous infectious illnesses (Brandt, 1950; Munsat *et al.*, 1969). In other cases there has apparently been a sudden increase in pre-existing weakness following an acute infection (Munsat *et al.*, 1969) or measles (Gardner-Medwin *et al.*, 1967). However, it is always difficult to assess the significance of such a history, particularly in the context of a genetically determined disorder, and to distinguish between a causal relationship between the two events and a mere coincidence in time.

One hypothesis that has attracted attention involves the normal process of cell death. Cell death has traditionally been looked upon as a relatively passive process, in response to some environmental toxin or other pertubation, resulting in the disorganized disintegration of the cell (necrosis). In contrast to this mechanism, the process of a programmed cell death has in recent years aroused much interest, both amongst biologists in relation to the normal processes of development and the physiological elimination of unneeded cells, and amongst pathologists trying to explain the pathophysiology of various degenerative disorders. The somewhat pedantic term, 'apoptosis' has been coined to describe the morphological features of this patterned cell death (Kerr *et al.*, 1972; Wyllie, 1981) and a characteristic cleavage or 'laddering' in the DNA of the cell that has been recognized (Wyllie *et al.*, 1984). Much has been contributed to this knowledge from the study of lowly animals, such as nematodes and insects, and alternative mechanisms of programmed cell death, differing from apoptosis and dependent on 'cell death' genes, have been identified (Schwartz, 1991).

Another component of this biological cell death model is the possible importance of nerve growth factor and other trophic factors in the survival of neurones and also the role of the end-organ in this process (Martin *et al.*, 1988; Thoenen, 1991). In an interesting series of experiments, Oppenheim (1991) showed that in the chick embryo 50% of spinal neurones undergo naturally occurring cell death by day 6. By removing the target tissue (limb bud) all the motor neurones die, whereas by increasing the amount of target tissue by implantation, the number of surviving neurones can be increased. This supports the hypothesis that target-derived neurotrophic factors may be important in the process of cell death or survival.

Further studies in the neonatal rat have shown that preventing interaction of the developing neurone or its target muscle results in the death of a large proportion of motorneurones (Greensmith and Vrbová, 1992). Experiments have also been designed to try and replace lost motoneurones by embryonic spinal cord grafts (Sieradzan and Vrbová, 1989, 1991).

PROGNOSIS AND MANAGEMENT ————

Severe form (type 1)

In the congenital form, with weakness already present at birth there is often sucking and swallowing difficulty in the immediate newborn period, necessitating tube feeding. These children also have difficulty in swallowing their salivary secretions and may need frequent aspiration of the pharynx. It is often difficult for the parents to cope with these problems at home so an initial period of hospitalization is necessary until the extent of the problem can be fully assessed.

These patients are also prone to repeated respiratory infections, which accounts for the poor prognosis for survival. The very severe group with onset before birth and difficulties already in the neonatal period (type 1.1) usually do not survive their first birthday, irrespective of the intensity of supporting therapy. In general, the earlier the onset the more severe the phenotype, and a recent survey of our patients with severe SMA included in the genetic linkage study showed a more severe course in those with onset in the first 3 months compared with those

with onset between 3 and 6 months of age, who had a variable survival up to about 2 years (Thomas and Dubowitz, 1994) (Figure 8-38).

Because the diaphragm is spared and still functions well, it is able to compensate for the marked intercostal weakness; consequently these infants are usually able to cope at birth (or whenever the onset) without significant respiratory deficit, until they have a superadded infection that can rapidly precipitate them into respiratory failure. One has to be extremely cautious about the use of ventilator support. It can rarely be successful as a transitory procedure to tide the infant over a respiratory crisis, and once the infant is on ventilator support he usually becomes ventilator-dependent.

It is remarkable how consistent the prognosis is in relation to type 1 SMA. In the genetic linkage study of Melki *et al.* (1990b) there were 39 infants who had died; the mean age of death was 7.2 months with a range of 1–23 months, so that all had died by 2 years. Of the ten cases I reviewed for the first edition of my Floppy Infant monograph (Dubowitz, 1969b), eight had died at ages less than 12 months, one at 17 months and one was still alive at 15 months. Affected siblings had all died under 12 months. Of the 36 cases of type 1 SMA (onset under 6 months and inability to sit unsupported) included in our gene linkage study, mean age at death was 9.6 months, the median 7 months, and all but one died by 2 years of age. The one long-term survivor was in his teens and on clinical review conformed to a borderline type 1/type 2 case (type 1.8; see above). In an analysis of this cohort by age of onset of symptoms (at birth, 0–1 months, 1–2 months, 2–3 months and 3–6 months), with cumulative mortality graphs of the proportion who had died in relation to age of onset, there was a steeper slope for those with onset within the first 3 months compared with after 3 months (Thomas and Dubowitz, 1994) (Figure 8-38).

In response to a questionnaire, distributed by the Parents Support Group for SMA (Jennifer Trust), on cases of severe SMA conforming to the criteria of age of onset under 6 months and inability to sit unaided, but also having the associated severe paralysis of the trunk and legs and associated intercostal weakness, 78 were completed; seven had already been included in the previous genetic cohort, one was incomplete, and the remaining 70 showed a remarkable similarity to our earlier cohort in the cumulative mortality graphs in relation to age of onset, with an even closer consistency within the overall cohort. All patients had died by 2 years of age and over 80% by 1 year (Thomas and Dubowitz, 1994) (Figure 8-38). An almost identical graph was produced by Ignatius (1994) on analysis of the Finnish cohort of patients with Type 1 (severe) SMA included in his gene linkage study.

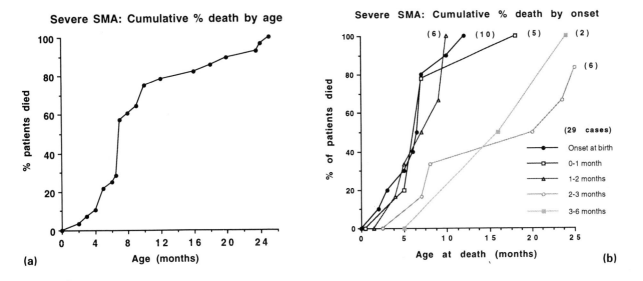

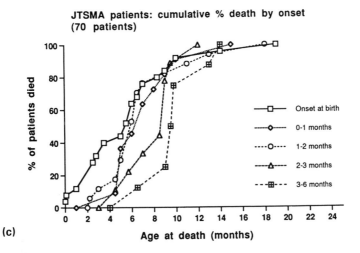

Figure 8-38a-c Prognosis in severe (type 1) spinal muscular atrophy. (a) Cumulative mortality for cohort of 29 cases from genetic linkage study. One patient who is still alive at 18 years has been excluded. He is of borderline to intermediate severity (type 1.9). In (b) the same data is subdivided by age of onset. (c) Corresponding data on a cohort of 70 cases obtained by questionnaire from the British parents support group for SMA (Jennifer Trust for SMA, JTSMA). From Thomas and Dubowitz (1994) with permission of *Neuromuscular Disorders*.

This data should prove extremely useful in relation to any future therapeutic trials in severe (type 1) SMA, where length of survival may be the most reliable index of benefit.

Intermediate form (type 2)

In these cases prolonged survival into adolescence is the rule. The ultimate prognosis is dependent on the degree of intercostal weakness and respiratory deficit. Many of these patients may remain free of respiratory complications. It is thus important to treat any respiratory infections that do occur intensively with antibiotics and physiotherapy.

The prevention of deformities. This is an important part of the management of these cases. Once these children achieve a sitting posture they are prone to develop scoliosis, which can be very rapidly progressive. In view of the variable severity within this intermediate group, some of these infants are more prone to severe scoliosis than others. This applies particularly to those infants at the more

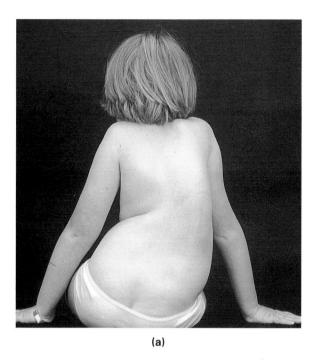
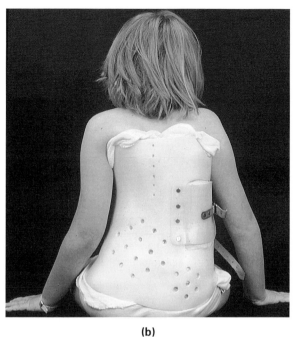

(a)   **(b)**

Figure 8-39a,b   Intermediate severity spinal muscular atrophy in an 8-year-old girl with polyethylene orthosis to try and prevent progression of scoliosis, which is commonly present at an early age and relentlessly progressive in these infants, particularly at the severe end of the intermediate spectrum (types 2.1 to 2.4).

severe end of the scale, who are just able to sit unsupported for short periods, but very floppy and unstable (type 2.1), through to those with better control but still unable to sustain the sitting posture for any length of time (types 2.2 to 2.4). Those infants who are able to sustain a sitting posture with a straight back for prolonged periods (type 2.5) are less likely to develop scoliosis, but still need close monitoring. Those even better than this (types 2.6 to 2.9), with increasing ability in addition to take weight on their legs, are correspondingly more stable and if one can get them standing in orthoses or a standing frame, this has an additional protective effect on the spine.

One should thus be able to get a reasonable idea of the risk of developing scoliosis in these intermediate severity infants at the time of the first assessment, and it is important to take active measures to prevent the development of scoliosis at an early stage. While the back is still straight, the children should be fitted with an appropriate lightweight support for the spine (Figure 8-39). Attention should also be paid to the posture of the back when they sit in a wheelchair or chair. The back should be vertical and also reclining slightly backwards. A wheelchair with a soft canvas back which gives support to the spine and prevents tilting to either side, or one of the specially moulded types of wheelchair to maintain upright support, is

ideal. The seat of the chair should, on the other hand, be firm to prevent tilting of the pelvis and secondary scoliosis.

Once scoliosis has developed, active measures should be taken to try to correct it and to prevent further progression (see Figures 8-5 and 8-39). There is usually considerable mobility in the scoliosis and in general it does not become completely fixed or rigid till the late stages. Some degree of correction can be achieved with some of the spinal supports, but there seems to be an inevitable progression of the scoliosis in most cases, and internal fixation may become necessary. One of the difficulties one often faces is that the scoliosis starts early and the child is still growing and has not yet had its growth spurt by the time the severity of the scoliosis already dictates surgical fixation. This has not yet been fully resolved but it seems practical to consider operation in cases needing it from about 8 years onward. The Luque and related procedures where the vertebrae are individually attached to the rod to spread the load, in contrast to the traditional Harrington rod which anchors at either end, also allows some growth of the vertebral column. Owing to the mobility of the spine one can also usually achieve a considerable degree of straightening of the spine at the time of fixation. Bone grafting is often used in addition to instrumentation to further stabilize the spine.

Promotion of ambulation. Efforts should be made to get these children with intermediate severity SMA standing and walking with callipers, particularly in the less severe ones with stable spines who are able to take some weight on their legs (Figures 8-40, 8-41). I think it is worth trying even at an early age. Initially, in the first year or two of life, one can try and get them standing in a standing frame which supports the trunk as well as the limbs. One can then assess whether they may have sufficient stability to manage with knee–ankle–foot orthoses (KAFOs) or whether they are too weak around the hips and trunk and may need extra trunk support and initially standing callipers.

Many of these children will show some actual increase in power in the limb muscles once one can get them into a standing position. If one is trying to achieve ambulation it is important that they have well-supporting knee–ankle–foot orthoses, allowing the ischia to rest on the lip of the orthosis and to maintain a lordotic posture. They usually swing the upper body from side to side with their broad-based ambulation and any attempt to fixate the spine is likely to put them off their feet.

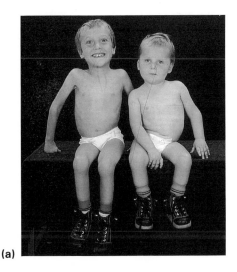

(a)

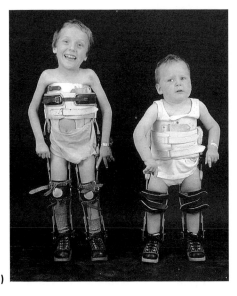

(b)

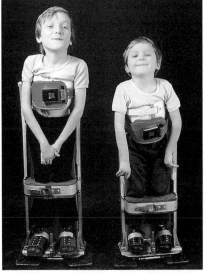

(c)

Figure 8-40a–c Spinal muscular atrophy of intermediate severity (type 2.4) in two brothers, aged 5 and 3 years. (a) Their severity was similar. They were able to sit at a normal age but not able to stand or take much weight on the legs. Early onset of scoliosis was noted and controlled with bracing. They were stood up in standing frames (b) and subsequently 'walked' in swivel walkers, aged 7 and 5 years (c). The older brother subsequently lost the ability to stand and developed contractures at the knees. He also had a progressive scoliosis which necessitated a Luque operation at 9 years. The younger brother also lost the ability to stand and died unexpectedly after an attack of pneumonia at 7 years.

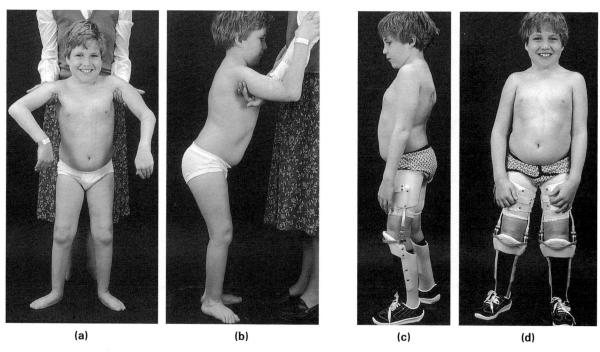

(a)   **(b)**   **(c)**   **(d)**

Figure 8-41a-d   Spinal muscular atrophy of intermediate severity (type 2.8). This boy's early milestones were normal. He sat unsupported but was not able to stand. He was diagnosed as 'Werdnig–Hoffmann disease' at 18 months and given a poor prognosis but did not deteriorate, and his power remained static. When assessed at 8 years of age he was unable to stand without support but could take some weight on his legs (a,b). He was mobilized in ischial weight bearing callipers (c,d) and a year later was still actively ambulant in his callipers and had shown some improvement. He subsequently remained ambulant through his puberty growth spurt until about 16 years when he had increasing difficulty, put on a lot of weight and lost mobility, but could still stand in his callipers. He had no scoliosis.

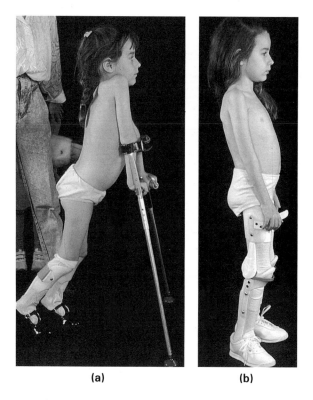

(a)   **(b)**

Figure 8-42a,b   Intermediate spinal muscle atrophy. This 7-year-old girl had never achieved independent standing or walking but was able to take some weight on her legs (type 2.7, 2.8). She had been fitted with inappropriate below-knee orthoses and with the aid of sticks had started 'walking' (a). However, this needed a forward stooping posture to prop herself on the sticks and she was only able to achieve a few laboured steps – almost four-legged. Following provision of conventional knee–ankle–foot orthoses, she was able to maintain a satisfactory upright lordotic posture and to achieve independent ambulation without the need for any sticks (b). She remained freely mobile through the ensuing 4 years, but has recently had increasing difficulty in association with a marked pubertal growth spurt.

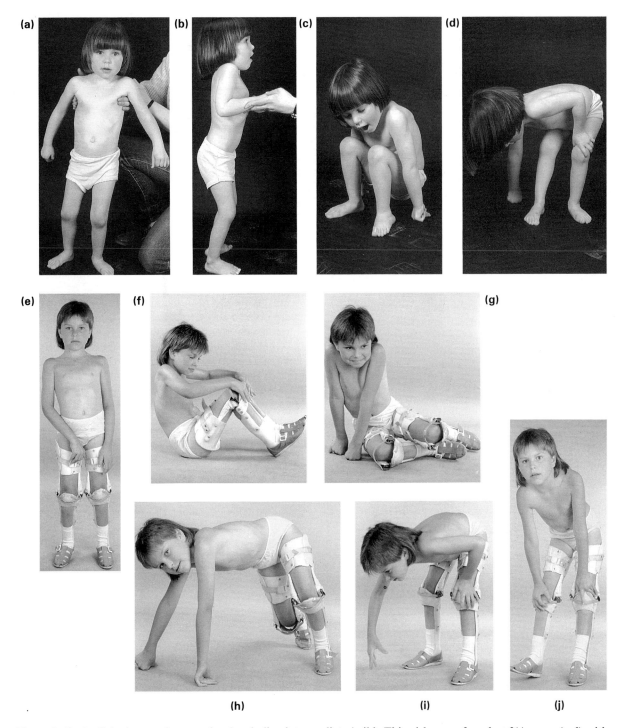

Figure 8-43a-j Spinal muscular atrophy; borderline intermediate/mild. This girl was referred at 3½ years (a-d) with inability to walk without support (type 3.0). She was able to get up unaided with a Gowers' manoeuvre. Her early milestones had been normal. She stood with support by 11 months and was cruising around furniture at 13 months. Onset of weakness was noted at 14 months with loss of ability to stand, and she reverted to crawling. She was fitted with below-knee ankle–foot orthoses at 2½ years and became more stable and walked with support. We provided her with knee–ankle–foot orthoses (KAFOs) and she became independently mobile. On annual review she remained fully mobile in her KAFOs and was improving and managing longer distances (e, 9 years). She was also able to take a few steps without callipers, to go up stairs with her callipers and to get up from the floor (f-j). She managed to remain mobile through her growth spurt and when recently reviewed at 13 years she was able to walk about a mile. Her mother described her KAFOs as her 'lifeline'.

If they need to use the arms for ambulation, a K-walker, with the arms behind the body, is better for a good upright posture than any form of sticks, which cause a forward stoop and loss of upright posture and balance (Figure 8-42).

If the child has already developed a scoliosis this can complicate one's efforts to promote ambulation. The fitting of a spinal brace may make it more difficult for the child to cope with callipers. On the other hand, if one does not treat the scoliosis it will become progressively worse. A compromise in some cases is to use the orthoses for ambulation and to wear the spinal brace whenever sitting.

Mild forms

In the Kugelberg–Welander syndrome the children are already ambulant and should be encouraged to remain so. Some cases who have barely achieved independent standing and can perhaps manage a few steps independently, but do not really have functional walking (type 3.1), can be benefited considerably by provision of knee–ankle–foot orthoses to establish efficient walking (Figure 8-43). Ambulation should be possible in all patients with spinal atrophy who have achieved the ability to stand without support, and intensive efforts should be directed at encouraging ambulation. As discussed earlier, they may have increasing difficulties with ambulation during their growth spurt and supportive help is particularly important to tide them through that period. Once they become chair-bound and develop scoliosis or contractures of the knee and hip flexors it will be much more difficult to re-establish ambulation (see Figure 8-20).

OTHER SYNDROMES THAT MAY MIMIC SMA

There have been numerous reports in the literature of cases of SMA with atypical features. These have included cerebellar hypoplasia, arthrogryposis, long bone fractures, diaphragmatic paralysis and congenital heart disease. I have always objected to these cases being referred to as infantile SMA, or at times even Werdnig–Hoffmann disease, as they usually differed quite radically from the classical clinical picture of SMA. I have preferred to designate these as cases of a different syndrome, with associated denervation or anterior horn cell disease. A number of these may well be quite distinct genetically. With the introduction by the international consortium on SMA of specific exclusion criteria, most of these

cases would not have passed the barrier for inclusion in the SMA clinico-genetic studies (Munsat and Davies, 1992).

ANTERIOR HORN CELL DISEASE WITH PONTOCEREBELLAR HYPOPLASIA

These infants may be mistaken for type 1 SMA as they are floppy and weak and there is certainly a superficial resemblance. However, they usually have associated developmental delay, are socially unresponsive, may have associated arthrogryposis, may have more generalized weakness rather than a proximal distribution, and do not show the differential weakness of the intercostals and sparing of the diaphragm. The pontocerebellar hypoplasia can be identified on brain imaging. In a study of two consecutive siblings in the same family (Figure 8-44), we were able to show that they had inherited different haplotypes for the 5q markers from each of their parents and thus proved that the disease is not related to the 5q locus of SMA (Dubowitz et al., 1995). Similar conclusions were drawn by Rudnik-Schöneborn et al. (1995) in a family where an affected and an unaffected sibling had the same haplotype for the 5q markers.

ANTERIOR HORN CELL DISEASE WITH CONGENITAL FRACTURES

This entity is characterized by multiple congenital, metaphyseal or epiphyseal long bone fractures, associated with large joint and digital contractures. It may include two separate conditions. In some families polyhydramnios, intrauterine growth retardation, hypomineralized bones and dysmorphic features are present. The pedigrees are consistent with autosomal recessive inheritance. In some families the pregnancy is uneventful, birth weight is normal and dysmorphic features are not prominent. Linkage analysis has been performed in one family (Lunt et al., 1992) and this disorder also appears to be unlinked to 5q.

ANTERIOR HORN CELL DISEASE WITH CONGENITAL HEART DEFECTS

Congenital heart defects occur in about 1% of births, septal defects being the most common. The incidence of ventricular septal defect is 2.5–5/1000 and atrial septal defect 1/1000 live births. A child presenting with both SMA and heart defect may thus

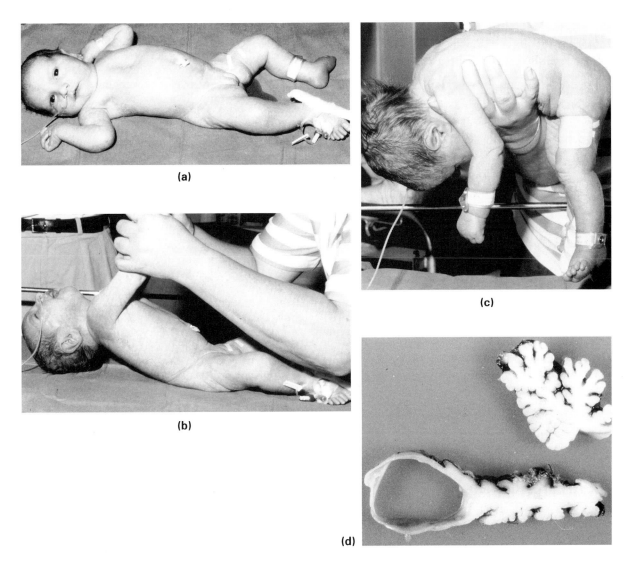

Figure 8-44a-d Anterior horn cell disease; pontocerebellar hypoplasia. This 10-day-old female infant was transferred to our newborn unit within 24 hours of birth with marked hypotonia and weakness from birth and a provisional diagnosis of severe spinal muscular atrophy (Werdnig–Hoffmann) (a-c). In addition to the trunk and limb weakness there was also fasciculation of the tongue. However, the respiratory function and absence of any intercostal weakness and costal recession seemed inappropriately good for an infant with severe (neonatal) spinal muscular atrophy. In addition, on routine neurological assessment she seemed surprisingly unresponsive to auditory and visual stimuli, in contrast to the normal alertness and responsiveness in Werdnig–Hoffmann disease. Routine ultrasound imaging revealed cerebellar hypoplasia, subsequently confirmed on cranial MRI. She showed little subsequent improvement, remained hypotonic and weak and also intellectually unresponsive, and died of pneumonia at 9 months. Autopsy confirmed cerebellar hypoplasia and cystic change (d) and associated degeneration of the anterior horn cells and atrophy of the anterior roots. (Reprinted from Dubowitz *et al.*, 1995, with permission of *Neuromuscular Disorders* and the publisher.)

represent a coincidence, but congenital heart defect (usually atrial septal defect) associated with SMA has been proposed as a distinct entity and has been observed among sibs. However, these patients do appear to have additional atypical features such as arthrogryposis, respiratory distress, bone fractures and at postmortem arrhinencephaly or partial agenesis of the corpus callosum. A heart defect associated with SMA should always prompt a search for additional atypical clinical features.

ANTERIOR HORN CELL DISEASE WITH ARTHROGRYPOSIS

When carefully studied, most patients described in the literature as having 'SMA and arthrogryposis' appear to represent one or other of the atypical entities above. Arthrogryposis associated with anterior horn cell disease in isolation seems to be very rare.

CONGENITAL HYPOMYELINATION NEUROPATHY

Congenital hypomyelination neuropathy may also mimic early onset severe SMA. This entity is rare and most cases described have been sporadic. The muscle biopsy may show grouped atrophy like SMA. The differential diagnosis is based on nerve conduction velocities which are extremely slow (<10 metres/second). This condition is probably inherited as an autosomal recessive and overlaps with HMSN III (see Chapter 9). The very severe cases may have almost amyelination, have a very slow motor nerve conduction velocity (<6 metres/second), and present at birth with severe respiratory problems and have a very poor prognosis.

PROGRESSIVE BULBAR PARALYSIS (FAZIO-LONDE DISEASE)

This is a rare hereditary condition with fewer than 20 reports in the literature. Although they were not the first to describe the condition, Fazio (1892) and Londe (1893) reported the first familial cases. Fazio described a 22-year-old woman and her 4-year-old son who had progressive bulbar paralysis, suggesting a dominant inheritance. The mother's symptoms only commenced at the age of 18 years. The two cases of Londe were brothers and a number of subsequent reports have included affected siblings with unaffected parents, suggesting an autosomal recessive inheritance. The age of onset of symptoms has ranged from 2 to 12 years. The most common initial symptoms are facial weakness, dysarthria or dysphagia and the condition tends progressively to affect other cranial nerves. The facial and hypoglossal nerves are consistently affected and in most cases also the vagus. Some, in addition, have involvement of the oculomotor nerves and the trigeminal. The course may be rapidly progressive with death within a matter of months, or may go on for several years.

In the first autopsy report on the condition Gomez *et al.* (1962) described a girl whose initial symptom was drooling soon after her first birthday, followed by a convulsion at 33 months and after that progressive right ptosis, bilateral facial weakness, inspiratory stridor, hoarse voice and croupy cough. At 38 months she developed left-sided ptosis and was unable to close her eyes tightly. She was also dysphagic. At 3½ years she had tracheostomy and she eventually died at 4 years 2 months. Autopsy revealed extensive changes in the nerve cells of the III, IV, VI, VII, X and XII cranial nerve nuclei, similar to those seen in the anterior horn cells in spinal muscular atrophy. Similar changes were also observed in the anterior horn cells of the cervical and upper thoracic spinal cord.

While this condition does bear some resemblance to severe spinal muscular atrophy, the onset is usually later, and in spinal muscular atrophy the cranial nerves are not as severely affected, although changes are frequently found at autopsy in the neurones of the cranial nerve nuclei of the oculomotor, facial and hypoglossal nerves. In progressive bulbar paralysis, however, there does not appear to be involvement of the skeletal musculature.

Two more cases have been documented in recent years (Alexander *et al.*, 1976; Della Giustina *et al.*, 1979) and also a subsequent sibling of the original Gomez *et al.* (1962) case (Benjamins, 1980). The age of onset of symptoms, usually stridor and dyspnoea, was at 25, 66 and 29 months respectively, with progressive involvement of other cranial nerves and death at 3.6, 7.6 and 3 years respectively.

X-LINKED SPINAL AND BULBAR MUSCULAR ATROPHY (KENNEDY DISEASE)

Spinal and bulbar muscular atrophy (SBMA) is characterized by the insidious onset of proximal muscle weakness, atrophy and fasciculations around age 30. There is involvement of the bulbar muscles, so that patients develop swallowing difficulty. Affected individuals often have recurrent aspiration by the sixth or seventh decade of life and may die from aspiration pneumonia.

In 1968, Kennedy *et al.* described the X-linked inheritance of SBMA. Subsequent clinical reports have defined the disorder clearly enough for it to be readily diagnosed in isolated patients without the X-linked family history (Harding *et al.*, 1982). Affected males may have gynaecomastia, testicular atrophy and reduced fertility, with normal or increased serum levels of testosterone. Some patients present with these signs of androgen insensitivity before the development of weakness.

MOLECULAR GENETICS ————————

In 1986, the SBMA gene was mapped to the proximal long arm of the X chromosome (Fischbeck *et al.*, 1986). Subsequently the androgen receptor gene was cloned and mapped to the same region (Brown *et al.*, 1989). This result, together with the androgen insensitivity in the disease and previous work which had demonstrated the presence of androgen receptors in spinal motor neurons (Sar and Stumpf, 1977) and a role for androgens in the control of motor neuron growth, development and response to injury in animals (Kurz *et al.*, 1986; Yu, 1989), made the androgen receptor gene a candidate gene for SBMA, and its association with Kennedy disease has now been confirmed (La Spada *et al.*, 1991). Although essentially a disease of adult life, the recognition of mutations in the androgen receptor gene should enable preclinical diagnosis in childhood cases and may reveal early clinical signs not hitherto recognized. The mutation has recently been identified as a gene expansion with an increased number of triplet repeats (La Spada *et al.*, 1991).

REFERENCES ————————————

Alexander, M.P., Emery, E.S. and Koerner, E.C. (1976) Progressive bulbar paresis in childhood. *Archives of Neurology* 33: 66–68.

Amick, L.D., Smith, H.L. and Johnson, W.W. (1966) An unusual spectrum of progressive spinal muscular atrophy. *Acta Physiologica Scandinavica* 42: 275.

Becker, P.E. (1966) Krankheiten mit hauptsächlicher Beteiligung von Pyramidenbahn, Vorderhorn und bulbären motorischen Kernen (Spastik, spinale Muskelatrophie und Bulbarparalyse). In: Becker, P.E. ed., *Humangenetik* Vol. 5, part 1. Stuttgart: Thieme, p. 314.

Beevor, C.E. (1902) A case of congenital spinal muscular atrophy (family type) and a case of hemorrhage into the spinal cord at birth, giving similar symptoms. *Brain* 25: 85.

Benjamins, D. (1980) Progressive bulbar palsy of childhood in siblings. *Annals of Neurology* 8: 203.

Brandt, S. (1950) Werdnig–Hoffmann's infantile progressive muscular atrophy. *Opera ex domo biologiae hereditariae humanae universitatis hafniensis*, Vol. 22. Copenhagen: Ejnar Munksgaard.

Brown, C.J., Goss, S.J., Lubahn, D.B. *et al.* (1989) Androgen receptor locus on the X chromosome: regional localization to Xq11-12 and description of a DNA polymorphism. *American Journal of Human Genetics* 44: 264–269.

Brzustowicz, L.M., Lehner, T., Castilla, L.H. *et al.* (1990) Genetic mapping of chronic childhood-onset spinal muscular atrophy to chromosome 5q11.2-13.3. *Nature* 344: 540–541.

Brzustowicz, L.M., Merette, C., Kleyn, P.W. *et al.* (1993) Assessment of nonallelic heterogeneity of chronic (type II and III) spinal muscular atrophy. *Human Heredity* 43: 380–387.

Byers, R.K. and Banker, B.Q. (1961) Infantile muscular atrophy. *Archives of Neurology (Chicago)* 5: 140–164.

Della Giustina, E., Ferriere, G., Evrard, P. *et al.* (1979) Progressive bulbar paralysis in childhood (Londe syndrome). A clinicopathological report. *Acta Paediatrica Belgica* 32: 129–133.

Dubowitz, V. (1964a) Infantile muscular atrophy. A prospective study with particular reference to a slowly progressive variety. *Brain* 87: 707–718.

Dubowitz, V. (1964b) Infantile muscular atrophy. A seven year study with particular reference to a slowly progressive form. *Revue Neurologique* 110: 558–563.

Dubowitz, V. (1967) Infantile muscular atrophy – a broad spectrum. *Clinical Proceedings of the Children's Hospital, Washington* 23: 223–239.

Dubowitz, V. (1969a) Hereditary proximal spinal muscular atrophy: single or multiple genes? In: Barbeau, A. and Brunette, J.R. eds, *2nd International Congress on Neurogenetics and Neuroophthalmology, Montreal, 17–23 September, 1967*. Amsterdam: Excerpta Medica, I.C.S. No. 175.

Dubowitz, V. (1969b) *The Floppy Infant.* Clinics in Developmental Medicine No.31. London: Spastics International Medical Publications/Heinemann.

Dubowitz, V. (1985) *Muscle Biopsy: A Practical Approach* 2nd edn. London: Baillière Tindall.

Dubowitz, V. (1991) Chaos in classification of the spinal muscular atrophies of childhood. *Neuromuscular Disorders* 1: 77–80.

Dubowitz, V. (1995) Chaos in the classification of SMA: a possible resolution. *Neuromuscular Disorders* 5: 3–5.

Dubowitz, V. and Brooke, M.H. (1973) *Muscle Biopsy: A Modern Approach.* London and Philadelphia: W.B. Saunders.

Dubowitz, V., Daniels, R.J. and Davies, K.E. (1995) Olivopontocerebellar hypoplasia with anterior horn cell involvement (SMA) does not localize to chromosome 5q. *Neuromuscular Disorders* 5: 25–29.

Dunne, P.B. and Chutorian, A.M. (1966) The relationship between infantile and juvenile spinal muscular atrophy. *Neurology (Minneapolis)* 16: 306.

Dyck, P.J., Thomas, P.J., Griffin, J.W. *et al.* (eds.) (1992) *Peripheral Neuropathy* 3rd edn. Philadelphia: W.B. Saunders.

Emery, A.E.H. (1971) The nosology of the spinal muscular atrophies. *Journal of Medical Genetics* 8: 481–495.

Fazio, F. (1892) Ereditarietà della paralisi bulbare progressive. *Riforma Medica* **4**: 327.

Fischbeck, K.H., Ionasescu, V., Ritter, A.W. *et al.* (1986) Localization of the gene for X-linked spinal muscular atrophy. *Neurology* **36**: 1595–1598.

Fried, K. and Emery, A.E.H. (1971) Spinal muscular atrophy type II. A separate genetic and clinical entity from type I (Werdnig–Hoffmann disease) and type III (Kugelberg–Welander disease). *Clinical Genetics* **2**: 203–209.

Gamstorp, I. (1967) Progressive spinal muscular atrophy with onset in infancy or early childhood. *Acta Paediatrica Scandinavica (Uppsala)* **56**: 408–423.

Gardner-Medwin, D., Hudgson, P. and Walton, J.N. (1967) Benign spinal muscular atrophy arising in childhood and adolescence. *Journal of the Neurological Sciences* **5**: 121–158.

Gilliam, T.C., Brzustowicz, L.M., Castilla, L.H. *et al.* (1990) Genetic homogeneity between acute and chronic forms of spinal muscular atrophy. *Nature* **345**: 823–825.

Gomez, M.R., Clermont, V. and Bernstein, J. (1962) Progressive bulbar paralysis in childhood (Fazio-Londe disease): report of a case with pathologic evidence of nuclear atrophy. *Archives of Neurology (Chicago)* **6**: 317–323.

Greensmith, L. and Vrbová, G. (1992) Alterations of nerve-muscle interactions during postnatal development influence motoneurone survival in rats. *Developmental Brain Research* **69**: 125–131.

Harding, A.E., Thomas, P.K., Baraitser, M. *et al.* (1982) X-linked recessive bulbospinal neuropathy: a report of ten cases. *Journal of Neurology, Neurosurgery and Psychiatry* **45**: 1012–1019.

Hausmanowa-Petrusewicz, I. (1970) Infantile and juvenile spinal muscular atrophy. In: Walton, J.N., Canal, N. and Scarlato, G. eds, *Muscle Diseases*. Proceedings, International Congress, Milan, 1969. Amsterdam: Excerpta Medica, I.C.S. No. 199, pp. 558–567.

Hausmanowa-Petrusewicz, I., Prot, J. and Sawicka, E. (1966) Le problème des formes infantiles et juvéniles de l'atrophie musculaire spinale. *Revue Neurologique* **114**: 295–306.

Hoffmann, J. (1893) Ueber chronische spinale Muskelatrophie im Kindesalter auf familiarer Basis. *Deutsche Zeitschrift für Nervenheilkunde* **3**: 427–470.

Hoffmann, J. (1897) Weitere Beiträge zur Lehre von der hereditären progressiven spinalen Muskelatrophie im Kindesalter. *Deutsche Zeitschrift für Nervenheilkunde* **10**: 292.

Hoffmann, J. (1900a) Ueber die hereditäre progressive spinale Muskelatrophie im Kindesalter. *Münchener Medizinische Wochenschrift* **47**: 1649–1651.

Hoffmann, J. (1900b) Dritter Beitrag zur Lehre von der hereditären progressiven spinalen Muskelatrophie im Kindesalter. *Deutsche Zeitschrift für Nervenheilkunde* **18**: 217–224.

Ignatius J. (1994) The natural history of severe spinal muscular atrophy – further evidence for clinical subtypes. *Neuromuscular Disorders* **4**: 527–528.

Kennedy, W.R., Alter, M. and Sung, J.H. (1968) Progressive proximal spinal and bulbar muscular atrophy of late onset. A sex-linked recessive trait. *Neurology (Minneapolis)* **18**: 671–680.

Kerr, J.F.R., Wyllie, A.H. and Currie, A.R. (1972) Apoptosis: a basic biological phenomenon with wide ranging implications in tissue kinetics. *British Journal of Cancer* **26**: 239–257.

Kohn, R. (1968) Postmortem findings in a case of Wohlfart-Kugelberg–Welander disease. *Confinia Neurologica (Basel)* **30**: 253–260.

Kugelberg, E. and Welander, L. (1986) Heredofamilial juvenile muscular atrophy simulating muscular dystrophy. *Archives of Neurology and Psychiatry (Chicago)* **75**: 500–509.

Kurz, E.M., Sengelaub, D.R. and Arnold, P. (1986) Androgens regulate the dendritic length of mammalian motoneurons in adulthood. *Science* **232**: 395–398.

La Spada, A.R., Wilson, E.M., Lubahn, D.B. *et al.* (1991) Androgen receptor gene mutations in X-linked spinal and bulbar muscular atrophy. *Nature* **352**: 77–79.

Lefebvre, S., Burglen, L., Reboullet, S. *et al.* (1995) Identification and characterisation of a spinal muscular atrophy-determining gene. *Cell* **80**: 155–165.

Londe, P. (1893) Paralysie bulbaire: progressive, infantile et familiale. *Revue de Médecine (Paris)* **13**: 1020–1030.

Lunt, P.W., Mathew, C., Clark, S. *et al.* (1992) Can prenatal diagnosis be offered in neonatally lethal spinal muscular atrophy (SMA) with arthrogryposis and fractures? *Journal of Medical Genetics* **29**: 282 (abstract).

Martin, D.P., Schmidt, R.E., Di Stefano, P.S. *et al.* (1988) Inhibitors of protein synthesis and RNA synthesis prevent neuronal death caused by nerve growth factor deprivation. *Journal of Cell Biology* **106**: 829–844.

Meadows, J. C., Marsden, C.D. and Harriman, D.G.F. (1969) Chronic spinal muscular atrophy in adults. Part 1. The Kugelberg–Welander syndrome. *Journal of the Neurological Sciences* **9**: 527–550.

Melki, J., Abdelhak, S., Sheth, P. *et al.* (1990a) Gene for chronic proximal spinal muscular atrophies maps to chromosome 5q. *Nature* **344**: 767–768.

Melki, J., Sheth, P., Abdelhak, S. *et al.* (1990b) Mapping of acute (type 1) spinal muscular atrophy to chromosome 5q12-q14. *Lancet* **336**: 271–273.

Moosa, A. and Dubowitz, V. (1973) Spinal muscular atrophy in childhood: two clues to clinical diagnosis. *Archives of Disease in Childhood* **48**: 386–388.

Moosa, A. and Dubowitz, V. (1976) Motor nerve conduction velocity in spinal muscular atrophy of childhood. *Archives of Disease in Childhood* **51**: 974–977.

Muller, B., Melki, J., Burlet, P. *et al.* (1992) Proximal spinal muscular atrophy (SMA) types II and III in the same sibship are not caused by different alleles at the SMA locus on 5q. *American Journal of Human Genetics* **50**: 892–895.

Munsat, T.L. (1991) Workshop report: International SMA collaboration. *Neuromuscular Disorders* **1**: 81.

Munsat, T. and Davies, K.E. (1992) Report on International SMA Consortium Meeting held in Bonn, Germany, June 1992. *Neuromuscular Disorders* **2**: 423–428.

Munsat, T.L., Woods, R., Fowler, W. and Pearson, C.M. (1969) Neurogenic muscular atrophy of infancy with prolonged survival. *Brain* **92**: 9–24.

Oppenheim, R.W. (1991) Cell death during development of the nervous system. *Annual Review of Neuroscience* **14**: 453–501.

Pearn, J.H., Carter, C.O. and Wilson, J. (1973) The genetic identity of acute infantile spinal muscular atrophy. *Brain* **96**: 463–470.

Roy, N., Mahadevan, M.S., McLean, M. *et al.* (1995) The gene for neuronal apoptosis inhibitory protein is partially deleted in individuals with spinal muscular atrophy. *Cell* **80**: 167–178.

Rowland, L.P., Schotland, D.L., Lovelace, R.E. and Layzer, R.B. (1967) Neurogenic muscular atrophies. In: Milhorat, A.T. ed., *Exploratory Concepts in Muscular Dystrophy and Related Disorders.* Amsterdam: Excerpta Medica, I.C.S. No. 147, pp. 41–45.

Rudnik-Schöneborn, S., Wirth, B., Röhrig, D. *et al.* (1995) Exclusion of the gene locus for spinal muscular atrophy on chromosome 5q in a family with infantile olivopontocerebellar atrophy (OPCA) and anterior horn cell degeneration. *Neuromuscular Disorders* **5**: 19–23.

Sar, M. and Stumpf, W.E. (1977) Androgen concentration in motor neurons of cranial nerves and spinal cord. *Science* **197**: 77–80.

Schwartz, L.M.: The role of cell death genes during development. *Bioessays* **15**: 389–395, 1991.

Sieradzan, K. and Vrbová, G. (1989) Replacement of missing motoneurones by embryonic grafts in the rat spinal cord. *Neuroscience* **31**: 115–130.

Sieradzan, K. and Vrbová, G. (1991) Factors influencing survival of transplanted embryonic motoneurones in the spinal cord of adult rats. *Experimental Neurology* **114**: 286–299.

Thoenen, H. (1991) The changing scene of neurotrophic factors. *Trends in Neurosciences* **14**: 165–170.

Thomas, N.H. and Dubowitz, V. (1994) The natural history of type I (severe) spinal muscular atrophy. *Neuromuscular Disorders* **4**: 497–502.

Werdnig, G. (1891) Zwei frühinfantile hereditäre Fälle von progressiver Muskelatrophie unter dem Bilde der Dystrophie, aber auch neurotischer Grundlage. *Archiv für Psychiatrie und Nervenkrankheiten* **22**: 437–481.

Werdnig, G. (1894) Die frühinfantile progressive spinale Amyotrophie. *Archiv für Psychiatrie und Nervenkrankheiten* **26**: 706–744.

Wohlfart, G., Fex, J. and Eliasson, S. (1955) Hereditary proximal spinal muscular atrophy — a clinical entity simulating progressive muscular dystrophy. *Acta Psychiatrica et Neurologica (Kjobenhavn)* **30**: 395–406.

Wyllie, A.H. (1981) Cell death: a new classification separating apoptosis from necrosis. In: Bowen, I.D. and Lockshin, R.A. eds, *Cell Death in Biology and Pathology.* New York: Chapman & Hall, pp. 9–34.

Wyllie, A.H., Morris, R.G., Smith, A.L. *et al.* (1984) Chromatin cleavage in apoptosis: association with condensed chromatin morphology and dependence on macromolecular synthesis. *Journal of Pathology* **142**: 67–78.

Yu, W.H. (1989) Administration of testosterone attenuates neuronal loss following axotomy in the brain-stem motor nuclei of female rats. *Journal of Neuroscience* **9**: 3908–3914.

Zellweger, H. (1971) The genetic heterogeneity of spinal muscular atrophy (SMA). In: Bergsma, D. ed. *The 2nd Conference of Clinical Delineation of Birth Defects, Original Article Series,* Vol. vii, No. 2. New York: The National Foundation, pp. 82–89.

Zellweger, H., Schneider, H.J., Schuldt, D.R. and Mergner, W. (1969) Heritable spinal muscular atrophies. *Helvetica Paediatrica Acta* **24**: 92–105.

CHAPTER 9

Disorders of the Lower Motor Neurone Hereditary Motor Neuropathies

This heterogeneous group of disorders has been based on a number of classical descriptions of clinical syndromes which usually still carry the eponymous titles of their authors. The application in recent years of more sophisticated techniques for quantification of motor as well as sensory involvement of the peripheral nerve, on clinical, electrophysiological and morphological grounds, lead to a more logical approach to their clinical classification. However, the advent of molecular genetic techniques over the past few years has provided a completely new perspective and orientation to these disorders, with the recognition of gene loci for many of them and also the recognition not only of some of the mutations in the genes but also the specific proteins involved. This revealed the presence of genetic heterogeneity, with several different genes producing a similar clinical syndrome, and also questioned the very existence of some of the time-honoured clinical entities.

HISTORICAL BACKGROUND

In order to provide an overall perspective I have retained a short historical introduction, followed by a description of the main clinical syndromes and finally the impact of molecular genetics in realigning the various syndromes on a sound genetic and biochemical basis. A few loose ends still await adequate resolution.

Charcot–Marie–Tooth disease

In 1886 Charcot and Marie, in Paris, described a specific variety of progressive muscular atrophy first affecting the feet and legs and later the hands. The condition often started in infancy and had a familial tendency, frequently affecting siblings and also successive generations (suggesting a dominant inheritance). Sensation was usually normal but sometimes affected. Fasciculation and reaction of degeneration were present in atrophic muscles. Vasomotor abnormalities were also noted. They thought the condition might be a myelopathy rather than a neuropathy.

In the same year, Tooth (1886) published an almost identical description of the peroneal type of progressive muscular atrophy in his Oxford MD thesis, highlighting the early age of onset, the familial pattern and the peripheral involvement of the legs. He thought the disease was in the peripheral nerves. These classical descriptions provided the basis of Charcot–Marie–Tooth disease.

Roussy–Lévy syndrome

In 1926 Roussy and Lévy described a dominantly inherited syndrome, resembling Charcot–Marie–Tooth disease, with talipes and distal weakness of the legs, some associated sensory loss and decreased response to galvanic or faradic stimulation. In addition, the cases in this kinship had a tremor of the hands, but no evidence of cerebellar disease. A similar syndrome was later documented in a large kinship by Yudell et al. (1965) under the eponymous title of Roussy–Lévy syndrome. It seemed likely that this syndrome was probably part of the clinical spectrum of Charcot–Marie–Tooth disease, rather than an independent disorder.

Dejerine–Sottas disease

Dejerine and Sottas (1893) described a syndrome in two siblings, with onset in infancy in the girl and at

14 years in her brother, characterized by clubfoot, kyphoscoliosis, distal weakness and atrophy beginning in the lower extremities and spreading to the upper, areflexia, marked sensory loss of all four extremities, incoordination of the arms, Rombergism, miosis and ataxia. The girl subsequently died at 45 years, having lost the ability to walk, and at autopsy her peripheral nerves showed marked thickening of the nerve trunk with demyelination and denuded axons and hypertrophy of the interstitial connective tissue.

The description of the hypertrophic nerves created for the Dejerine–Sottas syndrome a separate nosological entity but it is now recognized that, as with the pseudohypertrophy of Duchenne dystrophy, hypertrophic neuropathy is not a distinct entity in itself but common to a number of different disorders. In addition to cases of recessively inherited disorder as described by Dejerine and Sottas, and often with a raised cerebrospinal fluid protein, hypertrophic neuropathy has also been reported in dominantly inherited cases resembling Charcot–Marie–Tooth disease, in cases of relapsing polyneuropathy, and in Refsum's disease.

Refsum's syndrome

In 1946 Refsum described a recessively inherited syndrome of polyneuropathy associated with retinitis pigmentosa, ataxia and other cerebellar signs, an increased cerebrospinal fluid protein and frequently also hearing loss and cardiomyopathy. Irregular additional features include pupillary abnormalities, lens opacities, anosmia, skeletal malformations and ichthyosis. Klenk and Kahlke (1963) discovered the excess of phytanic acid, a fatty acid not detected before in humans. Steinberg (1972) designated Refsum's disease as an inborn error of metabolism, phytanic acid storage disease, due to an enzyme defect of α-oxidation of phytanic acid (and other β-methyl-substituted fatty acids). The enzyme defect was also demonstrated in cultured fibroblasts. Further studies in recent years have characterized Refsum's syndrome as one of the peroxisomal disorders.

HEREDITARY MOTOR AND SENSORY NEUROPATHIES (HMSN); CHARCOT-MARIE-TOOTH DISEASE (CMT)

In 1968 Dyck and Lambert (1968 a,b) reported a detailed clinical, genetic, electrophysiological and nerve biopsy study of patients with motor and sensory neurone disease with peroneal muscular atrophy. They were able to divide their patients into

two main groups: (1) those in whom motor and sensory conduction velocity was markedly reduced and in whom hypertrophic neuropathy was found; these were further subdivided into dominantly inherited Charcot–Marie–Tooth disease, and recessively inherited Refsum's disease and neuropathy of Dejerine–Sottas type; (2) those in whom the nerve conduction was normal or only slightly reduced and in whom hypertrophic neuropathy was not found; these were looked upon as neuronal degenerations and could be further subdivided into five clinical disorders: (a) a progressive muscular atrophy of Charcot–Marie–Tooth type with only lower motor neurone involvement; (b) a neuronal form of Charcot–Marie–Tooth disease in which both motor and sensory peripheral neurones were affected, with no hypertrophic neuropathy and normal conduction velocity in the upper limbs and slight reduction in the lower; (c) hereditary sensory neuropathy with peroneal muscular atrophy; (d) spastic paraplegia with peroneal muscular atrophy; and (e) various spinocerebellar degenerations with peroneal muscular atrophy.

With the advent of more sophisticated techniques for the quantification of sensory responses to graded stimuli and its correlation with the number and size of myelinated and unmyelinated nerve fibres (Dyck *et al.*, 1971), it became possible to demonstrate some degree of sensory involvement in a large proportion of these cases of motor neuropathy in the absence of any clinical signs thereof. For this reason Dyck (1975) suggested that this whole group of disorders be classified generically as hereditary motor and sensory neuropathies (HMSN) and subdivided into individual types, comparable with the recognized clinical syndromes, as follows:

Hypertrophic neuropathy
(peroneal muscular atrophy)
    (HMSN type I)

Neuronal type of peroneal muscular atrophy
    (HMSN type II)

Hypertrophic neuropathy of infancy
(Dejerine–Sottas)
    (HMSN type III)

Hypertrophic neuropathy with excess phytanic acid
(Refsum's disease)
    (HMSN type IV)

Peripheral neuropathy with spastic paraplegia
    (HMSN type V)

Although a bit of a jawbreaker, 'hereditary motor and sensory neuropathy' or 'HMSN' as a designation for the various individual diseases within this group has found fairly wide appeal among neurologists, although colloquially 'Charcot–Marie–Tooth' has persisted and has also been adopted by the geneticists for the designation of the various genetic subtypes (CMT1, CMT2, etc).

HYPERTROPHIC NEUROPATHY; PERONEAL MUSCULAR ATROPHY; DEMYELINATING NEUROPATHY (HMSN TYPE I)

This corresponds to the hypertrophic neuropathy of the Charcot–Marie–Tooth type delineated by Dyck and Lambert (1968a).

Clinical features

The earliest signs, usually in the first decade, are foot deformity and abnormality of gait (Figures 9-1 to 9-4). In affected families pes cavus or curling of the toes (hammer toes) may be noted in early childhood long before the onset of symptoms. The gait is often described as awkward or clumsy or the 'fairy walk'

and is associated with frequent tripping and a high steppage to compensate for foot drop. Subjects may also experience difficulty in standing still. Some patients may have normal arches to the feet in the early stages and only develop pes cavus later.

The peroneal muscles are affected early but there is also usually weakness of the intrinsic muscles of the feet and the dorsiflexors of the ankles. Later there is involvement of the hands, with difficulty in fine manipulations. The weakness, which is symmetrical, gradually involves other distal muscles of the limbs and moves proximally. The tendon reflexes become diminished or absent. Sensory impairment may be noted, especially in the feet and hands. This is often absent on routine clinical examination but can be demonstrated by quantified stimuli compared with controls. Some patients experience muscle pains or other sensory disturbances. The peripheral nerves may be palpably enlarged or excessively firm in about a quarter of cases. The nerves between shoulder and elbow are suitable but not the ulnar at the ulnar groove of the elbow where it may be thickened in normal subjects. Other nerves such as the great auricular may also be palpably affected.

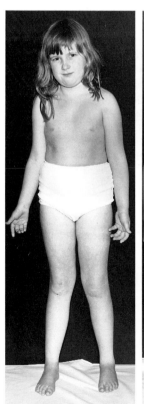 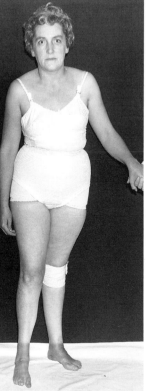

(a)   (b)

Figure 9-1a,b HMSN I. (a) 7-year-old girl with inversion of feet since she started walking at 21 months. There was no progression. There was mild pes cavus and varus deformity of feet. The tendon reflexes were sluggish. Motor nerve conduction velocity was markedly slowed: ulnar 13 m/s; posterior tibial 10 m/s. EMG of deltoid was normal; extensor digitorum brevis showed frequent fibrillation potentials at rest, and fasciculation potentials and large polyphasic motor units with reduced interference pattern on activity. Muscle biopsy of gastrocnemius was histologically normal but showed some fibre type grouping and isolated core/target fibres on histochemical preparations indicative of denervation/reinnervation. Her mother (b) had a similar problem from the age of 5 years. She also showed wasting and weakness of lower limbs distally and sluggish tendon jerks. The motor conduction velocity was very slow (ulnar 22 m/s; posterior tibial, impossible to get adequate motor response). EMG of the deltoid was normal, but first dorsal interosseous and tibialis anterior showed evidence of denervation. This conforms to the dominantly inherited demyelinating form of neuropathy (HMSN type I).

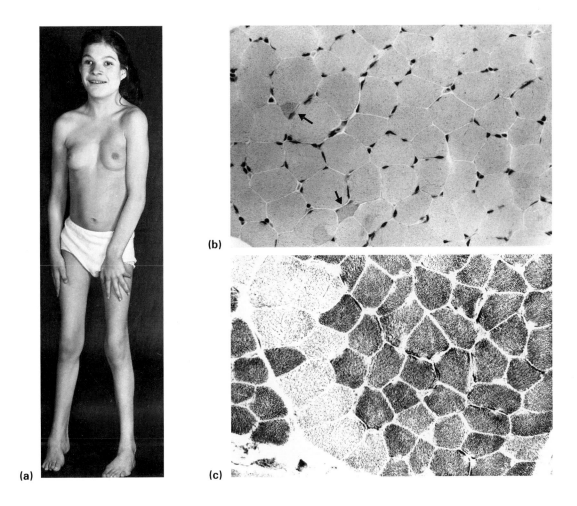

Figure 9-2a-c   HMSN I. (a) A 14-year-old girl with pes cavus from the age of 2 years, and weakness and wasting of legs from 8 years, with slow progression. She also has a mild scoliosis. All tendon reflexes were sluggish. There was slight weakness of hands and limited extension and supination of forearm. Motor conduction was markedly slowed: ulnar 11 m/s; posterior tibial 10 m/s. Her symptom-free mother also has slow conduction (ulnar 23 m/s). Two female siblings are normal. Mother's sister, father and grandfather have pes cavus. This family conforms to a dominantly inherited demyelinating neuropathy (HMSN type I) with subclinical involvement of the mother. Muscle biopsy (b) of gastrocnemius was essentially normal on routine stain apart from isolated atrophic fibres (H & E × 255). Histochemical preparation (c) showed fibre type grouping (NADH-TR × 255. Note large cluster of type 1 (dark-staining) fibres).

There may be an associated tremor of the hands. (The Roussy–Lévy syndrome is probably not a separate entity from the Charcot–Marie–Tooth disease.)

Muscle wasting is usually mild and not a striking feature (in contrast to the neuronal form of motor neuropathy; see below).

The prognosis is usually good, with a very slowly progressive or relatively static course and, commonly, a normal life expectancy. Ambulation should be encouraged and is usually not lost. Where indicated, corrective procedures may be needed for the foot deformities.

Genetics

The condition is dominantly inherited, with variable clinical expression. In affected families apparently symptom-free persons may be found to have some of the features, such as foot deformities or tremor, in isolation.

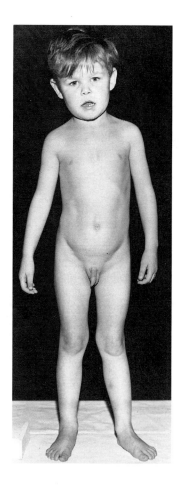

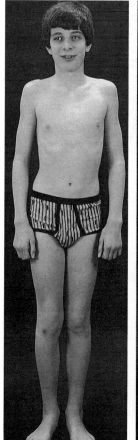

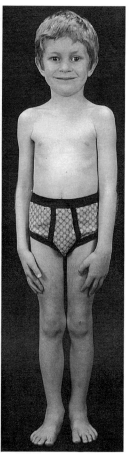

(a)

(b)

Figure 9-3 HMSN I. A 5-year-old boy with delay in motor and intellectual milestones. He walked at 16 months and had a tendency to recurrent falls since. He walked with a flat-footed gait. He had some difficulty getting up from floor. There was a positive Gowers' sign. Two older brothers and his parents were clinically normal. Motor conduction was markedly slowed: ulnar 14 m/s; posterior tibial 17 m/s. His father also had slow nerve conduction: right ulnar 20.5 m/s; left ulnar 23 m/s. Nerve conduction in his mother and brothers was normal. Muscle biopsy of gastrocnemius was histologically normal but showed fibre type grouping, indicative of denervation/reinnervation pattern. This is presumably a dominantly inherited, demyelinating neuropathy (HMSN type I), with sub-clinical involvement of father.

Figure 9-4a,b HMSN I. Two brothers, aged 14 and 5 years. Note the normal appearance and posture. The older brother (a) was seen initially at 5 years. He walked at 14 months, had difficulty in running and had frequent falls. He was able to stand and hop on one leg. He later developed tremor of the hands but the ECG showed normal baseline. Nerve conduction velocity (NCV) in the right and left ulnar was 17 and 15 m/s and in anterior tibial 11 m/s. The younger brother (b) was seen initially at 2½ years of age. He dragged his legs when running. NCV was 25 m/s in ulnar and 26 m/s in lateral peroneal. His condition subsequently remained steady. At 6 years of age his NCV in ulnar was 32 m/s. His father was also affected: NCV in right ulnar 18 m/s. NCV in mother normal (53 m/s). Dominant inheritance.

Conduction velocity

The markedly slow motor nerve conduction velocity is the hallmark of the disease. It is usually less than one-half the normal values and often less than 20 m/s. Sensory nerve conduction is also affected.

The slow conduction may also be demonstrated in cases without any clinical symptoms (Vanasse and Dubowitz, 1981). It is thus always worth testing the parents of any affected child. Occasionally, sporadic cases may be found with no evidence of involvement in any family members (Figure 9-5). Such cases may possibly have an autosomal recessive inheritance or represent new mutations of the dominant gene (see below).

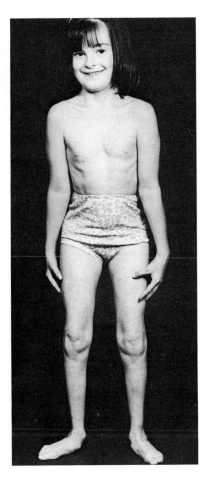

Figure 9-5 HMSN I ?, HMSN III ? Demyelinating peripheral neuropathy; sporadic or autosomal recessive. A 7-year-old girl with marked wasting and weakness of the distal part of the legs and also involvement of the hands. There was associated laxity of ligaments and hyperextensibility of joints. She stood holding on to furniture at 1 year, but did not walk independently until callipers were fitted at 6 years. There was bilateral dislocation of hips in infancy. Her parents and sibling were normal. Nerve conduction was very slow: ulnar 22 m/s. No motor response was obtained on supramaximal stimulus of anterior or posterior tibial nerves. Nerve conduction in both parents was normal.

Nerve biopsy

The transverse fascicular area of the nerve is increased but the number and diameter of the myelinated fibres are reduced and there is evidence of demyelination. The characteristic onion bulb formation of hypertrophic neuropathy may also be seen.

NEURONAL TYPE OF PERONEAL MUSCULAR ATROPHY (HMSN TYPE II)

This group resembles the HMSN Type I in its dominant inheritance and distribution of weakness in the extremities, but differs in the following respects: the onset of symptoms is usually later; peripheral nerves are not palpably enlarged; weakness of the small hand muscles is less severe and that of the plantar flexors of the ankles more severe; the degree of atrophy of muscles is much more striking and the nerve conduction velocity is not appreciably slowed; motor conduction velocities in the ulnar and median nerve are usually within the normal range, whereas the velocity of the peroneal nerve is usually slightly below or borderline (see Figures 9-6 to 9-11).

The commonest early symptom is difficulty with walking or inability to stand still. The onset may not be till middle age and the patient may have excelled at sports in his youth. Occasionally the onset is in the first two decades. Some patients experience cramps in the leg muscles or in the feet. Weakness of the hands is usually not a problem.

There is usually marked atrophy of muscles and some show the characteristic 'stork legs' (Figure 9-11). There may be an associated pes cavus (see Figure 9-6). The tendon reflexes are depressed in the legs but usually normal in the arms.

Mild sensory deficit may be present over the distal parts of the limbs. Some cases may not have any clinical or electrophysiological evidence of sensory involvement, suggesting they may have a pure motor neuropathy, but there is usually some evidence histologically of sensory nerve involvement.

Electromyography

This may show large motor unit potentials and fasciculations suggestive of anterior horn cell involvement. The nerve conduction is usually normal, or slightly depressed in the legs. Sensory nerve conductions are also normal.

Nerve biopsy

This shows no demyelination or hypertrophy but evidence of neuronal atrophy with a shift towards more small-sized fibres than normal.

Although considered to be an autosomal dominant condition, it is not possible to identify a symptom-free affected patient, since the nerve conduction velocity is normal. It is thus difficult to be sure whether cases of affected siblings but normal parents are autosomal dominant or possibly autosomal recessive in inheritance, especially where the parents are related (see Figure 9-9).

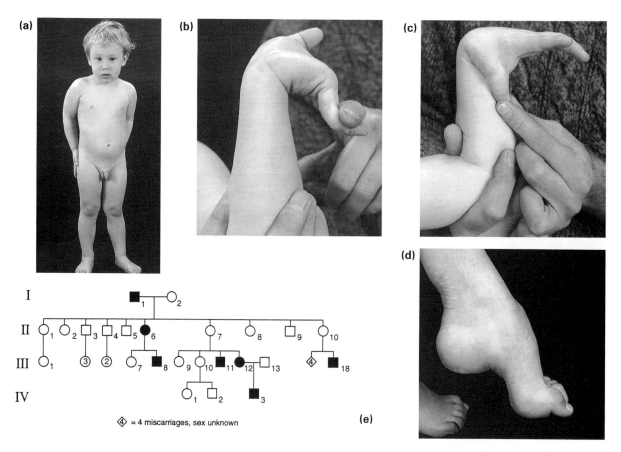

⬧ = 4 miscarriages, sex unknown

Figure 9-6a-e HMSN II. This 2½-year-old boy presented with minimal disability. He walked intermittently on his toes. He sat at 4 months, stood at 7 months and started walking at 8 months. Note reasonably normal muscle bulk and hyperextended knees (a). He had associated joint hypermobility (b, c). NCV 56 m/s (normal). EMG normal. His mother was also affected. Note the marked equinus posture of her feet (d). Her NCV was 41 and 44 m/s in the ulnar and median nerves (mildly slow). There was a positive family history through three generations (e), with a dominant pattern. It is of interest that, although his mother's (III,12) grandfather (I,1) was affected, her own mother (II,7) was symptom-free, as was her aunt (II,10) who had an affected son (III,18).

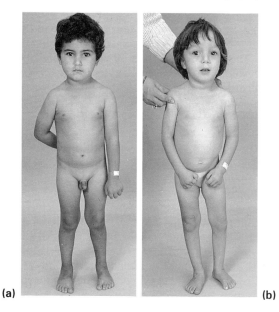

Figure 9-7a,b HMSN II. Two cousins, aged 3½ and 2 years of age, presented with mild motor disability. The older boy sat at 6 months and walked at 15 months. The younger boy sat at 9 months, stood at 18 months and at 2 years was still not walking independently. Note wasting of lower legs and eversion of feet with flat-footed posture (a, b). Ulnar nerve conduction velocities of 50 and 38 m/s were found in the two boys respectively. Their CKs were 215 and 115. Their fathers are brothers and are both affected. Nerve conduction velocity was not performed on the parents. Dominant inheritance.

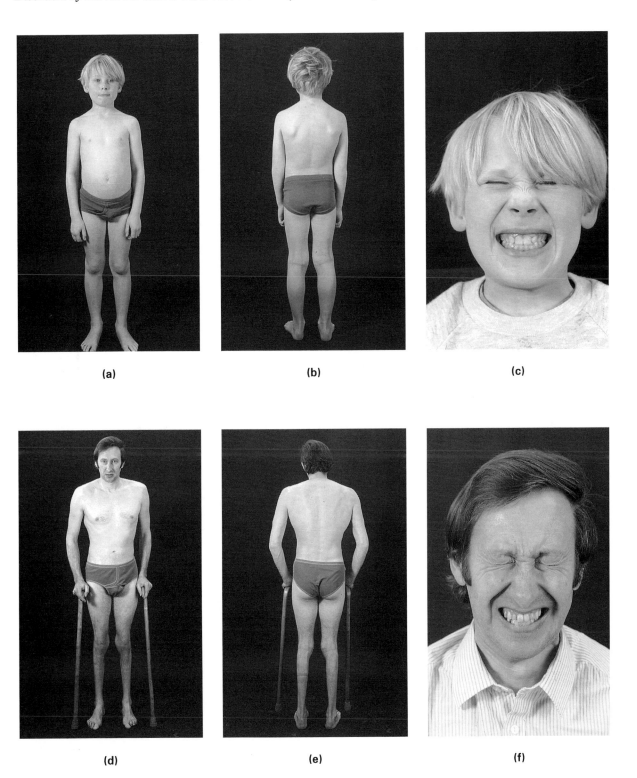

(a) (b) (c)

(d) (e) (f)

Figure 9-8a-f HMSN II. This 9-year-old boy (a,b) presented with minimal disability plus pain in the legs since 4 years of age. His facial muscles were normal (c). Peroneal NCV 49 m/s. His 39-year-old father had Charcot–Marie–Tooth disease, which was diagnosed at 29 years of age after gradual slowing of activity and cramps on exercise (d-f). He had associated sensory loss. Ulnar NCV 50 m/s, peroneal 43 m/s.

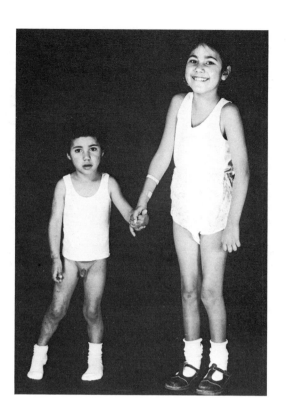

Figure 9-9 HMSN II. A girl of 9 years and brother aged 4 years with distal weakness of the legs. The girl was weaker than her brother but there was no fixed deformity. The boy had 5° fixed equinus of right foot. Weakness and wasting of distal muscles of arms were also present. Early motor milestones were normal, but his gait was abnormal from time of walking soon after 1 year. Associated sensory deficit present in hands and feet of both children. The parents are first cousins. No clinical abnormality in parents or two remaining male siblings. Ulnar nerve conduction normal: 56 m/s in girl; 43 m/s in boy. Unable to get any motor response to stimulation of anterior or posterior tibial nerve in either child. EMG showed fibrillation potentials at rest and recruitment of large polyphasic motor units. Phenotype consistent with neuronal form of neuropathy. Inheritance autosomal recessive or possibly dominant with one parent a non-manifesting heterozygote.

Figure 9-10a,b HMSN II. A 12-year-old girl with marked wasting of lower legs and fixed equinus of feet. She walked at 12 months, but had difficulty with getting up after falling from 18 months and toe-gait from 20 months. Arms were normal apart from 10° limitation of elbow extension. Nerve conduction was normal: ulnar 59 m/s; anterior tibial 48 m/s. EMG of tibialis anterior showed a normal interference pattern, no fibrillation potentials at rest, but rather large motor units on volition suggesting anterior horn cell lesion. Parents and four siblings were normal. Eight-year-old sister was said to have some stiffness of gait but on examination no abnormality was detected; nerve conduction: ulnar 58 m/s; anterior tibial 51 m/s. Surgical elongation of tendo Achillis led to improvement in gait but the shortening gradually recurred. She also tended to put on weight, which aggravated her walking problems. Power seemed static. This is probably a neuronal form of peripheral neuropathy. Possibly hereditary, but difficult to be sure in face of normal conduction velocities and no weakness in rest of family.

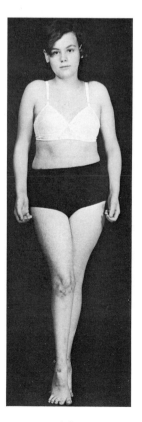

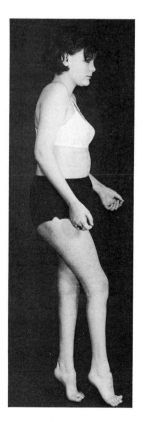

(a)   (b)

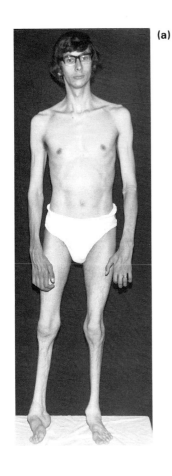

(a)

(b)

Figure 9-11a,b A 26-year-old man showing (a) classical 'stork' leg appearance with marked wasting of lower legs from the lower third of the thighs down. Note that from the mid-thigh upwards the muscle development is reasonably normal. (b) Associated wasting and weakness of the small muscles of the hands.

HMSN II is much less common than HMSN I. In a study of 227 cases of CMT, Harding and Thomas (1980a) found that only 54 had HMSN II and the majority of these had autosomal dominant inheritance.

HYPERTROPHIC NEUROPATHY OF INFANCY (DEJERINE–SOTTAS) (HMSN TYPE III)

This is a recessively inherited disorder with onset usually in infancy. There is delay in early motor milestones and walking may only be achieved by the third or fourth year (Figure 9-5). After an initial improvement in motor function there is subsequently a gradual decline and some patients may lose the ability to walk in adult life.

Weakness affects the hands as well, and in both lower and upper limbs may spread proximally. Atrophy is not a striking feature, but may be partly concealed by subcutaneous fat. The nerves are palpably enlarged.

The tendon reflexes are usually diminished or absent. Evidence of sensory loss may be found over the distal extremities, and also ataxia of the limbs or trunk. Associated features may include shortness of stature and scoliosis.

Nerve biopsy

There is an increase in the fascicular area together with segmental demyelination and onion bulb formation, as in the dominant form of hypertrophic neuropathy.

Electrophysiology

The conduction velocity is slow in both motor and sensory nerves. It is important to check the motor conduction velocity in other members of the family, as subclinical disease in siblings may be found and a slow conduction velocity in a symptom-free parent designates the dominantly inherited type.

HYPERTROPHIC NEUROPATHY WITH EXCESS PHYTANIC ACID (REFSUM'S DISEASE) (HMSN TYPE IV)

This recessively inherited hypertrophic neuropathy has a clinical motor and sensory neuropathy, similar to that of the Dejerine–Sottas type, in association with retinitis pigmentosa, ataxia and cerebellar signs, hearing loss, cardiomyopathy, pupillary abnormalities, lens opacity and skin changes resembling ichthyosis. The onset is usually insidious and varies from early childhood to the third decade. Sometimes the onset is fairly abrupt and may be precipitated by an infection. In some cases there is a tendency to exacerbation and remission. Some patients go on into adult life with little change, whereas others show steady progression. Sudden death may occur, presumably from the cardiomyopathy.

There is a consistent elevation of cerebrospinal fluid protein, the level of which seems to correlate with the clinical severity in relapsing cases or in those responding to a diet low in phytanic acid (Eldjarn *et al.*, 1966).

The syndrome may be difficult to diagnose clinically because none of the individual features is pathognomonic, but is readily confirmed by the high serum phytanic acid levels.

PERIPHERAL NEUROPATHY WITH SPASTIC PARAPLEGIA (HMSN TYPE V)

Several families with this dominantly inherited disorder have been documented since the original report of Strümpell (1883). The onset is usually in the second or later decades. The spastic paraplegia dominates the clinical picture and is slowly progressive. Distal limb weakness appears later and there may be EMG evidence of denervation in the lower limbs. Nerve conduction velocity is usually normal or only slightly depressed. Sensory neurones may also be affected.

THE IMPACT OF MOLECULAR GENETICS

With the application of modern molecular genetic techniques to the study of the hereditary motor and sensory neuropathies, the whole clinical classification has been turned on its head. Some of the traditional eponymous entities such as HMSN I and HMSN II have survived but, as expected, shown to

Table 9-1 Gene locations and candidate proteins in the hereditary neuropathies

			Chromosome	Protein
Hereditary motor and sensory neuropathies				
HMSN I	CMT1A	AD	17p11.2–12	PMP-22
	CMT1B	AD	1q22–23	P_0
	CMT1C	AD	unknown	unknown
	CMT1D	AR	8q	unknown
	CMTX	X–L	Xq13.1	unknown
HMSN II	CMT2A	AD	1p36	? PMP-2
	CMT2B	AD	unknown	unknown
HMSN III			??	?? (see text)
Hereditary neuropathy with pressure palsies				
HNPP		AD	17p11.2–12	PMP-22

be genetically heterogeneous. The recognition of specific protein abnormalities has made possible a more accurate designation of some of these individual entities, and also brought together some unlikely bedfellows, such as HMSN I and hereditary liability to pressure palsies, found to be due to different mutations in the same gene. Other time-honoured diseases, such as Dejerine–Sottas, are in the process of being eclipsed by the molecular revelations or possibly resurfacing under a different guise (see below and Table 9-1).

While things are currently still in a state of flux, and mild confusion, I thought it helpful to retain the above historical and traditional clinical background as a baseline for reviewing the recent advances in the molecular genetics and the reclassification that is now evolving.

HMSN I (CMT1)

Chromosome 1q (CMT1B)

In 1982, Bird *et al.* and Guiloff *et al.* independently reported linkage data suggesting that the Duffy (Fy) blood group on chromosome 1 was linked to CMT1. Further linked families were reported by Stebbins and Conneally (1982) and Dyck *et al.* (1983). Lebo *et al.* (1991) subsequently re-studied the family reported by Stebbins and Conneally, and found linkage of CMT1 to the FC γ-RII gene known to map near the Duffy locus in proximal 1q. Most families with CMT1, however, were found not to be linked to Duffy (Bird *et al.*, 1983; Griffiths *et al.*, 1988).

Families with CMT1 not linked to Duffy were designated as CMT1A; those linked to Duffy as CMT1B (Dyck *et al.*, 1993a).

Myelin protein zero (P_0) in CMT1B.

Hayasaka *et al.* (1991) have recently isolated and mapped the gene for myelin protein zero (MPZ, P_0) to chromosome 1q22-q23 in the region of the CMT1B locus. Myelin protein zero, a major structural protein of peripheral myelin, is an adhesive glycoprotein of the immunoglobulin superfamily and is thought to play a significant role in the compaction of myelin. Hayasaka *et al.* (1993a) subsequently investigated P_0 as a candidate gene in two pedigrees with CMT1B and demonstrated point mutations in the P_0 gene, involving a glutamate substitution for lysine 96 and for aspartate 90 respectively. The affected individuals were heterozygous for the normal allele and the mutant allele, thus confirming autosomal dominant transmission. The mutant allele was absent in unaffected persons in the two pedigrees and in 100 unrelated healthy controls. They concluded that the P_0 gene is responsible for CMT1B. Kulkens *et al.* (1993) subsequently documented a CMT1B family with a deletion of the codon for serine 34.

Chromosome 17p (CMT1A)

In 1989, Vance *et al.* detected linkage to two markers in the proximal short arm of chromosome 17 in six non-Duffy linked (CMT1A) families. Similar results were obtained by Raeymaekers *et al.* (1989), Middleton-Price *et al.* (1990), Patel *et al.* (1990) and Chance *et al.* (1990). Using multilocus analysis, Vance *et al.* (1991) narrowed the localization to band 17p11.2. The majority of pedigrees studied were found to map to chromosome 17p (Type 1A).

17p11.2 duplication in CMT1A.

Raeymaekers *et al.* (1991) and Lupski *et al.* (1991) independently discovered a DNA duplication in a large segment spanning a genetic distance of about 5 cM (centi-Morgan). The duplication was found to be associated only with CMT1A patients and was detected in several ethnic groups. Somewhat unexpectedly, it also emerged that the duplication can arise as a *de novo* event. Hoogendijk *et al.* (1992) found a *de novo* duplication of 17p11.2 in nine out of ten cases of sporadic CMT1A they studied. This may account for many isolated cases of CMT1 thought to be autosomal recessive. All inherited and *de novo* patients have given evidence for a novel fragment of approximately the same size. These findings strongly implicate the duplicated region in the molecular pathogenesis of CMT1A.

A small number of patients have also been identified who have total or partial trisomy of 17p, including band 17p11.2, the region of the DNA duplication in CMT1A patients (Bartsch–Sandhoff and Hieronimi, 1979; Magenis *et al.*, 1986; Feldman *et al.*, 1982). The consistent phenotypic features of these patients, who seem to have a separate syndrome, are mental retardation and multiple somatic anomalies, including micrognathia, hypoplastic low-set ears, and foot deformities. Chance *et al.* (1992a) detected features consistent with CMT1A in a 14-year-old patient with complete trisomy 17p, supporting the hypothesis that the DNA duplication in CMT1A can have phenotypic consequences through a gene 'dosage effect'. Lupski *et al.* (1992) reported a similar patient with trisomy 17p11.2-p12 and reduced motor nerve conduction velocities, suggesting the presence of demyelinating neuropathy.

The Trembler mouse: an animal model of CMT1A.

The mouse Trembler (Tr) mutation is a dominant disorder with a hypomyelinating neuropathy (Falconer, 1951; Aguayo *et al.*, 1977; Henry and Sidman, 1988) and is a murine model for CMT1A. The Tr locus maps to mouse chromosome 11 (Davisson and Roderick, 1978) which has homology with human chromosome 17p, in the region of the CMT1A locus (Buchberg *et al.*, 1988). Recently, a candidate gene for the Tr locus was identified when a point mutation was found in the peripheral myelin protein-22 (PMP-22) gene (Suter *et al.*, 1992), which is expressed in Schwann cells and is identical to the growth arrest-specific gene, gas3 (Manfioletti *et al.*, 1990; Spreyer *et al.*, 1991; Welcher *et al.*, 1991).

Peripheral myelin protein (PMP)-22 in CMT1A.

These observations in the Tr mouse suggested that the human PMP-22 gene might map to chromosome 17p11.2 in the region of the CMT1A gene, and might actually be the critical gene for CMT1A. To test this hypothesis and further characterize the DNA duplication associated with CMT1A, several laboratories constructed sets of overlapping yeast artificial chromosomes (YACs) in the region of the CMT1A locus on chromosome 17p11.2 and mapped PMP-22 to the CMT1A gene region (Patel *et al.*, 1992; Valentijn *et al.*, 1992a; Timmerman *et al.*, 1992; Matsunami *et al.*, 1992).

Many important questions still await resolution in CMT1A. Although PMP-22 maps to the duplicated region, implicating its role as a candidate gene in CMT1A, more direct proof of its role in CMT1A is needed. Given that there are three copies of the PMP-22 gene present, does the CMT1A phenotype actually result from overexpression of PMP-22? Lupski *et al.* (1992) studied an infant with a dysmorphic syndrome associated with a cytogenetically visible duplication of chromosome 17p11.2-p12, who had slow motor nerve conduction velocity. Molecular analysis showed that he was duplicated for all the DNA markers duplicated in CMT1A, as well as markers proximal and distal to the CMT1A duplication, thus supporting the hypothesis that the CMT1A phenotype can result from a gene dosage effect. Further support for a dosage effect came from the observation of an individual homozygous for the CMT1A mutation, who was more severely affected than the heterozygote parents and sibling (Lupski *et al.*, 1991). In addition, Yoshikawa *et al.* (1994) have recently shown elevated expression of mRNA for PMP-22 in biopsied peripheral nerve in CMT1A.

The mechanism generating the DNA duplication is also of interest. Unequal crossing-over is a possible mechanism for generating the DNA duplication in CMT1A (Tartof, 1988). As the duplication in CMT1A spans an estimated 1.5 Mb, two homologous regions, widely separated within chromosome 17p11.2, may be required for unequal crossing-over. Lupski's group (Pentao *et al.*, 1992) have identified a low-copy number repeat sequence mapping to the proximal and distal duplication breakpoint regions, which is present in three copies on the CMT1A duplicated chromosome.

Point mutations in PMP-22 gene.

CMT1A patients with point mutations have now been identified. Valentijn *et al.* (1992b) described a CMT1 pedigree mapping to 17p11.2 in which no duplication was present, suggesting that forms of CMT1A may exist with other mechanisms (e.g. point mutation). They detected a missense mutation within the PMP-22 gene in this non-duplicated pedigree. The point mutation in this family (a proline for leucine substitution in the first putative transmembrane domain) was identical to that in the Trembler-J mouse, a variant of Trembler.

Roa *et al.* (1993a) identified a point mutation in PMP-22 in a 10-year-old boy with CMT1 without a duplication, resulting in the substitution of cysteine for serine in a putative transmembrane domain of PMP-22. Analysis of family members revealed that the point mutation arose spontaneously and segregated with the CMT type 1 phenotype in an autosomal dominant pattern. The affected father and two sons had clinical and electrophysiological phenotypes similar to patients with the duplication. This supported the view that the PMP-22 gene has a causative role in CMT1A and can result from either a duplication or a point mutation involving the PMP-22 gene.

Roa *et al.* (1993b) subsequently identified a recessive PMP-22 point mutation in a female patient with severe CMT1 who turned out to be a compound heterozygote for a recessive PMP-22 point mutation and a 1.5Mb deletion in 17p11.2-p12. A son, heterozygous for the PMP-22 point mutation, had no signs of neuropathy, whilst two other sons, heterozygous for the deletion, had hereditary neuropathy with liability to pressure palsies (HNPP) (see below), suggesting that point mutations in PMP-22 can result in dominant and recessive alleles contributing to CMT1A.

A third locus (CMT1C)

Chance *et al.* (1992b) reported two clinically typical, autosomal dominant, CMT1 pedigrees which did not map to either the Duffy locus on chromosome 1 (CMT1B) or the proximal short arm of chromosome 17 (CMT1A), suggesting a possible third locus for CMT1. Pedigrees with autosomal dominant CMT1 not mapping to chromosome 1q or to 17p have been designated as CMT1C.

X-linked CMT (CMTX)

The existence of an X-linked form of CMT1 (CMTX) has been well established (Fryns and Van den Berghe, 1980). The clinical features comprise a demyelinating neuropathy, absence of male-to-male transmission, and a generally earlier onset and faster rate of progression of illness in males than females.

In a study of two large CMTX families Nicholson and Nash (1993) demonstrated the more severe clinical involvement in males than females and also an intermediate conduction velocity in females (45±9 m/s) compared with the males (31±6 m/s) which could be helpful clinically in distinguishing these families from CMT1A where both males (20±6 m/s) and females (22±8 m/s) had an equally marked slowing of nerve conduction velocity.

Xq linkage.

Gal *et al.* (1985) established a linkage to the proximal Xq region and the localization was subsequently refined to the region of Xq13-q21 (Fischbeck *et al.*, 1986; Ionasescu *et al.*, 1991; Mostacciuolo *et al.*, 1991), and a close linkage established to the gene for phosphoglycerate kinase (PGK) (Ionasescu *et al.*, 1992).

Connexin 32 in CMTX.

After further localization of the gene (Berghoffen *et al.*, 1993a; Fain *et al.*, 1994), the gene for connexin 32, which encodes a major component of gap junctions and is expressed at high levels in peripheral nerve, was found to map to the CMTX candidate region (Berghoffen *et al.*, 1993b) and an analysis of connexin 32 (CX32) in unrelated CMTX pedigrees showed multiple point mutations in association with the CMTX phenotype.

HMSN II (CMT2) ————————————————

Chromosome 1p35-p36

CMT2 appeared to be genetically distinct from all forms of CMT1 and Loprest *et al.* (1992) excluded linkage in three CMT2 pedigrees to either the CMT1A region in 17p11.2 or the CMT1B region in 1q2.

In a recent linkage study in six large autosomal dominant CMT2 families, Ben Othmane *et al.* (1993a) established linkage in three pedigrees to the distal short arm of chromosome 1 (1p35-p36) and designated this gene CMT2A. The other three families were unlinked to this locus, indicating genetic heterogeneity and suggesting at least one additional gene for CMT2 (CMT2B).

HMSN III ————————————————————

Does it exist?

In his original classification of the hereditary motor and sensory neuropathies, Dyck (1975) defined HMSN III as a severe, demyelinating motor and sensory neuropathy presenting in infancy, associated with a very slow motor nerve conduction velocity. An autosomal recessive form of HMSN I has been recognized by Harding and Thomas (1980b) and Gabreëls–Festen *et al.* (1992) and there has been debate as to whether the pathology of the nerves differs in the autosomal recessive and autosomal dominant forms (Ohnishi *et al.*, 1989; Gabreëls–Festen *et al.*, 1990, 1992) and also whether the type III was characterized by its striking hypomyelination and large onion-bulbs (Dyck, 1975; Ouvrier *et al.*, 1987).

It is now also important to exclude the possibility of *de novo* mutations in the CMT1A gene in isolated cases of demyelinating neuropathy (Hoogendijk *et al.*, 1992).

Gabreëls–Festen *et al.* (1994) recently undertook a review of five personal cases plus all those reported in the literature since the paper of Dyck and Lambert (1968a,b) outlining the clinical and morphological features of HMSN III, with a median motor nerve conduction velocity of less than 6 m/s and characteristic morphological features with thin myelin and large onion bulbs. They recognized three different pathological groups, classical onion bulbs, basal lamina onion bulbs and amyelination.

They concluded that a diagnosis of autosomal recessive HMSN type III could only reasonably be applied to the condition of hypomyelination/amyelination. An inherited basis for type III HMSN with classical onion bulbs is difficult to sustain as only sporadic cases have been described.

Hypomyelination/amyelination neuropathy

This is a severe congenital neuropathy, often with associated arthrogryposis, which presents with respiratory distress or swallowing difficulties and follows a fatal course in days or months. Six cases have been reported (Karch and Urich, 1975; Kasman *et al.*, 1976; Palix and Coignet, 1978; Hakamada *et al.*, 1983; Seitz *et al.*, 1986; Charnas *et al.*, 1988) and in one (Palix and Coignet, 1978) there was an affected sibling, suggesting an autosomal recessive inheritance. Nerve conduction velocity was unrecordable or severely delayed and morphological studies showed hardly any myelin and onion bulbs were usually absent.

Point mutations

Roa *et al.* (1993c) recently reported two patients fulfilling the clinical and morphological criteria of Dejerine–Sottas syndrome, in whom a point mutation was found in exon 3 of the peripheral myelin protein 22 (PMP-22), predicted to cause single amino acid substitutions Met69Lys and Ser72Leu respectively. Both patients were heterozygous for the mutation, suggesting an autosomal dominant gene. In the first patient the mutation was *de novo* as the parents were unaffected and did not carry it; in the second patient the mother had been similarly affected and died at 30 years, suggesting autosomal dominant transmission.

Since similar mutations may be responsible for cases of CMT1A (see above) and in the Trembler mouse, I still find it difficult to understand why these cases have not been classified as variants of CMT1A. In fact, the clinical severity of the first case of Roa *et al.* (1993c) is closer to that of CMT1A than to the Dejerine–Sottas phenotype, with no symptoms at birth, normal motor milestones with ambulation at 15 months, and subsequent development of abnormal gait, pes cavus and gradual decline, with loss of ambulation when assessed again at 18 years. The second patient, an 8-year-old boy, was more severely affected, with hypotonia and weakness at birth, delayed motor milestones and late achievement of ambulation in braces at 7 years. However, his motor nerve conduction velocity was 21 m/s, which is faster than the Dyck criteria.

In a parallel report in the same journal, Hayasaka *et al.* (1993b) documented two unrelated boys, aged 7 and 16 years respectively, with delayed motor development, hypotonia, muscle weakness and sensory loss, included as cases of Dejerine–Sottas syndrome in previous reports by Tachi *et al.* (1984) and Ouvrier *et al.* (1987) respectively, in whom they found different mutations in the P_0 gene. The first case had a cysteine substitution for serine 63 in the extracellular domain, the second an arginine substitution for glycine 167 in the transmembrane domain. The patients were genetically heterozygous for the normal allele and the mutant allele, which was absent in their parents and in 100 unrelated healthy controls. These results suggest that a *de novo* dominant mutation of the P_0 gene is responsible for some sporadic cases with a Dejerine–Sottas clinical phenotype. Once again this begs the question whether this clinical phenotype is merely a more severe variant of CMT1B.

Autosomal recessive demyelinating HMSN

In a recent study of four families with autosomal recessive HMSN with slow nerve conduction, hypomyelination and basal lamina onion bulbs, Ben Othmane *et al.* (1993b) were able to establish linkage to chromosome 8q. This variant was given a designation of CMT4A.

Once again this provides a conflict between this form of HMSN as a separate type on morphological grounds or whether it is another variant within the blanket of CMT1 but with a separate (recessive) genetic basis. It would seem more logical to designate it as CMT1D together with the other demyelinating neuropathies.

Hayasaka *et al.* (1993c) have localized the gene for P_2 (peripheral myelin protein-2; PMP-2) to this region, making P_2 a candidate for this autosomal recessive neuropathy. Further studies for linkage to 8q and mutations in this gene in Tunisian families, and also other reported families with autosomal recessive HMSN, would be of interest to establish possible genetic heterogeneity.

OTHER TYPES OF HMSN

Cases of HMSN have been recorded in association with optic atrophy and also with retinitis pigmentosa without excess phytanic acid. There may also be involvement of the motor and sensory neurones in association with various spinocerebellar degenerations, including Friedreich's ataxia (Figure 9-12). As the sensory rather than the motor neurones are predominantly involved they were classified by Dyck (1975) with the hereditary sensory neuropathies rather than the mixed ones. The gene for Friedreich's ataxia has been located on the proximal long arm of chromosome 9 (Chamberlain *et al.*, 1988, 1989), which could be helpful in the study of families with unusual presentation.

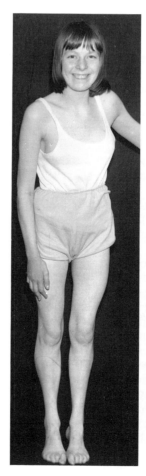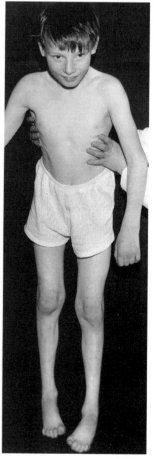

(a) (b)

Figure 9-12a,b Neuronal neuropathy/Friedreich's ataxia. (a) A 15-year-old girl with a 2-year history of walking on toes and unsteadiness of gait. There was no progression. There was tendency to clawing of hands but no difficulty with fine movements, and pes cavus and wasting of distal part of legs. Tendon jerks were absent in legs, sluggish in arms. Some sensory loss to painful stimuli in legs. Motor conduction normal in ulnar nerve: 63 m/s; in anterior and posterior tibial, supramaximal stimulus produced very small motor response, inadequate for measurement of latency. (b) A 13-year-old brother had classical Friedreich's ataxia with intellectual retardation, slurring of speech, ataxia and inability to walk since 6 years of age. Associated pes cavus, but no scoliosis. Tendon reflexes were absent, plantar response extensor. Three other siblings and the parents were normal. This is presumably a recessively inherited form of neuronal peripheral neuropathy, and illustrates the overlap clinically between the hereditary motor and sensory peripheral neuropathies and Friedreich's ataxia.

SCAPULOPERONEAL MUSCULAR ATROPHY

The scapuloperoneal syndrome is a heterogeneous one. Some cases have had a myopathic basis but others are neurogenic (Figure 9-13).

Kaesar (1965) described a family in which 12 members were affected in five generations, suggesting a dominant inheritance. The onset was usually in adult life and investigation revealed a neurogenic disorder.

A somewhat similar condition starting in infancy or childhood, but with a recessive inheritance or occurring sporadically, has been described in sporadic cases by Emery *et al.* (1968), Zellweger and McCormick (1968) and Feigenbaum and Munsat (1970) and in two sibs by Emery (1971), suggesting an autosomal recessive inheritance. Muscle weakness may be present at birth or occur in the first year of life. The anterior or posterior lower leg muscles are diffusely affected and there is often associated equinovarus deformity. Scapular involvement may

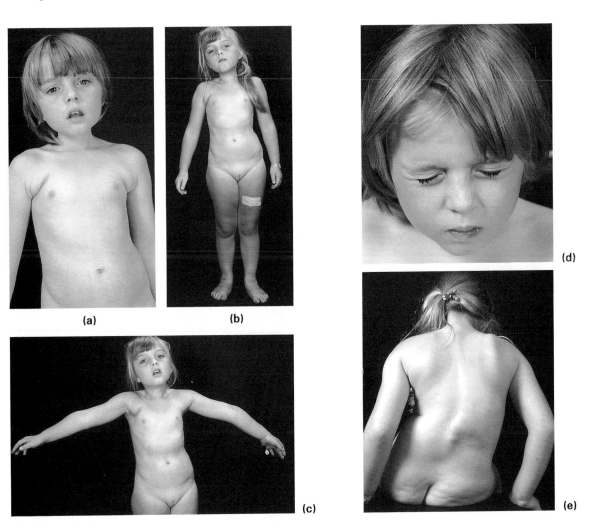

(a) (b) (c) (d) (e)

Figure 9-13a-e Facioscapuloperoneal muscular atrophy. This 7-year-old girl presented with difficulty in walking and other motor activities (a-c). She had sat unsupported at 6 months, stood at 18 months and walked at 2 years but was always reluctant to let go. She also had poor head control and had never crawled. Scoliosis was noted from 5 years of age. She was unable to run and had difficulty negotiating stairs. On examination there was weakness of the shoulder girdle with difficulty in raising her arms and wasting of pectoral muscles, with associated skin creases (c). There was also mild facial weakness with difficulty in screwing up eyes and burying eyelashes (d). She walked with a drop-foot gait and had weakness of the ankle dorsiflexors as well as asymmetrical weakness of the quadriceps. She also had an associated scoliosis (e). Peroneal NCV was normal (59 m/s). EMG showed evidence of denervation. Needle biopsy of quadriceps showed focal atrophy of fibres and type 1 predominance. Family history was negative. This neuropathy has a predominantly scapuloperoneal distribution plus involvement of the face and other muscle groups.

be present early or occur later. Electromyography and muscle biopsy reveal a neurogenic pattern.

In a family recorded by Mawatari and Katayama (1973) there were five affected male children in one generation, suggesting an X-linked recessive inheritance. In addition to the scapuloperoneal weakness there was evidence of cardiomyopathy in the cases and also in two symptom-free mothers.

HEREDITARY NEUROPATHY WITH LIABILITY TO PRESSURE PALSIES (HNPP) (TOMACULOUS NEUROPATHY)

Hereditary neuropathy with liability to pressure palsies (HNPP) was first described in a family in which three generations had recurrent peroneal neuropathy after digging potatoes in a kneeling posture (De Jong, 1947). It is associated with periodic episodes of pain, muscle weakness, atrophy and numbness, and may follow relatively minor compression or trauma to the peripheral nerves (Davies, 1954; Earl *et al.*, 1964; Staal *et al.*, 1965). Carpal tunnel syndrome and other entrapment neuropathies are frequent manifestations of HNPP. Electrophysiological studies may show mildly slowed motor and sensory nerve conduction velocity in clinically affected individuals as well as asymptomatic carriers. Peripheral nerves show segmental demyelination and remyelination with tomaculous or sausage-like, focal thickenings of the myelin sheath (Behse *et al.*, 1972; Bradley *et al.*, 1975; Madrid and Bradley, 1975).

Clinical features

From their own study and a review of 261 cases published in the literature, Meier and Moll (1982) proposed the following diagnostic criteria: autosomal dominant inheritance; clinical presentation of a recurrent mononeuropathy simplex or multiplex frequently related to trauma; significant slowing of motor and sensory conduction velocity in clinically affected but also unaffected nerves; characteristic morphological findings on sural nerve biopsy featuring 'tomaculous' or sausage-like swellings of myelin sheaths, transnodal myelination, and segmental demyelination.

The age of onset is within the first and second decade in about 50% of cases and clinical features may be apparent by 4 years. Many are not diagnosed until later, since a firm diagnosis is only possible after recurrent episodes in individuals without a clear family history.

Patients develop single or multiple mononeuropathies, usually of those nerves subject to pressure, such as the peroneal nerve at the fibula head, the ulnar nerve at the elbow, the radial nerve in the spiral groove of the humerus, and the median nerve at the carpal tunnel, but any nerve may be affected, including the digital, brachial plexus, sciatic or cranial nerves. Onset is usually associated with trauma, often trivial, such as sleeping on an arm, sitting cross-legged, or resting on an elbow. Patients, however, may not be able to identify the precipitating trauma. Episodes are usually painless.

On examination there is often weakness, with or without sensory loss, in the territory of the affected nerve. Recovery, usually complete, occurs over days to several weeks. Some patients, mainly older adults, show signs of a diffuse neuropathy, predominantly with distal limb weakness and wasting of the intrinsic muscles of hands and feet, and may develop progressive unremitting palsies. Most patients learn to avoid precipitating causes and are able to live normal lives.

17p11.2 deletion in HNPP

Chance and colleagues (1993) assigned the HNPP locus to chromosome 17p11.2 and detected a 1.5 Mb deletion associated with this disorder. All DNA markers known to map to the region in 17p11.2 associated with the CMT1A duplication, including the PMP-22 gene, are deleted in HNPP. The deletion breakpoints in HNPP map to the same chromosomal intervals in which the CMT1A duplication breakpoints map. It is also likely that the deleted chromosome 17 in HNPP and the duplicated chromosome 17 in CMT1A are the reciprocal products of unequal crossing over.

OTHER PERIPHERAL NEUROPATHIES

Peripheral neuropathy may occur in association with a wide variety of conditions, both acute and chronic, hereditary and acquired. Many of these cases may present with hypotonia or muscle weakness. The weakness tends to be distal more than proximal and in some cases there may be associated sensory deficit. The diagnosis of the neuropathy can be further confirmed by electrodiagnostic studies.

ACUTE INFLAMMATORY DEMYELINATING POLYRADICULONEUROPATHY (GUILLAIN–BARRÉ SYNDROME)

This syndrome is characterized by a fairly acute symmetrical paralysis, starting in the legs and gradually moving upwards to involve the trunk and upper limbs as well, often causing a marked flaccid quadriplegia. It frequently also affects the cranial nerves, particularly the facial. Some cases have associated respiratory paralysis, which can be life-threatening and may need tracheostomy and artificial ventilation. There may be associated sensory symptoms and signs and also at times evidence of autonomic dysfunction. Some young cases may also show meningeal irritation.

There is often a preceding, non-specific, prodromal illness, usually respiratory or gastrointestinal, within 4 weeks of the onset. The condition is thought to have an autoimmune basis, possibly triggered by a viral infection.

The evolution of the weakness may occur over a variable period of a few days to a few weeks, and in most cases reaches its maximum within 3 weeks. The disease then tends to remain fairly static for a few weeks before starting to recover. Recovery may be very slow and continue over several months.

The cerebrospinal fluid shows a characteristic picture of raised protein without increase in cells (usually under 10 mononuclears present). In the early stages the cerebrospinal fluid may be normal.

The peripheral neuropathy is of the demyelinating type and may be confirmed by the very slow motor nerve conduction velocity. This may not be manifest in the early stages in some cases but is usually found after a few weeks.

The pattern of improvement, both clinically and reflected in the nerve conduction velocity, tends to follow the same sequence as the evolution of the weakness, starting in the legs and progressing upwards. Resolution of the slow nerve conduction may take longer than the clinical recovery.

The overall prognosis is very good and more than 60% of patients show full recovery. Some may be left with residual disability, such as foot drop, pes cavus, weakness of the hands, or postural tremor. There is also a small mortality, usually as a result of respiratory paralysis in the acute phase.

Treatment

Given the overall good prognosis and tendency to resolution of the disease, the main treatment is supportive. Special attention needs to be paid, especially in young children, to the possibility of impending respiratory failure in the acute phase and appropriate supportive treatment instituted, including, where indicated, mechanical ventilation. If there is evidence of dysphagia or bulbar paralysis, appropriate action should be taken for feeding by nasogastric tube or gastrostomy.

The use of steroids, plasma exchange or more particularly intravenous gammaglobulin with worsening or unremitting disease, or with the chronic form of radiculopathy (see below), has been claimed to be beneficial, often dramatic, in individual case reports, but the overall value has been difficult to assess in controlled studies (Ouvrier *et al.*, 1990; Arnason and Soliven, 1993; Dyck *et al.*, 1993b).

No benefit was found in a controlled trial of prednisolone (Hughes *et al.*, 1978) or in a multicentric study of high-dosage, intravenous methylprednisolone (Hughes *et al.*, 1992). A North American multicentre, therapeutic trial of plasma exchange in severe Guillain–Barré syndrome showed its efficacy if given within 2 weeks of onset of illness (McKhann *et al.*, 1984). In a given comparative study of plasma exchange vs high-dose intravenous human immunoglobulin, a Dutch study showed greater benefit for the gammaglobulin group (Van der Meché, 1992). Recent open studies with intravenous gammaglobulin suggest a dramatic reversal of symptoms in some of the acute, deteriorating, childhood cases (Shahar *et al.*, 1994). A dramatic response has also been claimed in some of the more chronic and intractable cases (Cook and Galverston, 1994).

CHRONIC INFLAMMATORY DEMYELINATING POLYRADICULONEUROPATHY ————

This disorder has been distinguished from acute polyradiculoneuropathy on the basis of its more insidious onset and its progressive course. It usually takes longer than 2 months to reach its maximum weakness and the course may be steadily progressive, follow a stepwise progression, or have a relapsing course. As in the acute form, the process is a demyelinating one, the nerve conduction velocity is slowed and the cerebrospinal fluid shows an increase in protein, without an increase in cells (Dyck *et al.*, 1993b).

The condition needs to be distinguished from the hereditary demyelinating neuropathies (HMSN I), and a careful family history and assessment of nerve conduction velocity in the parents is important, with further help from some of the new advances in characterizing individual hereditary neuropathies at the molecular genetic level (see above).

Treatment

The chronic relapsing polyneuropathy is often steroid-sensitive, which remains the first line of treatment (Figure 9-14). Refractory cases may benefit from other forms of immunosuppression, from plasma exchange or from intravenous gammaglobulin.

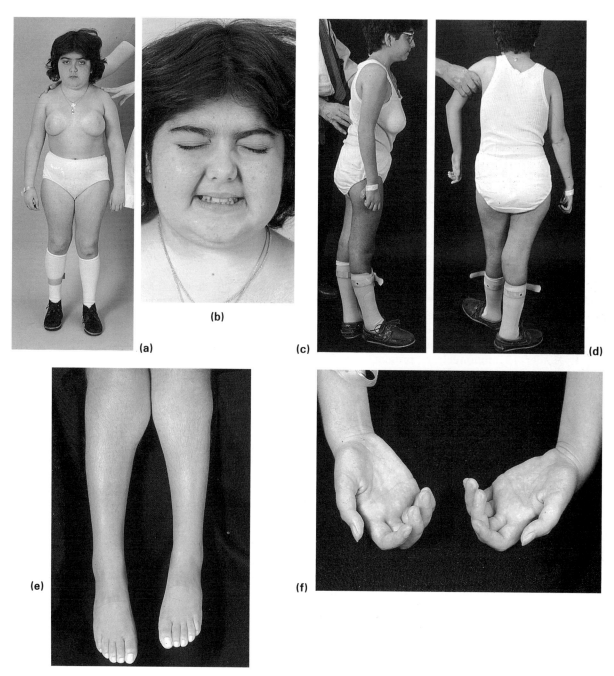

Figure 9-14a-f Chronic relapsing polyneuropathy. This girl was initially referred at the age of 9 years with a history of insidious onset of severe polyneuropathy at 7 years. This responded well to low-dosage steroids but she relapsed when the steroids were abruptly withdrawn after 6 months of continuous therapy. She improved again when the steroids were reintroduced but did not regain the previous function. The motor nerve conduction velocity was very slow (22 m/s in the ulnar and 10 m/s in the lateral popliteal nerves). There had also been an elevation in the CSF protein (102 mg/dl;n<40). She was still on a dose of daily prednisolone of 16 mg. In view of the marked cushingoid appearance and stunting of her growth, efforts were made to very gradually reduce the steroids by 1 mg every 2 weeks, but she once again relapsed and it was difficult to maintain her below 15 mg/day. Equal difficulty was subsequently found with trying to maintain her on an alternate-day regime (of 30 mg steroid) or to reduce the steroid under cover of associated azathioprine. At 14 years (a,b) she was still cushingoid and very stunted in growth from the continued steroid and was barely ambulant with the help of ankle-foot orthoses. By 16 years she had essentially lost independent ambulation (c,d). There was marked wasting and weakness of the lower legs affecting particularly the anterior tibial muscles (e) and of the hands (f) with associated flexion contractures of the fingers. She also had sensory loss of the distal arms and legs with a glove and stocking distribution.

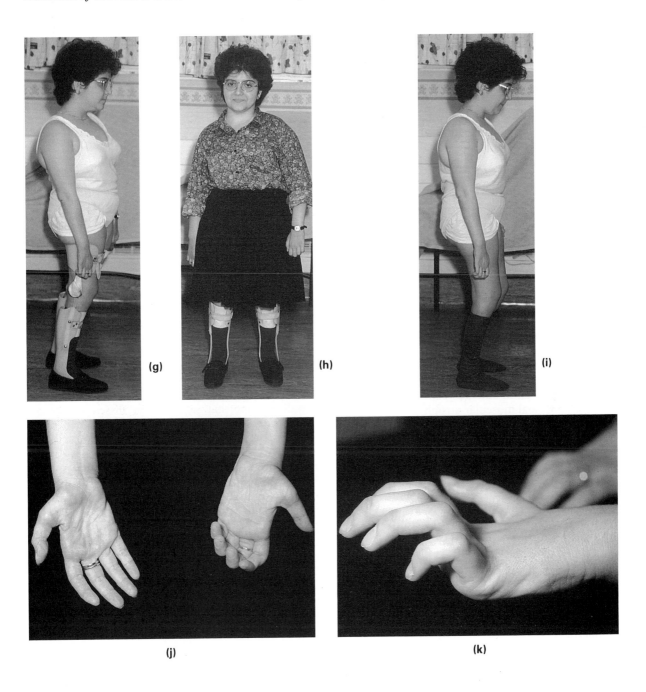

Figure 9-14g-k She became essentially wheelchair bound from that time for several years, but gradually responded to a succession of therapeutic efforts, particularly cyclophosphamide (which had to be stopped because of haemorrhagic cystitis) and cyclosporin. There was very little response to a series of six plasma exchanges. She was remobilized with knee-ankle-foot orthoses (g,h, 23 years) and once again achieved independent standing and walking without callipers (i). There was also improvement in hand function, but persistence in the contractures of the long finger flexors, especially of the left hand (j,k). She also developed marked general osteoporosis and DEXA scanning showed a reduction of 2–3 standard deviations below the mean in most of her bones. She also had a progressive S-shaped scoliosis, reaching a Cobb angle of 80°, which was partially controlled with a brace and became stable and relatively fixed. Although she was keen on operative treatment of the scoliosis to try and achieve increased length, this was considered inadvisable. Her respiratory function remained good.

POLIOMYELITIS

The advent of immunization has practically eradicated poliomyelitis in most developed countries, but the disease remains a scourge in underdeveloped countries.

It is usually suspected clinically on the basis of an acute onset, often with a prodromal illness associated with signs of meningeal involvement. The paralysis commonly has a rapid evolution reaching its maximum within a few days, and is characteristically asymmetrical. There is usually associated muscle spasm. The distribution is extremely variable. Some cases are fairly focal, others may have an almost total flaccid quadriplegia and there may also be proximal, bulbar and respiratory involvement which can be life-threatening.

The cerebrospinal fluid shows an increase in cells as well as protein.

Although the diagnosis is usually quite clear-cut, it may closely mimic severe spinal muscular atrophy (Werdnig–Hoffmann disease) if it has a fairly extensive weakness and occurs in the first year of life.

Electrodiagnostic studies and muscle biopsy show evidence of the denervation associated with anterior horn cell degeneration and are very similar to those of hereditary spinal muscular atrophy.

A very similar clinical picture to that of poliomyelitis may be produced by other viruses, particularly Coxsackie.

AMYOTROPHIC LATERAL SCLEROSIS (ALS); MOTOR NEURONE DISEASE

This is one of the more common neuromuscular disorders in adults and is characterized by a combined involvement of the corticospinal tracts and the motor nuclei of lower medulla and the anterior horn cells of the spinal cord. The weakness is usually asymmetrical and tends to start distally. Fasciculation of the tongue and skeletal muscles is often present. The tendon reflexes are usually brisk and there may be increased tone in the lower limbs as a result of the pyramidal tract involvement. The disease tends to follow a steadily downhill course, with death from respiratory paralysis and bulbar involvement in an average of about 3 years. Charcot (1874) coined the term 'amyotrophic lateral sclerosis' to highlight the pathological features. The condition is usually sporadic but may rarely be familial and then usually shows an autosomal dominant pattern of inheritance (Horton *et al.*, 1976).

In childhood, ALS is very rare and is very much milder than the adult form and has a more protracted course. In addition to the isolated cases that

have been documented (Kohn, 1971; Nelson and Prensky, 1972; Reif-Kohn and Mundel, 1974), familial cases have also been recorded with a presumptive autosomal recessive pattern of inheritance (Staal and Went, 1968; Gragg *et al.*, 1971).

FAMILIAL AMYOTROPHIC LATERAL SCLEROSIS (FALS)

The dominantly inherited familial form of ALS (FALS), estimated to account for about 10% of cases, is clinically similar to the sporadic form, although some cases may have earlier onset.

Recent advances at the molecular genetic level may have important implications, not only for amyotrophic lateral sclerosis itself but also for the pathogenesis and potential treatment of other neurodegenerative disorders. Siddique *et al.* (1991) showed that some pedigrees of FALS were linked to a gene on chromosome 21q, and recently Rosen *et al.* (1993) demonstrated a tight genetic linkage between FALS and a gene that encodes a cytosolic Cu/Zn-binding superoxide dismutase (SOD 1), a homodimeric metalloenzyme that catalyses the dissemination of the toxic superoxide anion to oxygen and hydrogen peroxide. They then investigated SOD 1 as a candidate gene in FALS and identified 11 different SOD 1 missense mutations in 13 different FALS families. This suggests a pathogenetic role of free radical toxicity in ALS, and possibly other neurodegenerative disorders. In addition to the cytosolic Cu/ZN SOD 1, the human genome encodes two other SOD proteins, a mitochondrial, Mn-dependent, SOD 2 (mapping to chromosome 6q25) and an extracellular SOD 3 (mapping to chromosome 4). These may be potential candidates for the non-chromosome 21 cases of FALS and for other neurodegenerative disorders. It also raises the possibility that either SOD itself, or compounds that may penetrate the central nervous system and decrease levels of free radicals, could have therapeutic possibilities.

PROGRESSIVE DEGENERATIVE DISORDERS OF THE CENTRAL NERVOUS SYSTEM

The lower motor neurone is consistently involved in some of the progressive degenerations of the central nervous system. In the demyelinating leucodystrophies, such as metachromatic leucodystrophy and globoid cell leucodystrophy (Krabbe's disease), there

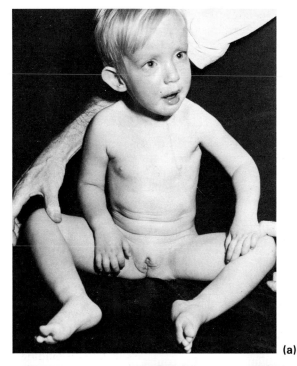

is an associated demyelination of the peripheral nerve with resultant marked slowing of the conduction velocity. The pattern of inheritance of these degenerative disorders is usually autosomal recessive.

METACHROMATIC LEUCODYSTROPHY (SULPHATIDE LIPIDOSIS)

The usual late infantile form presents in the second year of life with a deterioration in motor and intellectual function in a previously normal child. The motor symptoms are often the presenting ones and there is a tendency to loss of ability to stand and walk in association with hypotonia of the limbs and depression of the tendon reflexes (Figure 9-15 a,b). This is subsequently followed by deterioration in intellectual function, progressive optic atrophy and blindness, and finally a state resembling decerebrate rigidity (Figure 9-15 c,d).

(a)

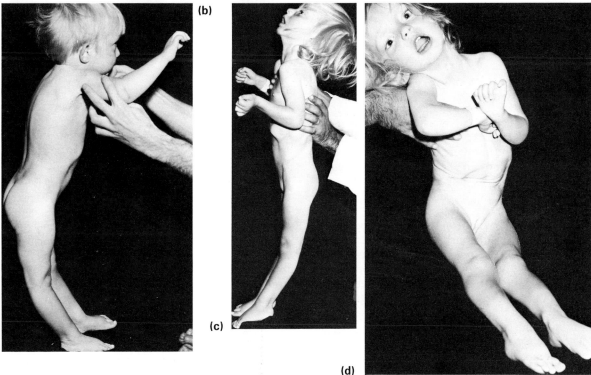

(b)

(c)

(d)

Figure 9-15a-d Metachromatic leucodystrophy. A girl aged 2 years and 3 months presented with hypotonia and difficulty with gait (a and b). Note the hyperextension of the knees. No associated intellectual problems at that stage. She subsequently had progressive deterioration of motor as well as intellectual function and developed marked rigidity of the muscles with associated extensor spasms (c and d). Nerve conduction velocity was very slow (ulnar 14.4 m/s, posterior tibial 10.7 m/s). Metachromatic material demonstrated intracellularly in deposits of freshly spun urine. Absence of the enzyme aryl sulphatase A was documented in the leucocytes.

In the early stages there is already a marked slowing of the motor nerve conduction velocity and the diagnosis can be confirmed by the demonstration of a marked reduction (or total absence) of the enzyme aryl sulphatase A in the leucocytes. There is a deposition of metachromatic material due to the accumulated sulphatide, which can be demonstrated in the sural nerve and also in nerves present in a muscle biopsy sample. Brain imaging, especially magnetic resonance imaging, will demonstrate the white matter changes.

The condition follows a steadily downhill course and usually leads to death by about the age of 5 years.

A more slowly progressive juvenile form also occurs, with a somewhat later onset, usually between 4 and 12 years, with decline in school performance, disturbance of gait and a more protracted course.

An adult form also exists, with onset in adolescence or early adult life.

The gene for aryl sulphatase A is located on chromosome 22q13.31-qter. Several different mutations have been identified in the DNA which relate to different clinical phenotypes (Kolodny, 1993).

Therapeutic efforts with bone marrow transplant (Krivit *et al.*, 1990) may be of some benefit in preclinical juvenile rather than the classical late infantile type and still await longer follow-up and appraisal.

GLOBOID CELL LEUCODYSTROPHY (KRABBE'S DISEASE)

This form of leucodystrophy usually presents in the second half of the first year of life with a deterioration of motor and intellectual function, following a more acute course than the metachromatic leucodystrophy and often leading to death within a matter of months. Late infantile, juvenile and adult cases have also been recognized.

The clinical diagnosis can again be supported by the demonstration of markedly slowed nerve conduction velocity. The recognition of a specific enzyme deficiency, galactocerebrosidase, has provided a means of confirming the diagnosis on leucocytes and also opened the way for prenatal diagnosis on cultured amniotic fluid cells and subsequently chorionic villus biopsy.

The gene for Krabbe's disease has been located on chromosome 14 (Zlotogora *et al.*, 1990). A number of animal models have also been identified, including the twitcher mouse (Duchen *et al.*, 1980; Kobayashi *et al.*, 1980), located on mouse chromosome 12, which has homology with human chromosome 14, as well as the dog, cat and monkey.

Therapeutic efforts with bone marrow transplant in the twitcher mouse apparently prolonged life but did not reduce neurological complications, and in the few human cases treated, the results have been disappointing (Wenger and Chen, 1993).

NEURAXONAL DYSTROPHY

This is also a progressive degenerative disorder of the central nervous system with onset in early infancy (Seitelberger, 1952; Huttenlocher and Gilles, 1967). A previously normal infant may present during the second year of life with muscle weakness and hypotonia, which may show a slowly progressive course. There is usually associated involvement of the corticospinal tracts, with increasing spasticity and decorticate posturing. These children subsequently develop bulbar signs, visual impairment and profound psychomotor retardation, and eventually die before reaching their teens.

The motor nerve conduction is not impaired (or may be slightly slowed). The characteristic histological abnormality on nerve biopsy is the presence of swellings along the course of the axon.

The condition appears to be clinically, as well as genetically, heterogeneous, and in one form a deficiency has been demonstrated by Schindler *et al.* (1989) of the lysosomal enzyme α-N-acetylgalactosaminidase, whose gene is located on chromosome 22q13-qter.

OTHER CENTRAL NERVOUS SYSTEM DISORDERS

Involvement of the lower motor neurone is a component of many of the other somewhat rare degenerative disorders of the nervous system. Marked slowing of motor nerve conduction and associated demyelination has been demonstrated in Cockayne's syndrome (Moosa and Dubowitz, 1970) and in some cases of Leigh's syndrome (Moosa, 1975). Hypotonia is a common component of the gangliosidoses, suggesting an associated involvement of the lower motor neurone, although there may be no overt abnormality in motor nerve conduction or electromyography. Hypotonia is also a common feature in familial dysautonomia and occurs as a non-specific manifestation of a wide variety of central nervous system disorders (see Chapter 12, The Floppy Infant Syndrome). In many of these conditions there is probably some functional disorder in the control of tone, rather than any direct involvement of the lower motor neurone itself.

REFERENCES

Aguayo, J.A., Attiwell, M., Trecarten, J. *et al.* (1977) Abnormal myelination in transplanted Trembler mouse Schwann cells. *Nature* **265**: 73–75.

Arnason, B.G.W. and Soliven, B. (1993) Acute inflammatory demyelinating polyradiculo-neuropathy. In: Dyck, P.J., Thomas, P.K., Griffin, J.W. *et al.* eds, *Peripheral Neuropathy* 3rd edn. Philadelphia: W.B. Saunders, pp. 1437–1497.

Bartsch-Sandhoff, M. and Hieronimi, G. (1979) Partial duplication of 17p. *Human Genetics* **49**: 123–127.

Behse, F., Buchthal, F., Carlsen, F. *et al.* (1972) Hereditary neuropathy with liabiity to pressure palsies: electrophysiological and histopathological aspects. *Brain* **95**: 777–794.

Ben Othmane, K., Middleton, L.T., Loprest, L.J. *et al.* (1993a) Localization of a gene (CMT2A) for autosomal dominant Charcot–Marie–Tooth disease type 2 to chromosome 1p and evidence of genetic heterogeneity. *Genomics* **17**: 370–375.

Ben Othmane, K., Hentati, F., Lennon, F. *et al.* (1993b) Linkage of a locus (CMT4A) for autosomal recessive Charcot–Marie–Tooth disease to chromosome 8q. *Human Molecular Genetics* **2**: 1625–1628.

Berghoffen, J., Trofatter, J. and Pericak-Vance, M.A. (1993a) Linkage localization of X-linked Charcot–Marie–Tooth disease. *American Journal of Human Genetics* **52**: 312–318.

Berghoffen, J., Scherer, S., Wang, S. *et al.* (1993b) Connexin mutations in X-linked Charcot–Marie–Tooth disease. *Science* **262**: 2039–2041.

Bird, T.D., Ott, J. and Giblett, E.R. (1982) Evidence for linkage of Charcot–Marie–Tooth neuropathy to the Duffy locus on chromosome 1. *American Journal of Human Genetics* **34**: 388–394.

Bird, T.D., Ott, J., Giblett, E.R. *et al.* (1983) Genetic linkage evidence for heterogeneity in Charcot–Marie–Tooth neuropathy (HMSN Type I). *Annals of Neurology* **14**: 679–684.

Bradley, W.G., Madrid, R., Thrush, D.C. *et al.* (1975) Recurrent brachial plexus neuropathy. *Brain* **98**: 381–398.

Buchberg, A.M., Brownell, E., Nagata, S. *et al.* (1988) A comprehensive genetic map of murine chromosome 11 reveals extensive linkage conservation between mouse and human. *Genetics* **122**: 153–161.

Chamberlain, S., Shaw, J., Rowland, L.P. *et al.* (1988) Mapping of mutation causing Friedreich's ataxia to human chromosome 9. *Nature* **334**: 248–250.

Chamberlain, S., Shaw, J., Wallis, J. *et al.* (1989) Genetic homogeneity at the Friedreich ataxia locus on chromosome 9. *American Journal of Human Genetics* **44**: 518–521.

Chance, P.F., Bird, T.D., O'Connell, P. *et al.* (1990) Linkage and heterogeneity in type I Charcot–Marie–Tooth disease (hereditary motor and sensory neuropathy I). *American Journal of Human Genetics* **47**: 915–925.

Chance, P.F., Bird, T.D., Matsunami, N. *et al.* (1992a) Trisomy 17p associated with Charcot–Marie–Tooth neuropathy I phenotype: evidence for gene dosage as a mechanism in CMT1A. *Neurology* **42**: 2295–2299.

Chance, P.F., Matsunami, N., Lensch, M.W. *et al.* (1992b) Analysis of the DNA duplication 17p11.2 in Charcot–Marie–Tooth neuropathy type 1 pedigrees: additional evidence for a third autosomal CMT1 locus. *Neurology* **42**: 2037–2041.

Chance, P.F., Alderson, M.K., Leppig, K.A. *et al.* (1993) DNA deletion associated with hereditary neuropathy with liability to pressure palsies. *Cell* **72**: 143–151.

Charcot, J.M. (1874) De la sclérose latérale amyotrophique. *Progrès Médical (Paris)* **2**: 325.

Charcot, J.M. and Marie, P. (1886) Sur une forme particulière d'atrophie musculaire progressive souvent familial débutant par les pieds et les jambes et atteignant plus tard les mains. *Revue Médicale (Paris)* **6**: 97–138.

Charnas, L., Trapp, B. and Griffin, J. (1988) Congenital absence of peripheral myelin: abnormal Schwann cell development causes lethal arthrogryposis multiplex congenita. *Neurology* **38**: 966–974.

Cook, J.D. and Galveston, T.X. (1994) Long-term experience with gamma globulin treatment of childhood chronic relapsing idiopathic polyneuropathy. *Annals of Neurology* **36**: 503 (abstract).

Davies, D.M. (1954) Recurrent peripheral nerve palsies in a family. *Lancet* **2**: 266–268.

Davisson, M.T. and Roderick, T.H. (1978) Status of the linkage map of the mouse. *Cytogenetics and Cell Genetics* **22**: 552–557.

De Jong, J.G.Y. (1947) Over families met hereditaire dispositie tot het optreden van neuritiden gecorreleerd met migraine. *Psychiatr Neurol Bull (Amst)* **50**: 60–76.

Dejerine, J. and Sottas, J. (1893) Sur la névrite interstitielle, hypertrophique et progressive de l'enfance. *Compte Rendu de la Société de Biologie* **45**: 63–96.

Duchen, L.W., Eicher, E.M., Jacobs, J.M. *et al.* (1980) Hereditary leucodystrophy in the mouse: the new mutant twitcher. *Brain* **103**: 695–710.

Dyck, P.J. (1975) Inherited neuronal degeneration and atrophy affecting peripheral motor, sensory, and autonomic neurons. In: Dyck, P.J., Thomas, P.K., Lambert, E.H. eds, *Peripheral Neuropathy* Vol.2. Philadelphia: W.B. Saunders, pp. 825–867.

Dyck, P.J. and Lambert, E.H. (1968a) Lower motor and primary sensory neuron diseases with peroneal muscular atrophy. Part I. Neurologic, genetic and electrophysiologic findings in hereditary polyneuropathies. *Archives of Neurology* **18**: 603–618.

Dyck, P.J. and Lambert, E.H. (1968b) Lower motor and primary sensory neuron diseases with peroneal muscular atrophy. Part II. Neurologic, genetic, and electrophysiologic findings in various neuronal degenerations. *Archives of Neurology* **18**: 619–625.

Dyck, P.J., Lambert, E.H. and Nichols, P.C. (1971) Quantitative measurement of sensation related to compound action potential and number and sizes of myelinated and unmyelinated fibres of sural nerve in health, Friedreich's ataxia, hereditary sensory neuropathy and tabes dorsalis. In: Cobb, W.A. ed., _Handbook of Electroencephalography and Clinical Neurophysiology_ Vol. 9. Amsterdam: Elsevier Publishing Co., p. 83.

Dyck, P.J., Ott, J., Breanndan, M.S. _et al._ (1983) Linkage evidence for genetic heterogeneity among kinships with hereditary motor and sensory neuropathy, Type I. _Mayo Clinic Proceedings_ 58: 430–435.

Dyck, P.J., Chance, P.F., Lebo, R.V. _et al._ (1993a) Hereditary motor and sensory neuropathies. In: Dyck, P.J., Thomas, P.K., Griffin, J.W. _et al._ eds, _Peripheral Neuropathy_ 3rd edn. Philadelphia: W.B. Saunders, pp. 1094-1136.

Dyck, P.J., Prineas, J. and Pollard, J. (1993b) Chronic inflammatory demyelinating polyradiculoneuropathy. In: Dyck, P.J., Thomas, P.K., Griffin, J.W. _et al._ eds, _Peripheral Neuropathy_ 3rd edn. Philadelphia: W.B. Saunders, pp.1498-1517.

Earl, C.J., Fullerton, P.M., Wakefield, G.S. _et al._ (1964) Hereditary neuropathy, with liability to pressure palsies. _Quarterly Journal of Medicine_ 33: 481–498.

Eldjarn, L., Try, K., Stokke, O. _et al._ (1966) Dietary effects of serum-phytanic-acid levels and on clinical manifestations in heredopathia atactica polyneuritiformis. _Lancet_ i: 691.

Emery, A.E.H. (1971) The nosology of the spinal muscular atrophies. _Journal of Medical Genetics_ 8: 481–495.

Emery, E.S., Fenichel, G.M. and Eng, G. (1968) A spinal muscular atrophy with scapuloperoneal distribution. _Archives of Neurology (Chicago)_ 18: 129–133.

Fain, P.R., Barker, D.F. and Chance, P.F. (1994) Refined genetic mapping of the X-linked Charcot–Marie–Tooth neuropathy locus. _American Journal of Human Genetics_ 54: 229–235.

Falconer, D.S. (1951) Two new mutants, 'Trembler' and 'Reeler' with neurological actions in the mouse (_Mus musculus_ L.). _Journal of Genetics_ 50: 192–201.

Feigenbaum, J.A. and Munsat, T.L. (1970) A neuromuscular syndrome of scapuloperoneal distribution. _Bulletin of the Los Angeles Neurological Society_ 35: 45–57.

Feldman, G.M., Baumer, J.G. and Sparkes, R.S. (1982) Brief clinical report: the dup(17p) syndrome. _American Journal of Medical Genetics_ 11: 299–304.

Fischbeck, K.H., Rushdi, N., Pericak-Vance, M. _et al._ (1986) X-linked neuropathy: gene localization with DNA probes. _Annals of Neurology_ 20: 527–532.

Fryns, J.P. and Van den Berghe, H. (1980) Sex-linked recessive inheritance in Charcot–Marie–Tooth disease with partial manifestations in female carriers. _Human Genetics_ 55: 413–415.

Gabreëls-Festen, A.A.W.M., Joosten, E.M.G., Gabreëls, F.J.M. _et al._ (1990) Congenital demyelinating motor and sensory neuropathy with focally folded myelin sheaths. _Brain_ 113: 1629–1643.

Gabreëls-Festen, A.A.W.M., Gabreëls, F.J.M., Jennekens, F.G.I. _et al._ (1992) Autosomal recessive form of motor and sensory neuropathy type I. _Neurology_ 42: 1755-1761.

Gabreëls-Festen, A.A.W.M., Gabreëls, F.J.M., Jennekens, F.G.I. _et al._ (1994) The status of HMSN type III. _Neuromuscular Disorders_ 4: 63–69.

Gal, A., Mucke, J., Theile, H. _et al._ (1985) X-linked dominant Charcot–Marie–Tooth disease: suggestion of linkage with a cloned DNA sequence from the proximal Xq. _Human Genetics_ 70: 38–42.

Gragg, G.W., Fogelson, M.H. and Zwirecki, R.J. (1971) Juvenile amyotrophic lateral sclerosis in two brothers from an inbred community-case report. _Birth Defects, Original Article Series_ 7: 222–225.

Griffiths, L.R., Zwi, M.B., McLeod, J.G. _et al._ (1988) Chromosome 1 linkage studies in Charcot–Marie–Tooth neuropathy Type I. _American Journal of Human Genetics_ 42: 756–771.

Guiloff, R.J., Thomas, P.K., Contreras, M. _et al._ (1982) Linkage of autosomal dominant type hereditary motor and sensory neuropathy to the Duffy locus on chromosome 1. _Journal of Neurology, Neurosurgery and Psychiatry_ 451: 669–674.

Hakamada, S., Kumagai, T., Hara, K. _et al._ (1983) Congenital hypomyelination neuropathy in a newborn. _Neuropediatrics_ 14: 182–183.

Harding, A.E. and Thomas, P.K. (1980a) Genetic aspects of hereditary motor and sensory neuropathy (types I and II). _Journal of Medical Genetics_ 17: 329–336.

Harding, A.E. and Thomas, P.K. (1980b) Autosomal recessive forms of hereditary motor and sensory neuropathy. _Journal of Neurology, Neurosurgery and Psychiatry_ 43: 669–678.

Hayasaka, K., Nanao, K., Tahara, M. _et al._ (1991) Isolation and sequence determination of cDNA encoding the major structural protein of human peripheral myelin. _Biochemical and Biophysical Research Communications_ 180: 515–518.

Hayasaka, K., Himoro, M., Sato, W. _et al._ (1993a) Charcot–Marie–Tooth neuropathy type 1B is associated with mutations of the myelin P_0 gene. _Nature Genetics_ 5: 31–34.

Hayasaka, K., Himoro, M., Sawaishi, Y. _et al._ (1993b) _De novo_ mutation of the myelin P_0 gene in Dejerine-Sottas disease (hereditary motor and sensory neuropathy type III) _Nature Genetics_ 5: 266–268.

Hayasaka, K., Himoro, M., Takada, G. _et al._ (1993c) Structure and localization of the gene encoding human peripheral myelin protein 2 (PMP-2). _Genomics_ 18: 244–248.

Henry, E.W. and Sidman, R.L. (1988) Long lives for homozygous Trembler mutant mice despite virtual absence of peripheral nerve myelin. _Science_ 241: 344–346.

Hoogendijk, J.E., Hensels, G.W., Gabreëls-Festen, A.A. _et al._ (1992) _De-novo_ mutation in hereditary motor and sensory neuropathy type I. _Lancet_ 339: 1081-1082.

Horton, W.A., Eldridge, R. and Brody, J.A. (1976) Familial motor neuron disease. Evidence for at least three different types. _Neurology_ 26: 460–465.

Hughes, R.A.C., Newsom-Davis, J.M., Perkin, J.D., Pearce, J.M. (1978) Controlled trial of prednisolone in acute polyneuropathy. _Lancet_ ii: 750–753.

Hughes, R.A.C. and the Guillain-Barré Syndrome Trial Group. (1992) Multicentre trial of high dose intravenous methylprednisolone in Guillain-Barré syndrome. _Journal of Neurology_ 239: S52.

Huttenlocher, P.R. and Gilles, F.H. (1967) Infantile neuraxonal dystrophy. _Neurology_ 17: 1174–1184.

Ionasescu, V.V., Trofatter, J., Haines, J.L. *et al.* (1991) Heterogeneity in X-linked recessive Charcot–Marie–Tooth neuropathy. *American Journal of Human Genetics* **48**: 1075–1083.

Ionasescu, V.V., Trofatter, J.L., Haines, J.L. *et al.* (1992) Mapping of the gene for X-linked dominant Charcot–Marie–Tooth neuropathy. *Neurology* **42**: 903–908.

Kaesar, H.E. (1965) Scapuloperoneal muscular dystrophy. *Brain* **88**: 407–418.

Karch, S.B. and Urich, H. (1975) Infantile polyneuropathy with defective myelination: an autopsy study. *Developmental Medicine and Child Neurology* **17**: 504–511.

Kasman, M., Bernstein, L. and Schulman, S. (1976) Chronic polyradiculoneuropathy of infancy: a report of three cases with familial incidence. *Neurology* **26**: 565–573.

Klenk, E. and Kahlke, W. (1963) Uber das Vorkommen der 3.7.11.15-Tetramethyl-hexadecansäure (Phytansäure) in den Cholesterinestern und anderen Lipoidfraktionen der Organe bei einem Krankheitsfall unbekannter Genese (Verdacht auf Heredopathia atactica polyneuritiformis (Refsum-Syndrom). *Hoppe-Seyler's Zeitschrift für physiologische Chemie* **333**: 133–139.

Kobayashi, T., Yamanaka, T., Jacobs, J. *et al.* (1980) The twitcher mouse: an enzymatically authentic murine model of human globoid cell leukodystrophy (Krabbe disease). *Brain Research* **202**: 479–483.

Kohn, R. (1971) Clinical and pathological findings in an unusual infantile motor neurone disease. *Journal of Neurology, Neurosurgery and Psychiatry* **34**: 427–431.

Kolodny, E.H. (1993) Metachromatic leukodystrophy and multiple sulfatase deficiency: sulfatide lipidosis. In: Rosenberg, R.N., Prusiner, S.B., DiMauro, S. *et al.* eds, *The Molecular and Genetic Basis of Neurological Disease*. Boston: Butterworth-Heinemann, pp. 497–503.

Krivit, W., Shapiro, E., Kennedy, W. *et al.* (1990) Treatment of late infantile metachromatic leukodystrophy by bone marrow transplantation. *New England Journal of Medicine* **322**: 28–32.

Kulkens, T., Bolhuis, P.A., Wolterman, R.A. *et al.* (1993) Deletion of the codon for serine 34 from the major peripheral myelin protein P_0 gene in Charcot–Marie–Tooth disease type 1B. *Nature Genetics* **5**: 35–39.

Lebo, R.V., Chance, P.F., Dyck, P.J. *et al.* (1991) Chromosome 1 Charcot–Marie–Tooth syndrome (HMSNIB) locus in FC gamma r II region. *Human Genetics* **88**: 1–12.

Loprest, L.J., Pericak-Vance, M.A., Stajich, J. *et al.* (1992) Linkage studies in Charcot–Marie–Tooth disease type 2: evidence that CMT1 and CMT2 are distinct genetic entities. *Neurology* **42**: 597–601.

Lupski, J.R., Montes de Oca-Luna, R., Slaugenhaupt, S. *et al.* (1991) DNA duplication associated with Charcot–Marie–Tooth disease type 1A. *Cell* **66**: 219–232.

Lupski, J.R., Wise, C.A., Kuwano, A. *et al.* (1992) Gene dosage is a mechanism for Charcot–Marie–Tooth disease type 1A. *Nature Genetics* **1**: 29–33.

McKhann, G. (the Guillain-Barré Study Group). (1985) Plasmapheresis and acute Guillain-Barré syndrome. *Neurology* (*Cleveland*) **35**: 1096–1104.

Madrid, R. and Bradley, W.G. (1975) The pathology of neuropathies with focal thickening of the myelin sheath (tomaculous neuropathy): studies on the formation of the abnormal myelin sheath. *Journal of the Neurological Sciences* **25**: 415–418.

Magenis, R.E., Brown, M.G., Allen, L. *et al.* (1986) De novo partial duplication of 17p [dup(17)(p12 p11.2)]: clinical report. *American Journal of Medical Genetics* **24**: 415–420.

Manfioletti, G., Ruaro, M.E., Del Sal, G. *et al.* (1990) A growth arrest-specific (gas) gene codes for a membrane protein. *Molecular Cell Biology* **10**: 2924–2930.

Matsunami, N., Smith, B., Ballard, L. *et al.* (1992) Peripheral myelin protein-22 gene maps in the duplication in chromosome 17p11.2 associated with Charcot–Marie–Tooth 1A. *Nature Genetics* **1**: 176–179.

Mawatari, S. and Katayama, K. (1973) Scapuloperoneal muscular atrophy with cardiopathy. *Archives of Neurology* **28**: 55.

Meier, C. and Moll, C. (1982) Hereditary neuropathy with liability to pressure palsies. Report of two families and review of the literature. *Journal of Neurology* **228**: 73–95.

Middleton-Price, H.R., Harding, A.E., Monteiro, C. *et al.* (1990) Linkage of hereditary motor and sensory neuropathy type I to the pericentromeric region of chromosome 17. *American Journal of Human Genetics* **46**: 92–94.

Moosa, A. (1975) Peripheral neuropathy in Leigh's encephalomyelopathy. *Developmental Medicine and Child Neurology* **17**: 621–620.

Moosa, A. and Dubowitz, V. (1970) Peripheral neuropathy in Cockayne's syndrome. *Archives of Disease in Childhood* **45**: 674–677.

Mostacciuolo, M.L., Muller, E., Fardin, P. *et al.* (1991) X-linked Charcot–Marie–Tooth disease: a linkage study in a large family using 12 probes of the pericentric region. *Human Genetics* **87**: 23–27.

Nelson, J.S. and Prensky, A.L. (1972) Sporadic juvenile amyotrophic lateral sclerosis. *Archives of Neurology* **27**: 300.

Nicholson, G. and Nash, J. (1993) Intermediate nerve conduction velocities define X-linked Charcot–Marie–Tooth neuropathy families. *Neurology* **43**: 2558–2564.

Ohnishi, A., Murai, Y., Ikeda, M. *et al.* (1989) Autosomal recessive motor and sensory neuropathy with excessive myelin outfolding. *Muscle and Nerve* **12**: 568–575.

Ouvrier, R.A., McLeod, J.G. and Conchin, T.E. (1987) The hypertrophic forms of hereditary motor and sensory neuropathy: a study of hypertrophic Charcot–Marie–Tooth disease (HMSN type I) and Dejerine-Sottas disease (HMSN type III) in childhood. *Brain* **110**: 121–148.

Ouvrier, R.A., McLeod, J.G. and Pollard, J.D. (1990) *Peripheral Neuropathy in Childhood*. New York: Raven Press.

Palix, C. and Coignet, J. (1978) Un cas de polyneuro-pathie périphérique neonatale par amyélinisation. *Pédiatrie* 33: 201–207.

Patel, P.I., Franco, B., Garcia, C. *et al.* (1990) Genetic mapping of autosomal dominant Charcot–Marie–Tooth disease in a large French-Canadian kindred: identification of new linked markers on chromosome 17. *American Journal of Human Genetics* 46: 801–809.

Patel, P.I., Roa, B.B., Welcher, A.A. *et al.* (1992) The gene for the peripheral myelin protein PMP-22 is a candidate for Charcot–Marie–Tooth disease type 1A. *Nature Genetics* 1: 157–165.

Pentao, L., Wise, C.A., Chinault, A.C. *et al.* (1992) Charcot–Marie–Tooth type 1A duplication appears to arise from recombination at repeat sequences flanking the 1.5 Mb monomer unit. *Nature Genetics* 2: 292–300.

Raeymaekers, P., Timmerman, V., DeJonghe, P. *et al.* (1989) Localization of the mutation in an extended family with Charcot–Marie–Tooth neuropathy (HMSN I). *American Journal of Human Genetics* 45: 953–958.

Raeymaekers, P., Timmerman, V., Nelis, E. *et al.* (1991) Duplication in chromosome 17p11.2 in Charcot–Marie–Tooth neuropathy type 1A. *Neuromuscular Disorders* 1: 93–97.

Refsum, S. (1946) Heredopathia atactica polyneuritiformis: a familial syndrome not hitherto described. *Acta Psychiatrica Neurologica* (Suppl) 38: 1–303.

Reif-Kohn, R. and Mundel, G. (1974) Second case of an infantile motor neuron disease. *Confinia Neurologica* 36: 23–32.

Roa, B.B., Garcia, C.A., Suter, U. *et al.* (1993a) Charcot–Marie–Tooth disease type 1A: Association with a spontaneous point mutation in the PMP22 gene. *New England Journal of Medicine* 329: 96–101.

Roa, B.B., Garcia, C.A., Pentao, L. *et al.* (1993b) Evidence for a recessive PMP22 point mutation in Charcot–Marie–Tooth disease type 1A. *Nature Genetics* 5: 189–194.

Roa, B.B., Dyck, P.J., Marks, H.G. *et al.* (1993c) Dejerine–Sottas syndrome associated with point mutation in the peripheral myelin protein 22 (PMP22) gene. *Nature Genetics* 5: 269–273.

Rosen, D.R., Siddique, T., Patterson, D. *et al.* (1993) Mutations in Cu/Zn superoxide dismutase gene are associated with familial amyotrophic lateral sclerosis. *Nature* 362: 59.

Roussy, G. and Lévy, G. (1926) Sept cas d'une maladie familiale particulière: trouble de la marche, pieds bots et aréfléxie tendineuse généralisée, avec accessoirement, légère maladresse des mains. *Revue Neurologique* 1: 427–450.

Schindler, D., Bishop, D.F., Wolfe, D.E. *et al.* (1989) Neuroaxonal dystrophy due to lysosomal α-N-acetylgalactosaminidase deficiency. *New England Journal of Medicine* 320: 1735.

Seitelberger, F. (1952) Eine unbekannte Form von infantiler lipoidspeicher Krankheit des Gehirns. *Proceedings of First International Congress of Neuropathology Rome* Vol. 3, Turin: Rosenberg and Sellier, p. 323.

Seitz, R.J., Wechsler, W., Mosny, D.S. *et al.* (1986) Hypomyelination neuropathy in a female newborn presenting as arthrogryposis multiplex congenita. *Neuropediatrics* 17: 132–136.

Shahar, E.M., Roifman, C.M., Shorer, Z., Barzilay, Z., Levi, Y., Brand, N. and Murphy, E.G. (1994) High dose intravenous serum gamma globulins are effective in severe pediatric Guillain-Barré syndrome: a prospective follow-up study of 23 cases. *Annals of Neurology* 36: 503 (abstract).

Siddique, T., Figlewicz, D.A., Pericak-Vance, M.A. *et al.* (1991) Linkage of a gene causing familial amyotrophic lateral sclerosis to chromosome 21 and evidence of genetic-locus heterogeneity. *New England Journal of Medicine* 324: 1381.

Spreyer, P., Kuhn, G., Hanemann, C.O. *et al.* (1991) Axon-regulated expression of a Schwann cell transcript that is homologous to a growth arrest-specific gene. *EMBO Journal* 10: 3661–3668.

Staal, A. and Went, L.N. (1968) Juvenile amyotrophic lateral sclerosis – dementia complex in a Dutch family. *Neurology (Minneapolis)* 18: 800.

Staal, A., De Weerdt, C.J. and Went, L.N. (1965) Hereditary compression syndrome of peripheral nerves. *Neurology* 15: 1008–1017.

Stebbins, N.B. and Conneally, P.M. (1982) Linkage of dominantly inherited Charcot–Marie–Tooth neuropathy to the Duffy locus in an Indiana family. *American Journal of Human Genetics* 34: 195A.

Steinberg, D. (1972) Phytanic acid storage disease: Refsum's syndrome. In: Stanbury, J.B., Wyngaarden, J.B. and Fredrickson, D. eds, *The Metabolic Basis of Inherited Disease* 3rd edn. New York: McGraw Hill, p. 833.

Strümpell, A. (1883) Zur kenntnis der multiplen degenerativen neuritis. *Archiv für Psychiatre und Nervenkrankheiten* 14: 339.

Suter, U., Welcher, A.A., Ozcelik, T. *et al.* (1992) Trembler mouse carries a point mutation in a myelin gene. *Nature* 356: 241–244.

Tachi, N., Ishikawa, Y. and Minami, R. (1984) Two cases of congenital hypomyelination neuropathy. *Brain Development* 6: 560–565.

Tartof, K.D. (1988) Unequal crossing over then and now. *Genetics* 120: 1–6.

Timmerman, V., Nelis, E., Van Hul, W. *et al.* (1992) The peripheral myelin protein gene PMP-22 is contained within the Charcot–Marie–Tooth disease type 1A duplication. *Nature Genetics* 1: 171–175.

Tooth, H.H. (1886) *The Peroneal Type of Progressive Muscular Atrophy*. Thesis. London: H.K. Lewis and Co. Ltd.

Valentijn, L.J., Bolhuis, P.A., Zorn, I. *et al.* (1992a) The peripheral myelin gene PMP-22/GAS-3 is duplicated in Charcot–Marie–Tooth disease type 1A. *Nature Genetics* 1: 166–170.

Valentijn, L.J., Baas, F., Wolteman, R.A. *et al.* (1992b) Identical point mutations of the peripheral myelin protein-22 in Trembler-J mouse and Charcot–Marie–Tooth disease type 1A. *Nature Genetics* 2: 288–291.

Vanasse, M. and Dubowitz, V. (1981) Dominantly inherited peroneal muscular atrophy (hereditary motor and sensory neuropathy type I) in infancy and childhood. *Muscle and Nerve* **4**: 26–30.

Vance, J.M., Nicholson, G.A., Yamaoka, L.H. *et al.* (1989) Linkage of Charcot–Marie–Tooth neuropathy type IA to chromosome 17. *Experimental Neurology* **104**: 186–189.

Vance, J.M., Barker, D., Yamaoka, L.H. *et al.* (1991) Localization of Charcot–Marie–Tooth disease type 1A (CMT 1A) to chromosome 17p11.2. *Genomics* **9**: 623–628.

Van Der Meché, F.G.A., Schmitz, P.I.M. and the Dutch Guillain-Barré Study Group. (1992) A randomized trial comparing intravenous immune globulin and plasma exchange in the Guillain-Barré syndrome. *New England Journal of Medicine* **326**: 1123–1129.

Welcher, A.A., Suter, U., De Leon, M. *et al.* (1991) A myelin protein is encoded by the homolog of a growth arrest-specific gene. *Proceedings of the National Academy of Sciences of the USA* **88**: 7195–7199.

Wenger, D.A. and Chen, Y.Q. (1993) Krabbe disease (globoid cell leukodystrophy). In: Rosenberg, R.N., Prusiner, S.B., DiMauro, S. *et al.* eds, *The Molecular and Genetic Basis of Neurological Disease.* Boston: Butterworth-Heinemann, pp. 485–495.

Yoshikawa, H., Nishimura, T., Nakatsuju, Y. *et al.* (1994) Elevated expression of messenger RNA for peripheral myelin protein 22 in biopsied peripheral nerves of patients with Charcot–Marie–Tooth disease type 1A. *Annals of Neurology* **35**: 455–450.

Yudell, A., Dyck, P.J. and Lambert, E.H. (1965) A kinship with the Roussy-Levy syndrome. *Archives of Neurology* **13**: 432–440.

Zellweger, H. and McCormick, W.F. (1968) Scapuloperoneal dystrophy and scapuloperoneal atrophy. *Helvetica Paediatrica Acta* **23**: 643–649.

Zlotogora, J., Chakraborty, S., Knowlton, R.G. *et al.* (1990) Krabbe disease locus mapped to chromosome 14 by genetic linkage. *American Journal of Human Genetics* **47**: 37–44.

CHAPTER 10

Myasthenia

INTRODUCTION

Myasthenia is characterized by an abnormal fatigue after repeated or sustained muscle activity and by improvement after rest. It has its peak incidence in young adults, but also occurs in infancy and childhood. One can recognize a number of separate clinical entities in the childhood period:

1. transient neonatal myasthenia in the infant born to a myasthenic mother;
2. congenital or infantile myasthenia in the child of a non-myasthenic mother;
3. juvenile myasthenia which is similar to the adult variety.

Myasthenia tends to affect muscles innervated by the cranial nerves as well as those of the neck, trunk and extremities. Respiration and swallowing may also be involved. Cardiac and smooth muscle are not affected.

HISTORICAL

The earliest clinical description of myasthenia can be traced back to Thomas Willis (1672), of circle fame (Viets, 1953). Two centuries later, Erb (1879) recognized its tendency to spontaneous remission and Goldflam (1893) the fluctuation in clinical symptoms. The name 'myasthenia gravis pseudo-paralytica' was suggested by Jolly in 1895 and he and Oppenheim (1887) first described the progressive failure of myasthenic muscle to respond to repeated faradic stimulation, the so-called 'myasthenic reaction'. At the turn of the century comprehensive reviews were produced by Campbell and Bramwell (1900) of Edinburgh and by Oppenheim (1901). The association with thymic tumour was already recognized in 1901 by Laquer and Weigert, and with thymic hyperplasia by Bell (1917). In 1934 Mary Walker recognized the similarity of myasthenia gravis to curare poisoning and suggested treatment with physostigmine. In the same year, Dale and Feldberg demonstrated the release of acetylcholine at the neuromuscular junction. Neostigmine was introduced in 1935 (Pritchard, 1935), pyridostigmine some 20 years later (Osserman, 1955).

In 1960 Simpson postulated an autoimmune basis for myasthenia gravis, and suggested that the disease might result from antibodies to a component of the postsynaptic membrane. In 1973 Patrick and Lindstrom demonstrated the development of weakness in rabbits immunized with the purified acetylcholine receptor from the electric organ of the eel. The character of the weakness and the improvement following administration of anticholinesterases suggested a similarity to human myasthenia gravis. Soon afterwards a deficiency of acetylcholine receptors was demonstrated in myasthenia gravis by Fambrough et al. (1973) and by 1977 the autoimmune nature of myasthenia gravis and the pathogenetic role of acetylcholine receptor (AChR) antibodies was firmly established by the demonstration of circulating antibodies to the ACh receptor in about 90% of patients with myasthenia gravis (Lindstrom et al., 1976), by the localization of immune complexes on the post-synaptic membrane (Engel et al., 1977), and by the beneficial effect of plasma exchange (Pinching et al., 1976; Dau et al., 1977). Therapeutic benefit has also been demonstrated with alternate-day steroids (Warmolts et al., 1970), with other immuno-suppressants such as azathioprine (Mertens et al., 1969) and with intravenous immunoglobulin (Cosi *et al.*, 1991). The first results of thymectomy were already documented by Blalock *et al.* in 1941.

The discovery of an immune basis for the common adult form of myasthenia gravis also helped to segregate those cases, particularly in childhood, in which an autoimmune basis could not be established. These were often genetically determined and presumably due to other mechanisms. Recent advances in the sophisticated technology for studying end-plate function have helped to define a number of important components in relation to neuromuscular transmission and have identified specific abnormalities of these several distinct syndromes. Andrew Engel and his group at the Mayo Clinic have contributed substantially to these advances (Engel, 1984, 1988, 1993).

PATHOPHYSIOLOGY ——————————————

Engel (1988) used the concept of the safety margin of neuromuscular transmission as a basis for understanding the pathogenesis in the various myasthenic syndromes, in each of which the safety margin may be compromised by one or more specific mechanisms. The safety margin of transmission is defined as the difference between the end-plate potential (EPP) amplitude and that required to trigger a muscle fibre action potential.

The neuromuscular junction comprises the nerve terminal separated from the postsynaptic region by the synaptic space. Acetylcholine (ACh) is stored in quantal packets (containing 6000–10 000 molecules) in synaptic vesicles in the nerve terminal, which can release the ACh into the synaptic space by exocytosis. The junctional folds in the postsynaptic region have acetylcholine receptor (AChR) molecules, at a density of some 10 000 sites/μm^2. Two ACh molecules bind to one AChR molecule with resultant opening of the AChR ion channel, which closes again when the ACh dissociates from the AChR. Acetylcholinesterase (AChE), which hydrolyses ACh, is distributed throughout the basal lamina of the synaptic space at a density of about 2500 sites/μm^2.

In the resting state, ACh quanta are randomly released into the synaptic space. The high ACh concentration saturates all nearby AChE sites so that most ACh molecules can reach the postsynaptic AChRs. Because of the high AChR packing density, the ACh needs to diffuse a very short distance before meeting all the AChR it can saturate. The resultant resting depolarizations of the muscle fibre are known as miniature end-plate potentials (MEPPs). When ACh dissociates from AChR it is hydrolysed by AChE to acetate and choline, which is taken up by the nerve terminal for synthesis of ACh.

The MEPP amplitude depends on the number of ACh molecules in the quantum, the number of available AChRs, the geometry of the synaptic space and the average depolarization generated by the opening of an AChR ion channel. The MEPP duration depends on the average channel open time, the functional state of AChE and the cable properties of the muscle fibre membrane.

Action potentials in the nerve terminal evoke transmitter release through the opening of Ca^{2+} channels. Transmitter release occurs in integral multiples of quantal packets of about 6000–10 000 ACh molecules each. Each packet is released independently of other packets in a very brief period of time (less than 0.2 ms). Under normal physiological conditions about 200 such packets are released with each nerve impulse, giving rise to an EPP which exceeds threshold for generation of an action potential in the muscle fibre. Occasionally a quantal packet of transmitter is released at random and gives rise to an MEPP.

The released ACh binds to AChRs on the postsynaptic membrane and is hydrolysed by AChE. About 250 000 AChRs, with bound molecules of ACh, open their channels for an effective duration of about 1 ms; Na^+, K^+, and to a lesser extent Ca^{2+}, pass through each open channel. There is a net influx of positive charge into the muscle cell, thus depolarizing it. If the muscle cell is sufficiently depolarized to produce an action potential, the muscle fibre contracts, the activated AChRs close their channels and lose their bound ACh.

Anticholinesterase inhibitor drugs (AChE inhibitors) are effective because they increase the number of ACh molecules available to bind to the AChR and the ACh molecules can spread over a wider area to compensate for the paucity of AChR. An overdose of AChE inhibitors may desensitize AChR by causing continued exposure of the same AChR molecules to ACh during physiological activity.

Molecular structure

The AChR in skeletal muscle membrane is a large glycoprotein made up of five homologous subunits that form a central core through which ions can flow. In adult innervated muscle over 95% of the AChRs are composed of α, α, β, δ and ε subunits; in embryonal and denervated muscle over 80% have the composition α, α, β, δ and γ; ACh binds predominantly to the two α subunits of the AChR.

In myasthenia gravis there are antibodies to the AChR, in Lambert-Eaton syndrome to the voltage-gated calcium channels and in neuromyotonia (Isaacs' syndrome) to voltage-gated K channels.

CHILDHOOD MYASTHENIAS

Although myasthenia gravis is predominantly a disease of adult life, a not insignificant proportion of cases of myasthenia do occur in adolescence, childhood and infancy. In a monumental review of 417 cases of myasthenia, Millichap and Dodge (1960) identified 16 cases with onset of symptoms in the neonatal period and 35 presenting between 1 and 16 years, whilst Osserman (1958), in a review of 217 cases of myasthenia in infancy, childhood and adolescence, had 34 cases with symptoms at or within a few days of birth and a further eight with onset before 2 years of age. More recently Rodriguez *et al.* (1983) reviewed a series of 157 cases of myasthenia with onset before 17 years of age, treated at the Mayo Clinic between 1932 and 1976. Eight had persistent symptoms before 1 year of age (congenital group), the remaining 149 (juvenile group) had an onset after 1 year of age. Eighty-five of the juvenile cases had a thymectomy because of disease severity, with a substantial increase in the remission rate compared with unoperated cases.

The earlier authors, of course, were not able to distinguish between the different types of myasthenia in childhood, other than on age of onset. Bundey (1972) undertook a detailed genetic study of infantile and juvenile myasthenia gravis based on available reports in the literature and cases from four London hospitals. She confirmed the mildness of the early onset (under 2 years) group and also noted a frequent occurrence of this form in sibs, suggesting an autosomal recessive pattern of inheritance. In contrast to the overall predominance of myasthenia in females, there was an excess of affected males in this early onset group.

Namba *et al.* (1971a,b) also recorded familial aggregation of cases and reviewed the occurrence of myasthenia in 21 pairs of twins of all ages. Six monozygotic twins had both members affected, eight sets only one member. There were seven sets of dizygotic twins reported with one member affected, and no dizygotic twins with both members affected. These data also supported an autosomal recessive inheritance.

Anti-AChR antibodies are detectable in the serum of about 85–90% of adult cases with generalized myasthenia gravis but only in about 50–60% of those with restricted ocular myasthenia. There is no direct correlation of disease severity with the absolute titre of antibody. Most childhood cases of myasthenia with postpubertal onset have AChR antibodies present, suggesting they are comparable with the adult autoimmune myasthenia gravis. They also show the same marked female predominance. At least half of prepubertal cases do not have antibodies to AChR, or a female predominance, suggesting that most of these are not autoimmune cases, and presumably various inherited forms. The situation, however, is not quite as clear-cut, since some of the adult autoimmune cases, particularly with predominantly ocular involvement, may not have antibodies present and may yet respond to plasma exchange or immunosuppressive therapy. Presumably this may apply to at least some of the prepubertal cases also. There is also a possibility that some autoimmune cases may have an association with certain HLA haplotypes and a familial incidence.

A higher incidence of myasthenia in childhood has been recorded in oriental races. In contrast to the usual childhood onset in about 10% of Caucasian cases (Millichap and Dodge, 1960; Osserman and Genkins, 1971; Batocchi *et al.*, 1990), Wong *et al.* (1992) found 103 individuals (54 girls and 49 boys) (39%) with onset of myasthenia before puberty (up to 16 years) out of 262 patients in an exhaustive survey covering 85% of the population of Hong Kong. The majority of these patients (71%) had restricted ocular myasthenia gravis. Similarly, Fukuyama *et al.* (1981) identified 418 patients under 15 years (29%) in a major epidemiological study of 1430 patients, distributed throughout 800 major hospitals in Japan.

A strong association with specific HLA haplotypes has also been documented in these oriental populations (Hawkins *et al.*, 1989; Matsuki *et al.*, 1990).

AUTOIMMUNE MYASTHENIA GRAVIS

Myasthenia gravis affects all races and the prevalence has been variably estimated at between 5 and 10 per 100 000. There is a marked preponderance of female cases (about 4:1).

CLINICAL FEATURES

The onset of the symptoms is often insidious, but at times the weakness comes on fairly acutely and may follow an acute febrile illness, an allergic episode or an emotional upset. The weakness may be focal or generalized (Figures 10-1 to 10-4).

The condition almost invariably affects the ocular muscles, and ptosis, with or without ophthalmoplegia, is usually present. The majority of cases will develop weakness of other muscle groups and in some cases these may be present at the outset. These include the face, the jaw, swallowing, speech, the neck, trunk and limbs. In the limbs, proximal muscles are affected more than distal and the upper limbs more than the lower.

The course tends to be a slowly progressive one, with marked fluctuation and tendency to relapse and remission. However, prolonged remissions are relatively uncommon and some cases may develop a fixed weakness, without fluctuation or remission. This tends particularly to occur in the ocular muscles but may also occur in the limb muscles and pose difficulties in clinical diagnosis (see case history, Figure 10-4).

A careful history will usually reveal some of the characteristic effects of muscle fatigue, such as diplopia brought on by continuous activity such as reading; progressive difficulty with chewing or swallowing in the course of a meal, and a tendency to support the jaw with one hand to prevent it hanging open; 'thickening' and slurring or weakening of speech after prolonged talking; and other episodes of fatigue associated with sustained use of particular muscles.

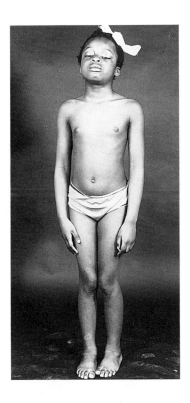

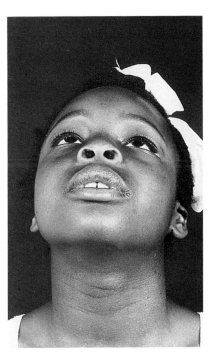

(a)   (b)

Figure 10-1a,b   ?Autoimmune myasthenia. This girl was normal until the age of 7 years, when she developed ptosis on waking in the morning which gradually progressed during the course of the day. She subsequently tired at school games and had to sit down. She also had difficulty with eating and had to hold her mouth to finish chewing. Her voice became very low and she could not blow up a balloon. She was diagnosed as myasthenic and treated with pyridostigmine 15 mg six times daily with definite improvement. The strength was still variable and definitely worse when she missed the tablets. The dosage was gradually increased. When examined in April 1976 at the age of 9½ years, she was taking pyridostigmine at a dose of 60 mg six times daily. She had a slight ptosis, and was able to sustain an upward gaze for only about 3 s. There was a slight convergent squint but the eye movements were full in all directions. No weakness was noted in any other muscles. When she was due for her next tablet the ptosis increased. A thymectomy was considered but deferred in view of her good control on anticholinesterase drugs. Voluntary tests of quadriceps strength showed a force of 12 kg on the right and 10 kg on the left, which was at the lower limit of the normal range. Muscle relaxation showed 5 per cent and 50 per cent loss of force at 68 and 138 ms respectively, which were both within the normal adult range. Repetitive ulnar stimulation at 1 Hz gave no change over 2½ min, at 3 Hz no change over 2 min and at 30 Hz 18% loss of force after 18 s (normal adult range 0–25%). There was thus no evidence of active myasthenia and the drug therapy was considered satisfactory. She has three normal siblings and the parents are normal and unrelated.

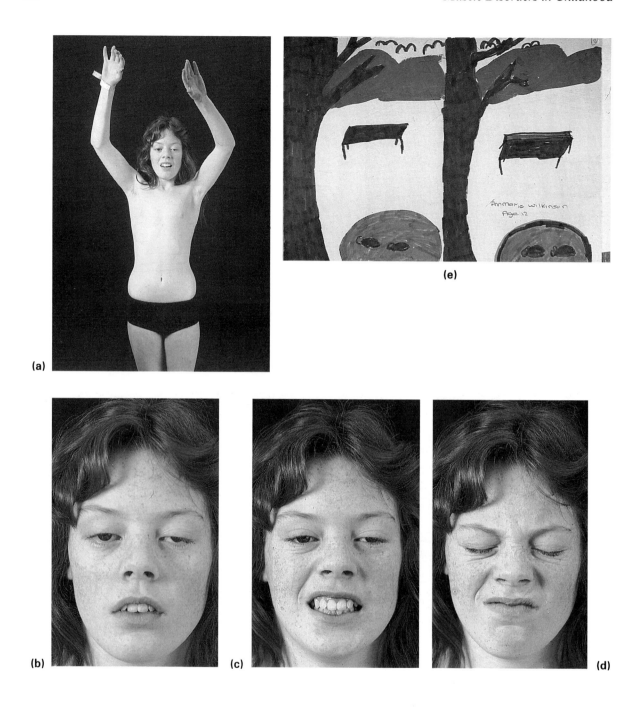

Figure 10-2a-e Autoimmune myasthenia. This 12½-year-old girl was referred with a 3-month history of difficulty with swallowing and weakness of the limbs with unsteadiness of gait. A diagnosis of myasthenia had been established and pyridostigmine was prescribed. She still had a marked weakness and was only able to raise her arms for about 45 seconds (a) and was barely able to stand on one leg. There was facial weakness and ptosis and the characteristic snarling smile and difficulty with eye closure (b-d). She experienced diplopia with upward gaze. She visualized a double image when drawing (e). She was also found to have respiratory muscle weakness and her peak flow was only 300 ml. Two plasma exchanges were done with marked improvement, followed by thymectomy a week later. She developed right lower lobe collapse postoperatively, requiring bronchoscopy and suction before she could be extubated. She became acutely weak 2 weeks later and was given three further plasma exchanges and started on alternate-day prednisolone and on azathioprine, in addition to her pyridostigmine.

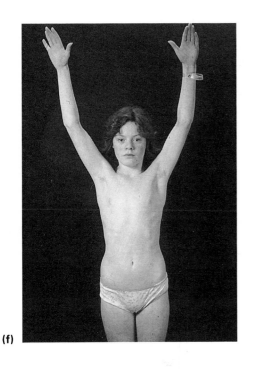

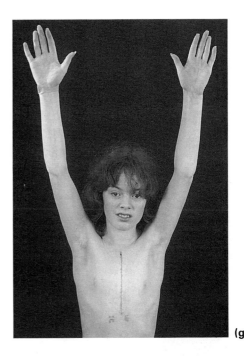

(f)

(g)

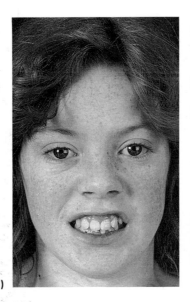

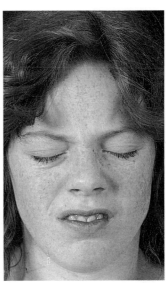

(h)

(i)

(j)

Figure 10-2f-j Her general strength and respiratory function gradually improved and she was allowed home 2 months after her operation (f-j). She subsequently had a somewhat stormy course with a number of acute myasthenic crises, which responded well to plasma exchanges. She also developed cholinergic symptoms with excessive salivation from increased pyridostigmine plus some overlay anxiety. She improved considerably with reduction in the pyridostigmine and efforts were made to gradually reduce her alternate-day steroids. Her anti-acetylcholine receptor level dropped fivefold, and single fibre EMG showed no abnormality of neuromuscular transmission. At 15 years she was coping well on 40 mg prednisolone on alternate days, 175 mg azathioprine/day and 15 mg pyridostigmine as required, about three to four times per day. Her condition then remained reasonably stable and the prednisolone was gradually tapered and completely stopped about 4 years after the thymectomy. She continued on azathioprine at 100 mg per day and subsequently also stopped her pyridostigmine. Towards the end of a pregnancy at age 18 she became weaker again and restarted pyridostigmine and her requirement gradually rose to 60 mg four or five times per day. During a second pregnancy she again became very weak at about 9 weeks and was admitted for plasma exchanges, with good result, and also recommenced on alternate-day prednisolone, 10 mg alternate days. When reviewed 2 months later her condition was stable but she still had some residual weakness.

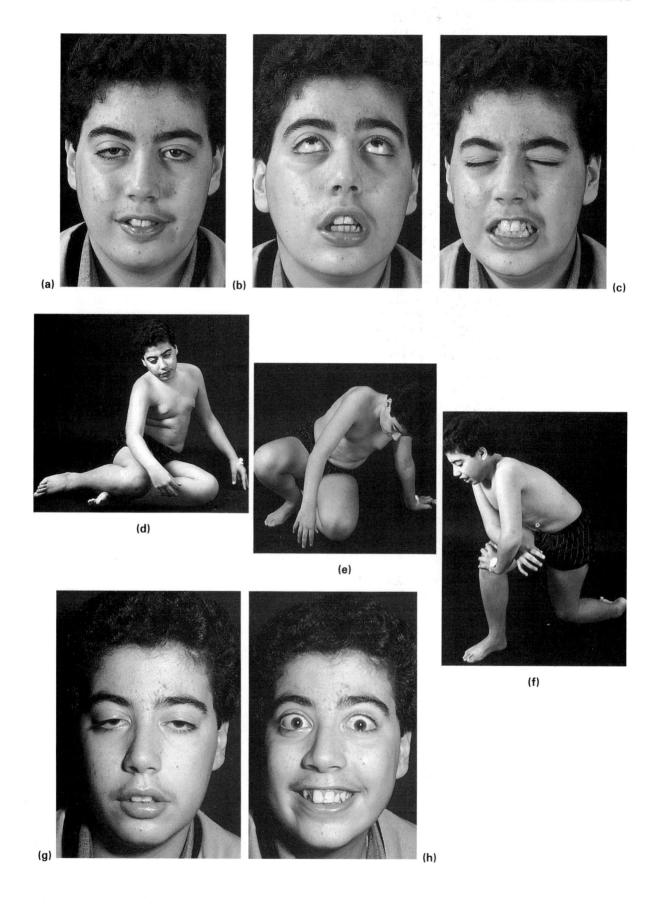

A careful history will also usually reveal that the patient is better when waking in the morning, or after a period of rest, and tends to fatigue more towards the end of the day. It is important to have a high degree of suspicion in any history suggestive of fatigue with effort. Myasthenia is often missed simply because it is not thought of.

On clinical examination the patient may show ptosis, often asymmetrical and associated with compensatory wrinkling of the forehead, ophthalmoplegia, an expressionless facies with a snarl on trying to smile, and inability to close the jaw, which may be compensated for by supporting the jaw with a hand. The tongue may show the characteristic triple longitudinal furrowing. As the myasthenic involvement can at times be fairly localized, careful assessment should be made of those muscle groups in which the patient is aware of fatiguability and weakness.

Associated diseases

As in adult cases, a higher incidence of other autoimmune disorders, such as thyroid disease, has been recorded in childhood cases. There have also been reports of associated diabetes and arthritis, single reports of a number of other associated disorders (which may be a coincidence), occasional reports of associated psychosis, and a somewhat unexpectedly high frequency of seizures in four of the 32 cases reviewed by Snead *et al.* (1980). Psychiatric disturbances, such as depression and emotional disorder, have been recorded with high frequency in some adult series (Magni *et al.*, 1988) but not in others (Cordess *et al.*, 1983). Thymoma, which occurs in about 10% of adult cases, is not a feature of the childhood-onset disease.

DIAGNOSIS OF MYASTHENIA ——————

Pharmacological

The usual method for confirmation of a suspected myasthenia is the response to an anticholinesterase drug. Edrophonium (Tensilon®) intravenously produces an almost instant response and should be evident within 30–60 seconds. At times it can be quite dramatic, with wide opening of previously droopy eyelids or a demonstrable change in muscle power in affected groups (Figure 10-3). It is fairly shortlived and the weakness will return after about 5–10 minutes. It may be difficult to assess a response and the ophthalmoplegia in particular may be unresponsive. Attempts should be made to quantitate objectively changes such as the degree of ptosis and the weakness in particular muscle groups.

Figure 10-3a-h *(facing page)* ?Autoimmune myasthenia. This 13-year-old boy presented with a history of progressive weakness over a period of 4 years. Initially the weakness was localized to the jaw and he tended to hold his mouth open. Over the past 6 months he had experienced some generalized weakness and noted progressive fatigue with activity. He was definitely worse towards the end of the day and in the mornings felt quite good. Also, he had noted difficulty with eating and this had become worse towards evening and he frequently had to support his lower jaw with his hand to help with chewing; swallowing food was difficult, particularly at night, although he had not experienced any episodes of choking. He had first noted the weakness after a particularly strenuous bout of swimming and had also become unable to walk uphill, which caused quite considerable fatigue, and he was experiencing difficulty going up stairs. On examination he had overt bilateral ptosis and an open mouth with a mildly myopathic looking facies and some limitation in full closure of his eyes (a,b,c). There was noticeable variability in his weakness during the course of the day. When we initially examined him in the afternoon he had no antigravity power in the shoulders or in most of the hip muscles and also marked ptosis. The following morning, however, he was able to raise his arms against gravity and his facial expression was much better. He also had antigravity movement in many of the hip muscles. He got up from the floor with an obvious Gowers' manoeuvre (d,e,f). A confident clinical diagnosis of myasthenia was confirmed with a marked reduction in motor action potential on repetitive stimulation of his median nerve at 4 Hz. He also showed a marked response to intravenous tensilon (total of 7 mg) with a striking improvement in his facies and also general improvement in his motor abilities (g,h). We prescribed 30 mg pyridostigmine 6-hourly, which was subsequently gradually increased to 45 mg 6-hourly, with a definite improvement. The anti-AChR antibody titre was negative but he was still considered to have autoimmune myasthenia. When reviewed a year later he still had residual weakness and a positive Gowers' sign. He also had evidence of respiratory muscle weakness with a forced vital capacity of 1.5 litres and a peak flow of only 230 ml. In view of his partial response to pyridostigmine he was considered a candidate for more intensive further treatment, either with thymectomy or steroids. He subsequently had a thymectomy with good result. Three months after thymectomy his dose of pyridostigmine, 30 mg five times daily, was reduced by 30 mg per day at one month intervals and completely stopped after 6 months. He remained symptom free and was later passed fit for army service.

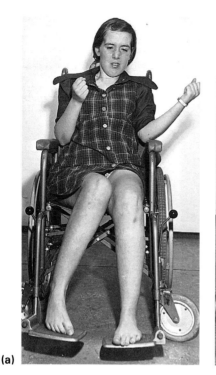
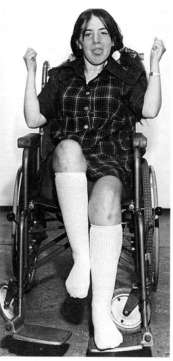
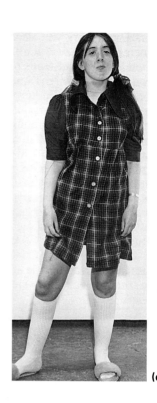

(a) (b) (c)

Figure 10-4a-c   ?Limb-girdle myasthenia. This girl was first seen at the age of 11 years with a history of bouts of weakness since the age of 10. Some days she was fine but on others she was unable to get on or off a bus. She also had recurrent bouts of 'collapsing' and falling to the floor and being unable to stand. On one occasion she had five such bouts in one evening. There was also a marked change in her temperament and she became emotionally labile, depressed and introverted. The family history was negative. On examination no weakness could be detected, nerve conduction and EMG were normal and there was no apparent fatigue on repetitive stimulation of the ulnar nerve. She was referred for psychiatric opinion for her depression and subsequently admitted for treatment to a long stay adolescent psychiatric unit. Over a period of a year there was a marked decline in her muscle ability and a neurologist found definite muscle weakness. There was a suggestion of increased fatigue, with improvement on edrophonium, but this could not be confirmed on detailed electrodiagnostic studies and there was no apparent response to a trial of pyridostigmine. A muscle biopsy was reported as showing some focal atrophy suggestive of denervation. She continued to show marked fluctuation from day to day and subsequently lost the ability to walk altogether. She had a number of bouts of difficulty with swallowing and choking on food and also developed a persistent ptosis and intermittent diplopia. When she was reassessed at the age of 14½ years she was chairbound and unable to stand without support (a). There was symmetrical weakness of the limbs, affecting the proximal muscles more than the distal and the arms more than the legs. There was also ptosis and a mild facial weakness. Nerve conduction was still normal and there was no decrement in response on repetitive stimulation of the ulnar nerve. EMG showed no fibrillation or fasciculation potentials to support a denervation but rather small units suggesting a myopathic pattern. A repetition of the edrophonium test produced a somewhat dramatic response with disappearance of her ptosis and ability to stand up from the wheelchair and walk unaided, for the first time in 18 months (b,c). The response persisted and six hours later she was still able to walk to the toilet at home, with some assistance. Her father noted that her voice that evening was much stronger, that she was not breathing as heavily as she usually did, and that although she needed to be carried upstairs to bed she was able to turn over in bed, which she had not done for a long time. The following day she was admitted for further assessment. The weakness had recurred. She showed no response to an intravenous placebo injection but a marked response as before to edrophonium. The improvement was maintained on pyridostigmine. She initially managed well on three tablets (60 mg) per day. She subsequently needed four, then five tablets per day. She showed no benefit from a larger morning dose of 75 mg. She continued to have difficulty going up steps and occasionally had swallowing difficulty and diplopia but remained ambulant all day. There was also a marked improvement in her temperament and she was no longer depressed. She subsequently had a severe respiratory infection necessitating tracheostomy and ventilation. Her general weakness gradually increased and she once again had difficulty with walking, as well as diplopia and dysphagia. Electrodiagnostic studies showed a marked decrement in amplitude of response on repetitive nerve stimulation. There was no improvement on injection of edrophonium, suggesting she might be having excess therapy, but also no improvement on subsequent reduction in anticholinesterase therapy. Thymectomy was considered but it was thought unlikely to benefit her. Her depression also returned. (*continued on facing page*)

The dosage of edrophonium varies with age. In infants under a year, 1 mg should be sufficient. In older children a small test dose of 1 or 2 mg should be given first to assess hypersensitivity and if there is no response within 30 seconds the remainder of the dose (0.2 mg/kg) can be given.

Neostigmine by intramuscular injection can also be used as a diagnostic test. Although slower in action, with response in perhaps 10 to 15 minutes or so, reaching a maximum in about 30 minutes, the action lasts longer, so that a more objective assessment of the response can be made. A dose of 0.125 mg is adequate in an infant and older children can be given 0.04 mg/kg. (A parallel injection of atropine can be given to counteract the undesirable side-effects due to stimulation of smooth and cardiac muscle and secretory glands.)

Electrophysiological

The fatiguability of the muscle can be demonstrated by a decrement in the muscle action potential (recorded by surface electrode) after repetitive stimulation of the nerve at a frequency of 3–5 Hz. One usually observes a decrement of 10% or more after the first four or five responses (Figure 10-5). A supramaximal stimulus is required and the ulnar or median nerve at the wrist is usually used with recording from a small muscle of the hand. Proximal muscles may also be studied.

More sophisticated studies, such as single-fibre electromyography which shows increased jitter, are also useful but usually impractical in children.

Circulating AChR antibodies

Anti-AChR antibodies can be detected in the serum of about 85–90% of patients with generalized myasthenia gravis and in about 50% of those with ocular myasthenia and provide a useful confirmation of the autoimmune disease. The level of the antibody titre is no index of clinical severity in the patient. The antibodies are usually assayed against human muscle AChRs which are labelled with iodinated α-bungarotoxin. The patients who are seronegative with this radioimmunoprecipitation assay are still considered to have autoimmune

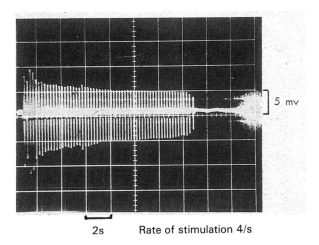

5 mv

2s   Rate of stimulation 4/s

Figure 10-5 Myasthenic response to repetitive ulnar stimulation at 4 Hz showing decrement of muscle action potential within 1–2 s.

myasthenia gravis on a number of grounds: infants with transient neonatal myasthenia have been born to seronegative mothers with severe myasthenia gravis; patients with seronegative myasthenia have responded to a course of plasma exchange, or to long-term immunosuppression for generalized disease.

MANAGEMENT ———————————————————

Although the onset of symptoms is usually insidious and focal, some patients may present acutely with life-threatening respiratory failure and will need the appropriate management, with intubation and ventilation as appropriate. Less severe cases may also deteriorate rapidly during a respiratory infection and need urgent ventilatory support.

In general, the objectives of treatment are to improve neuromuscular transmission, which is usually achieved by anticholinesterase drugs, and to prevent further destruction of the ACh receptors by intervening in the autoimmune lytic process and by preventing or slowing the synthesis of AChR antibodies. The latter objectives may be achieved by immunosuppressive therapy and thymectomy, and by plasma exchange as a rapidly effective tool in acute and severe crises.

Figure 10.4 (continued)   At 16½ years old she was still ambulant but having great difficulty getting about. Detailed studies of the quadriceps showed marked weakness with a maximum voluntary contraction of only about half the expected force. Repetitive stimulation of the quadriceps at 100 pulses/s produced a rapid decrement in force and a similar pattern after intravenous edrophonium. There was also a marked deficit in various respiratory function tests with only slight improvements in the peak flow rate after edrophonium. In view of her gradually deteriorating muscle function and resistance to anticholinesterase therapy, a thymectomy was performed at the age of 18. She died during the operation.

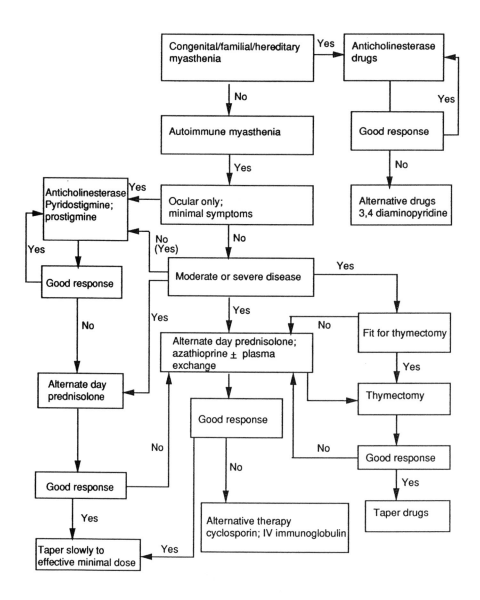

Figure 10-6 Management of childhood myasthenia. Flow diagram showing therapeutic options for congenital and autoimmune myasthenia. (Adapted from Newsom-Davis (1994) with permission.)

Most children with myasthenia gravis are given an initial trial of anticholinesterase drugs, and alternative or additional treatment is considered depending on the response. Most of the cumulative experience of treatment is based on adult cases and there is currently a body of opinion that severe cases of autoimmune myasthenia are best treated with thymectomy and immunosuppression rather than anticholinesterase drugs, which may at times aggravate the symptoms.

Newsom-Davis (1994) has drawn a flow diagram as a basis for reviewing various options of treatment, based on adult disease. I have tried to adapt this to

the paediatric age group (Figure 10-6). Most specialist centres dealing with the management of myasthenia have evolved their own protocols and dogma and there has been precious little in the way of controlled, comparative studies of different modes of treatment or different dosage schedules for individual treatments. It is also doubtful that experience in adult cases can be directly extrapolated to the childhood period. One of the additional difficulties in trying to critically assess the value of procedures such as thymectomy in childhood myasthenia is the complete absence of any detailed investigations, such as serum AChR antibody titres, in many of the series.

Anticholinesterase compounds

The two most widely used compounds are neostigmine bromide (Prostigmin®) and pyridostigmine bromide (Mestinon®). Both are given orally and the main difference is in the longer duration of the effect with pyridostigmine (up to 8 hours) compared with neostigmine (up to 4 or 6 hours). The size of the individual dose and the frequency of dosage has to be tailored to the individual patient. In older children this is relatively easy, since they will gradually be able to regulate their own need for the tablets. It is also important to tailor the needs of the child in relation to the physical activity through the day. Thus the initial dose should be given soon after waking in the morning and subsequent doses through the day may be spaced to coincide with the perceived need of the child when the previous dose wears off, rather than on a fixed clockwise basis. It is often more satisfactory to increase the frequency or adapt the timing of the dose, once an effective dosage level is established, rather than to increase the individual dose. In infants it may be more difficult to assess. The usual starting dose of pyridostigmine is 1.0 mg/kg by mouth every 4 hours (when awake) and of neostigmine bromide 0.3 mg/kg every 3 hours. In infants with swallowing difficulty neostigmine methyl sulphate by injection can be given before feeds and adjusted in dosage as required. The maximum response to the therapy may not necessarily be a complete remission of the weakness, so that patients may have to accept some degree of weakness without further improvement to avoid overdosage.

It may at times be difficult to decide whether increasing weakness in a child is due to under-treatment (myasthenic crisis) or overtreatment (cholinergic crisis). Some of the muscarine-like side-effects of the anticholinesterase, such as nausea, vomiting, cramps, diarrhoea and sweating or muscle fasciculations, may be present but are frequently not. One way of deciding is to withhold the drug for several hours and observe whether strength is increased or decreased.

Atropine may also be given for cholinergic crisis to counteract the muscarine-like side-effects.

Steroid therapy

Early trials of oral corticosteroid therapy in conjunction with anticholinesterase inhibitors were unfavourable and were often associated with exacerbation of the myasthenic symptoms within a few days of starting therapy (Millikan and Eaton, 1951; Grob and Harvey, 1952). However, Warmolts and Engel (1972) were more successful with an alternate-day, high-dosage, prednisone schedule, without anticholinesterase drugs, in two juvenile and five adult cases. Seybold and Drachman (1974) introduced a gradually incremental daily regime in the first two weeks of treatment and Brunner *et al.* (1976) combined a once-daily regime for the first month with an alternate-day regime after that. Authors still seem divided between either using a daily high-dosage initial regime, under close hospital supervision, with the possibility of some degree of worsening in the first 1–21 days of treatment in about half the patients, but the possibility of remission or marked improvement in about three-quarters of patients (Mann *et al.*, 1976); or, at the other extreme, using a very cautious, gradually incremental, low-dose alternate-day regime, building up over a prolonged period to an effective dose with a good response, and maintaining that dosage for about 3 months before starting gradual decrements of dose to find the minimum effective dose for long-term maintenance (Newsom-Davis, 1994); and various permutations between the two. Pulsed therapy with high-dosage intravenous methyl prednisolone as an alternative to oral prednisolone was introduced by Arsura *et al.* (1985) and tried in refractory childhood myasthenia by Sakano *et al.* (1989). Osawa *et al.* (1991) recently reported their favourable experience with intravenous methyl prednisolone at a dose of 30 mg/kg over a 3-hour period daily on three consecutive days in 16 children with myasthenia (13 ocular and three generalized), in comparison with oral prednisolone, which had been ineffective in 12 of the 13 cases of ocular myasthenia.

Other immunosuppressants

Azathioprine. At a dose of 2–3 mg/kg/day by mouth, azathioprine has been used in combination with steroids and has a steroid-sparing effect, allowing reduction in steroid dosage. It has also been used as a single therapy (Mantegazza *et al.*, 1988) but toxicity may be a problem in some cases (Hohlfeld *et al.*, 1988). Regular blood counts and assessment of liver function are necessary.

Cyclosporin. Cyclosporin has also been used, with variable therapeutic benefit, in a number of trials (Tindall *et al.*, 1987; Nyberg-Hansen and Gjerstad, 1988; Goulon *et al.*, 1989). Close monitoring for renal toxicity is important.

Intravenous gammaglobulin. Intravenous gammaglobulin has been tried in several trials over the past few years (Gajdos *et al.*, 1984; Ippoliti *et al.*, 1984; Arsura *et al.*, 1986; Arsura and Bick, 1988; Maruyama *et al.*, 1989; Sakano *et al.*, 1989). Most cases were adult but there were three children, aged 4, 7 and 11 years (Ippoliti *et al.*, 1984; Maruyama *et al.*, 1989;

Sakano *et al.*, 1989). The response rate was high but usually short-lived, with an average of about 30 days.

Plasma exchange

This is a valuable adjuvant therapy and may give a rapid improvement, which could last for 3–5 weeks. It can be used to prepare severely affected patients for thymectomy, for covering deterioration after thymectomy or during initiation of prednisolone treatment, and to control symptoms during an acute relapse while immunosuppressant drug therapy is being instituted.

Thymectomy

Although the potential value of thymectomy in myasthenia gravis was already documented by Blalock *et al.* in 1939, its exact place in the management of the myasthenia is still debated. Geoffrey Keynes (1954) was its major protagonist and showed that, if cases with thymoma were excluded, there was an improvement in 65% of his 200 personally operated cases. Simpson (1958) reviewed 404 London cases (including those of Keynes) and showed that the mortality in patients having thymectomy was lower than those treated medically, in spite of the hazards of the operation. Best results were in those operated on within 5 years of onset. In the large American series of Perlo *et al.* (1966) it was also established that thymectomy was of definite benefit and particularly in females under 40. In a review of 353 cases, Genkins *et al.* (1975) found the best results in association with early thymectomy in the milder stages of the disease.

In the early days of the operation there was an appreciable postoperative mortality, which has in recent years been considerably reduced by factors such as the assessment of respiratory function preoperatively with a view to a tracheostomy in patients with respiratory insufficiency, improvement of patients with acute symptoms by plasma exchange, and the stopping of all anticholinesterase therapy postoperatively to avoid cholinergic crises.

With the clearer demonstration of immunological aspects in recent years, thymectomy has been placed on a more secure and rational basis and seems to have two possible effects: (1) an immediate response from the removal of antibodies directly damaging the muscle, and (2) a more delayed response when depletion of T cells in the body prevents the abnormal response in other tissues.

Although most reports have dealt with adult cases, there were 21 children under 16 years in Keynes' (1954) series. Four died postoperatively and 16 showed improvement.

Fonkalsrud *et al.* (1970) reviewed their experience with thymectomy in 14 patients under 20 years over a 12-year period. There were no postoperative deaths, but one patient, aged 19, with a benign thymoma died after 2 years. Ten children had a good improvement, with reduction in anticholinesterase requirements, and one had an excellent result and was in remission without anticholinesterase therapy for 2 years before relapsing after an infection.

Geefhuysen *et al.* (1970) reported good results in two of three Bantu children who had been unresponsive to cholinesterase inhibitors. Ryniewicz (1975) analysed 37 cases of childhood myasthenia. Thymectomy was performed in 24, with resultant improvement in 17 cases (72%). Of these 17, five were still free of symptoms and off all therapy after 5 years.

Several other retrospective, non-randomized reports claimed a significant benefit for children undergoing thymectomy (Seybold *et al.*, 1971; Sarnat *et al.*, 1977; Ryniewicz and Badurska, 1977; Rodriguez *et al.*, 1983). Recently Adams *et al.* (1990) reviewed the results of thymectomy in 274 children with onset before 16 years, 250 coming from previous reports in the literature plus 24 personal cases. Although all the reported series claimed benefit from thymectomy, there were wide variations in response and remission rates of thymectomized versus non-thymectomized cases, making comparison of the different series difficult. Many of these cases were not adequately investigated for the presence or absence of AChR antibodies. A prospective, randomized, controlled study of thymectomy in childhood myasthenia would be extremely valuable in defining objectively the indications for thymectomy and the benefits.

In spite of the relatively low operative risk, and the potentially good long-term postoperative results, and the fact that thymectomy is probably more beneficial the earlier it is done, it is likely that for the present a trial of anticholinesterase drugs will continue to be the first line of therapy and thymectomy reserved for those cases failing to respond adequately, possibly also after a trial of steroid therapy (Figure 10-6).

Drugs to be avoided

Certain drugs may produce an exacerbation of myasthenia and are potentially hazardous. These include muscle relaxants such as curare and gallamine triethiodide (Flaxedil®); decamethonium and succinylcholine are better tolerated but also best avoided. Quinine, quinidine and neomycin may increase neuromuscular block. Procaine and derivatives also have a neuromuscular blocking action. Morphines may depress respiration and may be potentiated by anticholinesterase drugs.

LAMBERT–EATON MYASTHENIC SYNDROME

This is essentially a myasthenic syndrome of adult life associated with lung cancer but also occurring independently of an underlying malignancy. The primary defect is a reduction in the number of quanta released by nerve impulse, now thought to be secondary to an antibody-mediated reduction in the number of functional voltage-gated calcium channels at the motor nerve terminals. The diagnostic feature on electromyography is an increase in the amplitude of the muscle action potential following maximum voluntary contraction. Occasional cases have been recorded in childhood with a presynaptic defect resembling that of the Lambert–Eaton syndrome (Bady *et al.*, 1987; Vincent *et al.*, 1992).

TRANSIENT NEONATAL MYASTHENIA

This syndrome, first documented some 50 years ago (Strickroot *et al.*, 1942), occurs in about 10–15% of infants born to myasthenic mothers (Namba *et al.*, 1970; Wise and McQuillen, 1970) and is due to transplacental transfer of circulating anti-AChR antibodies from the myasthenic mother to the fetus (Keesey *et al.*, 1977). Most mothers have generalized myasthenia but the clinical severity in the mother bears no relation to the involvement in the neonate, and indeed the mother may be in remission at the time (Elias *et al.*, 1979). There also does not seem to be a consistent correlation between the clinical involvement in the infant and the antibody titre in the mother, and there has been much speculation on possible mechanisms to account for this, including a protective effect of specific anti-idiotypic antibodies (Lefvert and Osterman, 1983), which could not be verified by Tzartos *et al.* (1990); whilst Eymard *et al.* (1989) thought there was a correlation between the maternal antibody titre and the occurrence and severity of the disease in the newborn.

CLINICAL FEATURES

In most affected infants the symptoms appear within the first few hours of birth and certainly within the first day, although in occasional cases onset may be delayed for up to 3 or 4 days. Close monitoring of these infants in the first few days is thus essential. The cardinal features are feeding difficulty (80%), generalized weakness and hypotonia (70%), respiratory difficulties (65%), feeble cry (60%), facial weakness (55%) and, less frequently, ptosis (15%) (Figure 10-7).

DIAGNOSIS

This may be confirmed by a clinical response to edrophonium, given by either subcutaneous or intramuscular injection (1 mg) or by slow intravenous injection, with an initial test dose (0.03 mg/kg), followed by small fractional doses over a period of 3 or 4 minutes, with a total up to 0.15 mg/kg. If there is no obvious response to edrophonium then a test dose of intramuscular prostigmine (0.05 mg) or pyridostigmine (0.3 mg) can be tried, and a therapeutic trial over a few days may be worth giving in cases with equivocal results. The diagnosis can also be confirmed electrodiagnostically by demonstration of a response decrement on repetitive nerve stimulation at 2–5 Hz.

TREATMENT

This is largely supportive. Infants with profound weakness and respiratory insufficiency may need transient ventilator support. Nasogastric feeding may be necessary. The infants usually respond to cholinesterase inhibitors such as pyridostigmine bromide 4–10 mg by mouth or by gavage every 4 hours prior to feeds. In severely affected infants an exchange transfusion may be helpful (Donat *et al.*, 1981).

PROGNOSIS

The condition is self-limiting and most cases should resolve completely within 2 or 3 weeks, although occasional cases may persist longer. Once resolved, there is no risk of recurrence and these infants are also not at special risk of developing later myasthenia gravis (Pirskanen, 1977; Szobor, 1989). One can thus give parents a good long-term prognosis in even the most severely affected neonatal cases.

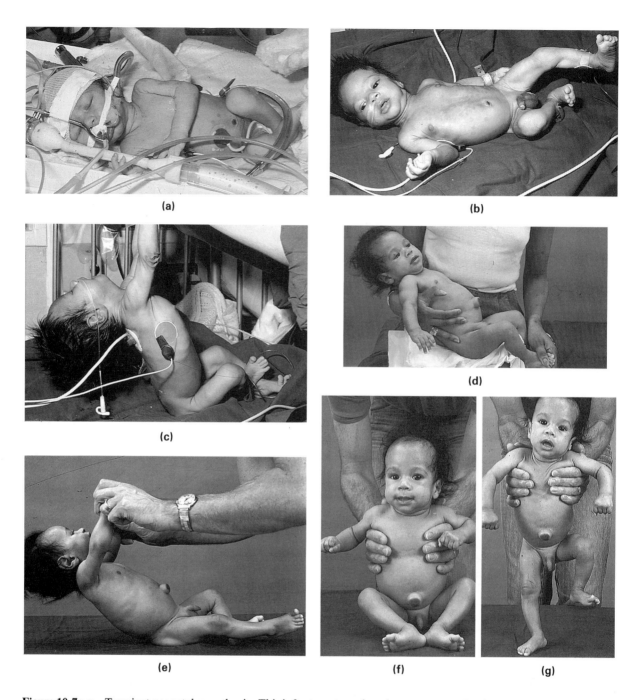

Figure 10-7a-g Transient neonatal myasthenia. This infant was transferred to our neonatal unit at 2 weeks of age with an unconfirmed diagnosis of neonatal myasthenia. He had been markedly hypotonic and ventilator-dependent from birth and the picture was further complicated by severe pneumonia and lung collapse (a). There was no obvious response to intravenous tensilon and response to intramuscular neostigmine was also equivocal. Repetitive posterior tibial nerve stimulation produced some decrement in motor potential. The diagnosis was confirmed by demonstrating an improvement in diaphragmatic function after neostigmine. The clinical diagnosis of myasthenia in the mother had also been questioned when her antibody titre was negative. Her anti-cholinesterase treatment was stopped postpartum and she had a respiratory arrest and needed resuscitation and intensive care and was left with a permanent tracheostomy. The child gradually improved in lung function and general mobility and was weaned off the ventilator on day 21 and the neostigmine tapered off. By 4 weeks he had good antigravity power in the legs (b) but head control was still poor (c). He continued to progress well and by 4 months had good head control (d,e), was sitting with support (f) and taking good weight on his legs (g). When reviewed at 10 months his development was quite normal.

NEONATAL MYASTHENIC ARTHROGRYPOSIS

In contrast to the relatively benign course of transient neonatal myasthenia, there have been several reports of infants born to myasthenic mothers with a much more severe syndrome, associated with arthrogryposis and respiratory distress, hydramnios during pregnancy, and a high stillbirth and neonatal death rate (Shepard, 1971; Holmes *et al.*, 1979; Pasternak *et al.*, 1981; Dulitzky *et al.*, 1987; Eymard *et al.*, 1989; Stoll *et al.*, 1991; Carr *et al.*, 1991; Dinger and Prager, 1993; Barnes *et al.*, 1995). In addition, there is a remarkable recurrence in siblings and AChR antibodies have been found in both the mother and the affected infant. Once again, there seems to be no direct correlation between the severity of the myasthenia in the mother and in the affected infant; indeed in two reports the diagnosis of myasthenia in the mother was not suspected until after the birth of an affected child (Dulitzky *et al.*, 1987), or until 18 months after the fourth affected child (Barnes *et al.*, 1995). The latter family was of particular interest as the diagnosis in the mother had not been made in spite of referral to a muscle centre specializing in myasthenia, and electrodiagnostic studies did not reveal a response decrement and repeated muscle biopsies were unhelpful. Following the suggestion by a medical geneticist of a possible maternal myasthenia to account for the recurrent arthrogryposis, the serum anti-AChR antibody titre was found to be 6000 nM (normal <0.2 nM). This illustrates once again how readily myasthenia can be missed when not specifically thought of, even by the well-initiated. The previous infants had been diagnosed as Pena–Shokeir syndrome. The first had died at 7 hours, the second had survived and had improved, the third had died at 7 weeks, and the fourth had severe asphyxia at birth and died at 20 minutes. The possibility of maternal myasthenia needs to be added to the list of possible causes of arthrogryposis in the newborn, and particularly in recurrent cases (see Chapter 13).

PATHOGENESIS

The involvement of four successive siblings in one family (Barnes *et al.*, 1995) makes it unlikely that this condition has a genetic basis and more likely that it is the direct result of the AChR antibodies in the mother. This is further supported by the therapeutic efforts of Carr *et al.* (1991) with steroids and serial plasma exchanges in a severely affected myasthenic woman, who had lost two previously affected neonates. In the treated pregnancy there was a fall in the anti-AChR antibody titre, an increase in fetal breathing movements, and the infant had a transient neonatal myasthenia, with normal pulmonary function and no limb deformity. Further experience will be needed to evaluate this potential treatment of recurrent intrauterine arthrogryposis in myasthenic women.

This syndrome is also reminiscent of the early experimental work of Drachman and Sokoloff (1966), producing arthrogryposis in the developing chick by paralysing the limbs with curare. A comparable human situation was reflected in the production of arthrogryposis in a fetus following the administration of muscle relaxants in a pregnant woman with tetanus (Jago, 1970).

CONGENITAL MYASTHENIC SYNDROMES

With the recognition and diagnosis of the auto-immune myasthenia gravis, it became possible to separate the group of so-called congenital myasthenic syndromes. These are genetically determined disorders. Although congenital in the sense of being born with the disorder, rather than acquiring it, only some patients may present in the neonatal period, whereas others may present later in childhood or even in adult life – a situation comparable with groups of congenital myopathies (Figures 10-8 to 10-11).

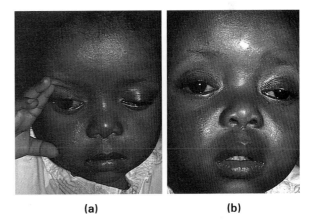

(a) **(b)**

Figure 10-8a,b Congenital myasthenia. This 2-year-old African child had myasthenia with marked ptosis and external ophthalmoplegia. She was unable to open her eyes and used her fingers to raise her eyelids (a). There was marked improvement after tensilon (b).

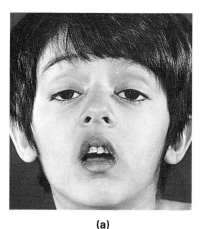
(a)

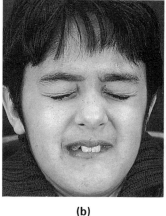
(b)

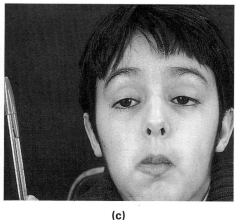
(c)

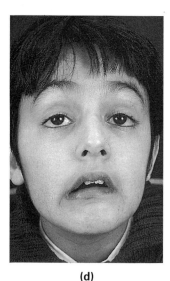
(d)

Figure 10-9a-d Congenital myasthenia. This child was referred at 4 years of age with a history of encephalitic illness at 2 years, with associated swallowing difficulty which persisted after the other symptoms had resolved. He had been normal in the neonatal period and sat at 6 months, cruised at 1 year and walked unsupported at 18 months. By 2 years his walking had not progressed further, and he was unable to run or climb stairs. His parents had also noted some ptosis in the first year. On examination he had obvious ptosis and also limited ocular movement and associated weakness of facial movement, an expressionless face, open mouth and with inability to close the eyes tightly (a). There was general hypotonia with joint laxity. He got up from the floor with a Gowers' sign and was unable to stand on one leg or to run. A diagnosis of myasthenia was confirmed by demonstrating response decrement to repeated ulnar nerve stimulation. A definite improvement in the ptosis and his ability to get up from the floor was noted after intravenous Tensilon®. He was treated with pyridostigmine with a definite improvement but with time he needed increase in the dose and frequency. His performance improved after each dose and tended to wane as the next dose became due. When reviewed at 7½ years he was taking 30 mg every 2–3 hours, with a higher dose of 45 mg at 8.00am and 1.30pm. There was no evidence of drug toxicity. He still had a Gowers' sign on rising from the floor, marked ptosis, external ophthalmoplegia and facial weakness (b-d). The parents are first cousins, so that this is probably a case of autosomal recessive infantile (congenital) myasthenia.

Although the exact delineation of the individual disorders requires sophisticated electrodiagnostic and associated investigations of appropriate biopsies, such as the intercostal muscle with available neuromuscular junctions, which are only currently available at a handful of specialized laboratories around the world, the general diagnosis of a congenital syndrome in an individual case is important in order to avoid unnecessary and inappropriate treatment with steroids, immuno-suppression and thymectomy. Most of them are sensitive to acetylcholinesterase inhibitors, with the exception of a few syndromes such as congenital acetyl cholinesterase deficiency or slow channel syndrome. As a group they show absence of anti-AChR antibodies, but in an individual case, particularly in later childhood, this in itself does not exclude the autoimmune disease, as a proportion of such cases can be negative for the antibody.

CLASSIFICATION

This is still evolving and a number of approaches have been suggested (Engel, 1993, 1994; Shillito *et al.*, 1993). One approach is to divide them into presynaptic or postsynaptic defects or a combination of the two. These can be further delineated into well-characterized and partially characterized syndromes. The factors that may compromise the safety margin of neuromuscular transmission (see pathophysiology above) can then be integrated into this framework in relation to the individual syndromes (Engel, 1994) (Table 10-1). If the neuromuscular junction is perceived as an engine driven by quanta of acetylcholine, a reduced safety margin can result from a defect in the quantal release mechanism, a decrease in quantal size or a reduction in quantal efficiency.

Table 10-1 Classification of congenital myasthenic syndromes

Presynaptic defects

Defect in ACh resynthesis or packaging ('familial infantile myasthenia')
Paucity of synaptic vesicles and reduced quantal release

Pre- and postsynaptic defects

End-plate AChE deficiency

Postsynaptic defects

Kinetic abnormalities of AChR with AChR deficiency
    Classic slow-channel syndrome
    Epsilon subunit mutations with prolonged open time
        and low conductance of the AChR channel
    AChR deficiency and short channel open time

Kinetic abnormalities of AChR without AChR deficiency
    High-conductance fast-channel syndrome
    Syndrome attributed to abnormal interaction of ACh with AChR

Partially characterized syndromes

AChR deficiency with paucity of secondary synaptic clefts
Other AChR deficiencies
Familial limb girdle myasthenia
Benign CMS with facial malformations

ACh: acetylcholine; AChE: acetylcholinesterase;
AChR: acetylcholine receptor; CMS: congenital myasthenic syndrome

From Engel (1994) with permission.

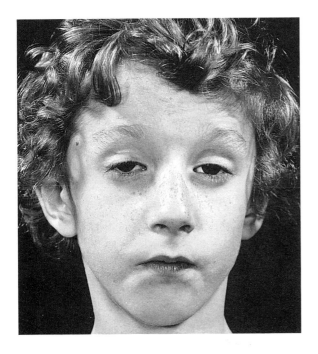

Figure 10-10 Congenital myasthenia. This 9-year-old boy had a history of reduced fetal movements *in utero*, birth asphyxia, poor sucking and a weak cry. On day 2 he had a seizure; between 4 months and 2 years he had several episodes of 'collapse'. Ptosis was first noted at 15 months. He responded dramatically to intravenous edrophonium at 2 years and was prescribed oral neostigmine with good effect. Recently the drug seemed less effective. Repetitive nerve stimulation had shown no apparent decrement in response. Currently he was managing most activities and able to walk 3 miles, but was aware of being less strong in his limbs than his peers. His neck tended to ache and his eyelids to droop but he had no diplopia. On examination he had intermittent and variable ptosis, with overactivity of the frontalis muscle (see fig), and a full range of eye movements, apart from some limited abduction on the right. There was mild facial weakness and inability to whistle. Power in his limbs seemed minimally reduced; he was able to sit up from the horizontal ten consecutive times without help. The reflexes were brisk in the lower limbs with sustained ankle clonus and an extensor plantar response. This may reflect upper motor neurone dysfunction in association with his perinatal asphyxia rather than his myasthenia. The test for anti-AChR antibodies was negative.

Table 10-2 Classification and features of the congenital myasthenic syndromes

	Probable inheritance	Typical onset	Extra-ocular weakness	Response to AChE	EMG response to single shock	MEPP amplitude	AChR	AChE staining
Presynaptic abnormalities								
Familial infantile myasthenia	Recessive	Neonatal	−	+	Single	↓ after stimulation	N	N
Paucity of synaptic vesicles	Recessive	Neonatal	−	+	Single	N(↓ QC)	N	N
Other putative presynaptic disorders	Recessive	Neonatal	−	+	Single	N(↓ QC)	N	N
Acetylcholinesterase abnormalities								
AChE deficiency	Recessive	Neonatal	+	−	Repetitive	Prolonged delay	N/↓	Absent
Postsynaptic abnormalities								
AChR deficiency	Recessive	<2 yr	+	+	Single	↓ at rest	↓	Elongated
Paucity of synaptic folds	Recessive	<2 yr	+	+	Single	↓ at rest	↓	Elongated
Abnormal ACh-AChR interaction	?	Neonatal/childhood	+/−	+/−	Single	↓ at rest	N/↓	Variable
Slow channel	Dominant	Childhood/adulthood	+	−	Repetitive	Prolonged delay	N/↓	Elongated
High conductance fast channel	?	Neonatal	+	−	Single	↑ at rest	N	N

N: normal; QC: quantal content; +: present; −: absent; ↓: decreased; ↑: increased.

From Shillito *et al.* (1993) with permission.

Quantal efficiency in turn can be affected by the geometry of the neuromuscular junction, the density and functional state of acetylcholinesterase, the density of AChR on the postsynaptic membrane, the affinity of AChR for ACh, and the kinetic properties of the AChR channel. Seen in the context of recognized syndromes, quantal release is reduced in a syndrome with paucity of synaptic vesicles and in congenital end-plate AChE deficiency; quantal size is reduced in familial infantile myasthenia; quantal efficiency is abnormal in a syndrome with abnormal interaction of ACh and AChR, the high-conductance and fast-channel syndrome, the slow-channel syndrome, and in other syndromes with prolonged open time or low conductance of the AChR channel. More than one mechanism may be involved in some individual disorders.

GENETICS

With the exception of the dominantly inherited slow-channel syndrome, these syndromes are probably all inherited through an autosomal recessive mechanism. As the molecular genetics in relation to these disorders unravels there may well turn out to be genetic heterogeneity in relation to some of these apparently individual syndromes.

CLINICAL PHENOTYPES

In the early days of the congenital myopathies the clinical phenotype was thought to be fairly non-specific in relation to the various individual structural disorders. With increasing experience, individual clinical phenotypes are now readily identified (see Chapter 3). The same evolution seems to occur at present in relation to these relatively rare congenital myasthenic syndromes (Table 10-2).

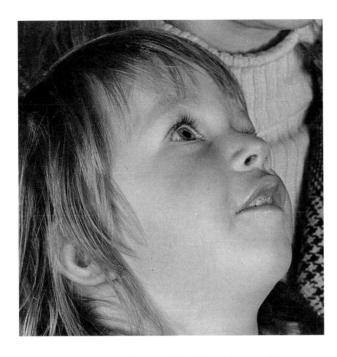

Figure 10-11 Congenital myasthenia. A classical history. This girl was born at 37 weeks gestation, birthweight 2.6 kg (5 lb 12 oz). She did not cry immediately, was kept on neonatal unit and developed some grunting respiration, which settled rapidly. Satisfactory progress but prone to vomiting and accumulation of mucus. Discharged home at 8 days, weighing 2.55 kg. At 8 weeks, mother noticed a series of episodes when she seemed unable to breathe and became still, associated with excessive mucus in the upper respiratory tract. No abnormalities were found on examination. These episodes continued until the age of 6 or 7 months. She was admitted to hospital at the age of 13 months with an episode of difficulty in breathing and eye rolling but no definite convulsion. She was noted to have increased nasal and pharyngeal secretion, but no other abnormality was found. Another similar episode occurred on the ward, and was thought to be due to respiratory obstruction. Her early milestones were slightly delayed with ability to sit unaided at 9 months, standing at 17 months and walking at 19 months. Her intellectual milestones were quite normal. Following this episode she recovered satisfactorily until about a year later, when she was again admitted with a similar episode. On admission, she had marked accumulation of pharyngeal mucus and considerable respiratory difficulty, which improved on aspiration. It was then noted that she also had a variable bilateral ptosis and tended to tire easily. In retrospect, the mother had noticed this for quite some time, possibly from about 6 months of age, and thought that it had become worse. There was also a tendency to drop her head. She also choked at times on medicine and had difficulty coughing up mucus.

The question of myasthenia was raised first at that stage and she had a dramatic response on two separate occasions to intravenous edrophonium (Tensilon®), with marked improvement in ptosis and general activity. She was then started on pyridostigmine with a very good response, and a deterioration when it was stopped after 5 days. She continued on pyridostigmine, 20 mg four times a day, and her mother commented that she was a completely different child. She then remained active and had no further episodes of obstruction.

When first assessed at our Muscle Clinic in September 1974 at the age of 2½ years, she had no particular problems and was coping well with all general activities. She was having 30 mg pyridostigmine three times per day, which seemed to control her satisfactorily. On examination we could find no evidence of weakness or fatigue and she seemed fully controlled. EMG study with repetitive stimulation of the nerve also showed no fatigue at frequencies from 3 to 50 H$_z$. She was subsequently reassessed after having stopped her pyridostigmine therapy that morning. When examined mid-morning, she was quite normal, but by 2pm, when she had missed two doses, she was much more unstable and had severe falls, and it was also apparent that her eyes were drooping slightly and not as widely open as normally, although there was no overt ptosis. Repetitive stimulation of the ulnar nerve, with recording of the muscle potentials from the hypothenar muscles, showed a definite decrement at frequencies of 3 per second after about a 10-s interval. This decrement was subsequently abolished after an intravenous injection of edrophonium. She also became somewhat 'gurgly' in the throat during this time, due to some mucus accumulation, which she had not previously experienced since starting the therapy. This unequivocally confirmed the diagnosis of myasthenia. She continued very well on pyridostigmine, 30 mg four times per day. About 6 months later she complained of diplopia and an intermittent squint was noted by her mother. Her pyridostigmine dosage was increased from 30 mg to 60 mg four times daily and the symptoms and signs resolved completely. During the following year she had no recurrence of symptoms. The mother had two previous pregnancies. The first ended in a stillbirth. The second child was born at term and subsequently died at 4½ months from bronchopneumonia and associated convulsions. She apparently stopped breathing, and in retrospect seems to have had a similar problem to the present child.

One of the limiting factors may be the difficulty of adequate investigation of these cases on a routine basis. The clinical dictum seems to be 'cure them first and diagnose them afterwards'. As many of them are sensitive to treatment with anticholinesterases, it is expedient to go ahead with treatment once a diagnosis of myasthenia is confirmed on the basis of the response decrement to repetitive nerve stimulation, a pretty routine and readily available investigation.

INVESTIGATION OF CONGENITAL MYASTHENIA

The complete investigation of a case of a congenital myasthenic syndrome requires a detailed correlation of the clinical, electrodiagnostic and serological assessment with morphological examination of the fine structure of the end-plate and *in vitro* electrophysiological studies to assess quantal release and the factors affecting the efficiency of the released quanta (see Table 10-3). To this may be added molecular genetic studies for possible mutations in the subunits of the AChR.

Table 10-3 Investigation of myasthenic syndromes

Clinical
History, examination, response to AChE inhibitor
EMG: conventional, stimulation studies, single fibre
  EMG
Serological tests (AChR antibodies)

Morphological studies
Routine histochemical studies
Cytochemical and immunocytochemical localizations of
  AChE, AChR, AChR subunits, lgG, C3, C9, MAC at
  the NMJ
Estimate of the size, shape and two-dimensional profile
  of AChE-reactive end-plates or end-plate regions on
  teased muscle fibres
Quantitative electron microscopy and electron
  cytochemistry

^{125}I-α-bungarotoxin binding sites/NMJ

In vitro **electrophysiological studies**
Conventional microelectrode studies: MEPP, MEPC,
  evoked quantal release (m, n, p)
Noise analysis; channel kinetics
Single-channel patch-clamp recordings

Molecular genetic analysis

AChE: acetylcholinesterase; AChR: acetylcholine receptor; EMG: electromyography; MAC: C5b-9 complement membrane attack complex; MEPP: miniature end-plate potentials; MEPC: miniature end-plate current; m: number of ACh quanta released by nerve impulse; n: number of readily releasable ACh quanta; NMJ: neuromuscular junction; p: probability of quantal release.

From Engel (1994) with permission.

TREATMENT

Most of these syndromes will respond fully or partially to acetylcholinesterase inhibitors, with the exception of the slow-channel syndrome and acetylcholinesterase deficiency, which may be worsened by it, and the high conductance, fast-channel syndrome cases, which respond incompletely to AChE inhibitors and may get additional benefit from 3,4-diaminopyridine, a potassium-channel blocking agent which increases transmitter release from the nerve terminal (Palace *et al.*, 1991).

OTHER MYASTHENIC SYNDROMES

MYASTHENIA WITH FACIAL MALFORMATION

A seemingly distinct autosomal recessive disorder has been described in ten Jewish families of Iraqi or Iranian origin (Goldhammer *et al.*, 1990), characterized by ptosis, facial and bulbar weakness and fatigue of speech, with onset in early childhood and associated with elongation of the face and high-arched palate. The underlying basis for the syndrome has not yet been characterized.

FAMILIAL LIMB-GIRDLE MYASTHENIA

McQuillen (1966) described an autosomal recessive syndrome of limb-girdle weakness with onset in childhood or early adult life, with no ocular or cranial involvement, and responsive to anti-AChE treatment (see also case history, Figure 10-4). Dobkin and Verity (1978) reported a similar case with an associated cardiomyopathy.

BOTULISM

This disease resembles myasthenia gravis, since the botulinum toxin also affects neuromuscular transmission. It may occur in early infancy with acute hypotonia, weakness, ptosis and dysphagia (Pickett *et al.*, 1976). There may also be signs of autonomic involvement, such as fixed dilated pupils. Although relatively common in the USA (Black and Arnon, 1977), the condition is practically unknown (or perhaps missed) in England (Turner *et al.*, 1978). There has been a suggestion that honey contaminated with *Clostridium botulinum* may have been a factor in a high proportion of infants with type B botulism affection (Arnon *et al.*, 1979).

REFERENCES

Adams, C., Theodorescu, D., Murphy, E.G. *et al.* (1990) Thymectomy in juvenile myasthenia gravis. *Journal of Child Neurology* 5: 215.

Arnon, S.S., Midura, T.F., Damus, K. *et al.* (1979) Honey and other environmental risk factors for infant botulism. *Journal of Pediatrics* 94: 331–336.

Arsura, E.L. and Bick, A. (1988) Effects of repeated doses of intravenous immunoglobulin in myasthenia gravis. *American Journal of Medical Science* 295: 438–443.

Arsura, E., Brunner, N.G., Namba, T. *et al.* (1985) High dose intravenous methylprednisolone in myasthenia gravis. *Archives of Neurology* 42: 1149–1153.

Arsura, E.L., Bick, A., Brunner, N.G. *et al.* (1986) High-dose intravenous immunoglobulin in the management of myasthenia gravis. *Archives of Internal Medicine* 146: 1365–1367.

Bady, B., Chauplannaz, G. and Carrier, H. (1987) Congenital Lambert-Eaton myasthenic syndrome. *Journal of Neurology, Neurosurgery and Psychiatry* 50: 476–478.

Barnes, P.R.J., Kanabar, D.J., Brueton, L. *et al.* (1995) Recurrent congenital arthrogryposis leading to a diagnosis of myasthenia gravis in an initially asymptomatic mother. *Neuromuscular Disorders* 5: 59–65.

Batocchi, A.P., Evoli, A., Palmisani, M.T. *et al.* (1990) Early-onset myasthenia gravis: clinical characteristics and response to therapy. *European Journal of Pediatrics* 150: 66–68.

Bell, E.T. (1917) Tumors of the thymus in myasthenia gravis. *Journal of Nervous and Mental Diseases* 45: 130.

Black, R.E. and Arnon, S.S. (1977) Botulism in the United States, 1976. *Journal of Infectious Diseases* 136: 829–832.

Blalock, A., Mason, M.F., Morgan, H.J. and Riven, S.S. (1939) Myasthenia gravis and tumors of the thymic region. *Annals of Surgery* 110: 544.

Blalock, A., Harvey, A.M., Ford, F.R. and Lilienthal, J.L. Jr (1941) The treatment of myasthenia gravis by removal of the thymus gland. *Journal of the American Medical Association* 117: 1529.

Brunner N.G., Berger, C.L., Namba, T. and Grob, D. (1976) Corticotropin and corticosteroids in generalised myasthenia gravis: Comparative studies and role in management. *Annals of the New York Academy of Science* 274: 577–595.

Bundey, S. (1972) A genetic study of infantile and juvenile myasthenia gravis. *Journal of Neurology, Neurosurgery and Psychiatry* 35: 41–51.

Campbell, H. and Bramwell, E. (1900) Myasthenia gravis. *Brain* 23: 277.

Carr, S.R., Gilchrist, J.M., Abuelo, D.N. *et al.* (1991) Treatment of antenatal myasthenia gravis. *Obstetrics and Gynaecology* 78: 485–489.

Cordess, C., Folstein, M.F. and Drachman, D.B. (1983) Quantitative psychiatric assessment of patients with myasthenia gravis. *Journal of Psychiatric Treatment and Evaluation* 5: 381.

Cosi, V., Lombardi, M., Piccolo, G. *et al.* (1991) Treatment of myasthenia gravis with high-dose intravenous immunoglobulin. *Acta Neurologica Scandinavica* 84: 81.

Dale, H.H. and Feldberg, W. (1934) Chemical transmission at motor nerve endings in voluntary muscle? *Journal of Physiology (London)* 81: 39P.

Dau, P.C., Lindstrom, J., Cassel, C.K. *et al.* (1977) Plasmapheresis and immunosuppressive drug therapy in myasthenia gravis. *New England Journal of Medicine* 297: 1134–1140.

Dinger, J. and Prager, B. (1993) Arthrogryposis multiplex in a newborn of a myasthenic mother: case report and literature. *Neuromuscular Disorders* 3: 335–339.

Donat, J.F.G.G., Donat, J.R. and Lennon, V.A. (1981) Exchange transfusion in neonatal myasthenia gravis. *Neurology* 31: 911.

Dobkin, B.H. and Verity, M.A. (1978) Familial neuromuscular disease with type 1 fiber hypoplasia, tubular aggregates, cardiomyopathy and myasthenic features. *Neurology* 28: 1135–1140.

Drachman, D.B. and Sokoloff, L. (1966) The role of movement in embryonic joint development. *Revue Biologique* 14: 401–420.

Dulitzky, F., Sirota, L., Landman, J. *et al.* (1987) An infant with multiple deformations born to a myasthenic mother. *Helvetica Pediatrica Acta* 42: 173–176.

Elias, S.B., Butler, I. and Appel, S.H. (1979) Neonatal myasthenia gravis in the infant of a myasthenic mother in remission. *Annals of Neurology* 6: 72.

Engel, A.G. (1984) Myasthenia gravis and myasthenic syndromes. *Annals of Neurology* 16: 519–534.

Engel, A.G. (1988) Congenital myasthenic syndromes. *Journal of Child Neurology* 3: 233–246.

Engel, A.G. (1993) The investigation of congenital myasthenic syndromes. In: Penn, A.S., Richman, D.P., Ruff, R.L. *et al.* eds, *Myasthenia Gravis and Related Disorders: Experimental and Clinical Aspects.* (*Annals of the New York Academy of Sciences* Vol 681. New York: The New York Academy of Sciences, pp. 425–434.

Engel, A.G. (1994) Myasthenic syndromes. In: Engel, A.G. and Franzini-Armstrong, C. eds, *Myology, Basic and Clinical* 2nd edn. New York: McGraw-Hill, pp. 1798–1835.

Engel, W.K., Lambert, E.H. and Howard, F.M. (1977) Immune complexes (IgG and C3) at the motor endplate in myasthenia gravis: ultrastructural and light microscopic localization and electrophysiological correlations. *Mayo Clinic Proceedings* 52: 267–280.

Erb, W. (1879) Zur Casuistik der bulbaren Lähmungen. *Archiv für Psychiatrie und Nervenkrankheiten* 9: 325.

Eymard, B., Morel, E., Dulac, O. *et al.* (1989) Myasthenie et grossesse: une étude clinique et immunologique de 42 cas (21 myasthenies neonatales). *Revue Neurologique Paris* 145: 696–701.

Fambrough, D.M., Drachman, D.B. and Satyamurti, S. (1973) Neuromuscular junction in myasthenia gravis: decreased acetylcholine receptors. *Science* 182: 293–295.

Fonkalsrud, E.W., Herrmann, C. Jr and Mulder, D.G. (1970) Thymectomy for myasthenia gravis in children. *Journal of Pediatric Surgery* 5: 157–165.

Fukuyama, Y., Hirayama, Y. and Osawa, M. (1981) Epidemiological and clinical features of childhood myasthenia gravis in Japan. In: Japan Medical Research Foundation, ed, *Myasthenia Gravis.* Tokyo: University of Tokyo Press, pp. 19–28.

Gajdos, Ph., Outin, H., Elkharrat, D. *et al.* (1984) High-dose intravenous gammaglobulin for myasthenia gravis. *Lancet* 2: 809.

Geefhuysen, J., Ronthal, M. and Rogers, M.A. (1970) Thymectomy for myasthenia gravis in Bantu children. *South African Medical Journal* 44: 239–241.

Genkins, G., Papatestas, A.E., Horowitz, S.H. and Kornfeld, P. (1975) Studies in myasthenia gravis: early thymectomy. Electrophysiologic and pathologic correlations. *The American Journal of Medicine* 58: 517–524.

Goldflam, S. (1893) Ueber einen scheinbar heilbaren bulbärparalytischen Symptomencomplex mit Betheiligung der Extremitaten. *Deutsche Zeitschrift für Nervenheilkunde* 4: 312.

Goldhammer, Y., Blatt, I., Sadeh, M. *et al.* (1990) Congenital myasthenia associated with facial malformations in Iraqi and Iranian Jews: a new genetic syndrome. *Brain* 113: 1291–1306.

Goulon, M., Elkharrat, D. and Gajdos, Ph. (1989) Traitement de la myasthenie grave par la ciclosporine: étude ouverte de 12 mois. *Presse Medicale* 18: 341–346.

Grob, D. and Harvey, A.M. (1952) Effect of adrenocorticotropic hormone (ACTH) and cortisone administration in patients with myasthenia gravis and report of onset of myasthenia gravis during prolonged cortisone administration. *Bulletin of the Johns Hopkins Hospital* 91: 124–136.

Hawkins, B.R., Yu, Y.L., Wong, V. *et al.* (1989) Possible evidence for a variant of myasthenia gravis based on HLA and acetylcholine receptor antibody in Chinese patients. *Quarterly Journal of Medicine* 70: 235–241.

Hohlfeld, R., Michels, M., Heininger, K. *et al.* (1988) Azathioprine toxicity during long-term immunosuppression of generalized myasthenia gravis. *Neurology* 38: 258.

Holmes, L.B., Driscoll, S. and Bradley, W.G. (1979) Multiple contractures in newborn of mother with myasthenia gravis. *Pediatric Research* 13: 486.

Ippoliti, C.G., Cosi, V., Piccolo, G. *et al.* (1984) High-dose intravenous gammaglobulin for myasthenia gravis. *Lancet* ii: 809.

Jago, R.N. (1970) Arthrogryposis following treatment of maternal tetanus with muscle relaxants. *Archives of Disease in Childhood* 45: 277–279.

Jolly, R. (1895) Ueber Myasthenia gravis pseudoparalytica. *Berliner klinische Wochenschrift* 32: 1.

Keesey, J., Lindstrom, J., Cokeley, H. *et al.* (1977) Anti-acetylcholine receptor antibody in neonatal myasthenia gravis. *New England Journal of Medicine* 296: 55.

Keynes, G. (1954) Surgery of the thymus gland. *Lancet* i: 1197.

Laquer, L. and Weigert, C. (1901) Pathologische-anatomischer Beitrag zur Erb'schen Krankheit (Myasthenia gravis). *Neurologisches Zentralblatt* 20: 594.

Lefvert, A.K. and Osterman, P.O. (1983) Newborn infants to myasthenic mothers: a clinical study and an investigation of acetylcholine receptor antibodies in 17 children. *Neurology* 33: 133–138.

Lindstrom, J., Seybold, M.E., Lennon, V.A. *et al.* (1976) Antibody to acetylcholine receptor in myasthenia gravis. *Neurology (Minneapolis)* 26: 1054–1059.

Magni, G., Micaglio, G.F., Lalli, R. *et al.* (1988) Psychiatric disturbances associated with myasthenia gravis. *Acta Psychiatrica Scandinavica* 77: 443.

Mann, J.D., Johns, T.R. and Campa, J.F. (1976) Long-term administration of corticosteroids in myasthenia gravis. *Neurology* 26: 729–740.

Mantegazza, R., Antozzi, C., Peluchetti, D. *et al.* (1988) Azathioprine as a single drug or in combination with steroids in the treatment of myasthenia gravis. *Journal of Neurology* 235: 449.

Maruyama, Y., Takeshita, S., Sekine, I. *et al.* (1989) High-dose immunoglobulin for juvenile myasthenia gravis. *Acta Pediatrica Japan* 31: 544–548.

Matsuki, K., Juji, T., Tokunaga, K. *et al.* (1990) HLA antigens in Japanese patients with myasthenia gravis. *Journal of Clinical Investigation* 86: 392.

Mertens, H.G., Balzereit, F. and Leipert, M. (1969) The treatment of severe myasthenia gravis with immunosuppressive agents. *European Neurology* 2: 321.

McQuillen, M.P. (1966) Familial limb-girdle myasthenia. *Brain* 89: 121–132.

Millichap, J.G. and Dodge, P.R. (1960) Diagnosis and treatment of myasthenia gravis in infancy, childhood, and adolescence. *Neurology (Minneapolis)* 10: 1007–1014.

Millikan, C.H. and Eaton, L.M. (1951) Clinical evaluation of ACTH and cortisone in myasthenia gravis. *Neurology (Minneapolis)* 1: 145–152.

Namba, T., Brown, S.B. and Grob, D. (1970). Neonatal myasthenia gravis: report of two cases and review of the literature. *Pediatrics* 45: 488–504.

Namba, T., Brunner, N.G., Brown, S.B., Muguruma, M. and Grob, D. (1971a) Familial myasthenia gravis. *Archives of Neurology* 25: 49.

Namba, T., Shapiro, M.S., Brunner, N.G. and Grob, D. (1971b) Myasthenia gravis occurring in twins. *Journal of Neurology, Neurosurgery and Psychiatry* 34: 531.

Newsom-Davis, J. (1994) Myasthenia gravis and related syndromes. In: Walton, J., Karpati, G. and Hilton-Jones, D. eds, *Disorders of Voluntary Muscle.* Edinburgh: Churchill Livingstone, pp. 761–780.

Nyberg-Hansen, R. and Gjerstad, L. (1988) Myasthenia gravis treated with ciclosporin. *Acta Neurologica Scandinavica* 77: 307–313.

Oppenheim, H. (1887) Ueber einen Fall von chronischer progressiver Bulbärparalyse ohne anatomischen Befund. *Virchow's Archive für pathologische Anatomie* 108: 522.

Oppenheim, H. (1901) *Die Myasthenische Paralyse.* Berlin: S. Karger.

Osawa, M., Hirasawa, K. and Fukuyama, Y. (1991) Myasthenia gravis in childhood. In: Fukuyama, Y., Kamoshita, S., Ohtsuka, C. *et al.*, eds, *Modern Perspectives of Child Neurology*. Proceedings II of the Joint Convention of 5th International Child Neurology Congress and 3rd Asian and Oceanian Congress of Child Neurology, Tokyo, 4–9 November 1990. Tokyo: The Japanese Society of Child Neurology.

Osserman, K.E. (1955) Progress report on Mestinon bromide (Pyridostigmine bromide). *American Journal of Medicine* 19: 737.

Osserman, K.E. (1958) *Myasthenia Gravis*. New York: Grune and Stratton.

Osserman, K.E. and Genkins, G. (1971) Studies in myasthenia gravis: review of a twenty year experience in over 1200 patients. *Mount Sinai Journal of Medicine* 38: 497–537.

Palace, J., Wiles, C.M. and Newsom-Davis, J. (1991) 3,4-Diaminopyridine in the treatment of congenital (hereditary) myasthenia. *Journal of Neurology, Neurosurgery and Psychiatry* 54: 1069–1072.

Pasternak, J.F., Hageman, J., Adama, M.A. *et al.* (1981) Exchange transfusion in neonatal myasthenia. *Journal of Pediatrics* 99: 644–646.

Patrick, J. and Lindstrom, J.M. (1973) Autoimmune response to acetylcholine receptor. *Science* 180: 871–872.

Perlo, V.P., Poskanzer, D.C., Schwab, R.S., Viets, H.R., Osserman, K. E. and Genkins, G. (1966) Myasthenia gravis: evaluation of treatment in 1,355 patients. *Neurology (Minneapolis)* 16: 431–439.

Pickett, J., Berg, B., Chaplin, E. *et al.* (1976) Syndrome of botulism in infancy: clinical and electrophysiologic study. *New England Journal of Medicine* 295: 769–772.

Pinching, A.J., Peters, D.K. and Newsom-Davis, J. (1976) Remission of myasthenia gravis following plasma exchange. *Lancet* ii: 1373–1376.

Pirskanen, R. (1977) Genetic aspect in myasthenia gravis. A family study of 264 Finnish patients. *Acta Neurologica Scandinavica* 56: 365.

Pritchard, E.A.B. (1935) The use of "prostigmin" in the treatment of myasthenia gravis. *Lancet* i: 432.

Rodriguez, M., Gomez, M.R., Howard, F.M. *et al.* (1983) Myasthenia gravis in children: long-term follow-up. *Annals of Neurology* 13: 504–510.

Ryniewicz, B. (1975) Miastenia dziecieca – obraz kliniczny i wyniki leczenia. *Neurologia, Neurochirurgia i Psychiatria Polska* 9 (25): 481.

Ryniewicz, B. and Badurska, B. (1977) Follow-up study of myasthenic children after thymectomy. *Journal of Neurology* 217: 133–138.

Sakano, T., Hamasaki, T., Kinoshita, Y. *et al.* (1989) Treatment for refractory myasthenia gravis. *Archives of Disease in Childhood* 64: 1191–1193.

Sarnat, H.B., McGarry, J.D. and Lewis, J.E. Jr. (1977) Effective treatment of infantile myasthenia gravis by combined prednisone and thymectomy. *Neurology (Minneapolis)* 27: 550–553.

Seybold, M.E. and Drachman, D.B. (1974) Gradually increasing dose of prednisolone in myasthenia gravis. *New England Journal of Medicine* 290: 81.

Seybold, M.E., Howard, F.M., Duane, D.D. *et al.* (1971) Thymectomy in juvenile myasthenia gravis. *Archives of Neurology* 25: 385–392.

Shepard, M.K. (1971) Arthrogryposis multiplex congenita in sibs. *Birth Defects* 7: 127.

Shillito, P., Vincent, A. and Newsom-Davis, J. (1993) Congenital myasthenic syndromes. *Neuromuscular Disorders* 3: 183–190.

Simpson, J.A. (1958) An evaluation of thymectomy in myasthenia gravis. *Brain* 81: 112.

Simpson, J.A. (1960) Myasthenia gravis: a new hypothesis. *Scottish Medical Journal* 5: 419–436.

Snead, O.C. III, Benton, J.W., Dwyer, D. *et al.* (1980) Juvenile myasthenia gravis. *Neurology (New York)* 30: 732–739.

Stoll, C., Ehret-Mentre, M-C., Treisser, A. *et al.* (1991) Prenatal diagnosis of congenital myasthenia with arthrogryposis in a myasthenic mother. *Prenatal Diagnosis* 11: 17–22.

Strickroot, F.L., Schaeffer, B.L. and Bergo, H.L. (1942) Myasthenia gravis occurring in an infant born of a myasthenic mother. *Journal of the American Medical Association* 120: 1207.

Szobor, A. (1989) Myasthenia gravis: familial occurrence. A study of 1100 myasthenia gravis patients. *Acta Medica Hungaria* 46: 13–21.

Tindall, R.S.A., Rollins, J.A., Phillips, J.T. *et al.* (1987) Preliminary results of a double-blind, randomized, placebo-controlled trial of cyclosporine in myasthenia gravis. *New England Journal of Medicine* 316: 719–724.

Turner, H.D., Brett, E.M., Gilbert, R.J. *et al.* (1978) Infant botulism in England. *Lancet* 1: 1277–1278.

Tzartos, S.J., Efthimiadis, A., Morel, E. *et al.* (1990) Neonatal myasthenia gravis: antigenic specificities of antibodies in sera from mothers and their infants. *Clinical Experimental Immunology* 80: 376.

Viets, H.R. (1953) A historical review of myasthenia gravis from 1672 to 1900. *Journal of the American Medical Association* 153: 1273.

Vincent, A., Newsom-Davis, J., Wray, D. *et al.* (1992) Clinical and experimental observations in patients with congenital myasthenic syndromes. *Annals of the New York Academy of Sciences* 681: 451–460.

Walker, M.B. (1934) Treatment of myasthenia gravis with physostigmine. *Lancet* i: 1200.

Warmolts, J.R. and Engel, W.K. (1972) Benefit from alternate-day prednisone in myasthenia gravis. *New England Journal of Medicine* 286: 17–20.

Warmolts, J.R., Engel, W.K. and Whitaker, (1970). Alternate-day prednisone in myasthenia gravis. *Lancet* ii: 1198.

Willis, T. (1672) *De anima brutorum*. Oxford: Theatro Sheldoniano, 404–406.

Wise, G.A. and McQuillen, M.P. (1970) Transient neonatal myasthenia. *Archives of Neurology* 22: 556.

Wong, V., Hawkins, B.R. and Yu, Y.L. (1992) Myasthenia gravis in Hong Kong Chinese. 2. Paediatric disease. *Acta Neurologica Scandinavica* 86: 68–72.

CHAPTER 11

Inflammatory Myopathies

There exist a number of disorders that are collectively grouped together as inflammatory. In some the cause is of known bacterial, parasitic or viral origin, whereas in others there is no specific aetiological agent and they approximate more closely to the connective tissue group of disorders, and may have an autoimmune basis.

DERMATOMYOSITIS/POLYMYOSITIS

HISTORICAL

In 1863 Wagner recorded a rapidly fatal case of generalized muscular disease associated with a skin eruption and coined the term polymyositis. In his review in 1887 Unverricht pointed out that all the recorded cases of polymyositis had associated skin changes and he subsequently suggested the term dermatomyositis (Unverricht, 1891). The first recorded case of polymyositis without skin involvement is probably that of Hepp (1887). In 1903 Steiner defined dermatomyositis as 'an acute, subacute or chronic disease of unknown origin, characterized by a gradual onset with vague and indefinite prodromata followed by oedema, dermatitis, and multiple muscle inflammation'. That is more or less how the disease still stands today.

As the literature expanded, the clinical picture became more complex and in recent times a number of attempts were made at classification. Eaton (1954) segregated polymyositis (without skin involvement) from dermatomyositis (with skin involvement) and further categorized those with associated disease, such as rheumatoid arthritis, lupus erythematosus or carcinoma. In addition the course of the disease might be acute, subacute or chronic. In their monograph on polymyositis, Walton and Adams (1958) adopted a similar approach but regrouped their cases to highlight the associated disorders. The four groups were:

1. polymyositis, which was subdivided into acute (with myoglobinuria) and subacute or chronic (with onset in childhood, early adult or middle and late adult life);

2. polymyositis with predominant muscular weakness but with some evidence of associated collagen disease or minimal skin changes;

3. severe connective tissue disease or florid skin changes with less marked muscle involvement;

4. polymyositis or dermatomyositis in association with malignant disease.

In any classification of this type there is bound to be overlap between individual categories based on the relative prominence of the muscle weakness or skin involvement, or associated collagen disorders. Whereas dermatomyositis is a fairly readily definable clinical condition with its characteristic dermal features plus muscle weakness, polymyositis in isolation is less clear-cut. More thorough investigation of muscle biopsies in recent years has shown that some cases of acute polymyositis are probably of viral origin. It is also possible that some cases designated as chronic polymyositis, usually on the basis of inflammatory cell infiltrates in the muscle biopsy, may be cases of muscular dystrophy, in which round cell infiltrates can also occur.

JUVENILE DERMATOMYOSITIS

In the childhood period the position is less complex. Dermatomyositis is a distinct and well defined disorder. It is not associated with underlying malignancy. There is probably an overlap with the collagen disorders, since features such as joint involvement are a common association with otherwise typical dermatomyositis. As there is considerable variability in the degree of skin involvement in idiopathic dermatomyositis, I prefer to look upon those cases with minimal skin involvement on the one hand and those with florid generalized skin involvement on the other as part of the same syndrome.

Bitnum *et al.* (1964) estimated that about one-third of the 1000-odd cases published in the world literature at that time were in the paediatric age group (under 16 years). They looked upon dermatomyositis as a syndrome closely related to other connective tissue diseases and having a wide clinical spectrum, involving primarily muscle at the one end, but presenting a more general disorder with skin and visceral involvement at the other.

In their classical study of the pathology of childhood dermatomyositis, Banker and Victor (1966) highlighted the consistent vascular abnormalities and suggested that childhood dermatomyositis is a distinct clinical entity, due to an underlying angiopathy, and best classified with the connective tissue disorders. This would also explain some of the other associated features, such as gastrointestinal ulceration.

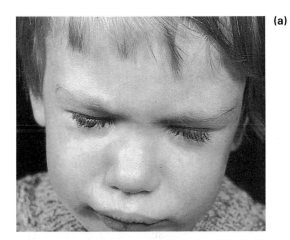

(a)

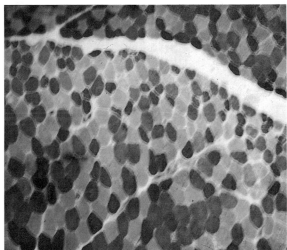

(b)

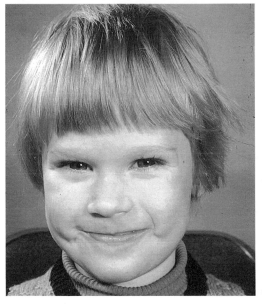

(c)

Figure 11-1a-c Acute dermatomyositis. This 3½-year-old boy presented with a 6-month history of listlessness, misery and tiredness and a week's history of redness of the eyes, increased misery and tearfulness, rash over the knees, elbow and knuckles, weakness of the limbs and joint pains (a). CK 405 iu/litre. Biopsy showed perifascicular atrophy with relative sparing of the rest of the muscle bundles and no obvious inflammatory response (b). He responded well within a week to steroid therapy (1 mg/kg), which was gradually tapered and stopped 1 year later (c). He continues well 10 years later and has had no relapse.

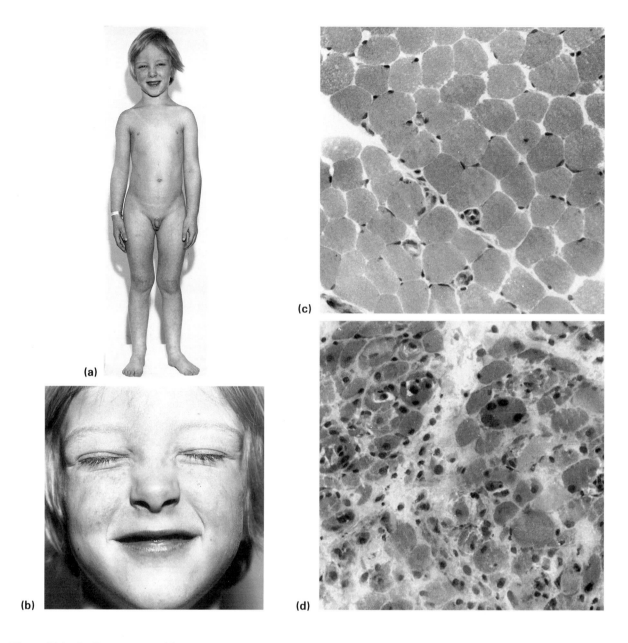

(a)

(b)

(c)

(d)

Figure 11-2a-d Dermatomyositis. This 6-year-old boy (a) had a 6-week history of 'slowing up' and difficulty walking home from school. He complained of inability to undress himself, climb on or off his bed, lift things off the floor or go to the lavatory on his own. He also complained of pains in his elbows, shoulders, knees and back and there was some swelling of the ankles and wrists. A rash was noted on his face and for 3 weeks prior to admission he had also been lethargic, miserable and anorexic. He had never had any previous similar problems. On examination he had marked weakness, with inability to get up from the floor or to raise his arms above his head, a waddling gait and also limitation of full flexion or extension of his elbows and knees and some pitting oedema around the ankles. There was a characteristic erythematous rash over the butterfly area of the face (b). A clinical diagnosis of dermatomyositis was made. His ESR was 38 mm and the CK was elevated at 330 iu/litre (normal <70). The SGOT at 45 units and SGPT at 18 units were normal; EMG showed a myopathic pattern of abnormality, and biopsy of the rectus femoris showed focal but unequivocal degenerative changes, whilst other areas were fairly normal (c,d). Prednisone was started at a dose of 30 mg/day and within 3 weeks he was considerably better, with ability to get up from the floor and to lift objects off the floor. He was also much improved in his general temperament and well-being. The CK was practically normal at 80 iu/litre and the ESR down to 25 mm/h. He was in complete remission 6 weeks later and the steroids were steadily reduced by 2.5 mg at half-weekly intervals. He had no further problems and the prednisone was subsequently stopped completely after retaining his final dose of 2.5 mg per day for a full month. He had no further relapse during the ensuing 2½ years of follow-up.

Cases in childhood of isolated 'polymyositis' without dermal manifestations may still be part of the dermatomyositis syndrome, but need thorough investigation to exclude other acute or chronic disorders, such as an acute myositis of viral origin and various hereditary myopathies.

CLINICAL FEATURES

There are three cardinal presenting features of dermatomyositis in childhood – muscle weakness, skin lesions and general symptoms. Muscle weakness is always present; in its absence it would be difficult to substantiate the diagnosis. Skin lesions may at times be florid, but more often they are inconspicuous and may go unnoticed. General symptoms in the way of malaise, listlessness and lethargy (or feeling 'one degree under') are an almost invariable accompaniment and may often be the main presenting complaint. There is often also an associated low grade fever. Since very few other neuromuscular disorders in childhood present with general symptoms in this way, it is a good rule of thumb that, until proved otherwise:

WEAKNESS + MISERY = DERMATOMYOSITIS

The onset is usually insidious and the diagnosis readily missed. It may occur at any age from the second year into adolescence.

The weakness is usually proximal and symmetrical and tends to start in the legs, but the arms and neck may also be involved. Some cases, particularly in the younger age group, tend to present with more generalized weakness. In rare cases the onset may be fairly acute, the weakness profound, and there may be an associated myoglobinuria with marked muscle necrosis.

A few patients may have associated difficulty with swallowing or respiratory distress, both of which are worrying features because of the greater risk of complications.

Pain and tenderness of muscles may occur but are not always present. There may also be a palpable induration of the muscle, and sometimes associated superficial oedema. Contractures, with limited extension of joints, are frequently present and may produce a toe-gait.

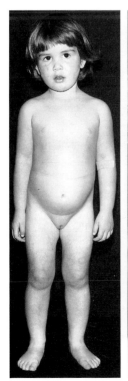
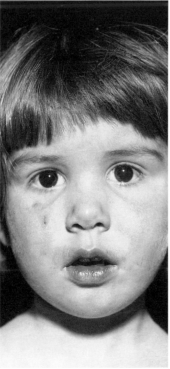

(a)   **(b)**

Figure 11-3a,b Dermatomyositis. This 3½-year-old girl was referred for investigation of possible muscular dystrophy. She had been admitted 2 months previously to hospital with joint pains and swelling and tenderness of both calves and arms 4 days after a sore throat. The ESR was 9 mm and ASO titre 625 units. The swelling subsided without any treatment after 9 days and she was discharged. At out-patient follow-up 3 weeks later, she had a waddling gait, difficulty in walking and a tendency to fall and was unable to get up from the floor. A diagnosis of muscular dystrophy was suspected but dismissed on the basis of the normal CK of 60 iu/litre. She was unchanged 3 weeks later and readmitted for further investigation, which proved negative. She was then referred to my muscle clinic. A diagnosis of dermatomyositis was made on the basis of her muscle weakness, her skin eruption over the butterfly area of the face and the erythematous violaceous discolouration over the knee joints and lateral malleoli of her ankles, and her general malaise and irritability. The CK and ESR were again normal; EMG and muscle biopsy were not done. Prednisone 20 mg/day was prescribed and when reviewed again as an outpatient 1 week later, she was considerably improved, both in muscle power and general temperament and enthusiasm for playing. After a further week at that dose there was further improvement and it was reduced to 15 mg/day. The prednisone was reduced by 2.5 mg decrements at intervals of about 2 weeks and completely stopped 6 months after starting. Although her skin changes persisted for some months she had no recurrence of muscle weakness and remained in complete remission during the subsequent 4 years of follow-up.

The skin manifestations are very variable. Usually there is violaceous discolouration of the upper eyelids and a slightly scaly erythematous eruption over the malar (butterfly) area of the face and possibly some periorbital oedema. There may also be erythematous areas over the metacarpophalangeal and interphalangeal joints of the fingers and an erythematous or violaceous scaly rash over the knee and elbow joints, the malleoli of the ankles or other pressure points. In addition to the erythema there may also be fine telangiectases over these various sites.

Usually the skin lesions are fairly focal, but occasionally they may be very florid and widespread, and affect the trunk as well as the face and extremities, and there may be associated oedema and also itch.

There is an infinite range in the relative severity of the muscle and skin manifestations. Some patients have marked weakness with only minimal skin manifestations, while others have marked skin manifestations with almost no muscle weakness; and in between are various permutations including patients with florid disease, either acute or chronic, with marked skin and muscle manifestations. The clinical features and treatment of a series of illustrative cases are included in Figures 11-1 to 11-16.

Figure 11-4a,b Dermatomyositis; depression. This 12-year-old schoolgirl was referred primarily for her depression. There was a 3-month history of shortness of breath on exertion, gradual loss of weight, aching of the shoulders when carrying a schoolbag, and a change in her gait, with walking on her toes. She also noted aching in the thighs and calves at times and an inability to straighten her elbows fully, with some associated pain in the elbow joint. Any activity beyond her routine led to rapid exhaustion. When examined, she tended to walk on her toes and was unable to walk on her heels (a). She was able to go up and down stairs, but refused to get up from the floor. The elbows showed about 10° limitation of extension, and some pain when trying to extend them. There was also some limitation of flexion of the spine. There was no joint swelling or tenderness. The muscles were not tender to palpation. The tendon reflexes were all present. A band of violaceous colour was present along the lower half of both eyelids, and there was also slight erythema of the malar region of the face (b).

On the basis of her general malaise in association with a suggestion of muscle weakness and the skin change, a diagnosis of dermatomyositis was made. The sedimentation rate was normal (10 mm/h), as was the serum CK (40 iu/litre). EMG showed fibrillation at rest and a myopathic pattern of small polyphasic potentials on volition. Muscle biopsy of the gastrocnemius (taken 2 days after treatment was started) appeared completely normal on histological and histochemical examination. Treatment was started immediately with prednisone 1 mg/kg daily in divided doses. Improvement started within 2 days and when reassessed a week later she was walking better, found it easier to dress herself, had an improved range of extension of the elbows, was able to go up and down steps without difficulty, and was able to get up from the floor, although with some difficulty still. In addition she was a changed personality, bright, cheerful and co-operative, and had also felt well enough to enter for her school examinations, from which she had previously had to withdraw because of her illness.

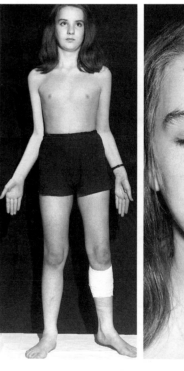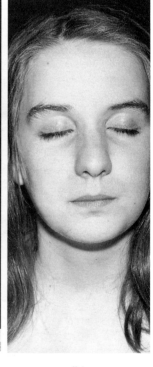

(a)   (b)

The prednisone was reduced by two decrements of 5 mg at 4-day intervals to 10 mg three times daily and after a further 2 weeks by 5 mg decrements at weekly intervals to 5 mg three times daily and then by 2.5 mg decrements at weekly intervals until it was completely stopped about 4 months after starting therapy. She was completely well and coping with both intellectual as well as physical activities. There was no recurrence of symptoms over the ensuing 3 years of follow-up.

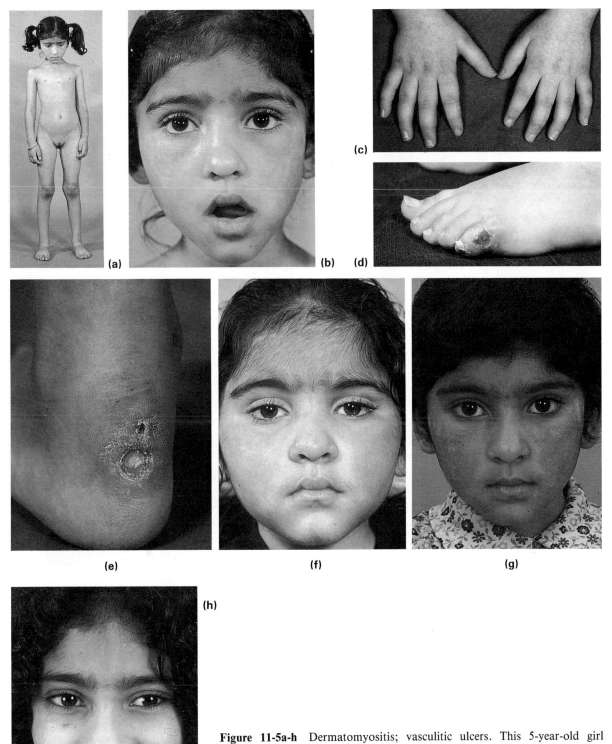

Figure 11-5a-h Dermatomyositis; vasculitic ulcers. This 5-year-old girl presented with weakness, irritability and skin rash (a-c). She responded well to steroid therapy and regained her power, but the rash persisted and she developed recurrent vasculitic ulcers and incipient gangrene of the toes (d), as well as calcinosis of the left forearm (e). These gradually resolved, as did the skin rash on the face (f,g), and after tapering and stopping the treatment she remained in remission and was discharged from further follow-up 2 years after presenting (h).

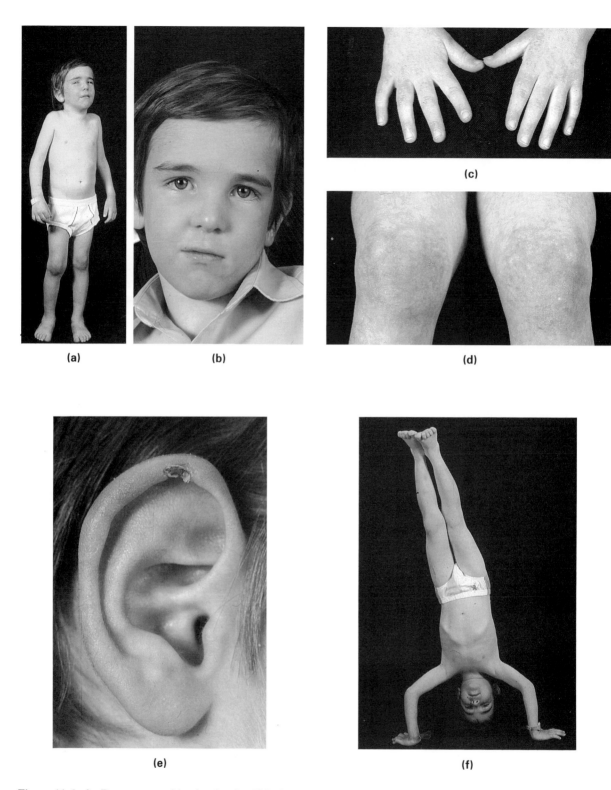

Figure 11-6a-f Dermatomyositis; dysphonia. This 5-year-old boy presented with a 7-month history of rash, misery, muscle pains and weakness, with difficulty in walking (a-d). There was associated dysphonia but no dysphagia. CK was normal (142 iu/litre). He responded well to low-dosage steroids, which were tapered and stopped. He regained his strength, but the skin lesions became more marked and vasculitic over the ears (e) and elbows. His muscle function remained normal (f).

Chronic disease

The chronic, unremitted case, either smouldering or burnt out, presents a fairly consistent and usually pathetic picture. The child is often chair- or bed-bound with generalized muscle wasting and severe contractures, particularly of the hip and knee flexors. The skin may also show chronic changes, with discolouration, desquamation and pigmentation, and there is often associated calcinosis. The skin over the knuckles and interphalangeal joints may become thickened and discoloured, the so-called Gotron's nodules. This form of disease may be the result of either inadequate treatment on the one hand, or overtreatment, with consequent complications of steroid and other therapy, on the other, and the resultant inadequate control of the disease.

OTHER SYSTEMS ————————————————————

There may be involvement of other systems, either in the early or later phases of the disease.

Joints

Some patients experience arthralgia of various joints but there is usually no clinical evidence of overt arthritis.

Reticuloendothelial

Some cases' may have lymphadenopathy and mild splenomegaly and hepatomegaly in the acute phase of the disease.

Respiratory

Apart from the respiratory muscle involvement which may be a component of the disease, some patients may present in acute respiratory distress due to involvement of the lung parenchyma itself (Dubowitz and Dubowitz, 1964).

Skin ulceration

Apart from the classical skin changes, some patients develop marked ulceration of the skin. This may be painful and also indolent, with slow resolution (see Figures 11-5, 11-6 and 11-7).

Gastrointestinal

Ulceration of the gastrointestinal mucosa, with associated haematemesis or melaena in some instances, has been recorded by many authors. It is noteworthy that there were vascular changes, ulceration and perforation in the oesophagus, stomach, small and large intestines in seven of the eight autopsies studied by Banker and Victor (1966), who looked upon the bowel involvement as part of the basic angiopathy of the disease (see Figure 11-16).

Cardiovascular

A few patients have cardiac murmurs or pericardial friction rubs and a high proportion show ECG changes. Some authors have put the incidence of cardiac involvement as high as 25%.

Renal

A few patients may show albuminuria or other signs of renal dysfunction. Bitnum *et al.* (1964) did six renal biopsies in their series of cases and found glomerular abnormality in all six.

Calcinosis

This unusual feature is characteristic of childhood dermatomyositis and much more common than in the adult disease (see Figures 11-11 and 11-12). The calcification occurs in the interstitial tissues of the muscle itself or in the subcutaneous tissue, and nodules of calcium may be extruded through perforations in the skin. It is readily visible on X-rays of the soft tissues. The incidence in early reports, before the therapeutic era, varied from about 25% (Wedgwood *et al.*, 1953) to 50% (Everett and Curtis, 1957) in most series, to as high as 60% (Cook *et al.*, 1963) or even 73% (Muller *et al.*, 1959), usually in patients surviving over long periods. For this reason calcinosis was looked upon as a good prognostic sign and presumably reflected chronicity of disease. Occasionally it may occur within a few months of the onset of symptoms and has continued to occur in patients undergoing long-term steroid therapy.

DIAGNOSIS ——————————————————————

The diagnosis is essentially a clinical one. Because of the insidious onset and often vague nature of the early symptoms the condition frequently goes undiagnosed for several months.

The blood sedimentation rate is often normal in the active phase of childhood dermatomyositis and the serum creatine kinase may be consistently normal as well, even in the face of severe clinical weakness. As in childhood rheumatoid arthritis, immunological studies are usually unhelpful and negative.

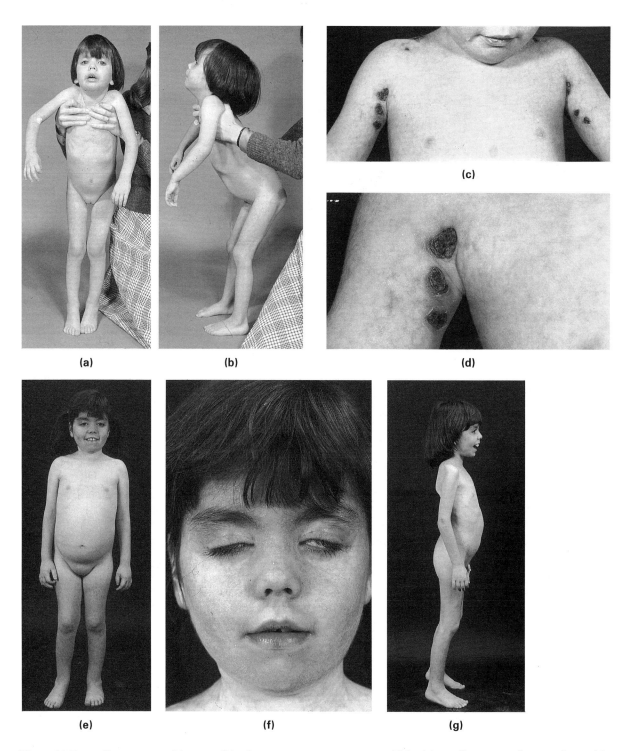

(a) (b) (c)

(d)

(e) (f) (g)

Figure 11-7a-g Dermatomyositis: vasculitic ulcers; recurrent contractures. This girl was first seen at 3 years of age with an 8-month history of weakness, skin rash and misery, with progressive flexion contractures of the hips (a,b). She responded well to steroids and was rehabilitated with active physiotherapy. She was readmitted from abroad 8 months later with marked vasculitic ulcers in the axillae, which gradually resolved (c,d). She later had recurrent relapses and remissions with adjustment of therapy. At 7 years of age she stopped walking after formation of a large haematoma in the right thigh. She was again rehabilitated with active physiotherapy (e). There was still active skin rash and some facial weakness with limited eye closure (f). She was still ambulant 15 months later but had considerable weakness and fixed equinus (g). She had also lost weight and had very little muscle bulk.

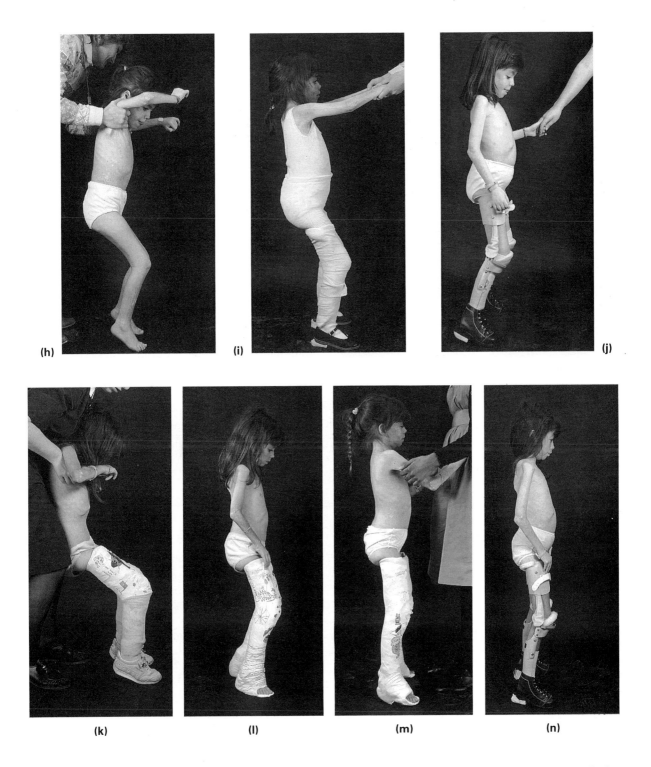

(h) (i) (j)

(k) (l) (m) (n)

Figure 11-7h-n Some 7 months later, aged 9 years, she was readmitted with inability to stand or walk and marked flexion contractures at the knees (h). Following intensive physiotherapy she was mobilized in callipers 2 months later (i,j). Eight months later she relapsed with even more marked fixed flexion of the knees of about 80° (k). This was treated with serial plasters and within 2 weeks there was marked improvement (l) and a month later the legs were almost straight (m). She was fitted with ischial weight-bearing callipers and became ambulant again in them (n). There was still fixed equinus at the ankle, but it was thought unwise to operate on the tendo Achilles. This case illustrates the importance of supportive physiotherapy and the rapid relapse when this is not maintained.

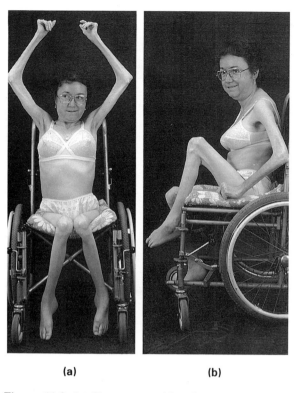

(a)　　　　　　　　**(b)**

Figure 11-8a,b Dermatomyositis. Contractures. This 26-year-old woman had acute dermatomyositis at 14 years of age, and although she responded well to steroid therapy she was not mobilized at that stage and developed contractures at her joints. She was never able to stand or walk again, although she had more than antigravity power in most of her muscle groups (a,b).

pathic pattern with small polyphasic potentials, and in addition signs of denervation such as fibrillation potentials at rest and positive sharp spikes.

Muscle ultrasound

This is another useful screening technique and characteristically in juvenile dermatomyositis may show little increase in echo but this becomes more marked with angulation of the probe (Heckmatt *et al.*, 1988). In more chronic cases there may be a marked and more diffuse increase in echogenicity.

Muscle biopsy

This may at times show a florid pathological picture, with degenerative change and inflammatory cellular response, but that is usually the picture of the long-standing case. More commonly the changes are minimal and may take the form of a perifascicular atrophy of fibres and possibly some focal degenerative changes (Dubowitz and Brooke, 1973; Dubowitz, 1985). Abnormalities of the small arterioles may be seen in some biopsies, but not with the consistency of the changes seen at autopsy by Banker and Victor (1966). Banker (1975) also described distinctive electron microscopic changes in the blood vessels in muscle biopsies from children with acute dermatomyositis.

Delayed diagnosis

There is a frequent reluctance on the part of physicians to make a clinical diagnosis without laboratory confirmation. In the case of juvenile dermatomyositis, where the investigations are often negative or minimally abnormal, this may lead to unnecessary delay, which may lead to deterioration and compromise treatment. As the clinical diagnosis is usually clearcut, particularly if the muscle weakness and skin changes are associated with general symptoms, one could readily institute treatment even without awaiting results of the laboratory investigations.

Electromyography

This is a useful diagnostic aid. It is almost invariably abnormal and will characteristically show a myo-

Immunocytochemistry

Immunocytochemical detection of HLA class I antigens is a useful diagnostic marker in inflammatory myopathies. Normal mature skeletal muscle fibres do not express class I or class II HLA antigens, but both are found on endothelial cells of blood vessels, and regenerating fibres express class I antigens (Appleyard *et al.*, 1985; Karpati *et al.*, 1988; McDouall *et al.*, 1989; Emslie-Smith *et al.*, 1989; Sewry and Dubowitz, 1994). In contrast, several fibres in polymyositis and dermatomyositis often express class I antigens. Although this may not be a universal feature, and areas within a biopsy may vary, it occurs in most cases of inflammatory myopathies. The only other condition where there is an abnormal expression of HLA class I antigens is in Duchenne and Becker muscular dystrophies (Appleyard *et al.*, 1985). HLA class I antigens have a role in the recognition of antigens by cytotoxic T-cells, but they may be expressed in the absence of an inflammatory reaction, and occasionally they may be the only apparent abnormality in a biopsy.

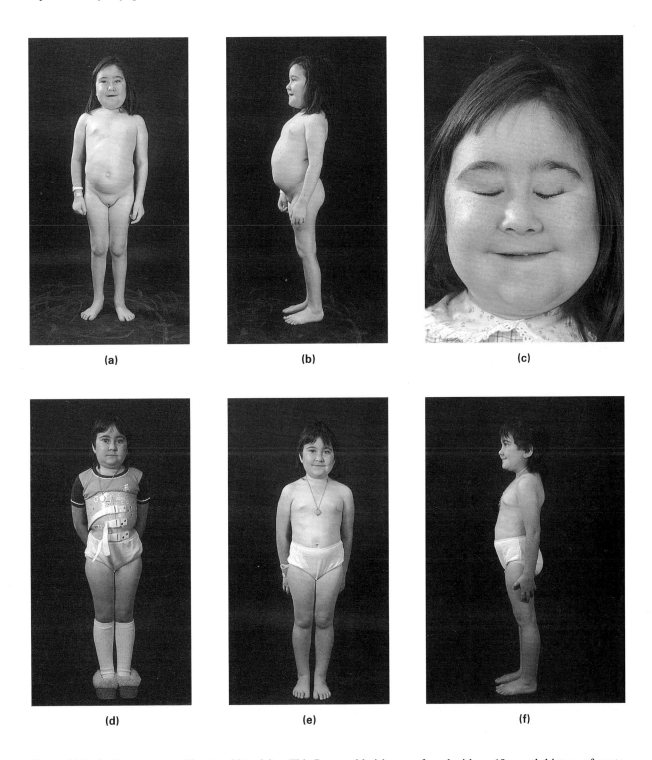

(a)   **(b)**   **(c)**

(d)   **(e)**   **(f)**

Figure 11-9a-f   Dermatomyositis; steroid toxicity. This 7-year-old girl was referred with an 18-month history of acute dermatomyositis, which was treated 5 months after onset with high-dosage steroids, with rapid tapering and cessation of treatment after 4 months, followed by relapse and further treatment with high-dosage steroids, followed by alternate-day, high-dose steroids and azathioprine. She had become markedly cushingoid, with associated hypertension and severe osteoporosis of the spine, with crush fractures of several vertebrae (a-c). She was fitted with a spinal jacket and gradually reduced to a low-dose, alternate-day schedule. Her general mobility increased and the osteoporosis gradually resolved (d-f). High-dosage steroid therapy does not produce a quicker or better response in childhood dermatomyositis, and has the disadvantages of more severe side-effects and taking longer to wean off, with more risk of relapse.

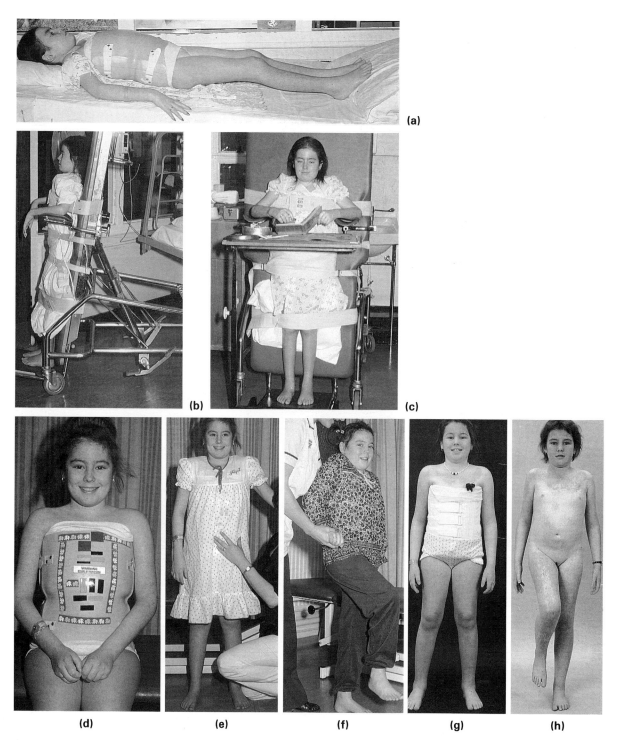

(a)

(b)

(c)

(d)

(e)

(f)

(g)

(h)

Figure 11-10a-n 'Terminal dermatomyositis'. Rehabilitation. This 11-year-old girl was admitted to our unit in December 1982 as a 'terminal' case of dermatomyositis. She had been bed-bound for 6 weeks, and had increasing muscle weakness and associated swallowing and breathing difficulties, despite increasing dosage of prednisolone to more than 2 mg/kg/day. Her illness had started in July 1981; treatment was begun with high-dosage steroid in October, with an initial improvement, but she relapsed in December, had a more severe relapse in July 1982, and failed to respond to increasing doses of prednisolone, i.v. methotrexate or chloroquine. On admission to Hammersmith Hospital she was almost totally immobile. There was excruciating pain of the spine with the slightest movement, due to severe osteoporosis from the high-dosage steroids. A plaster cast and subsequently a polypropylene jacket was fitted (a) to support the spine and to help mobilize her.

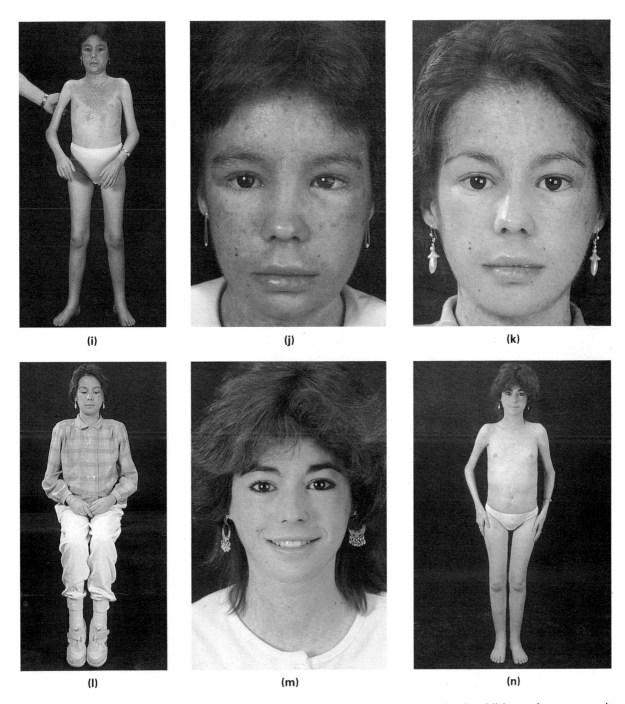

(i) (j) (k)

(l) (m) (n)

The steroids were gradually reduced, as it was thought she might have a steroid myopathy, in addition to the osteoporosis from the high-dose steroid therapy; she had about 20° fixed flexion at the hips and this was treated with gentle stretching, to which she strongly objected. Her bed was gradually tilted a few degrees at a time for increasing periods, as she was able to tolerate, until she could be transferred to a tilt table. With very gradual but steady increments we were able within a month to get her into a vertical position (b) and she soon managed long periods in this position (c). She then acquired the ability to sit with a jacket (d) and within 5 months was able to stand and take her first steps (e-f). A month later she was walking independently with a jacket (g) and after another month without a jacket (h). She progressed well until she relapsed 4 months later and never fully regained her strength with various permutations in steroid therapy, plus azathioprine or cyclophosphamide (i-l). Three years later she was still ambulant in callipers but much less active than before. She was then given cyclosporin, which markedly improved her chronic skin rash as well as her power, mobility and well-being (m,n), and she gradually returned to full activity.

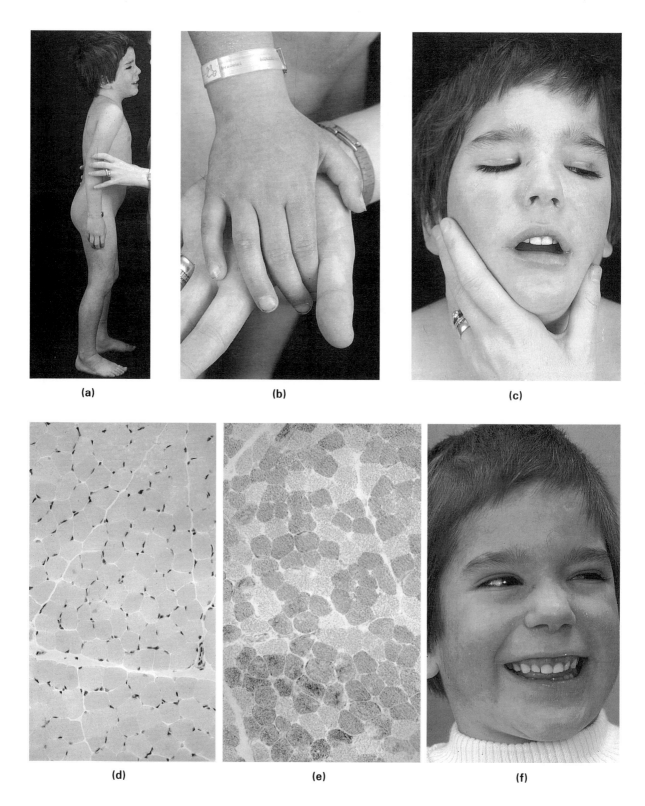

(a) (b) (c)

(d) (e) (f)

Figure 11-11a-f Dermatomyositis; calcinosis. This 4½-year-old boy presented with acute dermatomyositis with marked weakness, misery and facial and limb rash (a-c). His muscle biopsy was essentially normal (d) apart from some focal changes shown up on the oxidative reactions (e). He responded well to steroids and remained in remission after they were stopped (f).

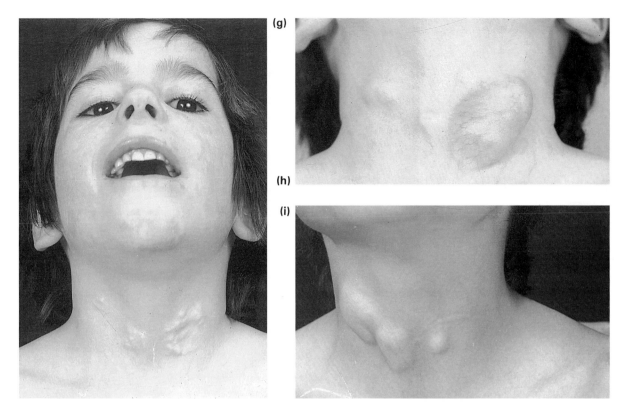

Figure 11.11g-i However, he later developed focal calcinosis, some of which caused discomfort and had to be removed surgically (g-i). Steroids were not recommenced and there was no suggestion of recurrence of the dermatomyositis.

Perifascicular atrophy

Perifascicular atrophy has long been recognized as a diagnostic feature in skeletal muscle from patients with dermatomyositis. The advent of immunocytochemistry and studies of myosin isoform expression have shown that many of the small perifascicular fibres express the developmetal, fetal isoform of myosin. These fibres often have other features of immaturity, including expression of desmin and HLA class I antigens, suggesting that many of them are regenerating fibres and not atrophic.

Associated viral infection

In a number of cases of typical dermatomyositis, as well as several atypical cases of 'myositis', patients have been found to have high antibody titres to the Coxsackie B group of viruses. It is difficult to appraise fully the relevance of these findings in the context of dermatomyositis in childhood but it would seem that in some of the classical cases the initial precipitating factor may be a viral infection, possibly damaging the muscle, or vessels to the muscle, and setting in train an autoimmune response.

Studies of Coxsackie viral titres in hereditary and other myopathies have also revealed occasional high titres. It is difficult to be sure whether this reflects an incidental infection with Coxsackie virus, as may occur in persons without any muscle disorder, or whether it may have played some part in the pathogenesis of the disease (see Figure 11-17).

Associated connective tissue disorders

Muscle involvement is common in the connective tissue disorders such as rheumatoid arthritis, systemic lupus erythematosus, scleroderma and periarteritis nodosa. The clinical presentation is extremely variable and may range from severe weakness and muscle pain and tenderness to complete absence of any clinical features.

In addition to the overlap between dermatomyositis and these various connective tissue disorders, joint manifestations such as arthralgia, but usually not overt arthritis, may occur in association with dermatomyositis (see Figure 11-14).

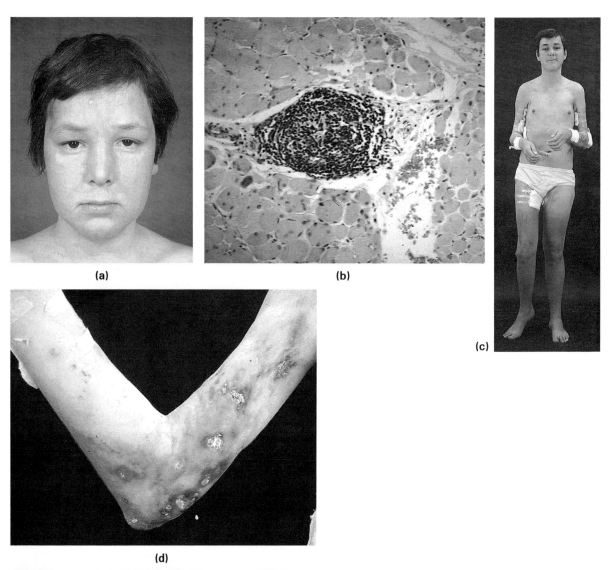

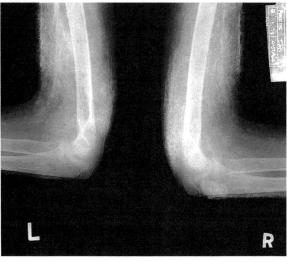

Figure 11-12a-e Dermatomyositis; calcinosis. This young man was first seen in 1976, aged 12 years, with an 8-month history of progressive weakness and disability, with loss of ability to stand or walk, and associated flexion deformities of the hips. He had a typical rash on the face (a). Muscle biopsy showed an active inflammatory myopathy with lymphorrhages (b). He responded well to steroid treatment and active physiotherapy and regained ambulation but subsequently had numerous relapses and remissions. He developed extensive calcinosis which spread palpably like a suit of armour down his arms and legs (c). This led to chronic discharge of calcium, particularly around the elbows (d,e) with occasional secondary infection needing antibiotic therapy. Over the years the calcinosis gradually lessened and he has remained active and mobile with regular physiotherapy support. Now in his late 20s he is coping in an academic position at university and has successfully completed a PhD thesis.

Figure 11-13a-b Dermatomyositis; unusual complications; vocal cord paralysis. This girl first presented at 3½ years with a 1-year history of abnormal gait, inability to run, a tendency to fall and difficulty going up steps (a). Her motor milestones had been normal and she walked at 15 months. On examination there was a waddling gait and lumbar lordosis, slight proximal weakness of the legs and a possible facial weakness with some degree of ptosis. A congenital myopathy was suspected. CK, EMG, nerve conduction velocity and quadriceps biopsy were all normal.

She was about the same 3 months later, although falling more frequently and complaining of fatigue with walking. Another 4 months after that she was possibly better in some respects but had more fatiguability and was exhausted by the end of the day. There was no evidence of myasthenia on electrophysiological studies.

In the next 2 months she improved, but then became weaker again and was more irritable. She had ptosis and was unable to go up steps. One day she seemed acutely worse, fell to the floor and was unable to get up and complained of aching of the legs, especially in the calves. She had also developed nocturnal enuresis after being dry for a year. On assessment at that time she was irritable and uncooperative, had great difficulty getting up from the floor and was generally hypotonic. There was no skin discolouration and a tentative diagnosis of polymyositis was made on the basis of 'misery + muscle weakness = dermatomyositis till proved otherwise'. A week later she was about the same, was still very irritable and weepy, and uncooperative. The EMG now showed a distinctly abnormal pattern of a myopathic type. Prednisone was commenced at a dose of 15 mg/day.

When reviewed 2 weeks later she was strikingly better, able to go up and down steps and to get up from the floor without difficulty. Her misery had also disappeared and the mother commented she was 'a different child'.

The prednisone was reduced by 2.5 mg every fourth day. She continued symptom-free until the dose was down to 2.5 mg/day for 2 days, when she became irritable and weepy again, although still able to get up from the floor without difficulty. On resuming 5 mg per day she was again symptom-free. She continued well till 2 weeks later when she developed a sore throat and difficulty going up steps. She fell twice but could get up from the floor without difficulty. She was given a 5-day course of oral penicillin and the prednisone increased to 7.5 mg/day.

In the following 2 weeks she was again irritable and started bed wetting again. There was some difficulty getting up from the floor. The prednisone was raised to 15 mg per day. Her mother thought she was back to her full strength again 2 weeks later and also temperamentally better. However, she had developed blotchy erythema over the upper eyelids and legs.

The following week she developed acute laryngo-tracheo-bronchitis, with marked respiratory-stridor, ptosis and general misery. She was admitted to hospital and treated with humidity and trimethoprim. Prednisone was continued at 15 mg/day. She steadily deteriorated and required tracheostomy 2 days later. Her post-tracheostomy condition was good and the tube removed 3 days later. She then continued well for 3 weeks when she had a recurrence of respiratory difficulty without stridor. She was re-

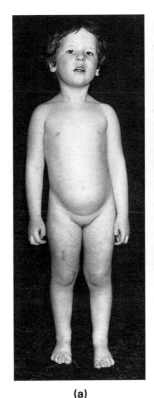
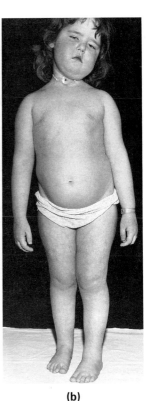

(a)   **(b)**

admitted with mild stridor 2 days later and after a sudden deterioration that evening a tracheostomy was again required. This improved her respiratory condition and although her general muscle power remained good, an initial injection of intravenous hydrocortisone and subsequently intramuscular cortisone was given until she was able to return to prednisone by mouth. It subsequently proved impossible to remove the tracheostomy tube owing to complete abductor paralysis of the cords (b).

Her general muscle power remained good and the prednisone was reduced to 5 mg twice daily and 2 months later to 7.5 mg/day. Her mother was coping well with the tracheostomy at home and there was no recurrence of muscle weakness.

In view of some anxiety on the part of the mother (as well as myself) about a risk of recurrence of her muscle weakness while on the tracheostomy, in spite of no evidence of muscle weakness, the prednisone was kept at the same dosage level for 3 months before reducing to 5 mg/day and then 6 months later to 2.5 mg and after a month to 2.5 mg alternate days for 2 weeks and then stopping it. She continued well apart from being a bit 'niggly and bad tempered' at times.

The vocal cords remained persistently adducted and it was impossible to remove the tube until 4 years later. The wound closed up and she continued well in the subsequent 2 years of follow-up review. She intermittently had bouts of slight muscle weakness, which responded well to short courses of prednisone.

The paralysis of the vocal cords was considered to be a complication of the tracheostomy and unrelated to the dermatomyositis.

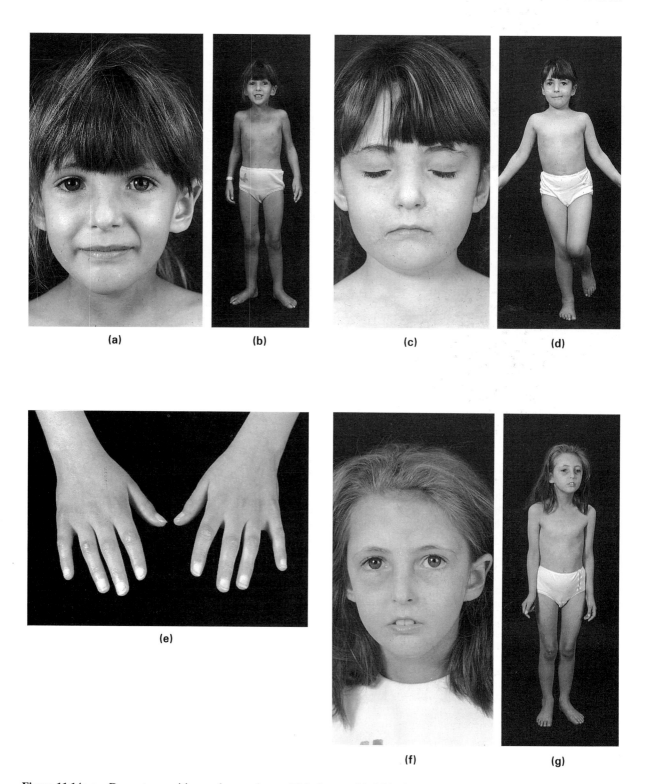

(a) **(b)** **(c)** **(d)**

(e)

(f) **(g)**

Figure 11-14a-g Dermatomyositis: overlap syndrome. This 6-year-old girl had a 1-month history of pains in the legs and weakness, malaise, tightness of the skin and dysphagia, dysphonia and dyspepsia (a,b). Her CK was grossly elevated (4435 iu/litre). She responded well to low-dosage steroids but had relapses 9 and 16 months later and was treated in addition with azathioprine and a 3-month course of cyclophosphamide. Her muscle power improved but she developed increasing tightness of the skin, a sclerodermatous facies and Raynaud's phenomenon and tapering fingers (c-g). These features suggest an 'overlap' syndrome. She also had marked ulceration over the knees and buttocks during her second relapse.

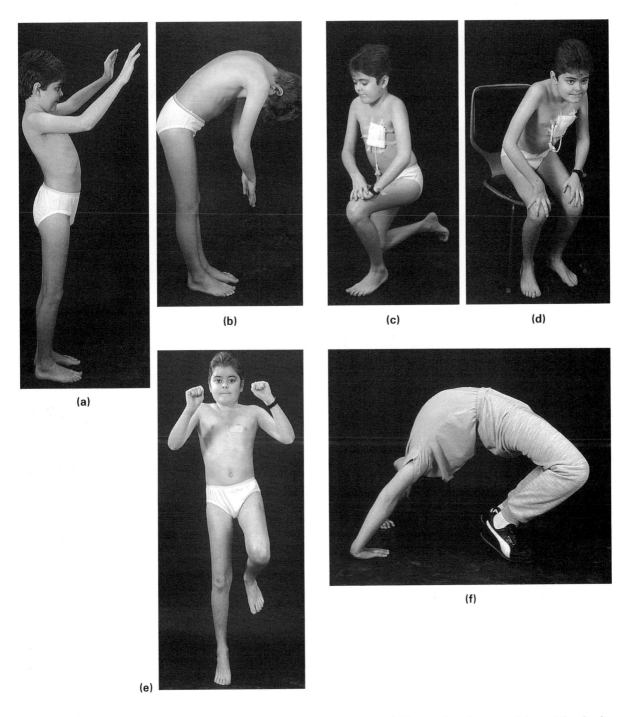

Figure 11-15a-f Polymyositis. This 10-year-old boy presented with a 3-month history of weakness, malaise and dysphagia. There was marked weakness but no obvious skin rash (a). He also had limitation of trunk flexion and elbow extension (b). He had difficulty getting up from the floor and from a chair (c,d). He responded poorly to low-dosage steroids and to increased dosage from 1 mg to 1.5 mg/kg/day, and had severe haemorrhagic cystitis after cyclophosphamide, which had to be stopped. He had a dramatic response to a course of five plasma exchanges and remained in full remission and no further exchanges were necessary. He was again able to hop on one leg (e) and to perform acrobatic feats (f). He was gradually weaned off prednisolone over 6 months and continued well at follow-up. However, a year after the original episode he began to experience some mild but definite weakness again and had some difficulty keeping up with his competitive sporting activities; once again the response to steroids was not striking. Azathioprine was added and subsequently cyclosporin, with good response, and return to full strength.

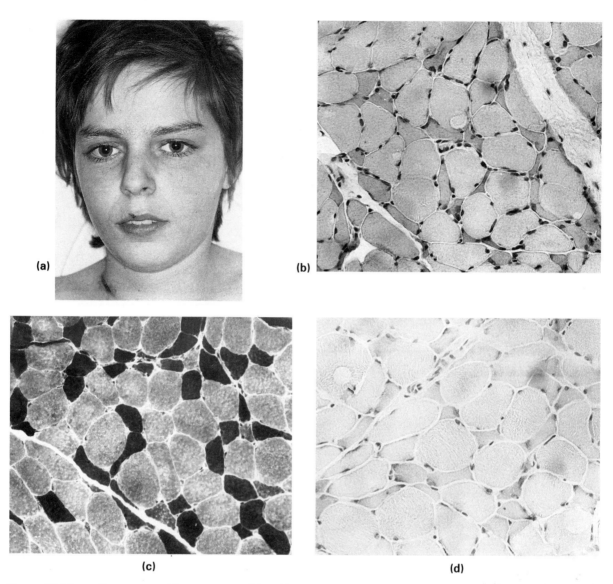

(a) (b)

(c) (d)

Figures 11-16a-g Dermatomyositis; severe vasculitis. This 14-year-old boy was admitted in March 1976 with a 1-month history of pain in the right knee for 6 days, followed by pain and swelling of the left jaw and subsequently generalized pains in most limb joints and inability to walk. His face then became swollen and his eyes puffy and partially closed. He also developed swelling of the hands. At another hospital soon after the onset he was found to have a persistent pyrexia. There was some focal lymphadenopathy but biopsy of a supraclavicular lymph node showed no specific pathology. The wound failed to heal (a). On admission to Hammersmith Hospital he was generally ill and miserable and had generalized tenderness and resented being handled. The face was puffy and there was a heliotrope discolouration of the eyelids (a). He was unable to stand and unable to raise his arms against gravity and there was marked weakness of all muscle groups of the limbs on testing. He had a persistently elevated temperature (around 38°C). His erythrocyte sedimentation rate was 96 mm/h. The CK was normal (19 iu/litre). A clinical diagnosis of dermatomyositis was made on the basis of his weakness, misery and skin changes. Nerve conduction velocity was normal and EMG of the quadriceps showed a myopathic pattern.

A muscle biopsy of the quadriceps showed a striking picture of selective type 2 fibre atrophy and, in addition, evidence of regeneration in these type 2 fibres (b-d) (b, H&E; c, ATPase 9.4; d, RNA, methyl green pyronin). He was started on treatment with prednisone 50 mg/day (1 mg/kg) and within 48 hours showed remarkable improvement. His temperament changed and he looked less toxaemic. His joint and muscle pains settled and there was marked improvement in muscle power. After 4 days he became able to stand and walk. The pyrexia subsided and his sedimentation rate dropped to 15 mm/h. The wound in his neck healed rapidly. The steroid dose was fairly rapidly tapered by 5 mg decrements half-weekly to 30 mg/day. He then showed no further improvement and had some residual muscle weakness, so it was raised to 35 mg/day and kept at that level. Over the next 2 months he had recurrent knee or wrist pain and felt generally unwell, although still ambulant.

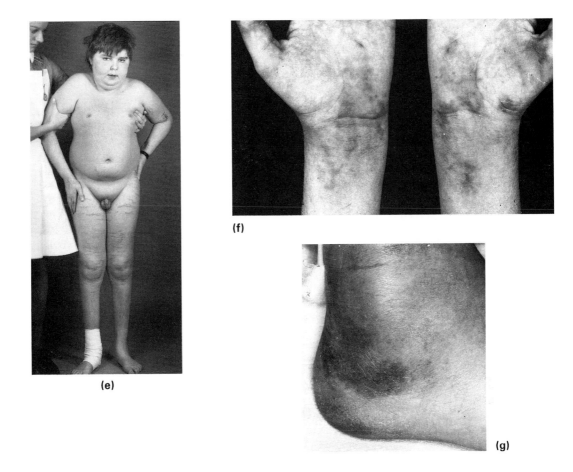

(e)

(f)

(g)

Figure 11-16f-g continued He also developed painful induration over the ventral aspect of the right wrist. At the beginning of June he was readmitted to his local hospital with increasing joint pains and general ill health and increase in weakness. The steroid dose at that time was 25 mg/day. His sedimentation rate was again up at 36 mm/h but the CK was consistently normal. He was discharged again at the same dose and given active physiotherapy. He subsequently developed 'violent' pains over his joints and a marked violaceous induration over both wrists and the left elbow. There was also Raynaud's phenomenon of the fingers and gangrene of the tip of the right fourth finger. Studies for autoantibodies and cryoglobulins were negative. He also complained of vague abdominal pain and was taking intermittent salicylates for his arthralgia. The prednisone was raised to 40 mg/day and subsequently tapered to 30 mg/day. In July he was admitted with haematemesis and melaena and needed blood transfusion. Barium studies revealed two gastric and one duodenal ulcers. It was uncertain whether the ulcers were due to his underlying vasculitis or the prednisone or aspirin, or a combination. All salicylates were stopped. The prednisone was raised to 40 mg/day. He subsequently had a very stormy and downhill course with marked general toxaemia and great misery from his pains. Cyclophosphamide was added to the regimen without apparent benefit and he was then given a series of plasmaphereses (to remove possible circulating immune complexes), with some possible temporary but unsustained benefit. The cut-down wounds of the arteriovenous anastomoses failed to heal and remained widely gaping. As a desperate resort, the steroid dose was raised to 100 mg/day, and in addition he was given 100 mg hydrocortisone intravenously. This produced a dramatic response and within 24 hours he was much improved and gradually returned to full mobility and ambulation again. It was difficult to reduce the high steroid dose appreciably and he subsequently developed crush fractures of several vertebrae. Repeat barium swallow studies showed partial healing of his ulcers. He was put on an alternate-day steroid regimen with a dose of 60 mg prednisone and no steroid on the intervening day. He remained reasonably ambulant on this regimen and lost part of his cushingoid features but his back remained troublesome (e). He also developed large ulcers on his ankles which were very slow to heal. He continued to develop focal areas of vasculitis on the fingers or various parts of the limbs (f,g). The alternate-day prednisone was raised to 70 mg. His Coxsackie B neutralization tests in March showed titres of 128, 128 and 16 for B_2, B_3 and B_4 respectively, and 6 weeks later showed titres of 32, 256 and 32 respectively. B_1, B_5 and B_6 were consistently <16. The significance of this was difficult to assess but suggested that a Coxsackie infection may have had a role in the development of his disease. The predominant pathology, however, seemed to be a widespread vasculitis. He subsequently died quite suddenly. A possible gastrointestinal haemorrhage was suspected but there was no confirmation of this or any specific cause of death at autopsy.

Graft-versus-host reaction

Polymyositis may also occur as a result of graft-versus-host reaction, for example, following bone marrow transplant for leukaemia (Pier and Dubowitz, 1983) (Figure 11-18).

COURSE AND PROGNOSIS ——————

The course is extremely variable and ranges from mild cases with complete spontaneous remission on the one hand, to acute severe fulminating disease with rapid death on the other. There is a tendency to remission followed by relapse and some patients follow a chronic progressive course, with development of severe deformities and disability.

In their exhaustive review of the literature Bitnum *et al.* (1964) were able to analyse 168 adequately documented paediatric cases. Approximately one-third of the patients died of the disease, one-third had recovered with no or only minimal sequelae, and about one-third were crippled to a moderate or severe degree. With a few exceptions, most of the cases included in their analysis antedated the steroid era. However, the mortality rates shown in several series published after the introduction of steroids still remained relatively high, despite the inclusion of treated patients: 11 of 19 (Everett and Curtis, 1957); 10 of 26 (Wedgwood *et al.*, 1953); 8 of 31 (Muller *et al.*, 1959); 2 of 8 (Thieffry *et al.*, 1967); 2 of 13 (Hill and Wood, 1970); 3 of 22 (Roget *et al.*, 1971); 6 of 22 (Ansell *et al.*, 1973).

TREATMENT ————————————

Steroids

A number of the early authors were initially dubious of the value of steroids, and in a comparative review of steroid versus non-steroid cases in the available literature, Bitnum *et al.* (1964) found an equivalent mortality and no striking difference in morbidity, and somewhat pessimistically concluded that although a striking and rapid improvement may occur with cortisone and ACTH in the acute and active stages of the disease, (1) the response is likely to be symptomatic only, (2) the response may be temporary and even those with dramatic initial improvement may die, and (3) the development of the disabilities and crippling effects of the disease may still occur.

Subsequent results were more encouraging and it seems likely that the bad early results may reflect overtreatment with steroids and the development of a superadded steroid myopathy in the place of the original myositis, or inappropriate schedules of treatment.

A number of fashions and dogmas seem to have evolved in relation to steroid therapy, based mainly on experience with adult patients, who probably have a less steroid-responsive disorder. These included the erroneous ideas that (1) high-dosage corticosteroid therapy is essential to produce remission; (2) initial high-dosage therapy needs to be continued until full remission is produced; (3) subsequent long-term low-dosage maintenance therapy is essential to prevent relapse; and (4) response to therapy can be monitored by the fall in serum enzyme levels. This approach was followed by most early authors (Thieffry *et al.*, 1967; Stögmann, 1971; Sullivan *et al.*, 1972; Vignos and Goldwyn, 1972; Benson and Aldo, 1973; Haas, 1973; Miller, 1973; Schaller, 1973; Rose, 1974).

However, it soon became obvious in clinical practice that one could obtain satisfactory remission of the active disease by a regimen of moderate dosage prednisone (about 1 mg/kg/day in contrast to the 2–3 mg usually recommended), of short duration, with gradual tapering of dosage once response begins, without waiting for full remission (Dubowitz, 1976). In this way one could usually stop the steroid therapy within 3–6 months, and it appears that if one can give just enough steroid to suppress the active condition for just long enough to reduce and stop the treatment safely and easily, the disease may go into sustained remission. Tapering of the steroid dosage can be done gradually but steadily, at weekly or 2-weekly intervals, and at the first sign of any failure of continued improvement can be stepped up by one increment to the previous level and retained there an extra week, before trying to steadily reduce it again.

Alternate-day steroid therapy

This came into vogue in cases where patients needed long-term steroids and has the advantage of preventing some of the severe side-effects of long-term corticosteroids, such as growth retardation and weight gain. It should not be used in the acute phase for suppression of the active disease, as it is not as effective as daily treatment and needs a much longer time for response. It should be reserved for those patients whom one cannot wean off the initial steroid regimen, and who may thus require a long-term steroid therapy to maintain remission, at varying levels of maintenance therapy.

Other immunosuppressive therapy

There has been cumulative experience over the past decade or so of a number of additional lines of treatment in juvenile dermatomyositis, including azathioprine, cyclophosphamide, methotrexate and cyclosporin, as well as intravenous gamma globulin and plasma exchange. These are no substitute for steroids in the acute phase, which remains the sheet anchor of treatment, but are extremely useful as second- and third-line therapies.

PERSONAL EXPERIENCE

Steroids

The vast majority of patients will respond to the lower dose steroid regime (1 mg/kg/day in divided doses) within 2–3 weeks and one can start to taper very carefully the dosage level, under close monitoring, at regular intervals of say 2 or 3 weeks. There is no advantage at all in using higher levels of initial steroid therapy and it carries the added risk of more severe side-effects and also more difficult in weaning. In a comparative study of patients undergoing low-dosage or high-dosage initial therapy (Miller *et al.*, 1983), we found no advantage in terms of response to the high dose and a much higher and more prolonged morbidity in those patients taking high doses.

Azathioprine

This does not appear to be effective in suppressing the active disease but is helpful in trying to wean steroid-dependent patients off steroids.

Cyclophosphamide and methotrexate

These are effective second-line drugs in suppressing acute or persistent disease and a good adjunct in patients either not fully responsive to steroids or who are becoming steroid-dependent and still not fully asymptomatic. Side-effects can be troublesome, especially haemorrhagic cystitis from cyclophosphamide. Careful monitoring of the blood count is also important for detecting marrow suppression.

Cyclosporin

This has proved to be an extremely valuable drug, particularly in patients who have developed complications of steroid therapy or have not fully responded and become chronic. We documented our early experience with 14 patients (Heckmatt *et al.*, 1989) and it is now my choice as a second line of treatment after steroids. If one monitors closely the blood levels and keeps them at a low therapeutic range, one can avoid the important side-effects of renal toxicity and hypertension.

Intravenous gammaglobulin

This is a rather 'hit-and-miss' type of therapy and our recent experience of its use in nine refractory cases over a 4-year period has shown marked variability in response, not only from patient to patient but also from one course to another in the same patient (Sansome and Dubowitz, 1995). Side-effects, such as headache, have been avoided by giving the same dose more slowly over a longer period. Its main disadvantage is its inconsistency and, until proved otherwise by properly controlled studies, I think its current place is still as a reserve in cases where patients fail to respond adequately to other therapy.

Plasma exchange

This is a drastic form of treatment and not very pleasant for the patient. We have used it in an occasional desperately ill and weak patient, usually in relapse on conventional therapy, with good effect. It is difficult to assess its efficacy in parallel with concurrent medical treatment and it may require several exchanges to achieve benefit.

A therapeutic regimen

I have tried to summarize in Table 11-1 our current therapeutic programme in relation to new patients who have not had any prior treatment. Every physician is likely to develop his own personal preferences and dogma, but I think there is an overall guiding principle in relation to the treatment of juvenile dermatomyositis, in that it is an extremely variable disease, both in its clinical manifestations and in its response to treatment, and each child needs to be treated individually and the treatment tailored to the needs of his disease. It also goes without saying that one needs to monitor very closely the response to treatment, particularly in the acute and active stage, at intervals of about 2–3 weeks, in order to adjust the treatment accordingly. It is quite foolhardy to think that one can simply write out a 3-month schedule of treatment and hope for the best; yet it is surprising how frequently this still happens in practice.

SUPPORTIVE MEASURES

These patients are very prone to develop muscle contractures, particularly in the early active phase of the disease, and also in the chronic phase if they are immobilized. It is important to encourage active movements even in the early stages of the disease, and once improvement starts the patient should be encouraged to maintain full activity within the limits

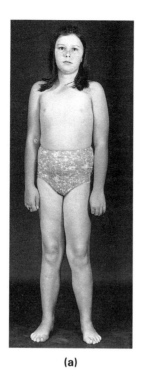

(a)

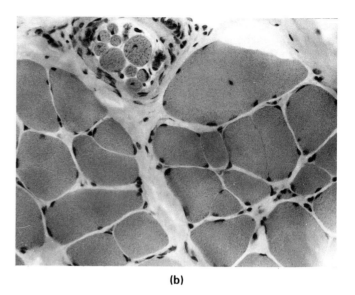

(b)

Figure 11-17a,b ? Polymyositis, ? Limb girdle dystrophy, ? Coxsackie infection. This 10-year-old girl (a) had normal motor milestones and no problems till the development of pain and swelling of the knees and elbows at the age of 9 years, diagnosed as rheumatoid arthritis and responsive to salicylates and physiotherapy. She subsequently had intermittent mild joint pains, followed by a severe attack of hip pains at the age of 9 years, responsive again to salicylates. The physiotherapist then noted weakness of the arms. The weakness progressed and she became unable to run, had difficulty climbing stairs and could not get up from the floor without help. There were no general symptoms of ill health, no change in temperament and no skin manifestations. When assessed at 10 years she had weakness affecting the legs more than the arms and the proximal muscles more than the distal. Ulnar conduction was normal (58 m/s), EMG of deltoid and quadriceps myopathic, and CK grossly elevated at 1690 iu/litre. On the basis of a clinical diagnosis of possible polymyositis, a course of prednisone (40 mg/day; 1 mg/kg) was given with a suggestion of some initial improvement but no sustained benefit. Biopsy of the quadriceps showed a picture compatible with a limb girdle dystrophy and no evidence of inflammatory response (b). Electron microscopy showed some inclusions suggestive of possible viral origin. Coxsackie viral titres showed a consistent elevation of B_2 and B_4 at 1:128 and 1:1024 respectively on three successive occasions at 3-monthly intervals. Routine rheumatoid immunological studies were all negative except for a raised antinuclear factor. There is a possibility that this child's current chronic myopathy may have been a sequel to an initial polymyositis which may have had a viral origin. Alternatively, she may have limb girdle dystrophy and the arthritis and Coxsackie titres may have been coincidental.

of his muscle power. Passive exercise and the use of night splints to maintain posture are useful in trying to prevent progression of the contractures. There is no need for confining these patients to bed in the acute phase, as long as they feel well enough to be mobilized (see Figure 11-8).

RESPONSE TO THERAPY

This is best judged on clinical grounds and the best parameter is the return of muscle power and motor function. Disappearance of the general malaise and misery is also a useful indication of response. The

return of these general symptoms is also a sensitive indication of incipient relapse.

Serum enzymes are an unreliable yardstick. In some cases they may be normal anyway, but even when elevated may lag behind the clinical improvement and one should not be tempted to treat the serum enzyme levels rather than the patient.

The skin manifestations often persist for a long time beyond the apparent remission of the active muscle symptoms. This is no indication for continued steroid therapy and is not indicative of a generally active or progressive disease. When troublesome, the skin eruption may respond well to cyclosporin.

Table 11-1 Current therapeutic regimen, in use in juvenile dermatomyositis

Drugs used, listed in order of preference and efficacy

1. Prednisolone

Dosage: 1 mg/kg/day in two or three divided doses.

This remains the most effective drug in juvenile dermatomyositis and the sheet-anchor of treatment.

Response usually occurs within 1–2 weeks and, once established, the dosage can be very gradually reduced, initially by 5 mg/day, at intervals of 2 weeks and, once one reaches a level of 30 mg/day, by 2.5 mg/day. After reaching 20 mg/day we prefer to reduce it more slowly, by 2.5 mg every alternate day. By giving it in divided doses it is easier to work out a schedule for the patient; thus for example reducing from 30 mg/day to 27.5 mg/day would be reducing from 10, 10, 10 to 10, 10, 7.5, and then to 10, 7.5, 7.5 and so forth. Similarly, reducing from 22.5 mg/day would be 7.5, 7.5, 7.5 to 7.5, 7.5, 5 on alternate days, and then 7.5, 7.5, 5 each day after a further 2-week interval.

It is important to monitor closely the progress, and if in any particular week the child is not as well as the previous week he should immediately revert to the previous week's dosage for a further 2 weeks before reducing it again.

Alternate-day prednisolone has no place in the acute phase and is reserved only for patients who become dependent on prednisolone and tend to relapse if reduced further and look set for a longer term need for maintenance of steroid.

Toxic effects: Weight gain, hypertension, and osteoporosis are the main side-effects of excessive and prolonged therapy and will gradually resolve on reduction of the dosage. These complications can be largely avoided and substantially reduced by the above low-dosage schedule with early and steady reduction in dosage.

2. Azathioprine

Dosage: 2.5 mg/kg/day in two or three divided doses. Can be increased up to 4 mg/kg/day.

Whilst not influencing the activity of the dermatomyositis itself, azathioprine has proved useful in trying to reduce the steroid dosage. One can maintain the same dosage of azathioprine until the steroid is completely stopped, or down to a small maintenance level. The azathioprine can then be reduced fairly rapidly by decrements of a third in three steps at intervals of about 2–3 weeks.

Toxic effects: Marrow suppression, liver toxicity, alopecia and aggravation of skin manifestation. Blood counts and liver function tests need regular checking.

3. Cyclosporin

Dosage: Initially 4 mg/kg/day. Can be increased up to 7 to 7.5 mg/kg/day depending on the trough blood level, which should be maintained at about 100 µg/l (range 80–120).

Toxic effects: Renal toxicity, hypertension.
Renal function should be assessed regularly by creatine clearance and other routine renal function tests at start of treatment and at 6-monthly intervals by excretion scanning with DMSO. Blood pressure and liver function also need monitoring. If any signs of toxicity develop, dosage can be reduced.

4. Gammaglobulin

Dosage: 2 mg/kg by slow intravenous infusion over 5 days.
Can be given in divided aliquots (1/5 of total dose) nightly over 8-hour period.

The infusion can be repeated after 21-day intervals for 3 months. We usually give three cycles of treatment.

Toxic effects: There are few toxic effects. Headache can be largely avoided by the slower infusion over a longer period. The main problems are its inconsistent effect, unpredictability and exorbitant cost.

5. Other immunosuppressant drugs

a) Cyclophosphamide

Dosage: 1 mg/kg/day by mouth.

Toxic effects: Haemorrhagic cystitis (may be prevented by increased fluid intake and mesna); suppression of bone marrow.

b) Methotrexate

Dosage: 2–3 mg/kg/dose orally or intravenously every 2 weeks (or 1 mg/kg every week).

Toxic effects: Bowel disturbance (mucositis); bone marrow suppression; side-effects of cytotoxic drugs generally: alopecia, nausea and vomiting; teratogenicity.

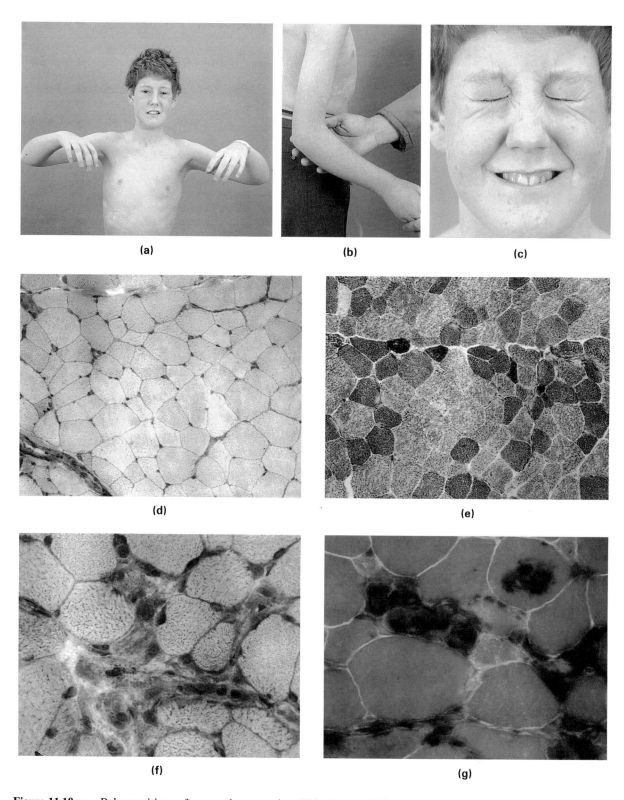

Figure 11-18a-g Polymyositis: graft-versus-host-reaction. This 11-year-old boy developed acute polymyositis as the only manifestation of chronic graft-versus-host disease 7 months after bone marrow transplant for acute leukaemia. There was weakness of the shoulder girdle and contractures at the elbows (a-c). Muscle biopsy showed variability in fibre size, focal necrosis and cellular response (d-g).

FOCAL MYOSITIS

This is a rare inflammatory disease of muscle that tends to present as a focal swelling or pseudotumour, and may be mistaken for a sarcoma or an abscess. It tends to be self-limiting and to resolve spontaneously. It has been documented in many different muscles, including upper and lower limb, abdominal rectus, neck, temporalis, tongue and masticatory muscles (Heffner *et al.*, 1977; Lederman *et al.*, 1984; Vercelli-Ratta *et al.*, 1988; Isaacson *et al.*, 1991; Moscovic *et al.*, 1991; Krendel *et al.*, 1992; Naumann *et al.*, 1993).

Changes in the muscle biopsy resemble those of polymyositis. Magnetic resonance imaging is helpful in identifying the location and extent of the lesion, and may recognize focal myositis in a muscle not palpable from the surface, and also help to document the resolution.

INCLUSION BODY MYOSITIS

As the name implies, this myopathy is characterized by its unusual inclusions and was initially thought to be an inflammatory 'myositis' because of its clinical resemblance to chronic polymyositis. Chou (1968) thought the inclusions resembled myxovirus, but a viral aetiology could not be substantiated and Yunis and Samaha (1971) suggested the inclusions might be distinctive and coined the term 'inclusion body myositis'.

Although most of the early cases seemed to be of late adult onset, some do occur in adolescence and early adult life and there have also been a few case reports in childhood. Mikol and Engel (1994) have recently done an exhaustive review of the fairly extensive literature of some 240 sporadic cases documented in recent years. Whilst most cases have been sporadic, there have recently been some reports of familial cases, with a particular prevalence among Iranian Jews (Sadeh *et al.*, 1993).

Clinical features

Clinically it presents with a slowly progressive weakness of variable distribution and severity, usually symmetrical and either predominantly distal, predominantly proximal or diffuse.

In contrast to polymyositis it has proved singularly resistant to treatment with steroids, immunosuppressive drugs and, apart from some anecdotal case reports, also to intravenous gammaglobulin.

Muscle biopsy

The diagnosis is made on the basis of the characteristic histological picture. At light microscopy, routine stains with haematoxylin and eosin reveal the presence of rimmed vacuoles, which have basophilic granular material around the vacuole and also within it. In addition there may be eosinophilic inclusions in the cytoplasm. There may also be degenerating and necrotic fibres present and an inflammatory response, predominantly of T lymphocytes.

On electron microscopy the characteristic features are the intranuclear and cytoplasmic filaments. Rimmed vacuoles have also been observed in some familial cases of distal myopathies (see Chapter 2).

Immunocytochemistry

A number of interesting immunocytochemical studies on inclusion body myositis in the past few years have shown the presence within the inclusions of amyloid deposits as well as ubiquitin, ß-amyloid protein, ß-amyloid precursor protein, α_1-antichymotrypsin, prion protein and apolipoprotein E (Askanas *et al.*, 1992, 1993a, b, c, 1994).

This has raised the interesting analogy between the strikingly similar features of the muscle in inclusion body myositis and the brain in Alzheimer's disease.

FAMILIAL INCLUSION BODY MYOSITIS

A familial form of inclusion body myositis, starting in early adult life, with a progressive, symmetrical weakness, affecting distal muscles more than proximal and sparing the quadriceps, has been documented in a number of families of Iranian Jewish origin (Argov and Yarom, 1984; Massa *et al.*, 1991; Sadeh *et al.*, 1993). Inheritance seems to be autosomal recessive. Some, but not all, of the immunocytochemical abnormalities noted in inclusion body myositis (see above) have also been found in the familial cases.

REDUCING BODY MYOPATHY

Brooke and Neville (1972) documented a severe and apparently progressive neuromuscular disease, with somewhat unusual pathological features, in two young girls. The disease was present from birth and both infants subsequently died, one at 9 months, the other at 2½ years. The pathological abnormality was

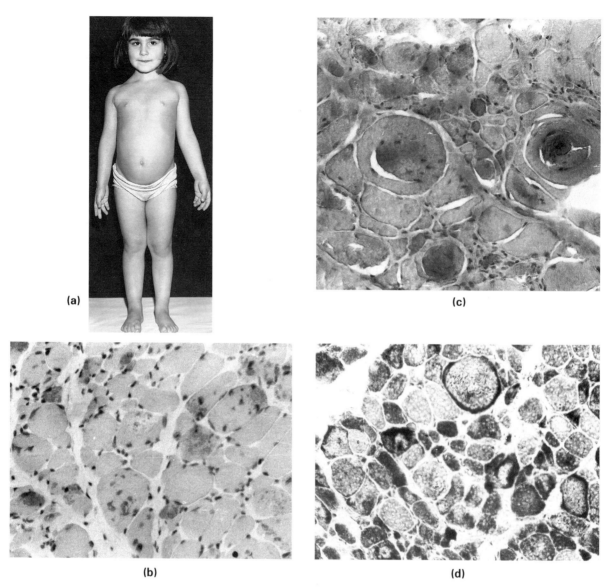

Figure 11-19a-g ? Myositis, ? Reducing body myopathy. This girl presented at 4 years of age with a 6-month history of progressive weakness and wasting of the right arm (a). (She had been immunized against poliomyelitis in infancy.) About 1 month prior to the onset she had measles, with no complications. There was no preceding history of muscle weakness, but she had walked with some flexion of the knees for about 2 years. On examination there was extensive wasting and weakness of all muscle groups of the right arm. In addition there was slight weakness of the left arm and neck muscles. Her gait was steady but she held the knees slightly flexed. She was able to get up from the floor and to ascend steps without difficulty. The distribution of weakness was reminiscent of poliomyelitis but EMG of the deltoid showed a typically myopathic pattern. The CK was moderately elevated (120–200 iu/litre) on repeated estimations. Muscle biopsy of the deltoid showed a strikingly pathological muscle, with variation in fibre size, several areas of predominantly atrophic fibres and many degenerating fibres. Eosinophilic inclusions were present within many fibres (b-f). A subsequent biopsy of the clinically unaffected quadriceps showed focal, and less extensive, similar changes.

the presence of inclusions within the muscle fibres capable, in histochemical preparations, of reducing tetrazolium salts in the presence of menadione without any substrate, hence the suggested name. On electron microscopy these bodies show a distinctive pattern with closely packed particles which could possibly be viral or ribosomal material (Neville, 1973).

Figure 11-19 illustrates an older child presenting with a progressive and subsequently fatal myopathy with similar histological features to the reducing body myopathy.

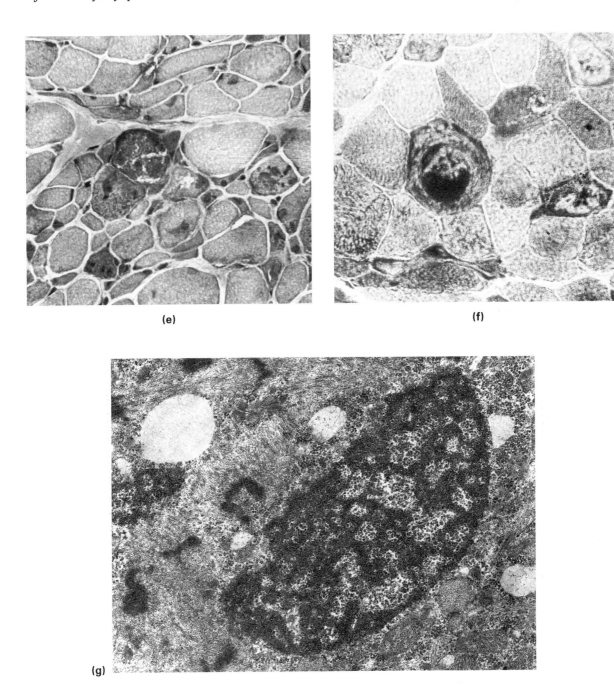

(e)

(f)

(g)

Figure 11-19 continued Electron microscopy of the deltoid and also quadriceps biopsy showed the inclusions to be non-membrane-bound and composed of tightly packed, rounded, electron-dense particles (g), thought to be of possible viral origin and resembling inclusions seen with Coxsackie infections. Specific anti-measles antibody studies failed to reveal any evidence of a measles antigen within the muscle. A consistently high blood titre of anti-Coxsackie B virus (1:512) suggested this might be the aetiological agent. Immunological studies showed no abnormality of her cellular or humoral mechanisms and there was no *in vitro* response to measles or Coxsackie virus. In the months after presentation she deteriorated markedly. On the grounds that she might have an unusual 'polymyositis', a course of prednisone was given for 4 months without effect. She was then given cyclophosphamide with apparent arrest of the progression for about a year, but then began to deteriorate again and subsequently lost the ability to walk. The relentless deterioration continued, despite various therapeutic trials of antiviral agents (amantadine), a second course of prednisone, methotrexate and also several courses of 'transfer factor' from packed white cells. She died of a respiratory infection 3 years after the onset of her illness. Autopsy was not done.

MYOSITIS OF KNOWN AETIOLOGY

Skeletal muscle may be affected in a wide variety of bacterial, parasitic and viral infections.

In some cases the involvement of the muscle is incidental to a more general disorder, and may in fact be clinically silent and only recognized at biopsy or autopsy. In others there is overt weakness of the musculature, or other symptoms referable to the musculoskeletal system.

BACTERIAL MYOSITIS

Pyomyositis

Normal muscle is resistant to bacterial infections, and suppurative myositis is rare, except in the tropics where patients may present with multiple acute abscesses of the muscle, usually of staphylococcal origin.

Gas gangrene

When muscle becomes devitalized as a result of trauma, there is a danger of clostridial invasion and resultant gas gangrene.

Tuberculosis

Muscle may also be involved in some of the more chronic infections. In tuberculosis there may be direct spread of a cold abscess into adjoining muscle, or haematogenous invasion in miliary tuberculosis.

Sarcoidosis

In sarcoidosis there is frequently involvement of the striated muscle, and muscle biopsy may be an effective way of establishing a diagnosis in a suspected case, even in the absence of overt weakness or other muscle symptoms (Myers *et al.*, 1952; Phillips and Phillips, 1956; Wallace *et al.*, 1958; Silverstein and Siltzback, 1969; Namba *et al.*, 1974). Weakness, if present, may be localized or more general, and there may be associated pain and tenderness. Nodules may at times be palpable in the muscle. Some patients may actually present with muscle weakness and thus resemble polymyositis or limb girdle dystrophy patients (Harvey, 1959; Crompton and MacDermot, 1961; Hinterbuchner and Hinterbuchner, 1964; Coërs and Carbone, 1966). Histologically there are the typical granulomatous lesions of sarcoidosis, with giant cells, histiocytes and variable inflammatory response. Although these lesions are predominantly in the supportive tissues, they may also be seen within the muscle fibres and there may be associated degenerative changes (Coërs, 1967).

VIRAL MYOSITIS

Epidemic pleurodynia (Bornholm disease, Devil's grip) has been recognized for over a century, initially being recorded in Iceland and subsequently in the Scandinavian countries (including Bornholm island) and in other parts of the world. The clinical and epidemiological aspects were reviewed by Sylvest (1934) in his classical monograph. The condition is a benign and self-limiting one, with general symptoms, such as fever and headache, associated with acute pain in the chest, mainly at the costal margins and substernal region, and aggravated by inspiration or cough. The intercostal muscles are often tender to touch.

It is now recognized that Coxsackie B virus is the causative agent and various strains of the B virus may be responsible (Kilbourne, 1950; Weller *et al.*, 1950; Patz *et al.*, 1953; Dalldorf, 1955).

In the past few years there have been a number of reports of a possible viral aetiology in cases of idiopathic polymyositis. These have been based mainly on the appearance of structures resembling viral inclusions within the nucleus or cytoplasm of the muscle fibre on electron microscopy. They have resembled either myxovirus (Chou, 1968; Carpenter *et al.*, 1970; Sato *et al.*, 1971; Yunis and Samaha, 1971) or picornavirus, possibly of the Coxsackie group (Chou and Gutmann, 1970; Mastaglia and Walton, 1971), while Norris *et al.* (1969) found virus-like particles in two cases of myositis associated with herpes zoster. Marcus and Bill (1976) documented an acute, rapidly resolving, myopathy in three brothers. Echo virus was cultured from the stool of two of them, but the muscle biopsy taken from one of them showed no viral particles on electron microscopy and culture for virus was also negative.

An acute myositis of varying severity, but usually mild, is probably a common component of influenza virus infections. It usually manifests with pain and tenderness of the muscles.

The possibility of a chronic polymyositis being due to a slow viral infection may be analogous to subacute sclerosing panencephalitis following infection with measles virus.

One problem in practice is the possible significance of a raised titre to Coxsackie B virus in the serum of a patient with muscle disease. We found this in a number of children, some of whom seemed to conform to limb girdle dystrophy or relapsing polyneuritis rather than a myositic problem. We were unable to identify the virus in electron microscopic preparations from these patients.

HIV MYOSITIS

An associated myositis has been well documented in recent years in patients infected with the human immunodeficiency virus (HIV), and also in those manifesting the acquired immunodeficiency syndrome (AIDS) (Dalakas and Pezeshkpour, 1986, 1988). A myopathy has also been directly linked with zidovudine, used in the treatment of AIDS, and shown to disturb mitochondrial function (Bessen *et al.*, 1988; Gorard *et al.*, 1988; Helbert *et al.*, 1988; Arnaudo *et al.*, 1991; Chariot and Gherard, 1991).

PARASITIC MYOSITIS

Trichinosis

A number of parasitic infections may affect muscle. The commonest is trichinosis, which is caused by ingesting the larvae of the nematode *Trichinella spiralis* in undercooked pork. The larvae mature in the human bowel, and the fertilized female penetrates the bowel mucosa and deposits large numbers of embryos, which enter the venules or lymphatics and are widely disseminated throughout the body. It is particularly in skeletal muscle that these larvae settle and persist, and may in time become calcified. During the invasive stage there may be general symptoms and an associated eosinophilia, together with variable pains and tenderness in the muscles. Muscle weakness may occasionally occur. In the chronic phase the condition is usually quiescent and only recognized by histological change, e.g. at routine autopsy.

Histologically the muscle may show, in addition to the presence of the encysted larvae, inflammatory response, degeneration and phagocytosis of muscle fibres, and connective tissue proliferation.

Cysticercosis

Other parasitic conditions which may produce encysted larvae in the muscle include cysticercosis, due to the pork tapeworm, *Taenia solium*. Although rare in Western countries, it is fairly common in India. It more usually affects the central nervous system, resulting in convulsions, intermittent hydrocephalus or dementia, but may rarely present with muscle enlargement, sometimes accompanied by weakness (Jolly and Pallis, 1971). At biopsy the tense cysts are readily apparent. The muscle itself is histologically normal.

Hydatid disease, which occurs in sheep-rearing countries, very rarely affects muscle.

Toxoplasmosis

Toxoplasmosis is due to a protozoan parasite and may occur as a congenital infection in the newborn infant of an affected mother, or as an acquired infection later in life. The congenital form has a predilection for the central nervous system but not for muscle. In the acquired form there are usually no associated muscle symptoms, but the parasites have been observed incidentally in the skeletal muscle (Callahan *et al.*, 1946; Andrus *et al.*, 1952). However, Rowland and Greer (1961) reported a case of toxoplasmosis presenting with polymyositis, and Chandar *et al.* (1968) diagnosed toxoplasmosis in a 7-year-old child who presented with general symptoms, cervical adenopathy and associated muscle weakness and tenderness. The muscle biopsy, which I had the opportunity of seeing, showed focal changes resembling a low grade polymyositis and only on careful search were parasites found. The toxoplasma dye test was positive at a titre of 1:4096 and the symptoms subsided on therapy with pyrimethamine plus sulphadimidine.

Sarcosporidiosis

Sarcosporidia (sarcocystis) are sporozoal parasites which are commonly found in the muscle of domestic animals, and also of various wild animals, but only very rarely in man (Darling, 1919; Feng, 1932). Usually the finding is incidental in a patient with no neuromusuclar symptoms, but Dastur and Iyer (1955) reported two patients with weakness and muscle pain and McGill and Goodbody (1957) documented a case with sarcosporidiosis associated with periarteritis nodosa.

REFERENCES

Andrus, K., Kass, E.H., Adams, R.D., Turner, F.C. and Feldman, H.A. (1952) Toxoplasmosis in the adult. *Archives of Internal Medicine* **89**: 759.

Ansell, B.M., Hamilton, E. and Bywaters, E.G. (1973) Course and prognosis in juvenile dermatomyositis. In: Kakulas, B.A. ed., *Clinical Studies in Myology*. Proceedings of the Second International Congress on Muscle Diseases. Perth, Australia, 1971, Part 2. Amsterdam: Excerpta Medica, I.C.S. No. 295.

Appleyard, S.T., Dunn, M.J., Dubowitz, V. *et al.* (1985) Increased expression of HLA ABC class I antigens by muscle fibres in Duchenne muscular dystrophy, inflammatory myopathy and other neuromuscular disorders. *Lancet* i: 361.

Argov, Z. and Yarom, R. (1984) "Rimmed vacuole myopathy" sparing the quadriceps: a unique disorder in Iranian Jews. *Journal of the Neurological Sciences* **64**: 33–43.

Arnaudo, E., Dalakas, M., Shankse, S. *et al.* (1991) Depletion of muscle mitochondrial DNA in AIDS patients with zidovudine-induced myopathy. *Lancet* **337**: 508–510.

Askanas, V., Engel, W.K. and Alvarez, R.B. (1992) Light- and electronmicroscopic localisation of ß-amyloid protein in muscle biopsies of patients with inclusion body myositis. *American Journal of Pathology* **114**: 31–36.

Askanas, V., Engel, W.K. and Alvarez, R.B. (1993a) Enhanced detection of congo-red positive amyloid deposits in muscle fibres of inclusion body myositis and brain of Alzheimer's disease using fluorescence technique. *Neurology* **43**: 1265–1267.

Askanas, V., Alvarez, R.B. and Engel, W.K. (1993b) Abnormal accumulations of ß-amyloid precursor epitopes in muscle fibres of inclusion body myositis. *Annals of Neurology* **34**: 551–560.

Askanas, V., Bilak, M., Engel, W.K., Alvarez, R.B., Tomé, F. and Leclerc, A. (1993c) Prion protein is abnormally accumulated in inclusion body myositis. *NeuroReport* **5**: 25–28.

Askanas, V., Mirabella, M., Engel, W.K., Alvarez, R.B. and Weisgraber, K.H. (1994) Apolipoprotein E immunoreactive deposits in inclusion body muscle diseases. *Lancet* **343**: 364–365.

Banker, B.Q. (1975) Dermatomyositis of childhood: ultrastructural alterations of muscle and intramuscular blood vessels. *Journal of Neuropathology and Experimental Neurology* **34**: 46.

Banker, B.Q. and Victor, M. (1966) Dermatomyositis (systemic angiopathy) of childhood. *Medicine* **45**: 261.

Benson, M.D. and Aldo, M. (1973) Azathioprine therapy in polymyositis. *Archives of Internal Medicine* **132**: 547.

Bessen, L.J., Greene, J.B., Louie, E. *et al.* (1988) Severe polymyositis-like syndrome associated with zidovudine therapy of AIDS and ARC. *New England Journal of Medicine* **318**: 708.

Bitnum, S., Daeschner, C.W., Travis, L.B., Dodge, W.F. and Hopps, H.C. (1964) Dermatomyositis. *Journal of Pediatrics* **64**: 101.

Brooke, M.H. and Kaplan, H. (1972) Muscle pathology in rheumatoid arthritis, polymyalgia rheumatica, and polymyositis. *Archives of Pathology* **94**: 101.

Brooke, M.H. and Neville, H.E. (1972) Reducing body myopathy. *Neurology (Minneapolis)* **22**: 829.

Callahan, W.P., Russell, W.O. and Smith, M.G. (1946) Human toxoplasmosis: a clinicopathologic study with presentation of 5 cases and review of the literature. *Medicine* **25**: 343.

Carpenter, S., Karpati, G. and Wolfe, L.S. (1970) Virus-like filaments and phospholipid accumulation in skeletal muscle. Study of a histochemically distinct chronic myopathy. *Neurology (Minneapolis)* **20**: 889.

Chandar, K., Mair, H.J. and Mair, N.S. (1968) Case of toxoplasma polymyositis. *British Medical Journal* i: 158.

Chariot, P. and Gherard, R. (1991) Partial cytochrome c oxidase deficiency and cytoplasmic bodies in patients with zidovudine myopathy. *Neuromuscular Disorders* **1**: 357–363.

Chou, S.M. (1968) Myxovirus-like structures and accompanying nuclear changes in chronic polymyositis. *Archives of Pathology* **86**: 649.

Chou, S.M. and Gutmann, L. (1970) Picornavirus-like crystals in subacute polymyositis. *Neurology (Minneapolis)* **20**: 205.

Coërs, C. (1967) The histological features of muscle sarcoidosis. *Acta Neuropathologica (Berlin)* **1**: 242.

Coërs, C. and Carbone, F. (1966) La myopathie granulomateuse. *Acta Neurologica et Psychiatrica Belgica* **66**: 353.

Cook, C.D., Rosen, F.S. and Banker, B.Q. (1963) Dermatomyositis and focal scleroderma. *Pediatric Clinics of North America* **10**: 979.

Crompton, M.R. and MacDermot, V. (1961) Sarcoidosis associated with progressive muscular wasting and weakness. *Brain* **84**: 62.

Dalakas, M.C. and Pezeshkpour, G.H. (1986) Neuromuscular complications of AIDS. *Muscle and Nerve* **9**: 92.

Dalakas, M.C. and Pezeshkpour, G.H. (1988) Neuromuscular diseases associated with human immunodeficiency virus infection. *Annals of Neurology* **235**: 88.

Dalldorf, G. (1955) Coxsackie viruses. *Annual Review of Microbiology* **9**: 277.

Darling, S.T. (1919) Sarcosporidiosis in an East Indian. *Journal of Parasitology* **6**: 98.

Dastur, D.K. and Iyer, C.G.S. (1955) Sarcocystis of human muscle. *Neurology Bulletin of the Neurological Society of India* **2**: 25.

Dubowitz, L.M.S. and Dubowitz, V. (1964) Acute dermatomyositis presenting with pulmonary manifestations. *Archives of Disease in Childhood* **39**: 293–296.

Dubowitz, V. (1976) Treatment of dermatomyositis in childhood. *Archives of Disease in Childhood* **51**: 494–500.

Dubowitz, V. (1985) *Muscle Biopsy: A Practical Approach* 2nd edn. London: Bailliere Tindall.

Dubowitz, V. and Brooke, M.H. (1973) *Muscle Biopsy: A Modern Approach*. London and Philadelphia: W.B. Saunders.

Eaton, L.E. (1954) The perspective of neurology in regard to polymyositis. A study of 41 cases. *Neurology* **4**: 245.

Emslie-Smith A.M., Arahata K. and Engel A.G. (1989) Major histocompatibility complex class I antigen expression, immunolocalization of interferon subtypes and T cell-mediated cytotoxicity in myopathies. *Human Pathology* **20**: 224.

Everett, M.K. and Curtis, A. (1957) Dermatomyositis. A review of nineteen cases in adolescents and children. *Archives of Internal Medicine* **100**: 70.

Feng, L.C. (1932) Sarcosporidiosis in man. Report of a case in a Chinese. *Chinese Medical Journal* **46**: 976.

Gorard, D.A., Henry, K. and Guiloff, R.J. (1988) Necrotising myopathy and zidovudine. *Lancet* **ii**: 689–690.

Haas, D.C. (1973) Treatment of polymyositis with immunosuppressive drugs. *Neurology* **23**: 55.

Harvey, J.C. (1959) A myopathy of Boeck's sarcoid. *American Journal of Medicine* **27**: 356.

Heckmatt, J.Z., Pier, N. and Dubowitz, V. (1988) Real-time ultrasound imaging of muscles. *Muscle and Nerve* **11**: 56–65.

Heckmatt, J., Saunders, C., Peters, A.M. *et al.* (1989) Cyclosporin in juvenile dermatomyositis. *Lancet* **i**: 1063–1066.

Heffner, R.R., Armbrustmacher, V.W. and Earle, K.M. (1977) Focal myositis. *Cancer* **40**: 302–306.

Helbert, M., Fletcher, T., Peddle, B. *et al.* (1988) Zidovudine-associated myopathy. *Lancet* **ii**: 689–690.

Hepp, P. (1887) Ueber einen Fall von acuter parenchymatoser Myositis, welche, Geschwülste bildete und Fluctuation, vortäuschte. *Berliner klinische Wochenschrift* **24**: 389.

Hill, R.H. and Wood, W.S. (1970) Juvenile dermatomyositis. *Canadian Medical Association Journal* **103**: 1152.

Hinterbuchner, C.N. and Hinterbuchner, L.P. (1964) Myopathic syndrome in muscular sarcoidosis. *Brain* **87**: 335.

Isaacson, G., Chan, K.H. and Heffner, R.R. (1991) Focal myositis, a new cause for the pediatric neck mass. *Archives of Otolaryngology, Head and Neck Surgery* **117**: 103–105.

Jolly, S.S. and Pallis, C. (1971) Muscular pseudohypertrophy due to cysticercosis. *Journal of the Neurological Sciences* **12**: 155.

Karpati, G., Pouliot, Y. and Carpenter, S. (1988) Expression of immunoreactive major histocompatibility complex products in human skeletal muscle. *Annals of Neurology* **23**: 64.

Kilbourne, E.D. (1950) Diverse manifestations of infection with a strain of Coxsackie virus. *Federation Proceedings* **9**: 581.

Krendel, D., Hedaya, E. and Gottlieb, A. (1992) Calf enlargement, S1 radiculopathy, and focal myositis. *Muscle and Nerve* **15**: 517–518.

Lederman, R., Salanga, V. and Wilbourn, A. (1984) Focal inflammatory myopathy. *Muscle and Nerve* **7**: 142–146.

Massa, R., Weller, B., Karpati, G. *et al.* (1991) Familial inclusion body myositis among Kurdish-Iranian Jews. *Archives of Neurology, Chicago* **48**: 519–522.

Marcus, J.C. and Bill, P.L.A. (1976) Acute myopathy in three brothers. *Neuropädiatrie* **7**: 101–110.

Mastaglia, F.L. and Walton, J.N. (1971) An ultrastructural study of skeletal muscle in polymyositis. *Journal of Neurological Sciences* **12**: 473.

McDouall, R.M., Dunn, M.J. and Dubowitz, V. (1989) Expression of class I and II MHC antigens in neuromuscular diseases. *Journal of the Neurological Sciences* **89**: 213.

McGill, R.J. and Goodbody, R.A. (1957) Sarcosporidiosis in man with periarteritis nodosa. *British Medical Journal* **ii**: 333.

Mikol J. and Engel A.G. (1994) Inclusion body myositis. In: Engel, A.G. and Franzini-Armstrong, C. eds, *Myology* 2nd edn. New York: McGraw-Hill.

Miller, G., Heckmatt, J.Z. and Dubowitz, V. (1983) Drug treatment of juvenile dermatomyositis. *Archives of Disease in Childhood* **58**: 445–450.

Miller, J.J. (1973) Late progression dermatomyositis in childhood. *Journal of Pediatrics* **83**: 543.

Moscovic, E., Fisher, C. and Westbury, G. (1991) Focal myositis, a benign inflammatory pseudotumor: CT appearances. *British Journal of Radiology* **64**: 489–493.

Muller, S.A., Winkelmann, R.K. and Brunsting, L.A. (1959) Calcinosis in dermatomyositis. Observations on course of disease in children and adults. *Archives of Dermatology* **79**: 669.

Myers, G.B., Gottlieb, A.M., Mattman, P.E., Eckley, G.M. and Chasan, J.L. (1952) Joint and skeletal muscle manifestations in sarcoidosis. *American Journal of Medicine* **12**: 161.

Namba, T., Brunner, N.G. and Grob, D. (1974) Idiopathic giant cell polymyositis. *Archives of Neurology* **31**: 27–30.

Naumann, M., Toyka, K.V., Goebel, H.H. *et al.* (1993) Focal myositis of the temporal muscle. *Muscle and Nerve* **16**: 1374–1376.

Neville, H.E. (1973) Ultrastructural changes in muscle disease. In: Dubowitz, V. and Brooke, M.H. eds, *Muscle Biopsy – A Modern Approach*. London and Philadelphia: W.B. Saunders, p.438.

Norris, F.H., Dramov, B., Calder, C.D. and Johnson, S.G. (1969) Virus-like particles in myositis accompanying herpes zoster. *Archives of Neurology* **21**: 25.

Patz, I.M., Measroch, V. and Gear, J. (1953) Bornholm disease, pleurodynia or epidemic myalgia: outbreak in Transvaal associated with Coxsackie virus infection. *South African Medical Journal* **27**: 397.

Pearson, C.M. (1961) Myositis: the inflammatory disorders of muscle. Chapter XV In: *Neuromuscular Disorders* Vol. 38. Research Publications, Association for Research in Nervous and Mental Diseases, pp. 422–477.

Phillips, R.W. and Phillips, A.M. (1956) The diagnosis of Boeck's sarcoid by skeletal muscle biopsy. *Archives of Internal Medicine* **98**: 732.

Pier, N. and Dubowitz, V. (1983) Chronic graft-versus-host disease presenting with polymyositis. *British Medical Journal* **286**: 2024.

Roget, J., Rambaud, P., Frappat, P. and Joannard, A. (1971) La dermatomyosite de l'enfant. Étude de 22 observations. *Pédiatrie* **26**: 471.

Rose, A.L. (1974) Childhood polymyositis. *American Journal of Diseases of Children* **127**: 518.

Rowland, L.P. and Greer, M. (1961) Toxoplasmic polymyositis. *Neurology (Minneapolis)* **11**: 367.

Sadeh, M., Gadoth, N., Hadar, H. *et al.* (1993) Vacuolar myopathy sparing the quadriceps. *Brain* **116**: 217–232.

Sansome, A. and Dubowitz, V. (1995) Intravenous gammaglobulin in juvenile dermatomyositis – four year review of nine cases. *Archives of Disease in Childhood* **72**: 25–28.

Sato, T., Walker, D.L., Peters, H.A., Reese, H.H. and Chou, S.M. (1971) Chronic polymyositis and myxovirus-like inclusions. Electron microscopic and viral studies. *Archives of Neurology (Chicago)* **24**: 409–418.

Schaller, J.G. (1973) Dermatomyositis. *Journal of Pediatrics* **83**: 699.

Sewry, C.A. and Dubowitz, V. (1994) Histochemical and immunocytochemical studies in neuromuscular diseases. In: Walton, J.N., Karpati, G. and Hilton-Jones, D. eds, *Disorders of Voluntary Muscle* 6th edn. Edinburgh: Churchill Livingstone.

Silverstein, A. and Siltzbach, L.E. (1969) Muscle involvement in sarcoidosis. Asymptomatic myositis and myopathy. *Archives of Neurology (Chicago)* **21**: 235.

Steiner, W.R. (1903) Dermatomyositis, with report of a case which presented a rare muscle anomaly but once described in man. *Journal of Experimental Medicine* **6**: 407–422.

Stögmann, W. (1971) Die Therapie der Dermatomyositis in Kindesalter. *Archiv für Kinderheilkunde* **182**: 264.

Sullivan, D.B., Cassidy, J.T., Petty, R.E. and Burt, A. (1972) Prognosis in childhood dermatomyositis. *Journal of Pediatrics* **80**: 555.

Sylvest, E. (1934) *Epidemic Myalgia: Bornholm Disease.* Copenhagen: Levin and Munksgaard.

Thieffry, S., Arthuis, M., Martin, C., Sorrel-Dejerine, J. and Benhamida, M. (1967) Dermatomyosite de l'enfant. Étude de huit cas personnels. *Annales de Pédiatrie* **14**: 554.

Unverricht, H. (1887) Polymyositis acuta progressive. *Zeitschrift für klinische Medizin* **12**: 533.

Unverricht, H. (1891) Dermatomyositis acuta. *Deutsche medizinische Wochenschrift* **17**: 41.

Vercelli-Ratta, J., Ardao, G. and De Cabrera, M. (1988) Focal myositis and its differential diagnosis. *Annals of Pathology* **8**: 54–56.

Vignos, P.J. and Goldwyn, J. (1972) Evaluation of laboratory tests in the diagnosis and management of polymyositis. *American Journal of the Medical Sciences* **263**: 201.

Wagner, E. (1863) Fall einer seltnen Muskelkrankheit. *Archiv Heilkunde* **4**: 282.

Wallace, S.L., Latter, R., Malia, J.P. and Raghan, C. (1958) Muscle involvement in Boeck's sarcoid. *Annals of Internal Medicine* **48**: 497.

Walton, J.N. and Adams, R.D. (1958) *Polymyositis.* Baltimore: Williams and Wilkins, p. 270.

Wedgwood, R.J.P., Cook, C.D. and Cohen, J. (1953) Dermatomyositis. Report of 26 cases in children with a discussion of endocrine therapy in 13. *Pediatrics* **12**: 447.

Weller, T.H. Enders, J.F., Buckingham, M. and Finn, J.J. (1950) The aetiology of epidemic pleurodynia: a study of two viruses isolated from a typical outbreak. *Journal of Immunology* **65**: 337.

Yunis, E.J. and Samaha, F.J. (1971) Inclusion body myositis. *Laboratory Investigation* **25**: 240.

CHAPTER 12

The Floppy Infant Syndrome

CLINICAL DIAGNOSIS

The floppy or hypotonic infant is a common diagnostic problem in paediatric practice, particularly in the newborn period and early infancy. The causes are many and a detailed review of the subject has been the basis of a separate monograph (Dubowitz, 1969, 1980).

A clinical diagnosis of hypotonia is usually suggested by three features:

1. bizarre and unusual postures of the infant;
2. diminished resistance to passive movements;
3. an excessive range of joint mobility.

In simple terms, the infant either looks floppy, or feels floppy, or has an excessive range of joint mobility. These infants are also usually relatively immobile. After the neonatal period they usually present with delay in motor milestones.

CHAOS IN TERMINOLOGY

Much of the early complexity and confusion in this subject was caused by the absolute chaos in terminology (Table 12-1). Although some of the early authors gave very clear and lucid descriptions of the diseases they were describing (e.g. Werdnig, 1891; Hoffmann, 1893), others did not (Oppenheim, 1900), and later authors tended to use the same nomenclature for different disorders with different prognosis, or different nomenclature for the same disorder. Fortunately this is now past history and nondescript terms such as 'amyotonia congenita', 'universal muscle hypoplasia' and 'benign congenital hypotonia' have been relegated to the archives as more careful investigation of these patients has enabled us to place the vast majority into a specific diagnostic compartment.

Table 12-1 Chaos in terminology (historical)

Infantile progressive spinal muscular atrophy	Werdnig (1891)
	Hoffmann (1893)
Myatonia congenita	Oppenheim (1900)
Amyotonia congenita	Collier and Wilson (1908)
Benign congenital myopathy	Batten (1903)
	Turner (1940)
Congenital universal muscular hypoplasia	Krabbe (1947)
Amyotonia congenita = infantile muscular atrophy	Greenfield and Stern (1927)
Amyotonia congenita = symptom complex	Brandt (1950)
Essential or primary hypotonia	Sobel (1926)
Benign congenital hypotonia	Walton (1956)

A PRACTICAL APPROACH TO DIAGNOSIS AND CLASSIFICATION ———

When assessing a floppy infant, the first decision to make is whether one is dealing with a neuromuscular problem or whether the hypotonia is symptomatic of a disorder in the central nervous system or some other system outside the neuromuscular; in other words, a weak or paralysed infant with associated hypotonia, or a hypotonic infant without significant weakness. This distinction is usually fairly easy in practice, on the basis of whether the infant has or has not got a significant degree of weakness in association with the hypotonia. Simple manoeuvres such as the ability to sustain the limbs against gravity, or the withdrawal response of a limb to a painful stimulus, are helpful in making the distinction. However, it is important to note that there are occasional exceptions to this general rule of thumb, such as cases of congenital myotonic dystrophy, when patients may be very floppy, with associated respiratory and swallowing difficulty, and yet have antigravity power in the limbs, or a case of early onset nemaline myopathy where the patient has difficulty swallowing, general hypotonia, mild facial weakness and good limb power.

Table 12-2 Paralytic conditions with incidental hypotonia

1. Infantile spinal muscular atrophy
     Severe and intermediate forms (types 1 and 2)

2. Congenital muscular dystrophy

3. Congenital myotonic dystrophy

4. Neonatal myasthenia/congenital myasthenia

5. Congenital myopathies
     (a) Myotubular myopathy
     (b) Nemaline myopathy
     (c) Congenital fibre type disproportion
     (d) Central core disease

6. Metabolic myopathies
     Glycogenoses (types II, III, (IV, V, VII))
     Mitochondrial myopathies
     Lipid storage myopathies
     Periodic paralysis

7. Neuropathies
     Hereditary motor and sensory neuropathies
     (types I, II, ?III)
     Congenital hypomyelination syndrome
     Acquired: Guillain-Barré syndrome
                      Poliomyelitis

8. Other neuromuscular disorders

HYPOTONIA OF NEUROMUSCULAR ORIGIN

If the hypotonia is of neuromuscular origin the main causes are likely to be spinal muscular atrophy, congenital myotonic dystrophy, congenital muscular dystrophy, one of the congenital myopathies, or other less frequent conditions (Table 12-2). (Illustrative cases have been included in the appropriate earlier chapters.)

The degree and distribution of weakness may help to distinguish between these causes. Careful assessment should also be made of associated features which can be helpful in pointing to some of the disorders.

Facial muscle involvement. This is common in some of the congenital myopathies and myotonic dystrophy but not present in spinal muscle atrophy.

Sucking and swallowing difficulty. This is a common feature of severe spinal muscular atrophy (with bulbar involvement), congenital myotonic dystrophy, myotubular myopathy, nemaline myopathy and neonatal myasthenia, as well as some of the non-neuromuscular disorders such as Prader–Willi syndrome and birth asphyxia.

Ocular muscle involvement. This is a feature of mitochondrial myopathy and also of some congenital myopathies such as myotubular myopathy and of myotonic dystrophy.

Contractures. The presence of skeletal deformities and contractures is common in congenital muscular dystrophy and congenital myotonic dystrophy.

INVESTIGATIONS ———

Routine nerve conduction and electromyography (EMG) are helpful in trying to establish a neuromuscular cause, either a denervation process or a myopathy. In all cases with weakness this should be followed by a needle biopsy (under local anaesthesia), which is the only accurate way of establishing a definitive diagnosis, since the serum enzymes as well as EMG may be completely normal in some of these floppy infants with congenital myopathies, even in the presence of marked weakness.

The muscle biopsy may reveal a recognizable structural abnormality, but a small proportion of floppy infants, with associated weakness and subsequent delay in motor milestones and no evidence of abnormality in other systems, show an essentially normal-looking biopsy, or one with only minimal change. I have suggested that these may conveniently be designated 'minimal change myopathy', somewhat in line with the pathological situation in childhood nephrotic syndrome (see Chapter 3). Some of these are probably cases of congenital muscular dystrophy. In cases with an essentially normal muscle biopsy, one should carefully assess joint mobility, as many of these floppy infants may have marked joint laxity and be variants of Ehlers–Danlos syndrome, and may give a clinical impression of actual muscle weakness (see Tables 12-3, 12-4 and Figures 12-1 to 12-5).

Table 12-3 Non-paralytic conditions: hypotonia without significant weakness

1. Disorders of the central nervous system
    (a) Non-specific mental deficiency
    (b) Birth trauma, intracranial haemorrhage, intrapartum asphyxia and hypoxia
    (c) Hypotonic cerebral palsy
    (d) Metabolic disorders: lipidoses; (leucodystrophies); mucopolysaccharidoses; aminoacidurias; Leigh's syndrome
    (e) Chromosomal abnormalities Down's syndrome

2. Connective tissue disorders
    Congenital laxity of ligaments
    Ehlers–Danlos and Marfan syndromes
    Osteogenesis imperfecta; arachnodactyly

3. Prader–Willi syndrome

4. Metabolic; nutritional; endocrine
    Organic acidaemias; hypercalcaemia; rickets; coeliac disease; hypothyroidism; renal tubular acidosis

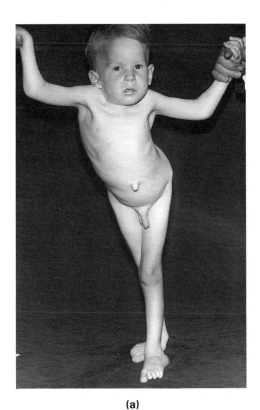

(a)

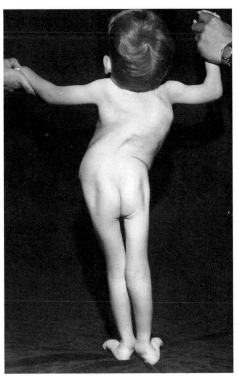

(b)

Figure 12-1a,b Hypotonia; laxity of ligaments; connective tissue disorder; ?Ehlers–Danlos syndrome. A 4-year-old boy presenting with delay in motor milestones and progressive scoliosis. Note associated calcaneo-valgus deformity and marked mobility of ankles. Muscle power, CK, nerve conduction and EMG normal.

HYPOTONIA ASSOCIATED WITH NON-NEUROMUSCULAR DISORDERS

There is a very wide range of disorders associated with many different systems that may have associated hypotonia, or indeed present with hypotonia and delayed motor milestones as a primary symptom (Table 12-3).

DISORDERS OF THE CENTRAL NERVOUS SYSTEM

These form the most common group of non-neuromuscular disorders associated with hypotonia. In every case presenting with hypotonia or delay in motor milestones, it is important to establish if the motor retardation is an isolated feature or whether there is also delay in other milestones, suggesting intellectual retardation, or the presence of other symptoms, such as convulsions. This would help to pinpoint a central nervous system disorder as a basis

for the hypotonia, and further distinction between various causes may result from specific clinical features. Thus the presence of brisk tendon reflexes and ankle clonus might point to a hypotonic cerebral palsy, the presence of characteristic stigmata to a chromosomal disorder such as Down's syndrome, and a history of a progressive deterioration in intellectual and other functions to a leucodystrophy or other progressive degenerative disorder of the nervous system. Slow nerve conduction velocity in leucodystrophies, which have an associated demyelinating peripheral neuropathy, is helpful in diagnosis, but other central nervous system disorders may have normal nerve conduction velocity and EMG pattern. Investigations should be aimed at the specific disorders within this group, including electrodiagnostic studies and brain imaging.

CONNECTIVE TISSUE DISORDERS

This is another important group of disorders which may present with hypotonia and delay in motor

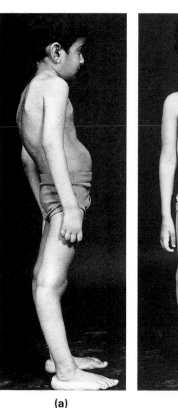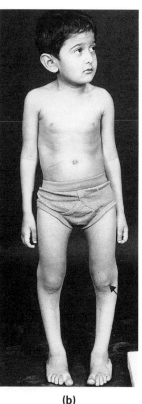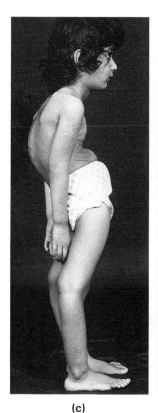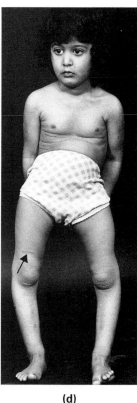

| (a) | (b) | (c) | (d) |

Figure 12-2 a-d   Ehlers–Danlos syndrome. This 4½-year-old boy (a,b) and his 3½-year-old sister (c,d) presented with a history of abnormal gait and delay in motor milestones. There was marked joint hypermobility with hyperextension of the knees, bowing of the legs and marked kyphosis. Both children also had wide parchment-like scars from old lacerations (arrows), suggesting Ehlers–Danlos syndrome. The CK, nerve conduction and EMG were normal and the muscle power was good.

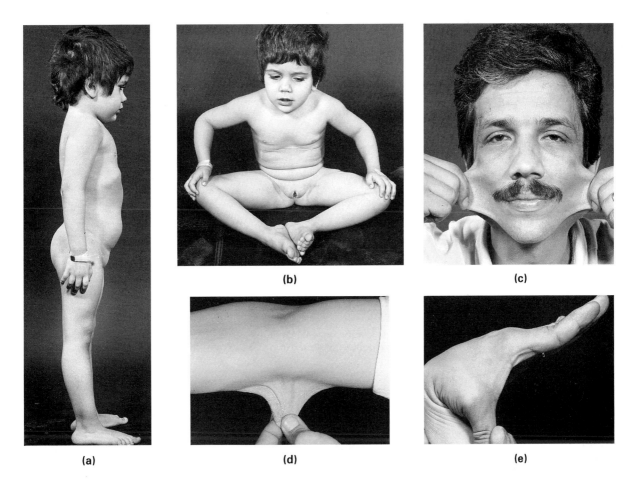

Figure 12-3 a-e Ehlers–Danlos syndrome/joint mobility. A 3-year-old girl with delay in motor milestones and increased joint mobility (a,b). Note valgus and everted posture of feet and slight hyperextension of knees. She also had bilateral congenital dislocation of the hips. She walked with support at 15 months but without support only at 2 years. There was slightly excessive elasticity of the skin. Her father had striking hyperelasticity of skin (c,d) and increased joint mobility (e).

milestones. In some cases there may be a close resemblance to disorders of the neuromuscular system, but careful assessment will usually reveal good muscle power, and the motor dysfunction is related to instability of joints, such as the knees or ankles, due to laxity of ligaments (Figures 12-1 to 12-5). The condition may be suspected because of an unusual range of joint mobility, such as hyperextending the metacarpophalangeal joints to 90°, approximating the thumb to the forearm or the dorsum of the foot to the front of the tibia, or abducting the hips, with little resistance, to 90°; or by the unusual posture of joints, such as hyperextension of the knees and eversion of the ankles

with standing, or the ability to do various contortions of the limbs. Many of these conditions are dominantly inherited and a history of 'double-jointedness' in one or other parent may provide a clue. Attention should also be given to the presence of other features such as blue scleral or hyperelastic skin in the patient or relatives and the occurrence of other connective tissue disorders such as osteogenesis imperfecta in the family.

This group of disorders has gained increasing prominence in recent years with the more accurate recognition of different syndromes, and subsyndromes, related to collagen structure (McKusick, 1972; Beighton, 1993; Royce and Steinmann, 1993).

Table 12-4 Subtypes of Ehlers–Danlos syndrome

Type	Special features/basic defect	Mode of inheritance
EDS I	Gravis type (severe basic features)	AD
EDS II	Mitis type (mild basic features)	AD
EDS III	Hypermobile type (predominantly joints)	AD
EDS IV	Vascular	
	IV-A acrogeric type	AD
	IV-B acrogeric type	AR
	IV-C ecchymotic type	AD
	IV-D others	
	(all forms have defect of type III collagen)	
EDS V	X-linked type	XL
EDS VI	Ocular-scoliotic type	AR
	VI-A decreased lysyl hydroxylase activity	
EDS VII	Arthrochalasis multiplex congenita (joint hypermobility, short stature, micrognathia)	
	VII-A structural defect of pro alpha 1(1) collagen	AD
	VII-B structural defect of pro alpha 2(1) collagen	AD
	(VII-C procollagen N-proteinase deficiency?)	AR
EDS VIII	Periodontitis type	AD
EDS IX	Vacant (formerly occipital horn syndrome; X-linked cutis laxa; now recategorized as a disorder of copper transport)	
EDS X	Fibronectin abnormality (normal skin texture; petechiae, striae, platelet aggregation)	AR
EDS XI	Vacant (formerly familial joint instability; recategorized with familial articular hypermobility syndromes)	

AD: autosomal dominant; AR: autosomal recessive; XL: X-linked.
After Beighton, 1993.

As in the case of the neuromuscular disorders, the new era of molecular genetics has had a major impact on the connective tissue disorders, and helped to define a molecular basis for many of these conditions, and has also helped to characterize some individual syndromes, such as the 11 different types of Ehlers–Danlos syndrome (Table 12-4).

The different clinical variants of Ehlers–Danlos syndrome are based predominantly on the associated features, in addition to the basic manifestations of joint hypermobility, skin hyperextensibility, dystrophic scarring of the skin and easy bruising, and connective tissue fragility (Beighton, 1993) (see Table 12-4).

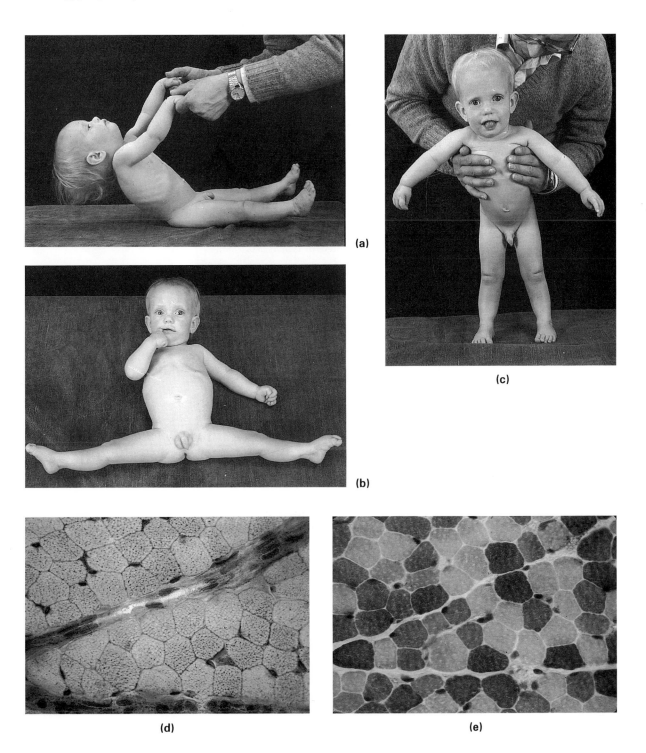

Figure 12-4a-e Joint laxity. This boy presented at 1 year with a history of marked hyotonia from birth, with delay in motor milestones, but a tendency to gradual improvement. He was still very floppy, with poor head control (a), and had marked joint hypermobility (b). He was able to take weight on his legs (c). In view of an impression of some associated weakness, a needle biopsy was done to exclude a congenital dystrophy. This was histologically and histochemically completely normal (d, Verhoeff–van Gieson; e, ATPase pH 9.4; serial sections). He walked unaided at 2 years and his tone and motor function continued to improve slowly. Currently at 6 years old, he manages at a normal school, although he still has some difficulty with mobility. This is the sort of patient who in the past might have been labelled as suffering from 'benign congenital hypotonia'.

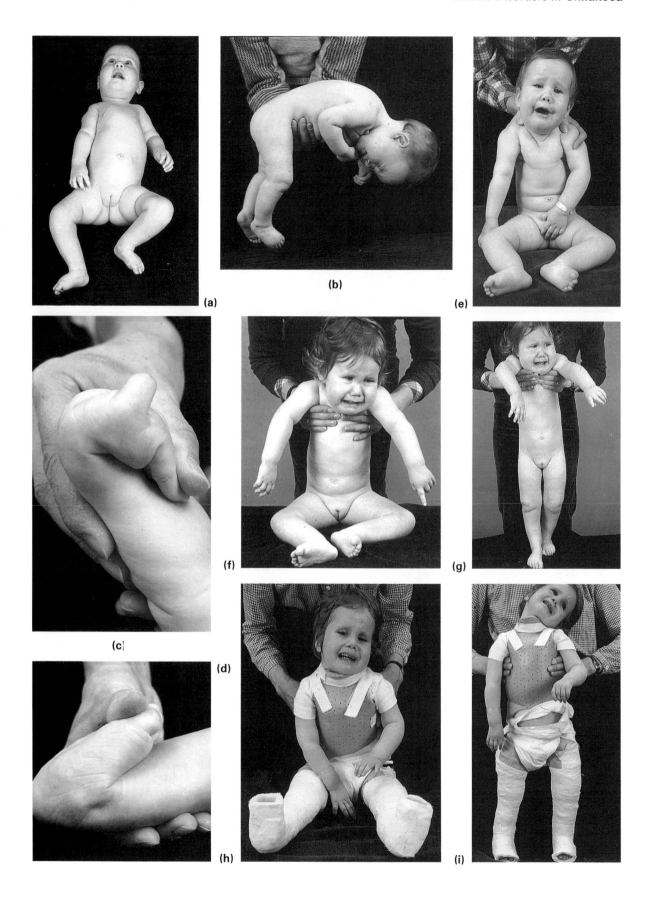

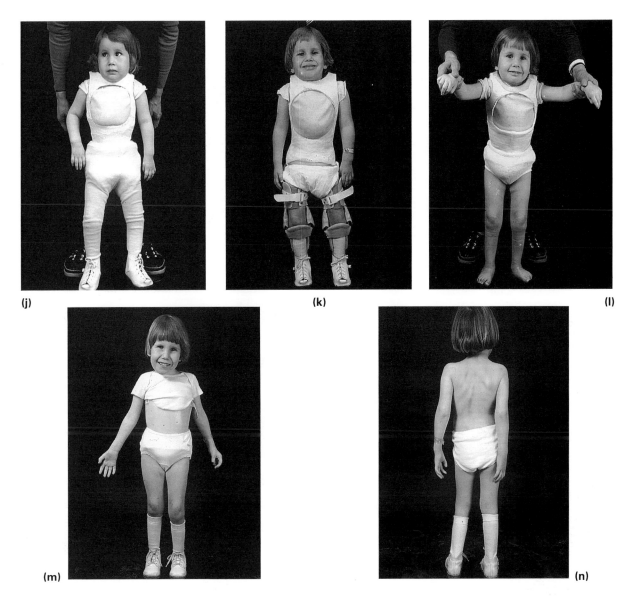

(j) (k) (l)

(m) (n)

Figure 12-5a-n Joint laxity mistaken for spinal muscular atrophy. This girl was referred for a second opinion at 6 months of age, with an established diagnosis of spinal muscular atrophy confirmed by muscle biopsy; a poor prognosis had been given. On examination the shape and movements of her chest seemed too good for an infant with SMA who had been floppy from birth and there also seemed to be relatively good movement of the legs (a) in spite of the hypotonic posture (b). There was a marked hypermobility of her joints, which was much more marked than that which usually accompanies the milder forms of SMA, with hyperextension of the wrists and fingers into approximation with the forearm (c) and also of the ankles with contact of the dorsum of the foot with the tibia (d). A diagnosis of laxity of ligaments was made, which was supported by normal conduction velocity with a good muscle action potential (unlike SMA) and a normal EMG. A repeat needle biopsy, to convince the parents, was also considered normal. A good prognosis was given. She showed slow but steady improvement in her motor function. At 9 months she was still extremely floppy and her condition had a superficial resemblance to SMA (e) but by 1 year she had better back posture (f) and was taking some weight on her legs (g). A plastazote jacket was made to control her incipient scoliosis (h). At 18 months she was sitting with minimal support (h) and efforts were made to get her standing in long-leg plaster casts (i). She still had poor head control (i). The scoliosis and spinal posture were better controlled with a plaster brace, and a year later, at about 2½ years of age, she was able to stand in gaiters (j). A few months later she walked in light-weight polyethylene callipers (k). By 3½ years she was standing well without leg supports (l) and was soon able to walk unsupported, although we advised continued use of the spinal brace to prevent progression of the scoliosis (m,n). At 6 years of age she is currently walking well and the scoliosis is unchanged. She still has joint hypermobility, but this is far less striking than originally. She also has subluxation of one hip but was advised against active treatment or surgical intervention.

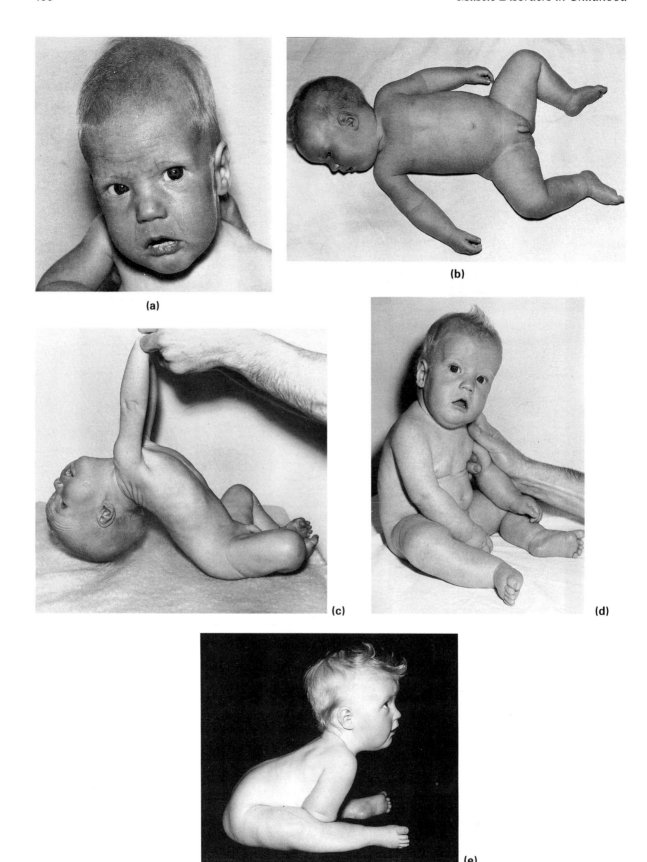

(a)

(b)

(c)

(d)

(e)

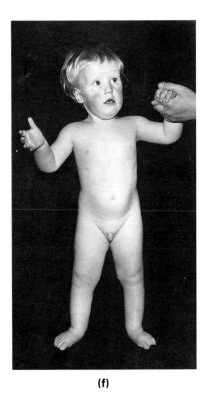
(f)

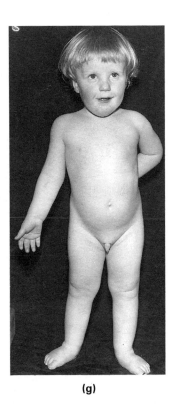
(g)

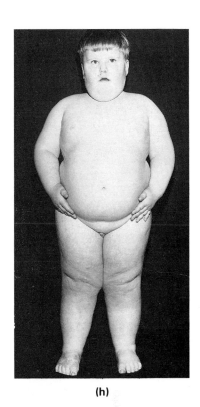
(h)

Figure 12-6a-h Prader–Willi syndrome. This infant was born at home, 3 weeks prematurely, with birthweight of 2490 g. During pregnancy, fetal movements were often absent for up to 3 days. He was admitted to hospital at 2½ hours with hypothermia (93°F, 34°C), profound hypotonia and immobility. He was unable to suck or swallow and had a very weak cry. Moro and grasp reflexes and all tendon jerks were absent. He was fair-haired and blue-eyed and had an unusual facies with high forehead, dolicocephalic-shaped head, small almond-shaped eyes and a small triangular-shaped mouth (a). The penis was small, the scrotum rudimentary and both testes undescended. At 2 weeks he was still grossly hypotonic, with severe head lag, but there were spontaneous limb movements. Initially, a diagnosis of 'benign congenital hypotonia' was made. By 5 weeks limb movements improved further and he was able to suck, but still needed tube feeding. He first smiled at 9 weeks. Knee jerks could first be elicited at 13 weeks and all tendon reflexes were present by 8 months. At 4 months he had some head control when supported in sitting position (a) but still had a frog posture (b) and marked head lag in supine (c). He subsequently showed a steady improvement and by 7 months was able to sit with support (d). At 11 months he was sitting without support (e) and was also able to stand unsupported. He was standing well and walking with one hand held by 20 months (f), and was able to walk unaided by 26 months (g). His weight remained below the third centile from birth to about 30 weeks, after which it rose to around the 80th centile by one year and remained at that level till about 3 years, when it increased precipitously and by 5 years had reached 42 kg, which was more than twice the 90th centile for this age (h). Height, in contrast, remained just below the 50th centile. Bone age was consistently retarded, and at 5 years was at about a 2-year level. Despite attempts at dietary restriction his weight continued to rise. Early intellectual development seemed reasonable and retardation seemed predominantly motor, but later he showed unequivocal delay in intellectual milestones and his intelligence quotient was found to be about 60. During a respiratory infection at 17 months he had two convulsions lasting about 5 minutes each. He had three further short convulsions at 3 years of age. Chromosome karyotype and glucose tolerance tests were normal. He died unexpectedly at home, aged 8 years. Autopsy did not show any structural or microscopic abnormality in the brain.

PRADER–WILLI SYNDROME ———————

This unusual syndrome was originally recognized by Prader, Labhardt and Willi (1956), who described five male and four female patients with adiposity, short stature, mental subnormality, undescended testes in the males, and a history of marked hypo-

tonia and feeding difficulty in the newborn period. Motor milestones were delayed but the hypotonia gradually decreased. Prader and Willi (1963) subsequently reviewed a series of 14 cases. I saw my first two cases presenting as floppy infants in early 1962, within a few weeks of each other (Figures 12-6 and 12-7).

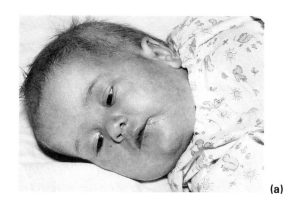

(a)

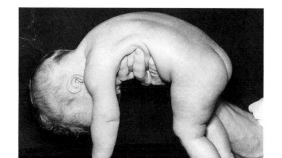

(b)

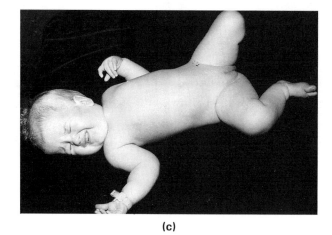

(c)

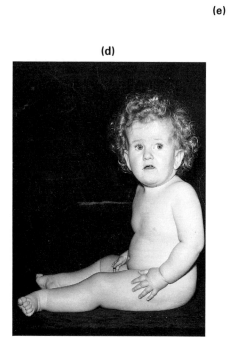

(d)

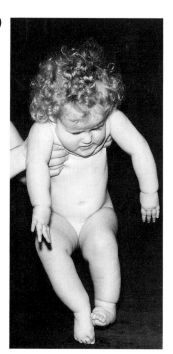

(e)

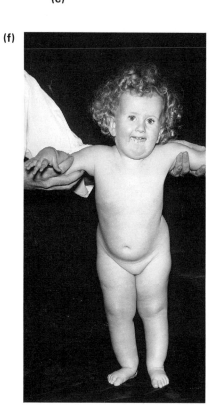

(f)

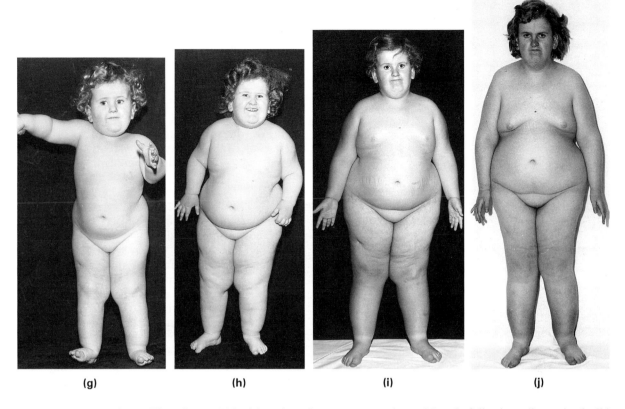

(g)   (h)   (i)   (j)

Figure 12-7a-j Prader–Willi syndrome. This girl was born by caesarean section at 36 weeks following a diagnosis of mild diabetes in the mother. Birthweight was 3430 g. She was very hypotonic at birth, slow to cry and was unable to suck or swallow. Her facies and dolicocephalic head (a) were strikingly similar to a previous patient (see Figure 12-6), seen a few weeks earlier. At 6 weeks she was still fed by tube (gavage) and had generalized hypotonia but good spontaneous limb movements (b,c). Note the characteristic Prader–Willi facies with crying (c). Knee and ankle jerks were easily elicited, but other tendon jerks were absent. By 10 weeks she was sucking normally, starting to smile, and taking an interest in her surroundings. At 15 weeks she could raise her head when prone. There was gradual improvement and by 9 months she was sitting with support, and by 1 year unsupported. At 15 months she was sitting quite steadily (d) but was still unable to support her weight standing (e). She was standing with support by 19 months (f) and at 2½ years was walking with one hand held (g). She did not walk without support till 3½ years. At 6 months she had several short episodes of unconsciousness, suggestive of convulsions, but these did not recur. Her weight remained around the 50th centile until 2 years but then rose precipitously (g,h) and by 4 years 4 months (h) was almost double the 90th centile at 34.5 kg. Her height, in contrast, was at the 10th centile and her bone age at a 2-year level. Weight continued to increase despite advice and efforts at dietary restriction, which was very difficult to enforce (i, aged 8 years; j, aged 15 years). Initially her intellectual development seemed reasonable and by 15 months she had a good vocabulary of simple words and good manipulative (motor) skills. However, she later had retardation of intellectual development and, despite speaking in full sentences, her comprehension was below normal and she experienced difficulty at school. Glucose tolerance curve was normal (at 5 years) and chromosome karyotype was normal.

The syndrome usually presents with profound hypotonia at birth and there is usually marked feeding difficulty, necessitating tube feeding, but no associated respiratory difficulties. The cry is often very weak and high-pitched. The infant is frequently also below 3000 g at term. There is a characteristic facies with a high forehead, dolicocephalic head, small almond-shaped eyes and an open triangular-shaped mouth. The hair is usually very fair and the eyes blue. The hands and feet are small. Another characteristic feature is the unusual appearance of the face with crying, which I think is quite pathognomonic in appearance (see Figures 12-7c and 12-8b).

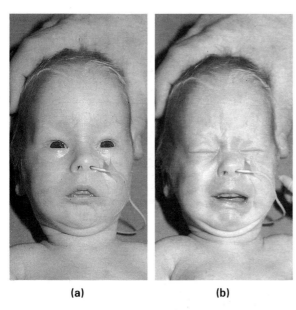

(a)   (b)

Figure 12-8a,b Prader–Willi syndrome. A 2-week-old infant presenting with marked hypotonia and feeding difficulty from birth. Note the characteristic facies (a) and the typical Prader–Willi facies with crying (b).

Although difficult to describe, essentially there is an unusual degree of screwing up and wrinkling of the face. Attempts can be made to make the infant cry by squeezing a toe or pinching the arm. They also seem to have a high threshold of response to painful stimuli.

The hypotonia gradually improves and eventually these children pass various motor milestones and achieve the ability to walk, usually after the age of 2 years.

There is a tendency to gross generalized obesity, which usually develops after the child starts walking but in some there is already a tendency earlier on. Once obesity becomes established, diet control is very difficult and there is an associated hyperphagia which is very difficult to handle in the older children. However, if one can condition these infants to a restricted food intake from early infancy, and try to avoid them crossing any centile lines for weight, one may succeed in maintaining a reasonable weight. Some of these infants do not seem to have a spontaneous hunger drive, but will eat any amount of food presented to them, whereas others will go searching for food and seem to have a hunger drive. They also seem to have no sense of satiety and can go on eating indefinitely without feeling full.

Growth is stunted and the majority are below the 50th percentile and also have retarded bóne age.

The males usually have undescended testes and a rudimentary scrotum, but do develop secondary sex characteristics. The testes are present intra-abdominally.

There is associated intellectual impairment and the IQ usually falls in the low normal to mildly retarded range. The deficit in intelligence is often less striking in early infancy.

Diabetes of the adult type tends to develop in adolescence and an abnormal glucose tolerance curve may be obtained in childhood on standard testing or with steroid provocation. This is probably a reflection of the obesity and overeating and can be prevented by adequate dietary control.

Associated features

There is a high frequency of associated convergent squint, convulsions, and behaviour problems, such as temper tantrums or rage reactions. Some may show an obsessive behaviour and be difficult to rationalize with in relation to these temper outbursts. There is also an associated scoliosis in some cases, which can be progressive, but rarely needs surgical treatment. Some patients seem to react adversely to minor infections and become unduly ill or even septicaemic. There is a tendency to obstructive apnoea and also a Pickwickian syndrome, with daytime hypersomnolence, which may partly relate to the associated obesity.

Administration of growth hormone to these children has produced a growth spurt and also improved the general appearance and body habitus in anecdotal reports. Controlled studies are currently in progress.

Genetic advances

Interest focused on the short arm of chromosome 15 following the discovery of unbalanced translocations involving this area in cases of Prader–Willi syndrome (Fraccaro et al., 1977; Kucerová et al., 1979; Berry et al., 1981) and the subsequent detection of deletions by high resolution chromosome banding techniques (Ledbetter et al., 1981). In a study of 19 of our cases (Fear et al., 1985), we found deletion to be present in about 50%. There was no apparent distinction in clinical phenotype between those with and those without the deletion. It was subsequently observed that the deletion seemed to be consistently in the paternal 15 chromosome (Butler and Palmer, 1983) and sophisticated studies with chromosome-specific DNA probes established that patients without a deletion usually had two copies of the maternal chromosome, and were missing the paternal contribution, an example of uniparental maternal disomy or genomic imprinting. Of interest was the additional discovery that in cases of Angelmann syndrome (which is clinically distinct from Prader–Willi syndrome) there is a similar deletion in chromosome 15q11-13, but involving the maternal contribution, and those patients without the deletion may be disomic for the paternal chromosome.

Further molecular studies have recently identified a possible candidate gene coding for a small nuclear ribonucleoprotein polypeptide N (SNRPN) (Ozcelik *et al.*, 1992) in the Prader–Willi syndrome critical region, which is absent in a mouse model of Prader–Willi syndrome (Cattanach *et al.*, 1992) and also shows maternal imprinting in the mouse (Leff *et al.*, 1992).

Genomic DNA probes are now available within the Prader–Willi deletion area which may help in the confirmation of clinical diagnosis by demonstrating a deletion at the molecular level.

METABOLIC DISORDERS ————————————

In recent years a number of metabolic disorders affecting the newborn or occurring in infancy have been recognized, which can produce a profound degree of hypotonia in the newborn period or later (Table 12-3). One such group is the organic acid-aemias, and any newborn infants with unexplained hypotonia should have a routine check of the blood gases and pH to detect a metabolic acidosis, which should be followed by lactic acid estimation, as there is often an associated lactic acidosis. The hypotonia in this condition, as with other metabolic disorders, responds to treatment of the underlying problem and presumably has a metabolic basis affecting the function of the neuromuscular system (Keeton and Moosa, 1976). The hypotonia in these infants is usually disproportionate to any underlying weakness and they will usually be able to sustain the limbs against gravity. I think they are thus best categorized under this general group of disorders, rather than the neuromuscular, since investigations should be aimed outside the neuromuscular system.

REFERENCES ————————————

Batten, F.E. (1903) Three cases of myopathy, infantile type. *Brain* **26**: 147.

Beighton, P. (1993) *McKusick's Heritable Disorders of Connective Tissue* 5th edn. St Louis: Mosby.

Berry, A.C., Whittingham, A.J. and Neville, B.G.R. (1981) Chromosome 15 in floppy infants. *Archives of Disease in Childhood* **56**: 882–885.

Brandt, S. (1950) Werdnig-Hoffmann's infantile progressive muscular atrophy. *Opera ex domo biologiae hereditariae humanae universitatis hafniensis* Vol. 22. Copenhagen: Ejnar Munksgaard.

Butler, M.G. and Palmer, C.G. (1983) Paternal origin of chromosome 15 deletion in Prader–Willi syndrome. *Lancet* **1**: 1285–1286.

Cattanach, B.M., Barr, J.A., Evans, E.P. *et al.* (1992) A candidate mouse model for Prader–Willi syndrome which shows an absence of *Snrpn* expression. *Nature Genetics* **2**: 270–274.

Collier, J. and Wilson, S.A.K. (1908) Amyotonia congenita. *Brain* **31**: 1.

Dubowitz, V. (1969) *The Floppy Infant*. Clinics in Developmental Medicine, No. 31. London: Spastics International/Heinemann.

Dubowitz, V. (1980) *The Floppy Infant* 2nd edn, Clinics in Developmental Medicine, No. 76. Cambridge: Cambridge University Press.

Fear, C.N., Mutton, D.E., Berry, A.C. *et al.* (1985) Chromosome 15 in Prader–Willi syndrome. *Developmental Medicine and Child Neurology* **27**: 305–311.

Fraccaro, M., Zuffardi, O., Buhler, E.M. *et al.* (1977) 15/15 translocation in Prader–Willi syndrome. *Journal of Medical Genetics* **14**: 275–276.

Greenfield, J.G. and Stern, R.O. (1927) Anatomical identity of Werdnig-Hoffmann and Oppenheim forms of infantile muscular atrophy. *Brain* **50**: 652.

Hoffmann, J. (1893) Ueber chronische spinale Muskel-atrophie im Kindesalter auf familiarer Basis. *Deutsche Zeitschrift für Nervenheilkunde* **3**: 427–470.

Keeton, B.R. and Moosa, A. (1947) Organicaciduria: a rare cause of the floppy infant syndrome. *Archives of Disease in Childhood* **51**: 636–638.

Krabbe, H. (1947) Kongenit generaliseret muskelaplasia. Dansk neurologisk selskabs forhandlinger. *Nordisk Medicin* **325**: 1756.

Kucerová, M., Strakova, M. and Polivková, Z. (1979) The Prader–Willi syndrome with a 15/3 translocation. *Journal of Medical Genetics* **16**: 234–235.

Ledbetter, D.H., Riccardi, V.M., Airhart, S.D. *et al.* (1981) Deletions of chromosome 15 as a cause of the Prader–Willi syndrome. *New England Journal of Medicine* **304**: 325–328.

Leff, S., Brannan, C.I., Reed, M.L. *et al.* (1992) Maternal imprinting of the mouse *Snrpn* gene and conserved linkage homology with the human Prader–Willi syndrome region. *Nature Genetics* **2**: 259–264.

McKusick, V. (1972) *Heritable Disorders of Connective Tissue* 4th edn. St Louis: Mosby, p. 687.

Oppenheim, H. (1900) Ueber allgemeine und localisierte Atonie der Muskulatur (Myatonie) im frühen Kindesalter. *Monatsschrift für Psychiatrie und Neurologie* **8**: 232.

Ozcelik, T., Leff, S., Robinson, W. *et al.* (1992) Small nuclear ribonucleoprotein polypeptide N (SNRPN), an expressed gene in the Prader–Willi syndrome critical region. *Nature Genetics* **2**: 265–269.

Prader, A. and Willi, H. (1963) Das Syndrom von Imbezillitat, Adipositas, Muskelhypotonie, Hypogonadismus und Diabetes Mellitus mit 'Myotonie'-Anamnese. In: *Verhand 2nd International Kongress der Psychiatrie und Entwicklungs-Storungen die Kindesalter, Vienna, 1961* Part 1. Basel and New York: Karger, p.353.

Prader, A., Labhardt, A. and Willi, H. (1956) Ein Syndrom von Adipositas, Kleinwuchs, Kryptorchismus und Oligophrenie nach myotonieartigem Zustand im Neugeborenenalter. *Schweizerische medizinische Wochenschrift* **86**: 1260.

Royce, P.M. and Steinmann, B. (1993) *Connective Tissue and its Heritable Disorders: Molecular, Genetic, and Medical Aspects.* New York: Wiley-Liss.

Sobel, J. (1926) Essential or primary hypotonia in young children. *Medical Journal and Record* **124**: 225.

Turner, J.W.A. (1940) The relationship between amyotonia congenita and congenital myopathy. *Brain* **63**: 163.

Walton, J.N. (1956) Amyotonia congenita: a follow-up study. *Lancet* **i**: 1023.

Werdnig, G. (1891) Zwei frühinfantile hereditäre Fälle von progressiver Muskelatrophie unter dem Bilde der Dystrophie, aber auch neurotischer Grundlage. *Archiv fur Psychiatrie und Nervenkrankheiten* **22**: 437–481.

CHAPTER 13

Disorders with Muscle Contracture and Joint Rigidity

Several conditions exist in which the predominant problem is not so much a weakness of the muscle but a limitation of the full range of movement of a joint as a result of permanent shortening of muscles. Although they comprise a rather heterogeneous group of clinical syndromes, I shall discuss them collectively in this chapter as they have a number of clinical features in common.

ARTHROGRYPOSIS

This is a symptom complex characterized by congenital rigidity of the joints, and is not a specific diagnostic entity (Greek: *arthron* – joint; *gryposis* – a bending). Although the title draws attention to the deformity of the joints, the underlying pathology is often in the muscles or supporting tissues rather than within the joint itself and any ankylosis of the joints is likely to be fibrous rather than bony. By definition, arthrogryposis involves multiple joints and the distal joints more than the proximal, so that the feet and ankles and the hands and wrists are likely to be more affected.

CHAOS IN TERMINOLOGY

Arthrogryposis has gone through much the same chaos in terminology as did the floppy infant syndrome (see Chapter 12), which had the effect of making a complex syndrome out of what is really a symptom complex occurring in several different disease situations.

A number of reports on rigidity of joints at birth appeared in the German and French literature of the second half of the nineteenth century and Rocher (1913) was able to review 31 reported cases and to delineate a clinical condition for which he suggested the title 'multiple congenital articular rigidity'. In 1923 Stern introduced the term 'arthrogryposis multiplex congenita' and subsequently Middleton (1934), in an exhaustive review of the subject, suggested 'myodystrophica congenita'. Sheldon (1932) looked upon the disease as a primary deficiency of muscle fibres, or whole muscles, and suggested the title 'amyoplasia congenita'. Later, Rossi (1947) capped it with 'arthromyodysplasia congenita'. The term 'arthrogryposis multiplex congenita' has been widely used, although 'amyoplasia congenita' has become popular in recent years, particularly amongst geneticists, with attempts to define a specific syndrome on clinical grounds.

PATHOGENESIS

Whilst some of the early authors drew attention to the pathological changes in the muscle, often of a dystrophic nature (Banker *et al.*, 1957; Pearson and Fowler, 1963), others documented evidence of denervation in the muscle and suggested abnormality of the anterior horn cells of the cord (Brandt, 1947; Wolf *et al.*, 1955; Byers and Banker, 1961; Krugliak *et al.*, 1978). It should be stressed that most cases of classical infantile spinal muscular atrophy (Werdnig–Hoffmann disease) tend to be floppy and the only common contractures seen are mild limitation of extension of the knees, or abduction of the hips and external rotation of the shoulders, and it is unusual to get fixed deformities of distal joints (see Chapter 8). This suggests that cases of arthrogryposis associated with anterior horn cell disease represent a different neurogenic syndrome. Hall and her colleagues (1982) tried to define and delineate various sydromes of arthrogryposis from a clinical and genetic point of view.

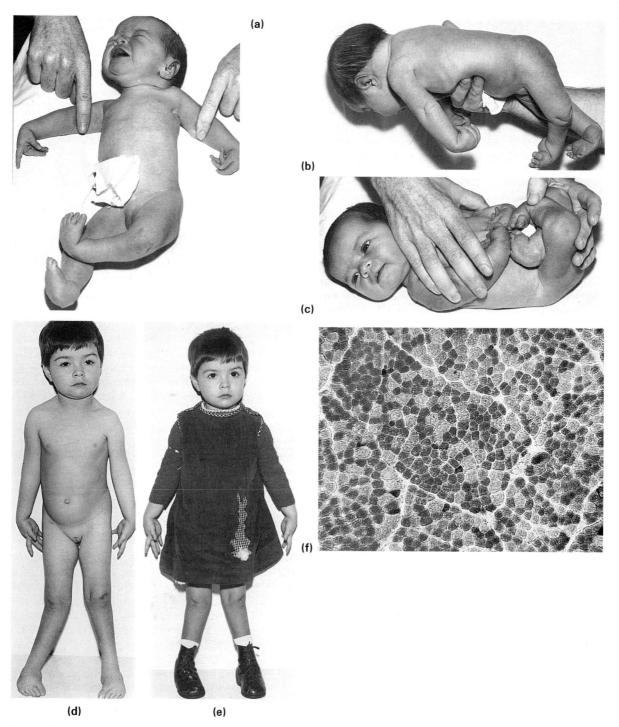

Figure 13-1a-f 'Arthrogryposis', ? cause. Following a normal pregnancy, during which there was no illness or drug therapy, this girl was born with striking deformities of the ankles, knees and wrists (a). She was bright and alert and her head and trunk control were good (b). She could be folded back into her presumptive intrauterine posture (c). There was associated bilateral dislocation of the hips. The deformities of the feet were partially corrected by passive stretching and splinting but subsequently required operative procedures. The hips were unstable and needed operative reduction. The wrists improved on passive and active exercises, but she was unable to extend them beyond the neutral position. The child was able to walk by the age of 2 years and in spite of her deformities subsequently coped well at an ordinary school (d,e). A biopsy obtained at the time of operative procedure on the feet showed a normal histological pattern and normal distribution of fibre types, with some variation in fibre size (f).

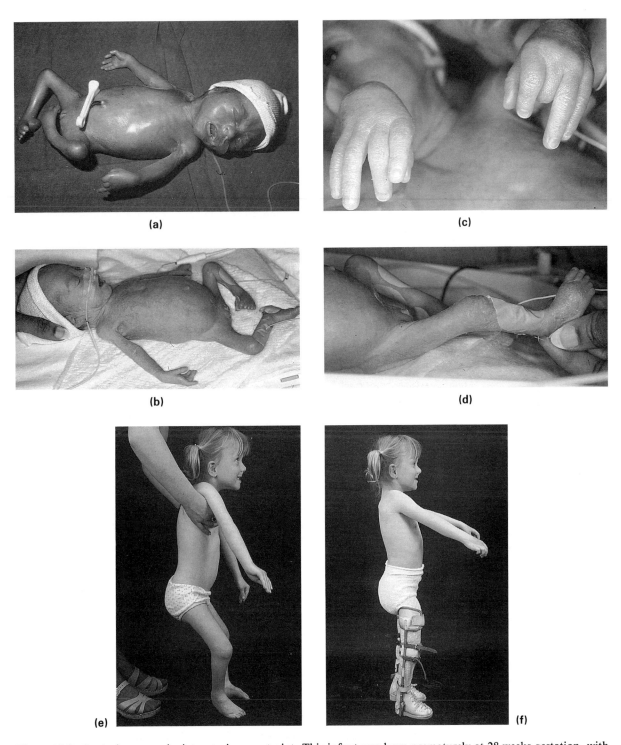

Figure 13-2a-f Arthrogryposis; intrauterine constraint. This infant was born prematurely at 28 weeks gestation, with severe contractures affecting all the joints of the lower limbs and to a lesser extent also the hands (a). She managed remarkably well without much respiratory support but needed tube feeding for several weeks. As she seemed to have good spontaneous movements of her limbs, it was thought unlikely that there was an underlying neuromuscular disorder, but that the arthrogryposis was probably due to intrauterine constraint, associated with a bicornuate uterus in the mother. Gentle passive exercises achieved a considerable increase in the range of movements of hands and legs within the first few weeks (b-d) and, following further surgical corrections, she subsequently achieved ambulation with callipers and support by 3 years and independently by 5 years (e,f).

If one looks upon arthrogryposis merely as a symptom complex, the common denominator in relation to the postural deformities is the presence of immobility of the limbs *in utero*. This could be the result of muscle paralysis, which could be caused by major problems within the central nervous system, such as myelomeningocoele or other syndromes with dysgenesis or malformation in the nervous system, or within the peripheral nervous system, including the anterior horn cells, the peripheral nerve, the neuromuscular junction or the muscle itself. In other cases, the neuromuscular system itself may be normal but the deformity results from crowding and immobilization of the fetus *in utero* from extraneous causes such as oligohydramnios, or uterine malformations such as bicornuate uterus (Figures 13-1, 13-2).

The deformities relate to the posture *in utero* and the infant can often be folded back into its *in utero* position (see Figures 13-1, 13-4). Thus, in most cases with the usual cephalic presentation and flexed position of the legs over the abdomen, the common deformity is an equinovarus of the feet and fixed flexion contractures at the knees and possibly the hips. The arms are usually flexed over the chest with the wrists against the chin, resulting in flexion deformities of the wrists and elbows, and possibly also producing hypognathia of the jaw (Figures 13-1, 13-4).

In contrast, the infant with a breech presentation and extended legs may have a calcaneovalgus deformity of the feet and fixed extension of the knees with limitation of flexion in association with fixed flexion contractures of the hips (Figure 13-3). Paradoxically, there may actually be hypotonia of muscles within their range of movement and at times an associated dislocation of the hips.

CLINICAL SYNDROMES ————————————

Central nervous system disorders

Arthrogryposis may be an associated feature of a wide range of syndromes associated with various developmental disorders, dysplasias and malformations in the central nervous system (Hageman *et al.*, 1987). It is of interest that in a recent review of 99 personal cases of arthrogryposis over a 25-year period, Banker (1994) classified 91 as neurogenic and only 8 as myopathic. A large proportion of the neurogenic cases had major disorders of the central nervous system, which probably reflects the more serious and potentially fatal disorders coming to the attention of a neuropathologist. The relative case load of myopathies in a paediatric muscle clinic may well be very different and the neonatologist is also more likely to meet with some of the myopathies and lower motor neurone disorders, once the major central nervous system cases are excluded.

Vuopala *et al.* (1995) recently reviewed 83 cases of lethal arthrogryposis, associated with either a stillborn fetus, a termination of pregnancy following a prenatal diagnosis, or death within 28 days postnatally. Sixty-seven cases were neurogenic in origin, including 41 with the so-called lethal congenital contracture syndrome, 15 with milder anterior horn cell involvement, and ten with dysgenesis and degeneration of the central nervous system. Congenital muscular dystrophy was seen in two cases, nemaline myopathy in one, and a non-neuromuscular cause was established in ten cases.

A complex syndrome that may present with arthrogryposis in the newborn period, in association with swallowing difficulties and later addition of developmental problems, hearing loss and epilepsy is associated with a migration disorder and central microgyria (Figure 13-4) (Kuzniecky *et al.*, 1989, 1993; Aicardi, 1991; Guerrini *et al.*, 1992) The muscle biopsy is normal.

Anterior horn cell disorders

Some cases of arthrogryposis of neurogenic origin may be associated with involvement of the anterior horn cells of the cord. These cases probably represent disorders distinct from classical severe infantile spinal muscular atrophy (SMA) (Werdnig–Hoffmann disease) and with the current resolution of the molecular genetic abnormality in spinal muscular atrophy and the recognition of consistent deletions in the gene area in the vast majority of cases (see Chapter 8) it should now be possible to exclude classical SMA in these cases.

Peripheral neuropathies

Congenital hypomyelination neuropathy, a severe and often fatal newborn disorder, which may represent a severe variant of autosomal recessive, hereditary motor and sensory neuropathy type III (see Chapter 9), is often associated with severe arthrogryposis (Karch and Urich, 1975; Seitz *et al.*, 1986; Charnas *et al.*, 1988; Gabreëls-Festen *et al.*, 1994). Other forms of peripheral neuropathy may also present with arthrogryposis (Figure 13-5).

Neonatal myasthenia

Infants with severe arthrogryposis may be born to myasthenic mothers and the recurrence in sequential pregnancies suggests that this is a severe variant of neonatal myasthenia (see Chapter 10).

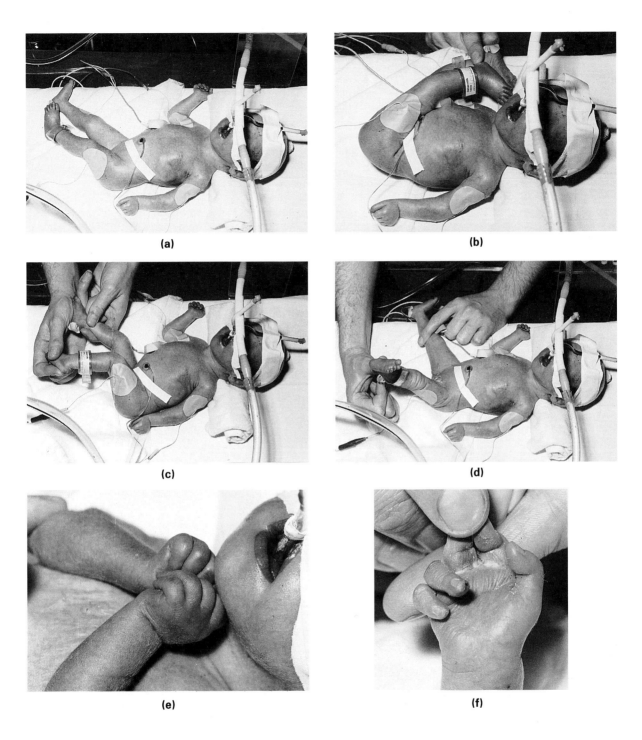

Figure 13-3a-f Arthrogryposis; extended breech; ? congenital muscular dystrophy. One-day-old infant born by caesarian section following spontaneous onset of labour at 34 weeks, because of neonatal death at 30 minutes of first infant born at term by breech with extended legs. Associated respiratory problems needing ventilator support (a). She could readily be folded back into the *in utero* breech position (b). Note the extended legs, with hyperextended knees and fully flexed hips. This was associated with limitation in flexion of the knees and of extension and abduction of the hips (c,d). The arms were folded into a flexed position on the chest, with wrists extended and fingers flexed (e). Note the difficulty in opening the hands and extending the fingers (f). Needle biopsy of the quadriceps showed an unequivocally pathological picture, with retention of bundle pattern but marked variation of fibre size and focal degenerative change, compatible with a congenital muscular dystrophy. She died on the second day.

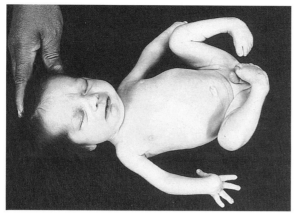

(a)

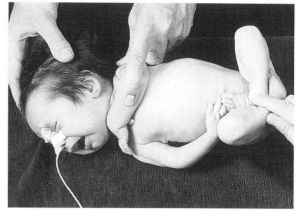

(b)

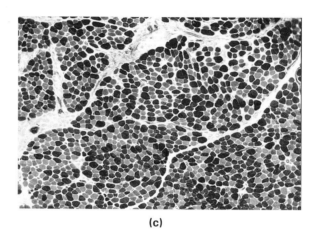

(c)

(d)

(e)

(f)

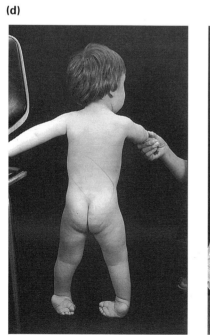

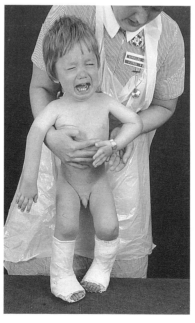

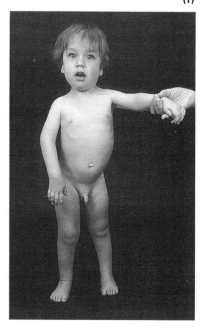

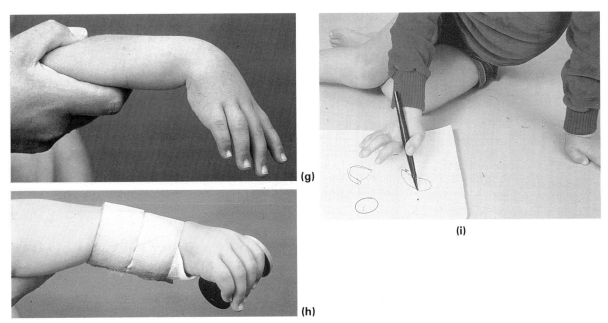

(g)

(i)

(h)

Figure 13-4a-i Arthrogryposis; central polymicrogyria. This child was born with severe deformities of feet and hands (a) and could readily be folded back into his intrauterine posture (b). A provisional diagnosis of congenital dystrophy was made at his referral hospital, on the basis of an open biopsy of quadriceps, and a poor prognosis was given. However, the biopsy was considered within the normal range apart from some variability in fibre size (c) and a guardedly good prognosis was suggested. Surgery was deferred. At 2 years of age, once he was able to stand well with support, his feet were corrected (d-f), following which he stood and walked well. The deformities of his hands improved with passive stretching, but he had persistent wrist-drop and function was helped by a dynamic splint (g-i). Associated severe swallowing difficulty from birth with submucosal cleft palate was overcome gradually from 10 months of age, with a programme of active 'forced' feeding. He also had associated hearing loss and speech delay. He continued to walk well and showed a slow but steady improvement in his speech and comprehension. At age 12 he unexpectedly developed convulsions and magnetic resonance imaging of the brain showed a migration abnormality with microectopic foci of cortex (central polymicrogyria).

(a) **(b)**

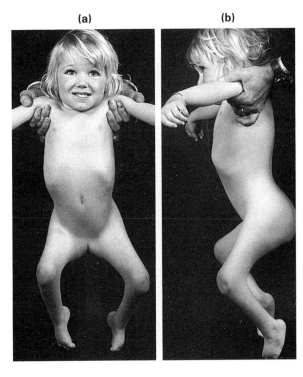

Figure 13-5a,b Arthrogryposis. Peripheral neuropathy. This 3-year-old child was born by breech delivery at 38 weeks and had stiff joints with contractures at the hips, knees and wrists from birth (a,b). During pregnancy mother thought movements were sparse. She took no drugs of note. The early motor milestones were normal and the child sat by a year. Her intellectual development was normal. The hands improved spontaneously but she needed operations for straightening of the knees and ankles at 2 years. She still had weakness of the shoulder girdle and legs. CK was normal (94 iu/litre). The ulnar nerve conduction velocity was very slow (21 m/s). She was uncooperative for EMG examination. ECG showed a tremulous baseline as in spinal muscular atrophy. Biopsy was deferred pending further corrective procedures. Nerve conduction in the parents was normal. The underlying pathology seems to be a demyelinating peripheral neuropathy, either sporadic or of recessive inheritance.

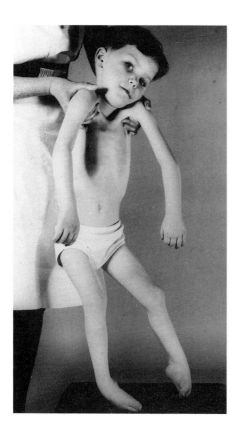

Figure 13-6 Arthrogryposis. Congenital muscular dystrophy. This child was born by normal delivery at term. He was hypotonic from birth, a slow feeder and subsequently delayed in motor milestones. He was able to sit by 7 months, but unable to roll over and never able to crawl or stand. When assessed at 6 years he still had generalized hypotonia, with muscle wasting and weakness and poor head control and was unable to support his body weight. There was fixed equinus of both feet of about 40°, fixed flexion of hips of 30° and of the knees of 20°. CK was normal (46 iu/litre), the EMG myopathic and the ulnar nerve conduction normal (55 m/s). Muscle biopsy (rectus femoris) showed a dystrophic picture, with variation in fibre size and proliferation of fat and connective tissue, compatible with congenital muscular dystrophy.

Myopathies

Arthrogryposis is a common manifestation in a number of individual myopathies presenting at birth, such as the severe X-linked form of myotubular myopathy, congenital myotonic dystrophy and congenital muscular dystrophy (Figure 13-6). These have been reviewed in the appropriate sections relating to these diseases. It may also be a less frequent association in other congenital myopathies.

Medication during pregnancy

Various medications given to the mother during pregnancy may have a direct effect on the peripheral nerve, the neuromuscular junction or the muscle itself, producing weakness and possibly an associated arthrogryposis. Jago (1970) described a newborn infant with arthrogryposis, whose mother had been treated with curare derivatives for tetanus around the tenth to twelfth week of gestation. This seems analogous to the neonatal arthrogryposis in infants of myasthenic mothers with the autoimmune disease. Philpot *et al.* (1995) documented an infant with symmetrical brachial plexus weakness and postural abnormality of the hands, whose mother had been treated for nausea and renal tract infection in early pregnancy with Debendox (Bendectin) and nitrofurantoin, both of which can cause peripheral neuropathy. A careful history of potentially significant medication during pregnancy is important in all cases of arthrogryposis.

Miscellaneous syndromes

Arthrogryposis may be an incidental feature of complex syndromes of chromosomal or genetic origin, such as trisomy 18, which is often associated with postural abnormality of the feet and flexion deformities with overlap of the fingers, and Pena–Shokeir syndrome(s), where arthrogryposis is but one manifestation of a multisystem, dysmorphic syndrome (Pena and Shokeir, 1974a,b).

Constraint in utero

In some cases of arthrogryposis the muscle is surprisingly normal on biopsy and this would account for the absence of specific weakness and the relatively good prognosis in many of them. It is possible that congenital absence or underdevelopment of some muscle groups may be a factor in some cases, but again this could be secondary to immobility *in utero*. Bizarre deformities of the joints are a regular feature of Potter's syndrome, with renal agenesis in the fetus and associated severe oligohydramnios, which accounts for the immobility of the fetus *in utero*.

Arthrogryposis is also a feature of oligohydramnios of other causes, such as leakage of liquor following premature rupture of membranes, and there is also a higher incidence following diagnostic amniocentesis in the first trimester.

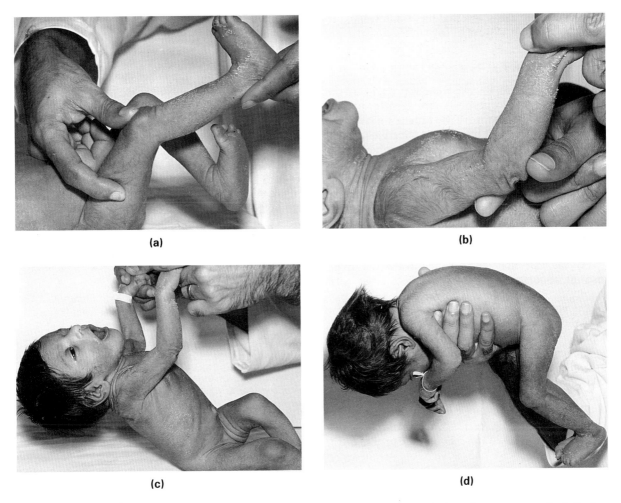

(a) (b)

(c) (d)

Figure 13-7a-d Benign congenital contractures. This low-birthweight (2.5 kg) infant, born at term, had flexion contractures at the knees and elbows, with limitation of full extension (a,b). Head and trunk control seemed reasonable and there was no associated neuromuscular problem (c,d). The contractures took 15 months to resolve and were ascribed to poor mobility *in utero*, possibly associated with oligohydramnios. The subsequent motor development continued normally.

Mild degrees of isolated limitation of full extension of joints such as the hips, knees or elbows are fairly frequently seen in the neonatal wards in otherwise normal infants (Figure 13-7). These usually resolve in time but may on occasion take several months to achieve a full range of movement, even with regular passive exercises (see below).

ANIMAL STUDIES

Arthrogryposis with an autosomal recessive inheritance has long been recognized in the newborn sheep (Roberts, 1929) and considered to be myopathic in origin (Middleton, 1934). On the other hand, in the calf, arthrogryposis was associated with malform-

ations in the central nervous system (Whittem, 1957; Hartley and Wanner, 1974). In guinea-pigs Edwards (1971) demonstrated the occurrence of arthrogryposis in newborn pups following hyperthermia during pregnancy, apparently associated with abnormalities in the spinal cord. In an interesting series of experiments Drachman and his colleagues produced arthrogryposis in the chick by various procedures *in ovo*, such as the infusion of tubocurare (Drachman and Coulombre, 1962), the infusion of decamethonium or botulinum toxin, the extirpation of the lumbosacral spinal cord, or the injection of Coxsackie virus (Drachman and Sokoloff, 1966; Drachman *et al.*, 1976). The common factor in all these studies was the paralysis or immobility of the muscles and the deformities of the joints seemed to be dictated by the posture of the embryo *in ovo*.

MANAGEMENT

Irrespective of cause, the two basic approaches to the treatment of arthrogryposis are gentle passive stretching, to try to improve the range of movement of the apparently fixed joints, and selective surgical intervention to correct residual deformities. It is often advisable to defer orthopaedic consultation in these cases until later, as early surgical intervention is unnecessary and may indeed be counterproductive and result in repeated operations for recurring deformity. One should also be cautious about immobilization of the joints in casts, either as a therapeutic approach to try to correct deformity or postoperatively, as this may further aggravate the fixed postural abnormality in some of these cases with neuromuscular disorders. It has been my policy over several years to defer any correction of the foot deformities in particular, however severe, until the child has reached a stage of being able to take weight on the legs. If one then corrects the deformity surgically, the child can maintain the corrected position when standing and the tendency to recurrence of the deformity is then much less. One often gets away with a single surgical corrective procedure in these cases (see Figure 13-4). Deformities of the hands and wrists often pose a complex problem for correction and need the advice of orthopaedic surgeons particularly skilled in dealing with hand deformities.

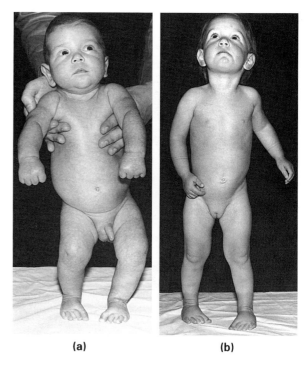

(a)   **(b)**

Figure 13-8a,b Congenital 'club foot'. Two siblings (a,b) with congenital equinovarus deformity of feet (mainly forefoot varus). Power and motor milestones were normal; EMG and nerve conduction were normal. Biopsy was not done. They had no appreciable functional disability.

CONGENITAL CLUB FOOT

This is a common condition, which usually occurs as an isolated phenomenon and may be bilateral or unilateral. The commonest deformity is a talipes equinovarus but occasionally other deformities such as calcaneo-valgus may be found.

Many cases are mild and readily reducible with no fixed equinus and will respond to passive stretching and splintage in a corrected posture.

A careful examination should be made for evidence of weakness or depressed reflexes and, where suspected, or where the deformity is more severe and fixed, investigations with nerve conduction and electromyography (EMG) are worth doing as a routine to exclude overt neuromuscular disorder. In cases not responding to treatment, or with recurrence, a muscle biopsy should also be performed to try to establish a more accurate diagnosis and give an

appropriate prognosis as well as guidance on the potential value of orthopaedic manoeuvres.

Familial cases should also be investigated as they are more likely to have a genetically determined underlying disorder such as a motor neuropathy or congenital myopathy (Figure 13-8).

'CONGENITAL' CONTRACTURE OF THE QUADRICEPS

This condition is usually not congenital (as originally thought), but acquired and often the sequel of multiple injections (e.g. penicillin) into the quadriceps muscle, a commonly used site in paediatric practice. After a variable latent period the quadriceps muscle becomes progressively shortened and limited in its full relaxation, so that there is limited flexion of the knee (but a full range of extension) (Figure 13-9). Eventually this causes difficulty with gait and other activities. EMG is normal, and muscle biopsy usually is normal but at times shows some focal degeneration and fibrosis. The muscle power is good and the condition can be cured by an ortho-

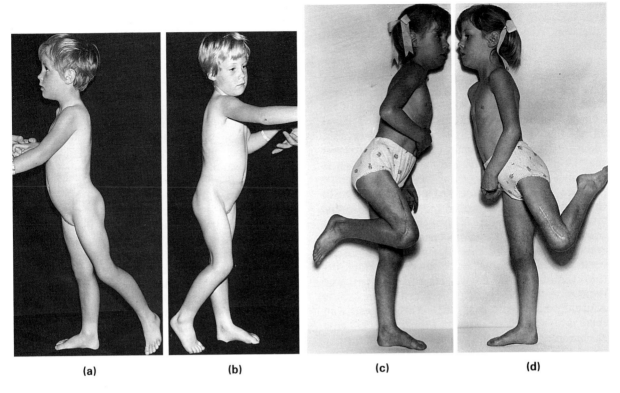

(a)   (b)   (c)   (d)

Figure 13-9a-d Progressive contracture of the quadriceps. This child was admitted with severe pneumococcal meningitis with associated coma and convulsions at 3 months of age. She was treated with intramuscular penicillin, 1 million units 4-hourly. This cured her meningitis but 4 years later she developed bilateral contractures of the quadriceps, with progressive limitation of flexion of the knees (a,b). The condition was completely cured by a lengthening procedure of the lower tendinous part of the quadriceps and she has no residual disability (c,d). Biopsy from the right vastus internus at the time of operation showed increased variability in fibre size but a normal histochemical distribution of fibre types. The left vastus internus showed a number of foci with atrophic fibres and associated proliferation of connective tissue.

paedic procedure for lengthening the quadriceps muscle. The condition does not recur if adequately treated.

The primary pathology is probably in the supportive connective tissue rather than in the muscle itself. The condition occasionally develops spontaneously, and familial cases have also been recorded.

BENIGN CONGENITAL CONTRACTURES

These are seen in newborn infants without associated neuromuscular problems and commonly affect the hip flexors, with marked limitation of extension, the elbow flexors and the knee flexors. They are pre-sumably related to relative immobility in a flexed posture *in utero*. They usually resolve completely but in some infants whose progress I have followed they have taken up to 15 or 18 months to do so (Figure 13-7). Regular passive movements of the joints probably promote the recovery process and can be undertaken by the parents.

CONGENITAL TORTICOLLIS ('STERNOMASTOID TUMOUR')

This is a common and usually benign condition. There is limited rotation of the head in one direction, due to shortening of the sternomastoid muscle on that side, with a full range of movement in the other direction. As with other conditions associated with muscle contractures, the power within the range of movement appears normal.

In the early stages there are usually no abnormal features but with time, if not corrected, asymmetry of the face and skull will develop as a result of the child's habitually lying with the head rotated to one side. A few cases may already show asymmetry at the onset of the problem, suggesting that the deformity may be of some duration and have had its onset *in utero*.

There is usually an associated localized swelling of the shortened sternomastoid muscle, the so-called 'sternomastoid tumour'. This is thought to arise by organization and fibrosis of a haematoma, probably resulting from trauma either during the birth process itself or possibly earlier on *in utero*. Histologically the 'tumour' area shows marked fibrosis and replacement of muscle tissue. The rest of the muscle is usually histologically normal. This suggests that there is no underlying disease of the muscle but that the pathological changes observed are secondary.

TREATMENT

This consists of passive rotation of the head to the affected side to encourage a full range of movement. If this is done frequently each day by the mother one can expect an almost 100% complete cure rate. As a result of the experience with a particular infant some 10 years ago (see case history below) I now routinely advise that the exercises be undertaken in a prone rather than in the traditional supine position. This has the added advantage that if the infant is encouraged to lie prone, with his head rotated towards the limited side, he will be providing his own physiotherapy most of the time.

Surgical treatment should rarely be needed and usually indicates failed or inadequate medical treatment. This may partly reflect an attitude in some textbooks of paediatrics that the outlook is good and no specific treatment is required. Unless one gives active physiotherapy and specifically shows the mother what to do, a proportion of these cases will not recover and will thus provide work for the surgeon and biopsy material for the pathologist. In cases with permanent shortening of the sterno-mastoid the ideal operative procedure would be a lengthening of the sternomastoid muscle. As this is not often practical, surgeons usually resort to a transection and release of the sternomastoid muscle, which can be done at the proximal attachment rather than in the region of the actual swelling itself.

Case history. The infant of a trained nurse was found to have limitation of rotation of the head to the right of about 60° compared with the left. An associated sternomastoid tumour was palpable. The mother was advised to take the head to its maximal range of rotation to the affected side several times daily and told that the prognosis for full recovery was good.

When she returned a month later for reassessment the condition was no better and possibly slightly worse. When questioned about the frequency and thoroughness of the exercises, she conceded that she had stopped doing them after a few days as they seemed to be painful and to upset the child and she could not bear the expression of pain on his face.

I suggested to her that perhaps if she did not see the child's face, by putting him in the prone rather than in the supine position, it might be advantageous to her and the child. For the first time I tried the manoeuvre with the child in the prone position and found that it was in fact much easier to do and better tolerated than in the supine. A month later the torticollis had completely resolved.

In 10 consecutive cases that I subsequently treated with the child in the prone posture, the results were consistently good. This seems to provide a distinct advantage over the standard supine approach since the child is essentially providing its own rotation in the required direction when the head is partly turned into that direction.

RIGID SPINE SYNDROME

The predominant feature in this condition is a marked limitation in flexion of the whole dorso-lumbar and cervical spine. The range of extension is not restricted and the power of the extensor muscles is good. This suggests that the main problem is a shortening or contracture of the spinal extensors without undue weakness. There may be limitation in movement of other joints as well, the most consistent being limited extension of the elbows.

Because these patients usually have difficulty with walking and going up steps in infancy they are readily misdiagnosed as having muscular dystrophy. The condition tends to be non-progressive except for the development of scoliosis and associated deformities (Dubowitz, 1965).

For want of a better name I suggested the descriptive title 'rigid spine syndrome' to highlight the central problem of limited spinal flexion (Dubowitz,

1971, 1973). There appeared to be an underlying myopathic process, since the creatine kinase (CK) tended to be moderately elevated, EMG of spinal muscles showed a myopathic pattern (and 'palpable' fibrosis on insertion of the needle) and muscle biopsy showed marked fibrosis and replacement of muscle by connective tissue, with associated cellularity and variation in fibre size.

The condition somewhat resembled some of the features of congenital muscular dystrophy, which also tends to have contractures that affect the elbows but not usually the spine, and also has a non-progressive dystrophic pattern in the muscle, but usually with much more adipose tissue than in the rigid spine syndrome.

The first four cases I saw were all male (see Figures 13-10 to 13-12) but I subsequently saw a similar condition in an occasional female. In one boy who died the central and peripheral nervous systems were normal.

This condition was not a chronic myositis and there was no improvement on steroid therapy in the one case in whom I tried it on the grounds of cellularity in the muscle biopsy.

With hindsight, the majority of these early, isolated male cases would probably conform to the Emery–Dreifuss muscular dystrophy (Emery and Dreifuss, 1966) which was not yet fully characterized in the early 1960s (see Chapter 2, p.105). The recent isolation and cloning of the Emery–Dreifuss gene and characterization of its novel protein, emerin (Bione *et al.*, 1994), should enable one in future to identify mutations in the gene in these cases or abnormalities in relation to the protein.

Meanwhile an extensive literature has grown over the past two decades in relation to the rigid spine syndrome, with the publication of over 50 papers, including a number of reviews (Bertini *et al.*, 1986; Van Munster *et al.*, 1986; Merlini *et al.*, 1989; Morita *et al.*, 1990). It is clearly a heterogeneous disorder and the frequent association of nocturnal hypoventilation and potential respiratory failure has been well documented, and also the association of cardiomyopathy in some cases. Numerous female cases have also been recorded. Apart from the cases that resemble the Emery–Dreifuss phenotype, some conform more to a congenital muscular dystrophy pattern with early onset of weakness and a tendency to contractures of various limb muscles and also the spinal extensors (see Chapter 2, p.93 and Figure 2-53). Recent advances in relation to the merosin (α2 laminin) gene and merosin deficiency associated with some cases of congenital muscular dystrophy, and potential further developments in relation to the merosin-positive cases, should help in future to establish the possible association of congenital muscular dystrophy with rigid spine syndrome.

Some patients with rigid spine syndrome have an early onset of symptoms with a striking rigidity of the spine and early respiratory failure (Figure 13-13), in association with reasonably good function of the skeletal muscles, which on biopsy show a minimal-change myopathy. The possible relation of this particular phenotype to congenital muscular dystrophy is currently also still unclear.

Unexpected associations I have observed with a rigid spine syndrome include an ambulant young boy with type 2 glycogenosis who subsequently went into respiratory failure (see Chapter 4, Figure 4-6) and a teenage boy with dominantly inherited type 2 Charcot–Marie–Tooth disease, who had a marked compensatory hyperextension of his neck to maintain a vertical posture.

MANAGEMENT

Careful evaluation of respiratory and cardiac function is essential in all cases to detect any associated respiratory deficit or cardiomyopathy, both of which can be life-threatening. The scoliosis tends to be progressive and if it is difficult to control with bracing, surgical intervention may be indicated. In contrast to other neuromuscular disorders associated with progressive scoliosis, such as spinal muscular atrophy, in which there is associated hypotonia and usually excessive mobility of the spine from side to side to maintain ambulation, the spine in rigid spine syndrome is, by definition, rigid and spinal fixation is thus unlikely to have any material effect on the ability to walk independently.

In cases where the contractures of the cervical extensors become marked and result in a hyperextended posture of the neck because of the marked limitation of flexion, even to a vertical position, the patient may adopt a forward-stooping posture, with marked hip flexion, to compensate for this and maintain a vertical alignment of the head in order to be able to look forward. If one tries to extend the hips, the face will then be looking upwards at the ceiling as a result of the limited flexion. As one cannot improve this situation by either active physiotherapy or by surgical efforts to release some of the shortened extensor muscles, Giannini *et al.* (1988) devised a very effective surgical procedure of opening the interspinous spaces from C2 to C7 through a capsulotomy and then stabilizing the cervical spine in a corrected posture with bone grafts fixed to the spinous processes. This enables the patient to achieve an upright posture and to look forward without any compensatory posturing of the hips. As C1 and C2 are left unfused this also allows some residual flexion and extension of the head.

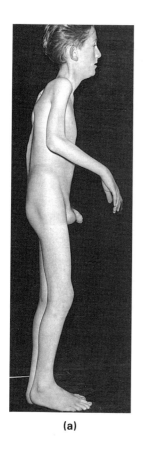

(a)

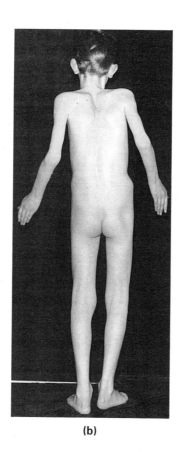

(b)

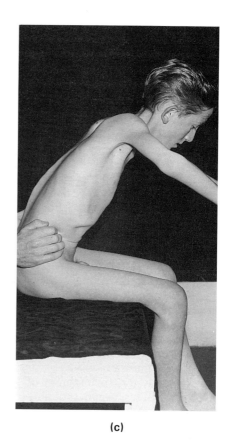

(c)

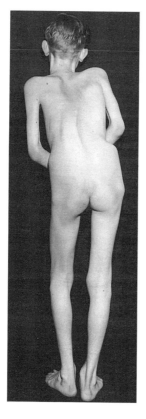

(d)

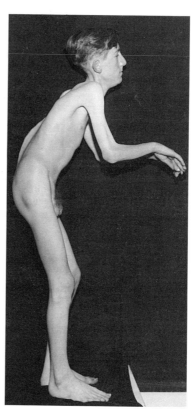

(e)

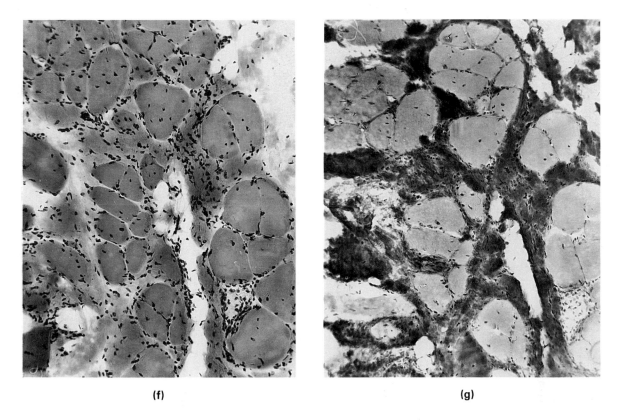

(f) (g)

Figure 13-10a-g Rigid spine syndrome. This was my first patient with rigid spine syndrome, whom I saw in the early 1960s. He was the only child of healthy parents. After a normal neonatal period he was late in his motor milestones. He never crawled, but shuffled on his bottom, did not stand till about 18 months, and walked at about 2 years. He tended to walk on his toes, had difficulty going up steps and was never able to run. At 4 years a paediatrician diagnosed Duchenne dystrophy. There was no subsequent deterioration in his motor ability but he developed scoliosis. When first examined at the age of 13 (a-c), he had a stable gait with a somewhat forward stoop. There was striking limitation of flexion of his cervical as well as dorso-lumbar spine, and also of rotation and lateral flexion of the cervical spine. Extension of the spine was normal. There was an associated dorsolumbar scoliosis, and also limitation of extension of both elbows beyond 90°, but full flexion. There was some associated weakness of the neck flexion (power MRC 3), and also of the shoulder girdle muscles (power MRC 3 to 4). The tendon reflexes were all sluggish. There was no fasciculation of the tongue or other muscles. At subsequent follow-up he showed no change in muscle power but had increasing disability owing to progression of his scoliosis and a tendency to hyperextension of his neck (d,e, aged 15 years). He was walking with an increasing flexion of the hips and hyperextension of his neck, to maintain the head in a vertical position (e). Biopsy of the biceps and brachialis muscles, taken at the time of an attempted lengthening procedure, showed similar changes. There was a myopathic pattern with marked variation in fibre size, with numerous giant fibres up to 150–200 µm in diameter, and fibres as small as 20–30 µm (f, H & E). Many fibres had internal nuclei. A few fibres were undergoing necrosis and phagocytosis. There was no inflammatory cell response. There was striking proliferation of the perimysial and endomysial connective tissue, which was more marked in the brachialis than in the biceps (g, Verhoeff-van Gieson, serial section). Histochemical enzyme reactions showed a normal distribution of fibre types and no structural changes within the fibres.

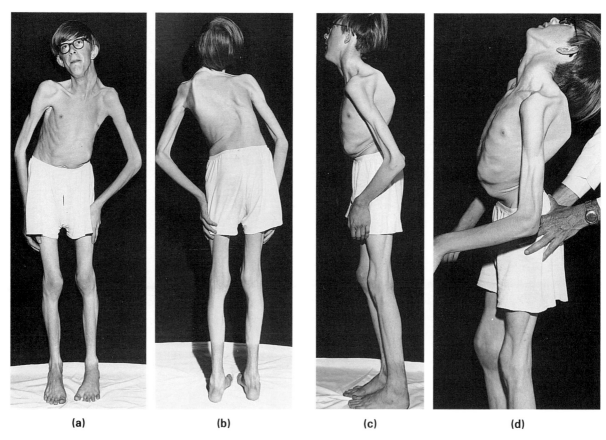

| (a) | (b) | (c) | (d) |

Figure 13-11a-d Rigid spine syndrome. This 15-year-old boy (a-d) gave an almost identical history to the previous case, with a waddling gait and difficulty going up steps after he started walking at 14 months, and a provisional diagnosis of muscular dystrophy. He subsequently had elongation of the tendo Achillis at 18 months and at 9 years. From an early age he had difficulty flexing his neck and back and for about 4 years had a marked progression of his scoliosis. He also had fixed deformities of his elbows. He had no difficulty getting up from the floor, or hopping on one leg. Despite his poorly developed musculature, the power was good. Note the striking wasting of his upper arm muscles (d). Serum CK was elevated at 360 iu/litre. His nerve conductions were normal. Radiographs of the spine showed no ankylosing spondylitis or other disorder. Over the ensuing 2 years his scoliosis progressed further and a fusion operation of the spine was advised. Muscle biopsy of the sacrospinalis (at time of operation) showed a myopathic pattern with marked variation in fibre size, degenerating fibres and proliferation of connective tissue and fat.

Figure 13-12a-f (*facing page*) Rigid spine syndrome; late onset. This boy presented at 8 years of age with a 1-year history of progressive limitation of flexion of his neck and trunk (a-c). His early motor milestones and subsequent course had been normal until the present symptoms. In addition to the marked limitation of flexion of the spine there was also wasting of the right calf with some shortening of the tendo Achillis and fixed equinus of about 10°. His CK ranged from 105 to 380 iu/litre (N <70). EMG of the sacrospinalis as well as the gastrocnemius and deltoid showed a myopathic pattern, with a full interference pattern and low amplitude polyphasic units. Muscle biopsy of the sacrospinalis and gastrocnemius were taken under general anaesthesia. Pentobarbitone-scoline produced no relaxation at all of the spinal extensors or gastrocnemius, excluding any state of spasm of the muscle. The sacrospinalis showed very extensive fibrosis and replacement of muscle, whereas the gastrocnemius showed a myopathic pattern with variation in fibre size and some increased cellularity, but no striking fibrosis. Over the next 4 years there was a slight increase in the lordosis of his spine and also in the equinus of the right foot, which was corrected surgically. He subsequently showed very little progression (d-f, aged 14 years).

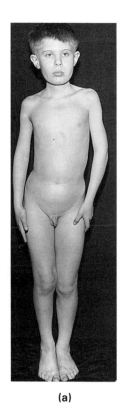

(a)

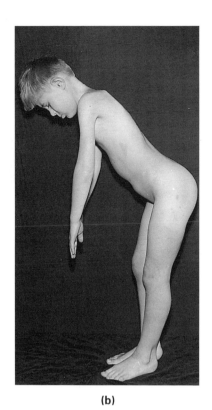

(b)

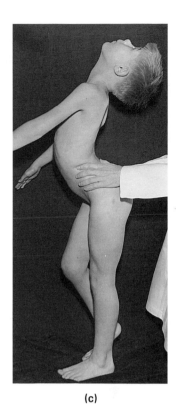

(c)

(d)

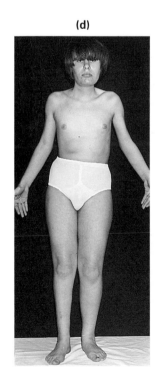

(e)

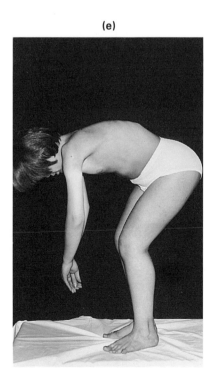

(f)

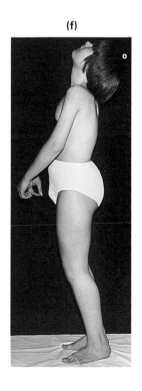

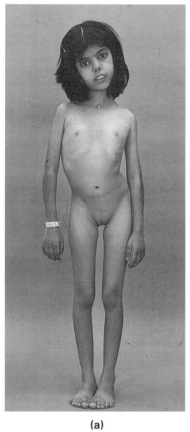

(a)

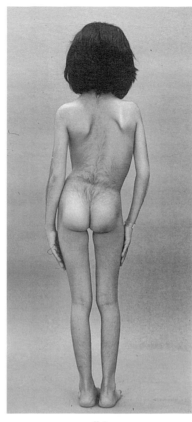

(b)

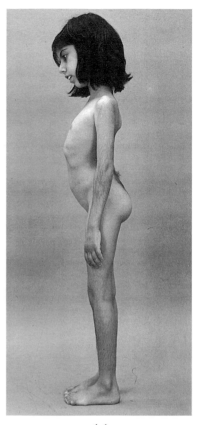

(c)

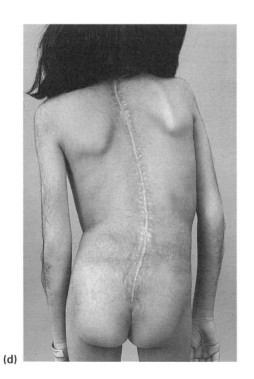

(d)

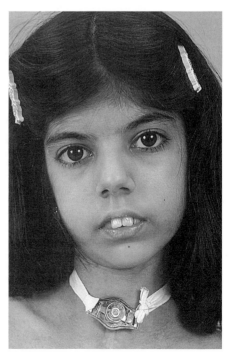

(e)

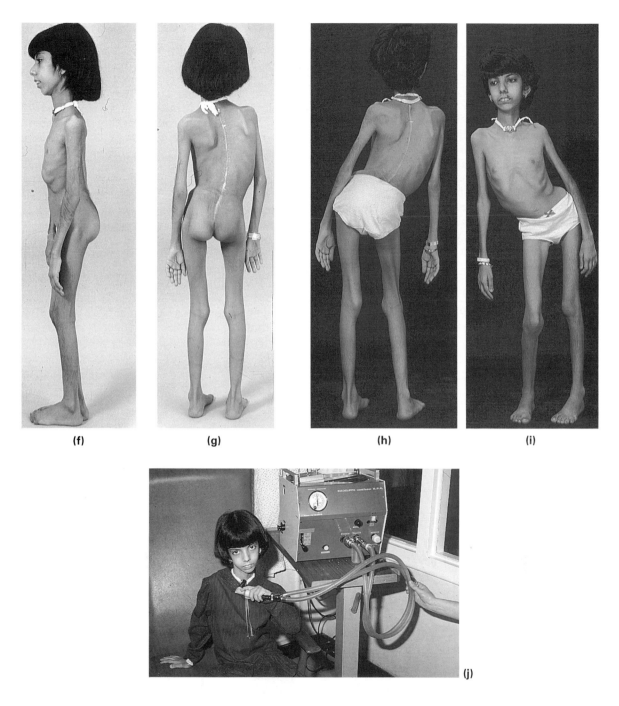

(f)   (g)   (h)   (i)

(j)

Figure 13-13a-j Rigid spine syndrome; minimal change myopathy; respiratory failure. This child was referred at 9 years with a progressive scoliosis (a-c). In addition she also had evidence of nocturnal hypoventilation, and sleep oximetry showed prolonged periods of apnoea. When her mother was told of the presence and significance of this problem, she said that she had in fact noted for some time that the child stopped breathing during her sleep, and that she had been keeping a close vigil on her and would shake her whenever this happened, which was effective in stimulating breathing again. As it was impossible at the time to fit her with a small enough cuirass-type ventilator, and mask ventilation had not yet come into vogue, a tracheostomy was done at the time of her spinal surgery and a portable ventilator provided for night time use (d,e). She subsequently managed extremely well and was able to manage her ventilator herself. On annual review her spine seemed reasonably stable (f,g, 10 years). However, during her growth spurt she subsequently developed a marked increase in the curvature , with an associated compensatory tilting of the pelvis (h,i, 12 years). She was still coping well with her ventilator support at night (j).

FIBRODYSPLASIA OSSIFICANS PROGRESSIVA (MYOSITIS OSSIFICANS)

This unusual condition is characterized by the deposition of bone in the supportive tissues of the muscle. Although traditionally called 'myositis ossificans' since the early descriptions in the mid-eighteenth century, it has been recognized in recent years that the primary pathology is not in the muscle but in the connective tissue, and may involve not only the interstitial fibrous tissue but also tendons, ligaments, fasciae and even the skin. It has thus qualified for inclusion among the heritable disorders of connective tissue and McKusick (1972) favoured the title 'fibrodysplasia ossificans progressiva'. There have been a number of comprehensive reviews of the condition in recent years (Smith *et al.*, 1976; Rogers and Geho, 1979; Schroeder and Zasloff, 1980; Connor and Beighton, 1982; Connor and Evans, 1982a,b; Connor, 1983).

CLINICAL FEATURES

The condition usually manifests in childhood with the appearance of palpable subcutaneous swellings in the region usually of the neck and back, particularly in the scapular area. They may initially feel cystic but become firm as they become ossified. They may occur spontaneously or be precipitated by trauma. The ossification gradually increases and bony bars and bridges are formed which gradually limit mobility of the chest as well as various joints as the limbs also become involved (Figures 13-14 to 13-16). This may lead to rigidity and postural abnormality in the spine and also of the limbs, as the tendons, fascia or ligaments become affected. The extent of the ossification can readily be demonstrated on radiography or with computerized tomography scanning.

A frequently associated feature, which is very helpful with diagnosis in the early stages, is shortening of the great toes and to a lesser extent also of the thumbs. The toes subsequently also tend to develop a hallux valgus deformity (Figures 13-15 and 13-16).

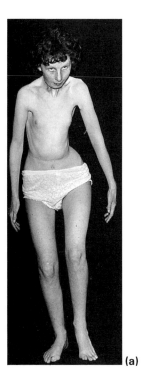
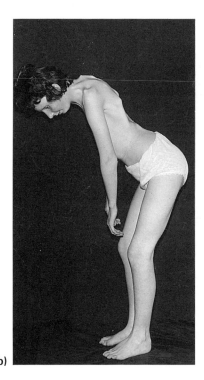
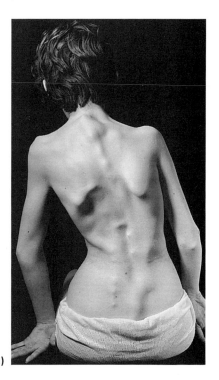

(a) (b) (c)

Figure 13-14a-c Fibrodysplasia ossificans progressiva. Aged 18 years. Onset in early childhood with progressive involvement over the years, predominantly affecting neck and trunk muscles. Note the extreme wasting of trunk muscles and the reduced size of the chest (a), the marked limitation of flexion of the trunk (b) and the visible bridges of bone between muscles (c). She also had marked reduction and associated hallux valgus deformity of the great toes (a).

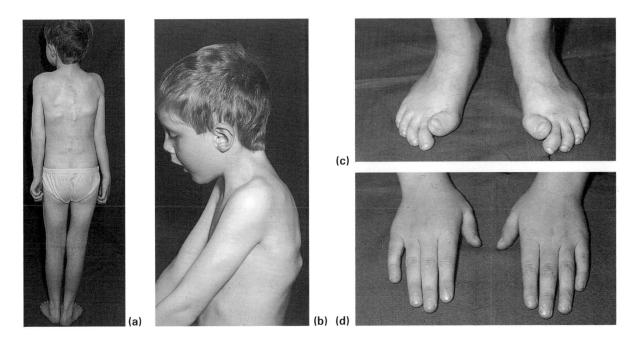

Figure 13-15a-d Fibrodysplasia ossificans progressiva. A 6-year-old boy with multiple bony swellings over back of trunk (a). Note limited neck flexion (b) and associated shortness and valgus deformity of the big toes (c) and small thumbs (d).

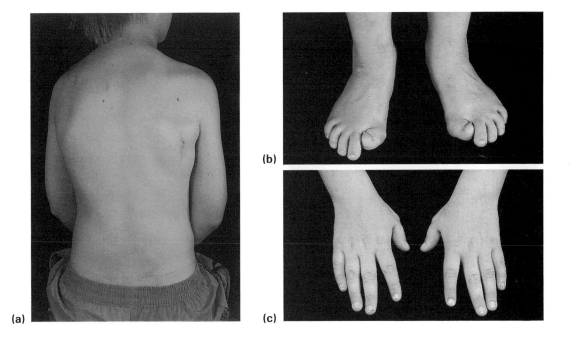

Figure 13-16a-c Fibrodysplasia ossificans progressiva. A 7-year-old boy with multiple bony swellings in the scapular region (a) and associated abnormalities of the big toes (b) and the thumbs (c) Note similarity to Fig. 13-15.

LABORATORY INVESTIGATIONS

Biochemical investigations such as serum calcium, phosphorus and alkaline phosphatase are normal. Biopsy procedures of muscle or soft tissues are best avoided as they may precipitate further ossification. Respiratory function studies may reveal restricted ventilation. Cardiac function is not usually affected.

MANAGEMENT

There is currently no effective therapy for the disorder, although a wide variety of therapeutic agents have been tried, including beryllium (for its inhibitory effect on alkaline phosphatase), corticosteroids, vitamins B and E, penicillamine and chelating agents. Diphosphonates have been in vogue for some time and have not been completely disbanded, although objective evidence for their beneficial effect is still not convincing. Geho and Whiteside (1972) documented the treatment of a large cohort of patients, 52 of whom had undergone at least 6 months treatment, and were encouraged by its apparent stabilization of the condition and suggestion of exacerbation after withdrawal. However, whilst possibly reducing calcification of ectopic bone matrix, diphosphonates may also have a detrimental effect on normal skeletal development (Wood and Robinson, 1976; Rogers *et al.*, 1977).

Surgical intervention in trying to correct disabling deformity and improve limb function has a very limited role and one should proceed with extreme caution because of the risk of precipitating more ossification and aggravation of the condition.

As pneumonia can be life-threatening in this condition, vigorous treatment of any respiratory infection is important, as is the use of anti-influenzal and other vaccines.

GENETICS

The condition is considered to have a dominant inheritance with variable penetration. Occasional families have been documented with multiple affected cases, including parent and offspring, and there have also been records of affected monozygotic twins. More frequently other members of the family may exhibit minor manifestations such as small great toes or thumbs. As affected patients are severely disabled and unlikely to reproduce, most cases probably result from new mutations. A gene locus for the disease has not yet been identified.

ANIMAL MODELS

Several sporadic cases have been documented in cats (Warren and Carpenter, 1984) and a dominantly inherited form in pigs (Seibold and Davis, 1967).

LOCALIZED MYOSITIS OSSIFICANS

This is a focal form of the disease, related directly to trauma. It is rare in childhood. Most cases have been in young adults and related to their particular occupation, e.g. 'riders' bone' in the adductors of the thighs in jockeys; ossification of the pectoralis or deltoids of infantrymen from the trauma of the rifle butt. Localized ossification can also follow a single severe localized trauma, such as a kick from a horse or a sudden exertion or strain, presumably as a result of calcification and ossification in a haematoma. As it is a rare event, there is presumably some additional predisposing factor in these cases.

REFERENCES

Aicardi, J. (1991) The agyria-pachygyria complex: a spectrum of cortical malformations. *Brain and Development* **13**: 1–8.

Banker, B.Q. (1994) Congenital deformities. In: Engel, A.G. and Franzini-Armstrong, C. eds, *Myology: Basic and Clinical* 2nd edn. New York: McGraw-Hill, pp. 1905–1937.

Banker, B.Q., Victor, M. and Adams, R.D. (1957) Arthrogryposis multiplex due to congenital muscular dystrophy. *Brain* **80**: 319.

Bertini, E., Marini, R., Sabetta, G. *et al.* (1986) The spectrum of the so-called rigid spine syndrome: nosological considerations and report of three female cases. *Journal of Neurology* **233**: 248–253.

Bione, S., Maestrini, E., Rivella, S. *et al.* (1994) Identification of a novel X-linked gene responsible for Emery–Dreifuss muscular dystrophy. *Nature Genetics* **8**: 323–327.

Brandt, S. (1947) A case of arthrogryposis multiplex congenita anatomically appearing as a foetal spinal muscular atrophy. *Acta Paediatrica* **34**: 365.

Byers, R.K. and Banker, B.Q. (1961) Infantile muscular atrophy. *Archives of Neurology (Chicago)* **5**: 140–164.

Connor, J.M. (1983) *Soft Tissue Ossification*. Berlin: Springer-Verlag, pp. 54–74.

Connor, J.M. and Beighton, P. (1982) Fibrodysplasia ossificans progressiva in South Africa: case reports. *South African Medical Journal* **61**: 404–406.

Connor, J.M. and Evans, D.A. (1982a) Genetic aspects of fibrodysplasia ossificans progressiva. *Journal of Medical Genetics* **19**: 35–39.

Connor, J.M. and Evans, D.A. (1982b) Fibrodysplasia ossificans progressiva: the clinical features and natural history of 34 patients. *Journal of Bone and Joint Surgery* **64**: 76–83.

Charnas, L., Trapp, B. and Griffin, J. (1988) Congenital absence of peripheral myelin: abnormal Schwann cell development causes lethal arthrogryposis multiplex congenita. *Neurology* **38**: 966–974.

Drachman, D.B. and Coulombre, A.J. (1962) Experimental clubfoot and arthrogryposis multiplex congenita. *Lancet* ii: 523.

Drachman, D.B. and Sokoloff, L. (1966) The role of movement in embryonic joint development. *Developmental Biology* **14**: 401.

Drachman, D.B., Weiner, L.P., Price, D.L. *et al.* (1976) Experimental arthrogryposis caused by viral myopathy. *Archives of Neurology* **33**: 362.

Dubowitz, V. (1965) Pseudo muscular dystrophy. In: Research Committee of the Muscular Dystrophy Group of Great Britain: *Research in Muscular Dystrophy*. Proceedings of the Third Symposium, London: Pitman Medical, p.57.

Dubowitz, V. (1971) Recent advances in neuromuscular disorders. *Rheumatology and Physical Medicine* **11**: 126–130.

Dubowitz, V. (1973) Rigid spine syndrome: a muscle syndrome in search of a name. *Proceedings of the Royal Society of Medicine* **66**: 219.

Edwards, M.J. (1971) The experimental production of arthrogryposis multiplex congenita in guinea-pigs by maternal hyperthermia during gestation. *Journal of Pathology* **104**: 221.

Emery, A.E.H. and Dreifuss, F.E. (1966) Unusual type of benign X-linked muscular dystrophy. *Journal of Neurology, Neurosurgery and Psychiatry* **29**: 338.

Gabreëls-Festen, A.A.W.M., Gabreëls, F.J.M., Jennekens, F.G.I. *et al.* (1994) The status of HMSN type III. *Neuromuscular Disorders* **4**: 63–69.

Geho, W.B. and Whiteside, J.A. (1972) Experience with disodium etidronate on diseases of ectopic calcification. In: Frame, B., Parfitt, A.M. and Duncan, H. eds, *Clinical Aspects of Metabolic Bone Disease*. Proceedings of the International Symposium on Clinical Metabolic Bone Diseases, New York: American Elsevier, pp. 506–511.

Giannini, S., Ceccarelli, F., Granata, C. *et al.* (1988) Surgical correction of cervical hyperextension in rigid spine syndrome. *Neuropediatrics* **19**: 105–108.

Guerrini, R., Dravet, C., Raybaud, C. *et al.* (1992) Neurological findings and seizure outcome in children with bilateral opercular macrogyric-like changes detected by MRI. *Developmental Medicine and Child Neurology* **34**: 694–705.

Hageman, G., van Ketel, B.A. and Verdonck, A.F.M.N. (1987) The pathogenesis of fetal hypokinesia. A neurological study of 75 cases of congenital contractures with emphasis of cerebral lesions. *Neuropaediatrics* **18**: 22–33.

Hall, J.G., Reed, S.D. and Greene, G. (1982) The distal arthrogryposes: delineation of new entities – review and nosologic discussion. *American Journal of Medical Genetics* **11**: 185–239.

Hartley, W.J. and Wanner, R.A. (1974) Bovine congenital arthrogryposis in New South Wales. *Australian Veterinary Journal* **50**: 185.

Jago, R.H. (1970) Arthrogryposis following treatment of maternal tetanus with muscle relaxants. *Archives of Disease in Childhood* **45**: 277.

Karch, S.B. and Urich, H. (1975) Infantile polyneuropathy with defective myelination: an autopsy study. *Developmental Medicine and Child Neurology* **17**: 504–511.

Krugliak, L., Gadoth, N. and Behar, A.J. (1978) Neuropathic form of arthrogryposis multiplex congenita: report of 3 cases with complete necropsy, including the first reported case of agenesis of muscle spindles. *Journal of the Neurological Sciences* **37**: 179–185.

Kuzniecky, R., Andermann, F., Tampieri, D. *et al.* (1989) Bilateral central macrogyria: epilepsy, pseudobulbar palsy, and mental retardation – a recognisable neuronal migration disorder. *Annals of Neurology* **25**: 547–554.

Kuzniecky, R., Andermann, F., Guerrini, R. *et al.* (1993) Congenital bilateral perisylvian syndrome: study of 31 patients. *Lancet* **341**: 608–612.

McKusick, V. (1972) *Heritable Disorders of Connective Tissue*, 4th edn. St. Louis: Mosby, p.687.

Merlini, L., Granata, C., Ballestrazzi, A. *et al.* (1989) Rigid spine syndrome and rigid spine sign in myopathies. *Journal of Child Neurology* **4**: 274–282.

Middleton, D.S. (1934) Studies on prenatal lesions of striated muscle as a cause of congenital deformity. *Edinburgh Medical Journal* **41**: 401–442.

Morita, H., Kondo, K., Hoshino, K. *et al.* (1990) Rigid spine syndrome with respiratory failure. *Journal of Neurology, Neurosurgery and Psychiatry* **53**: 782–784.

Pearson, C.M. and Fowler, W.G. (1963) Hereditary nonprogressive muscular dystrophy inducing arthrogryposis syndrome. *Brain* **86**: 75.

Pena, S.D.J. and Shokeir, M.H.K. (1974a) Syndrome of camptodactyly, multiple ankyloses, facial anomalies and pulmonary hypoplasia: a lethal condition. *Journal of Pediatrics* **85**: 373–375.

Pena, S.D.J. and Shokeir, M.H.K. (1974b) Autosomal recessive cerebro-oculo-facio-skeletal (COFS) syndrome. *Clinical Genetics* **5**: 285–293.

Philpot, J., Muntoni, F., Skellett, S. *et al.* (1995) Congenital symmetrical weakness of the upper limbs resembling brachial plexus palsy: a possible sequel of drug toxicity in first trimester of pregnancy? *Neuromuscular Disorders* **5**: 67–69.

Roberts, J.A.F. (1929) The inheritance of a lethal muscle contracture in the sheep. *Journal of Genetics* **21**: 57.

Rocher, H.L. (1913) Les raideurs articulaires congenitales multiples. *Journal de Médecine de Bordeaux* **43**: 772.

Rogers, J.G. and Geho, W.B. (1979) Fibrodysplasia ossificans progressiva: a survey of forty-two cases. *Journal of Bone and Joint Surgery* **61**: 909–914.

Rogers, J.G., Dorst, J.P. and Geho, W.B. (1977) Use and complications of high-dose disodium etidronate therapy in fibrodysplasia ossificans progressiva. *Journal of Pediatrics* **91**: 1011–1014.

Rossi, E. (1947) Le syndrome arthromyodysplasique congenital. *Helvetica Paediatrica Acta* **2**: 82.

Schroeder, H.W. and Zasloff, M. (1980) The hand and foot malformations in fibrodysplasia ossificans progressiva. *Johns Hopkins Medical Journal* **147**: 73–78.

Seibold, H.R. and Davis, C.L. (1967) Generalized myositis ossificans (familial) in pigs. *Veterinary Pathology* **4**: 79–88.

Seitz, R.J., Wechsler, W., Mosny, D.S. *et al.* (1986) Hypomyelination neuropathy in a female newborn presenting as arthrogryposis multiplex congenita. *Neuropediatrics* **17**: 132–136.

Sheldon, W. (1932) Amyoplasia congenita. *Archives of Disease in Childhood* **7**: 117–136.

Smith, R., Russell, R.G.G. and Woods, C.G. (1976) Myositis ossificans progressiva: clinical features of eight patients and their response to therapy. *Journal of Bone and Joint Surgery (Br)* **58**: 48–57.

Stern, W.G. (1923) Arthrogryposis multiplex congenita. *Journal of the American Medical Association* **81**: 1507–1510.

Van Munster, E.T.L., Joogsten, E.M., Van Munster-Uijtdehaage, M.A.M. *et al.* (1986). The rigid spine syndrome. *Journal of Neurology, Neurosurgery and Psychiatry* **49**: 1292–1297.

Vuopala, K., Leisti, J. and Herva, R. (1994) Lethal arthrogryposis in Finland – A clinico-pathological study of 83 cases during 13 years. *Neuropediatrics* **25**: 308–315.

Warren, H.B. and Carpenter, J.L. (1984) Fibrodysplasia ossificans in three cats. *Veterinary Pathology* **21**: 495–499.

Whittem, J.H. (1957) Congenital abnormalities in calves: arthrogryposis and hydranencephaly. *Journal of Pathology and Bacteriology* **73**: 375.

Wolf, A., Roverud, E. and Poser, C. (1955) Amyoplasia congenita. *Journal of Neuropathology and Experimental Neurology* **14**: 112.

Wood, B.J. and Robinson, G.C. (1976) Drug induced bone changes in myositis ossificans progressiva. *Pediatric Radiology* **5**: 40–43.

CHAPTER 14

Disorders of Movement

There is a wide variety of central nervous system disorders which are associated with involuntary movements. These may take the form of chorea, athetosis, dystonia, tics and tremor and a full review is beyond the scope of this book.

In most of these disorders the involuntary movements are an incidental component of a neurological syndrome. There are, however, a number of conditions in which the muscle dysfunction is likely to be the main or only presenting problem, with referral to a muscle clinic. A review of some of these conditions thus seemed appropriate in a book on neuromuscular disorders.

TORSION DYSTONIA (DYSTONIA MUSCULORUM DEFORMANS)

This condition often starts in childhood and presents with dystonic movements or posture. These are sustained, irregular, uncontrolled movements, often of a writhing or twisting character, which initially are often focal and may affect either the limbs or the axial skeleton. Equinus deformity of the foot or torticollis are common presenting features. The disorder is considered to reflect abnormality in the basal ganglia. The diagnosis is essentially clinical, since there are no consistent biochemical or pathological features. The condition is readily confused with hysteria and indeed emotional and psychological factors appear to precipitate or aggravate the symptoms. As in the case of the muscular dystrophies, attempts were made to define different clinical entities on the basis of the age of onset, the severity and the pattern of inheritance.

HISTORICAL

Oppenheim (1911) coined the term 'dystonia musculorum deformans', while in the same year Flatau and Sterling (1911) suggested 'progressive torsion spasms of childhood', which is perhaps less cumbersome and also a more accurate description. In his comprehensive review of the subject, Eldridge (1970) favoured the use of the term 'torsion dystonias' for the various forms of this disorder. As long ago as 1908 Schwalbe had already reported three affected siblings in a Jewish family, which highlighted the genetic basis and the tendency of the disease to occur with a much higher frequency in Ashkenazic Jews (Zilber *et al.*, 1984). Zador (1936) first stressed the apparent differences in the disease affecting Jewish and non-Jewish patients, the Jewish form tending to have an earlier onset and to affect the limbs more than the trunk.

CLINICAL FEATURES

The onset may be very insidious and often focal so that it may be difficult to confirm clinically in the early stages. Common presenting symptoms are torticollis, clumsiness in the use of the hands, or deformity of a foot (Figure 14-1). It is often revealing to watch the child walking barefoot and also writing with both the left and right hand.

Although broad clinical distinctions have been drawn between the autosomal recessive and autosomal dominant form, it may be impossible to assign a single isolated affected individual to one or other category on clinical grounds alone.

According to Eldridge (1970), the recessive form tends to have an earlier onset, within a range of about 4 to 16 years, with an average of about 10

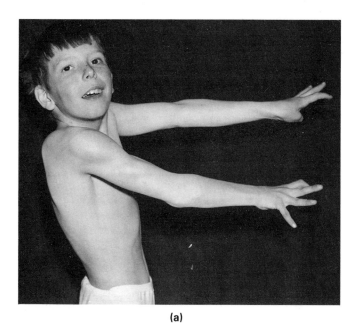

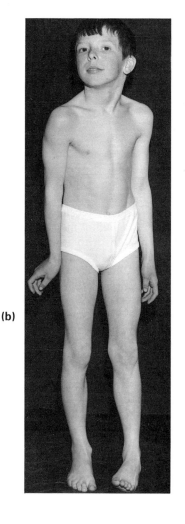

(a)

(b)

Figure 14-1a,b Torsion dystonia. The patient was a 10-year-old boy. Note the postural abnormality of the outstretched hands (a) and the torticollis and equinovarus deformity of left foot (b).

years. It also tends to be more severe and show a more rapid progression, particularly in the early stages. With time these patients tend to become more deformed and disabled and may become completely bedridden. After adolescence the condition usually becomes less progressive and may even improve. However, a number of patients with recessive inheritance have been described as having a milder form of disease and not progressing to complete debility. Of 42 cases reviewed by Marsden and Harrison (1974), 21 showed progression to a generalized torsion dystonia, whereas 21 remained localized. Generalized dystonia was more likely to occur in those cases with onset in early childhood than in those with adolescent or adult onset.

The dominant form has a much wider variability in age of onset (5 to 40 years) and also in clinical severity. As in other dominantly inherited disorders, its clinical expression may vary within the same family and there may be a low penetrance of the gene in some families. Some sporadic cases may be new mutations of the dominant gene.

Cranial nerves are usually spared but in addition to torticollis there may be grimacing of the face and at times difficulty with chewing, swallowing and speech. There may be an associated upset in the sleep rhythm with a tendency to insomnia. During sleep, dystonic symptoms tend to subside. Many authors have commented on the unusually high intellect of children with torsion dystonia and this was substantiated by Eldridge (1970) in a comparative study of 12 patients, 25 siblings and a series of matched controls.

It is also possible that many documented cases of spasmodic torticollis may indeed be examples of torsion dystonia and careful examination may reveal involvement of other muscle groups as well.

PATHOPHYSIOLOGY

There has been a remarkable expansion of knowledge and understanding over the past decade of disorders associated with the basal ganglia, both in relation to the neural pathways as well as to the neuropharmacology. For further details some of the recent reviews should be consulted (Rothwell *et al.*, 1983; Penney and Young, 1983; Alexander and Crutcher, 1990; DeLong, 1990; Hallet, 1993).

GENETICS

Torsion dystonia may be inherited through an autosomal dominant, an autosomal recessive and also an X-linked mechanism. Although earlier reports highlighted the autosomal recessive inheritance in many families, recent segregation analysis studies suggest that many may have an autosomal dominant inheritance with low penetrance (Bressman *et al.*, 1989; Pauls and Korczyn, 1990). A linkage has been established for a dominantly inherited dystonia gene (DYT-1) to chromosome 9q34.

An unequivocal autosomal recessive inheritance has been documented in four families of Spanish gypsies, three of which were consanguineous (Gimenez-Roldan *et al.*, 1988).

An X-linked form of dystonia, with a later, adult onset, some Parkinsonian features, and progression to severe generalized dystonia, has been documented in the Phillipines (Kupke *et al.*, 1990). A locus has been established for the X-linked gene (DYT-3) at Xq13.

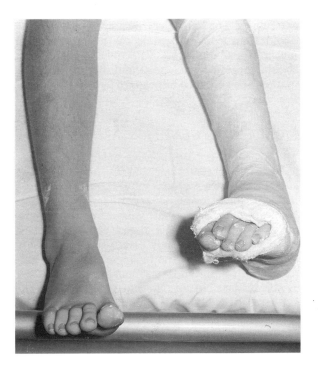

Figure 14-2 Torsion dystonia. Attempt to maintain a corrected posture of the foot with a plaster cast in a 14-year-old girl with torsion dystonia, initially thought to have some conversion overlay, with aggravation of the postural abnormality.

TREATMENT

One of the early approaches to treatment was an attempt at mechanical control of localized dystonia. Metal bands were used for torticollis and orthopaedic casting for involved limbs. Such casting may help correct an abnormal limb posture but it is usually not well tolerated by the patient (Figure 14-2).

Many drugs have been tried and recent advances in the neuropharmacology of the basal ganglia and understanding of the role of the various neurotransmitters has inspired a more rational approach to treatment.

To date, results overall have still been disappointing. Therapeutic approaches have included anticholinergic and antidopaminergic drugs as well as carbamazepine, benzodiazepines, and baclofen. Botulinum toxin has also been tried in focal dystonia in adults.

With more enthusiastic medical treatment, stereotactic surgical techniques with either neuroablative or neuroaugmentative procedures have declined in vogue but may still have a place in selective cases.

HEREDITARY PROGRESSIVE DYSTONIA WITH DIURNAL FLUCTUATION (SEGAWA SYNDROME)

This hereditary dystonia with a striking diurnal fluctuation, with alleviation on waking in the morning and aggravation towards evening, and a remarkable response to levodopa, was originally recognized by Segawa and his colleagues (1971, 1976), who suggested the title. Nygaard *et al.* (1988) subsequently defined as a potentially separate syndrome, dopa-responsive dystonia, but later considered the clinical features to be similar to those of hereditary progressive dystonia with diurnal fluctuation (Nygaard *et al.*, 1993a).

CLINICAL FEATURES

The onset of symptoms is usually in the first decade and the first manifestation is often a dystonic posture of the foot that gradually spreads to other extremities. The course is progressive in the first two decades but tends to become static thereafter. The diurnal fluctuation with worsening in the evening should suggest the diagnosis and there is usually a marked and sustained response to levodopa with few side-effects.

MOLECULAR GENETICS

The gene for dopa-responsive dystonia has been localized to chromosome 14q by Nygaard *et al.* (1993b). Segawa's group subsequently confirmed the same locus for hereditary progressive dystonia with diurnal fluctuations, suggesting these conditions comprise a single disease. In a systematic molecular biological study of tetrahydrobiopterin-synthesizing enzymes, the Japanese group were able to establish a chromosomal localization for GTP cyclohydrolase I to chromosome 14q22.1-q22.2 and subsequently to identify mutations in the GTP cyclohydrolase I gene in patients with hereditary progressive dystonia (Ichinose *et al.*, 1994). This is the first causative gene to be identified in the hereditary dystonias.

CONTINUOUS MUSCLE FIBRE ACTIVITY (ISAACS' SYNDROME)

This unusual disorder, in which the muscle is in a state of continuous contraction, was first described by Isaacs (1961, 1967). The appearance is vaguely reminiscent of myotonia, with inability of the muscle to relax, and led Mertens and Schocke (1965) to suggest the title 'neuromyotonia', but this has not found wide acceptance. It has occurred in childhood in some cases but mostly has been in adults. Isaacs drew an analogy in the appearance of the patient to an armadillo. There may be associated muscle twitching or myokymia, excessive sweating and increased metabolic rate.

The diagnosis can be confirmed on electromyography (EMG), which shows continuous discharge of normal potentials of the muscle at 'rest' and no silence at all. The discharges are not myotonic. The continuous firing on EMG is not abolished by peripheral nerve block, spinal anaesthesia or general anaesthesia, but can be abolished with curare, suggesting its origin within the terminal arborization of the nerve at the motor end plate. Isaacs (1961) first recorded the successful treatment with phenytoin and later suggested that the condition might be cured with long-term therapy (Isaacs and Heffron, 1974).

Although some 50 cases have been documented (Rowland, 1985), only one involved an infant and the response to phenytoin was poor and the course more severe, with a fatal outcome (Black *et al.*, 1972). Thomas *et al.* (1994) recently recorded another two infants who were severely affected, responded poorly to phenytoin and carbamazepine and died of respiratory failure.

A recent report of clinical and laboratory evidence supporting an autoimmune basis for this syndrome suggested a possible reduction in functional potassium channels, leading to increased nerve excitability (Sinha *et al.*, 1991). This also raised the possibility of immunosuppressant treatment in adults but it seems more likely the infantile form results from a congenital defect with an autosomal recessive inheritance.

The muscle is histologically normal but may show depletion of glycogen (Dubowitz and Brooke, 1973) or type 1 fibre predominance with 'moth-eaten' fibres (Scarlato *et al.*, 1974).

RIPPLING MUSCLE DISEASE

In this unusual disorder the muscles are abnormally irritable to mechanical stimulation and either pressure or percussion initiates a rolling wave of contraction that spreads laterally across the muscle like a ripple (Torbergsen, 1975; Ricker *et al.*, 1989).

A similar effect can result spontaneously after voluntary muscle contraction. Percussion may also produce a local mounding of the muscle, so-called myoedema. The condition is not particularly disabling and the patient usually has a sensation of muscle stiffness, together with cramps, during the contraction. Relaxation of the muscle seems normal. The muscle is electrically silent during the contraction.

The pathophysiology is not fully understood, but is thought to relate to an exaggerated release of calcium from the sarcoplasmic reticulum following mechanical deformation.

The condition may occur sporadically or follow an autosomal dominant pattern of inheritance. Stephan *et al.* (1994) have recently located a gene at chromosome 1q41 in a single large 44-member Oregon family. A further study of two previously documented German families did not show linkage to this locus, suggesting genetic heterogeneity.

STIFF MAN SYNDROME

In 1956 Moersch and Woltman described 14 cases from the Mayo Clinic, collected over 30 years, of a syndrome of progressive stiffness and rigidity of the muscles of the neck and trunk, with superimposed attacks of muscle spasm. Spasms were often precipitated by a sudden movement or stimulus. All patients were adult and the majority male. Price and Allott (1958) found that the rigidity was abolished by sleep and general anaesthesia. They were unable to identify any biochemical abnormality apart from raised inorganic phosphate in the blood during attacks. Gordon *et al.* (1967) wrote a critical review of this strange disorder and tried to lay down specific diagnostic criteria. Lorish *et al.* (1989) provided a further update on the syndrome from the Mayo clinic, with the addition of a further 13 cases since the original description. Asher (1958) described 'a woman with the stiff man syndrome' and more recently a number of reports documented a hereditary 'stiff-baby syndrome', with congenital onset and apparently dominant inheritance (Klein *et al.*, 1972; Sander *et al.*, 1980; Lingam *et al.*, 1981). This may overlap clinically with another inherited neonatal disorder, startle disease or hyperexplexia (Markand *et al.*, 1984).

Although the pathogenesis of this unusual disorder still remains obscure, recent studies have implicated a possible autoimmune mechanism and involvement of GABA mediated central inhibition of neurones (Solimena *et al.*, 1988, 1990). Some therapeutic benefit may be obtained from diazepam, but high dosages may be required.

There has also been a report of a family affected by a severe generalized muscle hypertonia during wakefulness, with autosomal recessive inheritance and death when only a few months old (Cantu and Cuellar, 1974). Recently Lacson *et al.* (1994) documented a somewhat similar autosomal recessive, fatal, infantile 'hypertonic muscular dystrophy' in 11 Canadian Aboriginal infants, normal at birth, with a rapidly progressive rigidity of skeletal muscles and early respiratory insufficiency and death before 18 months of age. This syndrome may overlap clinically with the syndrome of continuous muscle fibre activity in infancy (see above; Thomas *et al.*, 1994).

Satoyoshi (1978) documented an unusual syndrome of severe muscle spasms in association with alopecia totalis and diarrhoea. Onset was in childhood, with female predominance and also a tendency to early closure of epiphyses and stunting of growth. Creatine kinase (CK) was elevated after spasms but muscle biopsy was normal.

SPASTIC PARAPARESIS

These cases are at times referred to the muscle clinic as suspected cases of muscular dystrophy, usually because of a toe-gait and associated lordosis that may superficially resemble Duchenne dystrophy (Figure 14-3). The diagnosis of pyramidal tract involvement is usually made on the increased tone and associated fixed deformities of the ankles or hips, and the increased tendon jerks and extensor plantar responses.

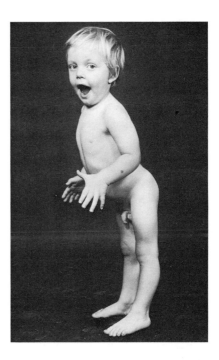

Figure 14-3 Spastic paraparesis. This 3-year-old boy was referred as a possible case of muscular dystrophy. He had a waddling toe-gait, fixed flexion deformity of hips (about 30°) and fixed equinus of feet. When standing with feet flat there was backward angulation of ankles and compensatory hyperextension of the knees. The tendon reflexes were brisk, plantar response extensor. The arms were normal; CK normal. X-ray and myelogram of spine were suggestive of diastematomyelia.

Hereditary spastic paraparesis, which is inherited through an autosomal dominant gene, may start in early childhood and usually shows a slowly progressive course. The arms may also be affected and the involvement is usually symmetrical.

HYSTERICAL (NON-ORGANIC) DISORDERS OF MOVEMENT; CONVERSION DISORDERS

Most physicians feel confident that they can recognize a hysterical disorder when they see one; yet they often lack the courage of their convictions and in order to exclude organic disease will embark on a battery of unnecessary and often painful, invasive and potentially hazardous investigations, which in turn may aggravate and further reinforce the patient's symptoms.

This is perhaps understandable, since the distinction between whether or not a particular illness is organic can at times be difficult. In a follow-up study by Slater (1965) of 85 adult patients diagnosed as having hysteria, an organic disease was subsequently found in no less than 28 (33%). In a similar review of 28 prepubertal children referred over a 22-year period with a diagnosis of hysteria, Caplan (1970) found that 13 (46%) had an organic basis for their presenting symptom on discharge or at later follow-up.

From my experience with a number of children presenting with hysterical disorders of gait, it became apparent that in each case hysterical symptoms were superimposed on an initial organic illness. The problem was thus not so much the distinction as to whether the disorder was 'organic' or 'hysterical' but rather to what extent the presenting features reflected the original illness or were due to psychogenic or 'functional' overlay.

Semantics. The term 'hysteria' is often used very loosely in medical circles and to the lay mind (and to that of some doctors) often carries an implication of absence of disease – a sort of 'non-problem' – which can create difficulties in the management.

Mildred Creak (1938) classified hysteria in childhood into three groups: first, true conversion hysteria, where neurological symptoms were due to conversion of anxiety into somatic manifestations; second, hysterical prolongation of a symptom originally part of an organically determined disease; and third, undoubted organic disease in which nervous (psychological) accompaniment plays an important part. She subsequently drew attention to some of the difficulties in diagnosis and treatment of such patients and made the point that 'hysterical symptoms command both sympathy and unrewarding investigations, which inevitably fail to clarify and so prolong the clinical picture' (Creak, 1969).

CLINICAL FEATURES

In a study of five consecutive cases of hysterical disorder of motor function, there seemed to be a number of clinical features in common (Dubowitz and Hersov, 1976). In the first four cases, the initial illness seemed to be associated with general symptoms, such as sore throat or gastrointestinal upset or fever, in association with either myalgic or arthralgic pain. In the fifth case the pain in the muscles seemed to be related to possible trauma, but this may have been a coincidence.

In all five cases a diagnosis of a non-organic disorder of gait could be made on the basis of the bizarre character of the gait and the disproportion of the disability to any objective evidence of muscle weakness. Three of the patients also demonstrated what I have come to regard as a very useful sign of hysterical paralysis, namely an inability to raise the foot off the floor when attempting to hop on one leg, almost as if the foot were glued to the floor ('glued to the floor' sign). The effort is always associated with exaggerated movements and contortions of the other limbs.

In two of the cases the symptoms may well have been consolidated and perpetuated by a battery of investigations, many of which involved injections.

There was no overt evidence of any particular gross psychopathology in the background of any of the patients and in each instance the condition followed an undoubtedly organic but relatively mild illness.

For some reason, which was not always apparent, the child seemed to need to continue in the 'sick role' situation, and rapid resolution followed once the parents and the child were reassured that the condition had a good prognosis and was in the process of resolution, and that complete normality could be anticipated.

MANAGEMENT

The current paediatric literature contained very little on the management of such patients. Indeed, some series of case reports made no mention of any treatment at all (Sebastianpillai and Wijesinghe, 1972). Neurologists seemed keen to pass the buck to their psychiatric colleagues (Ford, 1966): 'This is a psychiatric problem and if the neurologist is not prepared to undertake this responsibility, he should place the patient and the parents in the hands of the best psychiatrist available. It is my custom to follow this course and to wish both the patient and the psychiatrist the best of luck'.

Standard paediatric texts contained much about diagnosis of hysteria and the way patients can be made to reveal the hysterical basis of their paralysis by trick manoeuvres, but very little on treatment (Nelson *et al.*, 1969). Much was also made of 'la belle indifférence' – the apparent disconcern of the patient for his illness – as a pathognomonic feature, probably passed down from the time of Charcot. It was absent in all our five cases.

Three essentials of management in these cases seemed self-evident:

1. To stop any further investigations beyond the minimum that might possibly be necessary to assure the physician that there was no residual neuromuscular abnormality, e.g., an EMG or possibly a muscle biopsy.
2. To institute without delay a well-planned programme of physical rehabilitation with graduated physical activities. We found the use of an exercise bicycle and treadmill useful in this programme.
3. To involve the psychiatric team (psychiatrist, clinical psychologist and social worker) in assessing and dealing quickly with any important precipitating and aggravating psychological stresses in school or at home. The objective of treatment was to help the patient to give up his 'sick role' and to alter the parents' perception of their child as a chronic invalid to one of potential health and normal development. Once parents are clear that their child is basically healthy, they can throw their weight and influence into supporting his 'escape with honour' from the situation without feeling confused and guilty.

In the medical management, it is essential that the patient is able to form a liaison with one particular doctor, who is in the best position to co-ordinate the whole programme and whom the patient can confide in and regularly turn to for help or advice. It is also advantageous to have continuity of care by the same physiotherapist.

These cases are best managed by a combined approach of the physician and psychiatrist. Equal attention needs to be paid to the physical rehabilitation, which should be started immediately, and the psychological back-up can then go hand in hand with this treatment.

Although a few patients may reveal some psychopathology in their background personality, which may be triggered off by a factor such as an organic illness into the conversion phenomena, the majority seem to show no notable previous psychological abnormality and are perfectly normal once the condition resolves. It is thus important to proceed with treatment of the symptoms even in the absence of any proven basis for the functional overlay.

The relative roles of the physician and the psychiatrist may vary considerably from one patient to the next and it is quite likely that in some cases the condition may respond very rapidly to physical rehabilitation and associated reassurance by the physician before the psychiatrist has arrived on the scene. Others may need a lot more support from the psychiatrist.

The following detailed case reports of two of our five cases (Dubowitz and Hersov, 1976) illustrate the main clinical features and response to treatment.

Case history. This 10-year-old boy was completely well until January 1974, when he developed pain in the feet which was so severe that he found it difficult to stand. His general practitioner diagnosed 'fallen arches' and prescribed exercises. After 3 weeks he returned to school but did not participate in games. Within a few days he had a gastrointestinal upset and recurrence of the pains. He was referred for orthopaedic opinion. A series of X-ray films of the spine and legs was normal. He was measured for plastic inserts to support the arches. The following week the pain in the legs became so severe that he was unable to walk and even resented the jarring when being carried up and down stairs. The pain was mainly in the feet, but also in the thighs and lumbar region. He was admitted to hospital and placed on traction for 2 weeks, with no apparent benefit.

He was then seen by a paediatrician, who instituted a series of investigations, including blood studies for infection, CK and serological studies and routine cerebrospinal fluid (CSF) examination, all of which proved normal. He was discharged home 3 weeks later. The pains in the legs were unchanged and a few days later he woke one morning with weakness of one arm, followed later that morning by weakness of the other arm. He also complained of double vision (in all directions). He was readmitted to the paediatric unit for investigation of a possible intraspinal neoplasm and had a further series of blood studies, and a routine lumbar puncture plus myelogram, all of which were normal. The possibility of some 'supratentorial overlay' was raised. He was then referred to a neurologist who advised a muscle biopsy and EMG and the child was transferred to the adult neurology ward.

A muscle biopsy from the right deltoid, processed by formalin fixation with routine stains only, showed 'mild non-specific changes'; EMG, with 'widespread sampling' (at least eight sites), showed a normal pattern in all muscles, except the biceps and vastus lateralis, which were considered to show some evidence of 'primary myopathy'.

A presumptive diagnosis of polymyositis was made and he was placed on treatment with prednisolone. The dramatic improvement which was anticipated within 2–3 weeks did not occur and after 5 weeks the prednisolone was stopped.

He was discharged home in May 1974 and at that stage was able to walk with support. After 4 days he developed diarrhoea and vomiting, with associated pyrexia and was generally lethargic and unresponsive. He was readmitted and put back on steroid therapy for a further 2 weeks and given active physiotherapy. He was given a wheelchair at the time of discharge, which he continued to use till the end of June. During July he was much improved and played with other children.

In August the family moved to another town and although well and ambulant the boy still complained intermittently of pain in the legs. He had a further episode of pyrexia and gastrointestinal upset with associated lethargy 2 weeks later and was unable to move his arms. Steroids were prescribed again by his general practitioner and within 24 hours the arms returned to normal. However, he continued to have difficulty with walking and went up and down the stairs on his bottom. At that stage he was referred to Hammersmith Hospital.

On admission he had a bizarre gait, with a rolling movement from side to side. He was able to stand on one leg, with some difficulty, but when asked to hop on one leg made bizarre motions, with his foot 'glued to the floor'. The responses to testing individual muscle groups were variable but there was no overt and consistent weakness and he was able to sustain straight-leg raising in supine for 2 minutes. The tone in the limbs appeared to be normal and tendon reflexes were present and symmetrical. He still complained of blurring of vision and intermittent diplopia, but no abnormality could be detected.

A diagnosis of 'functional' weakness, probably following on a viral illness, was made. The steroid therapy was stopped. In view of the results of previous investigations, the EMG was repeated on the left deltoid and right rectus femoris and found to be completely normal; CK was normal at 32 iu/litre. Repeat muscle biopsy or other investigations were considered unnecessary and potentially harmful. He had one sister who attended an ophthalmologist for a squint, which may be relevant to his own visual symptoms. Both children were adopted.

A programme of active rehabilitation was started and he and his parents were reassured that there was no residual underlying muscle pathology, that his EMG was completely normal and that his 'weakness' should steadily resolve.

The tactics of return to school were discussed with the boy's mother and also with his headmaster, who was very willing to help. A date was fixed for the boy to return home, with the aim that he spend only half the day at school for the first week. If all went well

this would increase to a full day the next week. He was discharged after 10 days, and 2 weeks later he was fully ambulant again and started school. Regular contact was maintained by telephone between his mother and the psychiatric social worker. There was no subsequent recurrence of any pain, motor disability or visual symptoms and when assessed at outpatient follow-up after 4 months he was completely normal. There was no further problem in the 2 years of follow-up after that, and he subsequently remained completely well and fully active.

The following case history is very similar to the above and again highlights the possible iatrogenic effect of medical intervention, with unnecessary investigations.

Case history. This 10-year-old boy was well until February 1974 when he had a pyrexial illness with headaches, for which his general practitioner prescribed aspirin. The pyrexia subsided after 48 hours but the headaches recurred. He had a further bout of fever, associated with a sore throat, 2 weeks later.

At the end of March he developed pain in his neck and still complained of persistent headaches. He was referred to a paediatrician who saw him on two domiciliary visits and found some limitation in movement of his neck; the boy also limped with the right leg and there was some calf tenderness. As the family was in the process of moving house, the boy was admitted to hospital for investigations, instead of their being done on an outpatient basis. X-ray of his cervical spine, chest and pelvis and an intravenous pyelogram were all normal, as were routine examinations of urine and cerebrospinal fluid. The blood count and sedimentation rate were normal, and so were the anti-streptolysin (ASO) titre and antinuclear factor, CK, blood culture, agglutination tests for *Brucella*, complement fixation tests for a wide range of viruses, and the urinary vanillyl mandelic acid (VMA) level.

A tentative diagnosis of a rheumatoid disorder was made and he was referred to a rheumatologist, who diagnosed juvenile ankylosing spondylitis and transferred him on 19 May to a long-stay rheumatology unit. The normal sedimentation rate was thought to be unusual for this condition, but clinically he had limitation of movement of his spine and tenderness of both subacromial and acromioclavicular joints and the iliac crests. Prior to his transfer from the paediatric unit, one of the nursing staff explained to him that there were children in the rheumatology unit for up to a year or more with chronic heart disease or locomotor problems. It may also be relevant that a child with severe brain damage occupied the bed opposite his on the paediatric ward.

On the rheumatology ward he was put on complete bed-rest and told by the nursing staff that if he wanted moving he should call them. The oxyphenbutazone (Tanderil®) prescribed by the paediatrician was continued. He became depressed, with loss of appetite, and would not chat with his parents. Investigations included routine blood studies for rheumatoid arthritis and further X-rays of the cervical spine, lumbar spine, hands, feet, pelvis and chest. Attempts were made at active mobilization but he was reluctant to stand or move.

On 30 May he complained of acute anterior chest pain, aggravated by breathing. The chest was clear and pulse and temperature were normal. A pleuritic pain or referred root pain was diagnosed and analgesics prescribed. During the first week of June he still complained of the chest pain and on assessment still had marked limitation of dorsolumbar movements and straight-leg raising, as well as some tenderness over the costochondral junctions and left iliac crest. He was still considered to have juvenile ankylosing spondylitis, complicated by a 'marked but obscure behaviour problem' and was referred for psychiatric opinion. Further attempts at physiotherapy and mobilization were advised. The oxyphenbutazone was stopped and indomethacin was prescribed.

He was seen by several doctors and by a second paediatrician, who found no abnormality in the central nervous system but thought a peripheral neuropathy might be a possibility in view of some reduction in response to cotton-wool sensation over his lower limbs. He also drew attention to the opinion of the nursing and teaching staff that the boy's relationship with his family appeared to be abnormal, suggesting that the boy's condition might be a psychological problem. However, he thought it important to exclude a neuroblastoma and advised repetition of the VMA and associated tests.

Over the next 4 weeks there was no appreciable change in the boy's clinical condition. The sedimentation rate remained normal. The following week there was an improvement in the mobility of his spine and straight-leg raising. An incidental drop in haemoglobin was noted, and investigations of blood iron, folate, B$_{12}$, and full cell-count were undertaken. However, the haemoglobin rose again spontaneously.

At the end of July he complained of earache but no local abnormality was found by the Ear, Nose and Throat surgeon. He was discharged home on 1 August, and prescribed indomethacin and aspirin. He was still awaiting consultation with a psychiatrist and further action was deferred pending the psychiatrist's report.

At that time he was making efforts to walk with support but remained housebound throughout August. At the end of August he developed a ptosis of the left eye and was seen again by his original paediatrician. He was still unable to walk without support. An edrophonium test for myasthenia was negative.

There was little subsequent change in his symptoms and on 29 September he was referred to Hammersmith Hospital for investigation. On admission he was found to have a completely bizarre gait. He was reluctant to take any steps without support and his feet remained 'glued to the floor' when making efforts to move. With support, he kept the feet together, leaned forward and made short shuffling movements. There was no detectable weakness of any muscle groups on formal assessment and the tendon reflexes were normal and symmetrical.

The 'ptosis' was still present, but was variable in degree and involved a 'screwing up' of the whole eye with raising of the lower lid. There was no deficit in any of the cranial nerves and further examination of the central nervous system and other systems was normal. He complained of pain in the thighs and calves but there was no consistent tenderness.

A diagnosis of hysterical paralysis (conversion disorder) was made and a programme of rehabilitation started, with strict avoidance of further investigations of any description. He was referred for psychiatric advice and both he and his parents were assured that his weakness, which appeared to have followed on his original febrile illness, had a good prognosis and should respond well to therapy and completely resolve. While on the ward he subsequently related in vivid detail all the various procedures he had undergone, including 26 venepunctures and three enemas ('which were horrible'). He also took an interest in the diagnostic aspects of other children on the ward.

No apparent problems were present in the family background. He had previously been doing well at school, was top of his class and also good at games. An older sister and brother were normal. The parents were also normal, although the mother had suffered a rheumatoid illness 5 years previously, with no residual problems.

A treatment programme was begun, aimed at overcoming the boy's resistance to physical activity. This included gradually increasing his range of movements in physiotherapy sessions and on the ward, allied to a system of rewards and reinforcements for progress, which was set up and supervised by the clinical psychologist, after discussion with nurses and physiotherapists. The patient and his parents were seen by a psychiatrist and a social worker, respectively, and the boy's mother played an important role in maintaining and rewarding progress over weekends, and later when the boy returned home.

Within a week the 'ptosis' disappeared, although it recurred at times when he was being observed or under tension. His gait was slower to improve, and after the initial 2 or 3 weeks he seemed to become static again and still needed a lot of support with walking. He was doing much better on an exercise bicycle and on a treadmill than with ordinary walking. On 7 November he walked without support and 6 days later he was able to go up and down steps with his mother.

On 18 November, about 6 weeks after admission, he went home for the weekend and walked around on the railway station. The following weekend he was home again and went out shopping. On his return he spoke enthusiastically of his achievements. His gait was still somewhat shuffling and it was debated whether he was ready to be discharged. On 28 November it was decided to let him home for a 3-week trial period. His response was so enthusiastic that he got off his bed and walked spontaneously to the telephone to let his father know.

When seen at outpatient follow-up on 19 December he was maintaining progress. He was walking longer distances but still was not back to full activity. However, he was playing hockey with his brother and sister and was eager to go back to school (after 9 months absence). His gait was still somewhat shuffling when observed, but when he was walking in the hospital grounds out of (conscious) view it was quite normal. He was discharged from regular hospital follow-up, but telephone communication was maintained with his mother and there was no further problem in the 2 years after discharge. He subsequently became a sports enthusiast and excelled at competitive athletics.

Postscript

Since the early experience in managing these patients, I have had the opportunity of treating many children presenting with a wide range of conversion phenomena, mainly involving loss of motor function. The pattern of background clinical history usually followed a remarkably similar sequence to the above case histories. The management always followed the same principles:

1. Make a positive clinical diagnosis of conversion disorder.
2. Avoid any further investigations, except possibly some relatively non-invasive procedures that may be 'therapeutic' in helping to confirm normality of function.

3. Start forthwith on a programme of physical rehabilitation and reassure the patient and his parents that the original organic disorder has now resolved but that the muscles need re-educating in order to regain function. It is important to convey to the family that you are aware that there has been an underlying organic disorder and that the whole condition is not simply 'psychological' or 'non-existent'. The symptoms the patient experiences are always real, whatever the mechanism.
4. Enable the patient and his family, to 'escape with honour', so that there is no feeling of guilt or embarrassment at giving up the 'sick role' situation that has become firmly entrenched.

Many physicians still feel uneasy about making a diagnosis of conversion disorder without the inevitable battery of (unnecessary) investigations to exclude organic disease. My response to this attitude is 'cure it first, and diagnose it afterwards'.

REFERENCES

Alexander, G.E. and Crutcher, M.D. (1990) Functional architecture of basal ganglia circuits: neural substrates of parallel processing. *Trends in Neuroscience* **13**: 266–271.

Asher, R.A. (1958) A woman with the stiff-man syndrome. *British Medical Journal* **i**: 265.

Black, J.T., Garcia-Mullin, R., Good, E. *et al.* (1972) Muscle rigidity in a newborn due to peripheral nerve hyperactivity. *Archives of Neurology* **27**: 413–424.

Bressman, S.B., de Leon, D., Brin, M.F. *et al.* (1989) Idiopathic dystonia among Ashkenazi Jews: Evidence for autosomal dominant inheritance. *Annals of Neurology* **26**: 612–620.

Cantu, J.M. and Cuellar, A. (1974) Congenital severe generalised muscle hypertonia during wakefulness: a distinct autosomal recessive disorder. *Clinical Genetics* **6**: 32–35.

Caplan, H. (1970) *'Hysterical' Conversion Symptoms in Childhood*. M. Phil. Thesis, University of London.

Creak, M. (1938) Hysteria in childhood. *British Journal of Children's Disorders* **35**: 85.

Creak, M. (1969) Hysteria in childhood. *Acta Paedopsychiatrica* **36**: 264.

DeLong, M.R. (1990) Primate models of movement disorders of basal ganglia origin. *Trends in Neuroscience* **13**: 281–285.

Dubowitz, V. and Brooke, M. H. (1973) *Muscle Biopsy: A Modern Approach*. London and Philadelphia: W. B. Saunders.

Dubowitz, V. and Hersov, L. (1976) Management of children with non-organic (hysterical) disorders of motor function. *Developmental Medicine and Child Neurology* **18**: 358–368.

Eldridge, R. (1970) The torsion dystonias: literature review and genetic and clinical studies. *Neurology* **20**: 178.

Flatau, E. and Sterling, W. (1911) Progressive Torsionspasmus bei Kindern. *Zeitschrift fur die gesemte Neurologie und Psychiatrie* **7**: 586.

Ford, F.R. (1966) *Diseases of the Nervous System in Infancy, Childhood and Adolescence* 5th edn. Springfield, Illinois: Charles C. Thomas.

Gordon, E.E., Janusko, D.M. and Kaufman, L. (1967) A critical survey of the stiff-man syndrome. *American Journal of Medicine* **42**: 582.

Gimenez-Roldan, S., Delgado, G., Marin, W. *et al*. (1988) Hereditary torsion dystonia in gypsies. *Advances in Neurology* **50**: 73–81.

Hallett, M. (1993) Physiology of basal ganglia disorders: An overview. *Canadian Journal of Neurological Science* **20**: 177–183.

Ichinose, H., Ohye, T., Takahashi, E. *et al*. (1994) Hereditary progressive dystonia with marked diurnal fluctuation caused by mutations in the GTP cyclohydrolase I gene. *Nature Genetics* **8**: 236–242.

Isaacs, H. (1961) A syndrome of continuous muscle-fibre activity. *Journal of Neurology, Neurosurgery and Psychiatry* **24**: 319–325.

Isaacs, H. (1967) Continuous muscle fibre activity in an Indian male with additional evidence of terminal motor fibre abnormality. *Journal of Neurology, Neurosurgery and Psychiatry* **30**: 126.

Isaacs, H. and Heffron, J.J.A. (1974) The syndrome of "continuous muscle fibre activity" cured: further studies. *Journal of Neurology, Neurosurgery and Psychiatry* **37**: 1231–1235.

Klein, R., Hadow, J.E. and DeLuca, C. (1972) Familial congenital disorder resembling stiff-man syndrome. *American Journal of Diseases of Childhood* **124**: 730–731.

Kupke, G.E., Lee, I.V., Viterbo, G.H. *et al*. (1990) X-linked recessive dystonia in the Philippines. *American Journal of Medical Genetics* **36**: 237–242.

Lacson, A.G., Seshia, S.S., Sarnat, H.B. *et al*. (1994) Autosomal recessive, fatal infantile hypertonic muscular dystrophy among Canadian natives. *Canadian Journal of Neurological Science* **21**: 203–212.

Lingam, S., Wilson, J. and Hart, E.W. (1981) Hereditary stiff-baby syndrome. *American Journal of Diseases of Children* **124**: 730–731.

Lorish, T.R., Thorsteinsson, G. and Howard, F.M. Jr. (1989) Stiff-man syndrome up-dated. *Proceedings of the Mayo Clinic* **64**: 629.

Markand, O.N., Garg, B.P. and Weaver, D.D. (1984) Familial startle disease (hyperexplexia): electrophysiologic studies. *Archives of Neurology* **41**: 71.

Marsden, C.D. and Harrison, M.J.G. (1974) Idiopathic torsion dystonia (dystonia musculorum deformans). A review of forty-two patients. *Brain* **97**: 793–810.

Mertens, H.-G. and Schocke, S. (1965) Neuromyotonie. *Klinische Wochenschrift* **43**: 917.

Moersch, F. P. and Woltman, H. W. (1956) Progressive fluctuating muscular rigidity and spasm (stiff-man syndrome). *Proceedings of the Mayo Clinic* **31**: 421.

Nelson, W.E., Vaughan, V.C. and McKay, R. J. (1969) *Textbook of Paediatrics* 9th edn. Philadelphia: W.B. Saunders.

Nygaard, T.G., Marsden, C.D. and Duvoisin, R.C. (1988) Dopa-responsive dystonia: Clinical characteristics and definition. In: Fahn, S., Marsden, C.D. and Caine, D.B. eds, *Advances in Neurology* Vol 50. New York: Raven Press, pp. 377–384.

Nygaard, T.G., Snow, B.J., Fahn, S. *et al*. (1993a) Dopa-responsive dystonia: Clinical characteristics and definition. In: Segawa, M. ed. *Hereditary Progressive Dystonia with Marked Diurnal Fluctuation*. Camforth, UK: Parthenon, pp. 21–35.

Nygaard, T.G., Wilhelmsen, K.C., Risch, N.J. *et al*. (1993b) Linkage mapping of dopa-responsive dystonia (DRD) to chromosome 14q. *Nature Genetics* **5**: 386–391.

Oppenheim, H. (1911) Uber eine eigenartige Krampfkrankheit des kindlichen und jugendlichen Alters (dysbasia lordotica progressiva, dystonia musculorum deformans). *Neurologisches Zentralblatt* **30**: 1090.

Pauls, D.L. and Korczyn, A.D. (1990) Complex segregation analysis of dystonia pedigrees suggests autosomal dominant inheritance. *Neurology* **40**: 1107–1110.

Penney, J.B. Jr and Young, A.B. (1983) Speculations on the functional anatomy of basal ganglia disorders. *Annual Review of Neurosciences* **6**: 73–94.

Price, T.M.L. and Allott, E.H. (1958) The stiff-man syndrome. *British Medical Journal* i: 682–685.

Ricker, K., Moxley, R.T. and Rohkamm, R. (1989) Rippling muscle disease. *Archives of Neurology* **46**: 405.

Rothwell, J.C., Obeso, J.A., Day, B.L. *et al*. (1983) Pathophysiology of dystonias. *Advances in Neurology* **39**: 851–863.

Rowland, L.P. (1985) Cramps, spasms and muscle stiffness. *Revue Neurologique* **141**: 261–273.

Sander, J.E., Layzer, R.B. and Goldsobel, A.B. (1980) Congenital stiff-man syndrome. *Annals of Neurology* **8**: 195–197.

Satoyoshi, E. (1978) A syndrome of progressive muscle spasm, alopecia and diarrhea. *Neurology* **28**: 458–471.

Scarlato, G., Schoenhuber, R. and Valli, G. (1974) Particolarità istoenzimologische in un caso di neuromiotonia. *Acta Neurologica (Napoli)* **29**: 383–393.

Schwalbe, W. (1908) Eine eignetümliche tonische Krampform mit hysterischen Symptomen. *Medicin und Chirurgie*. Berlin: Universitats-Buchdruckerei von Gustav Schade.

Sebastianpillai, F.J.Y. and Wijesinghe, C.P. (1972) Hysterical paralysis. *Ceylon Medical Journal* **17**: 75.

Segawa, M., Ohmi, K., Itoh, S. *et al*. (1971) Childhood basal ganglia disease with remarkable response to L-dopa, hereditary basal ganglia disease with marked diurnal fluctuation. *Shinryo (Tokyo)* **24**: 667–672.

Segawa, M., Hosaka, A., Miyagawa, F. *et al*. (1976) Hereditary progressive dystonia with marked diurnal fluctuation. In: Eldridge, R. and Fahn,, S. eds, *Advances in Neurology* Vol 14. New York: Raven Press, pp. 215–233.

Sinha, S., Newsom-Davis, J., Mills, K. *et al.* (1991) Autoimmune aetiology for acquired neuromyotonia (Isaacs' syndrome). *Lancet* **338**: 75–77.

Slater, E. (1965) Diagnosis of hysteria. *British Medical Journal* i: 1395.

Solimena, M., Folli, F., Denis-Donini, S. *et al.* (1988) Autoantibodies to glutamic acid decarboxylase in a patient with stiff-man syndrome, epilepsy, and type 1 diabetes mellitus. *New England Journal of Medicine* **318**: 1012.

Solimena, M., Folli, F., Aparisi, R. *et al.* (1990) Auto-antibodies to GABA-ergic neurons and pancreatic beta cells in stiff-man syndrome. *New England Journal of Medicine* **322**: 1555.

Stephan, D.A., Buist, N.R.M., Chittenden, A.B. *et al.*

(1994) A rippling muscle disease gene is localised to 1q41: Evidence for multiple genes. *Neurology* **44**: 1915–1920.

Thomas, N.H., Heckmatt, J.Z., Rodillo, E. *et al.* (1994) Continuous muscle fibre activity (Isaacs' syndrome) in infancy: a report of two cases. *Neuromuscular Disorders* **4**: 147–151.

Torbergsen, T. (1975) A family with dominant hereditary myotonia, muscular hypertrophy, and increased muscular irritability, distinct from myotonia congenita Thomsen. *Acta Neurologica Scandinavica* **51**: 225.

Zador, J. (1936) Le spasme de torsion: paralléle des tableaux cliniques entre la race juive et les autres races. *Revue Neurologique* **66**: 365.

Zilber, N., Korczyn, A., Kahana, E. *et al.* (1984) Inheritance of idiopathic torsion dystonia among Jews. *Journal of Medical Genetics* **21**: 13–20.

CHAPTER 15

Genetics

INTRODUCTION

A detailed description of the intricacies of molecular genetics is beyond the scope of this book; in the first place I would not be able to provide it, and second I would not wish to turn my clinical readers off with too much blinding science. For an overview of the subject, readers are referred to the excellent publication by Trent (1993).

However, some general basic knowledge and understanding in relation to the everyday clinico-genetic problems we have to face in relation to neuromuscular disorders is essential, and I have tried accordingly to concentrate on a few of these practical aspects.

There can hardly be a subject in the whole field of medicine that has seen so much advance on the molecular genetic front as the neuromuscular disorders, and hardly a month passes without some new discovery being made, either in the location of the gene for a particular muscle disorder, or in the characterization of the gene or of its protein product. In order to provide a comprehensive overview, I have included a copy of the gene table, up to date at the time of going to press, which has been a regular feature of *Neuromuscular Disorders*, the bimonthly journal which I edit (Table 15.1). I am extremely grateful to Professor Jean-Claude Kaplan and Dr Bertrand Fontaine, keepers of the gene table, for their agreement for me to reproduce it in this book, and to the publishers, Elsevier Science/Pergamon

Press. I have amended it somewhat, mainly in relation to the clustering and sequence of various neuromuscular disorders, to provide a more pertinent pattern in relation to the neuromuscular disorders of childhood. I am also grateful to Dr Serenella Servidei, for her agreement for me to also include the recently added table of the mitochondrial genome, which she has prepared (Table 15.2). For future update on the molecular genetics of individual disorders, the reader should consult the current issue of the journal, *Neuromuscular Disorders*.

I have also provided a listing (Table 15-3) of gene locations by chromosome in the context of known neuromuscular diseases, and also of proteins that may have a relevance to muscle, which has proved of value in relation to candidate genes for individual proteins at the same locus as the gene for a particular disease.

Finally I have also included a glossary of some of the commonly used terms in everyday molecular genetics (Table 15.4) and a table for reference of the three-letter and one-letter codes for the amino acids, frequently used when referring to genetic mutations (Table 15.5).

Having frequently been bemused by the highly original, but usually totally incomprehensible, symbols that fledgling residents are prone to introduce into their pedigree charts, I thought it might be useful to illustrate the standard symbols used, as well as the well-recognized patterns of Mendelian plus mitochondrial/maternal inheritance (see Figures 15.1–15.5).

Table 15-1 Neuromuscular disorders: molecular genetics

Disease	Mode of inheritance [a]	Gene location [b]	Symbol [c] (gene product)	MIM [d]	Key references
A. Muscular dystrophies					
Duchenne/Becker	XR	Xp21.2	DYS (DMD) (*dystrophin*)	310200	Monaco *et al.* (1986) Burghes *et al.* (1987) Koenig *et al.* (1987, 1988) Hoffman *et al.* (1987, 1988)
Limb-girdle, dominant	AD AD	5q ?	LGMD1A LGMD1B	159000	Speer *et al.* (1992)
Limb-girdle, recessive	AR	15q	LGMD2A	253600	Beckmann *et al.* (1991) Young *et al.* (1992)
	AR	2p	LGMD2B	253600	Bashir *et al.* (1994)
('SCARMD')	AR	13q12	LGMD2C	253700	Ben Othmane *et al.* (1992) Matsumura *et al.* (1992) Azibi *et al.* (1993)
('SCARMD')	AR	17q12–q21	LGMD2D (*adhalin*)	253700	Passos-Bueno *et al.* (1993) Romero *et al.* (1994) Roberds *et al.* (1994)
	AR	?	LGMD2E		
Congenital muscular dystrophy (CMD)					
Fukuyama CMD	AR	9q31–33	FCMD	253800	Toda *et al.* (1993)
CMD (merosin deficient)	AR	6q	LAMM (*merosin*)	?	Tomé *et al.* (1994) Hillaire *et al.* (1994)
CMD (merosin normal)	AR	?			
Emery–Dreifuss	XR	Xq28	EMD (*emerin*)	310300	Hodgson *et al.* (1986) Romeo *et al.* (1988) Bione *et al.* (1994)
Facio-scapulo-humeral	AD	4q35	FSHD	158900	Wijmenga *et al.* (1990, 1991, 1992, 1993) Upadhyaya *et al.* (1990, 1992) Wright *et al.* (1993)
	AD	?	FSHD2	158900	Gilbert *et al.* (1993)
B. Congenital myopathies					
Myotubular myopathy	XR	Xq28	MTM1 (or MTMX)	310400	Thomas *et al.* (1987)
Central core disease	AD	19q13.1	CCD = MH (*ryanodine receptor*)	117000	Kausch *et al.* (1991) Zhang *et al.* (1993) Quane *et al.* (1993)
Nemaline myopathy	AD	1q21–q23	NEM1 (α-*tropomyosin*)	161800	Laing *et al.* (1992) Laing *et al.* (1995)
Congenital fibrosis of the extraocular muscles	AD	12 cen	CFEOM	135700	Engle *et al.* (1994)

continued

Table 15-1 *continued*

Disease	Mode of inheritance [a]	Gene location [b]	Symbol [c] (gene product)	MIM [d]	Key references
C. Ion channel muscle diseases					
Myotonia congenita, dominant (Thomsen's disease)	AD	7q35	**CLC-1** (*muscle chloride channel*)	160800	Koch *et al.* (1992b) George Jr *et al.* (1993)
Myotonia congenita, recessive (Becker disease)	AR	7q35	**CLC-1** (*muscle chloride channel*)	255700	Koch *et al.* (1992b)
Hyperkalaemic periodic paralysis	AD	17q13.1-13.3	**SCN4A** (*sodium channel α-subunit*)	170500	Fontaine *et al.* (1990) Ptacek *et al.* (1991a) Rojas *et al.* (1991)
Paramyotonia congenita	AD	17q13.1–13.3	**SCN4A** (*sodium channel α-subunit*)	168300	Ebers *et al.* (1991) Koch *et al.* (1992a) McClatchey *et al.* (1992) Ptacek *et al.* (1991b)
Hypokalaemic periodic paralysis	AD	1q31-q32	**CACNL1A3** (*calcium channel = dihydropyridine receptor*)	170400	Fontaine *et al.* (1994) Ptacek *et al.* (1994) Jurkat-Rott *et al.* (1994)
Episodic ataxia/myokymia	AD	12p	**EA = KCNA1** (*voltage gated potassium + channel*)	160120	Browne *et al.* (1994)
Malignant hyperthermia	AD	19q13.1	**MHS1** (*ryanodine receptor*)	145600	MacLennan *et al.* (1990) McCarthy *et al.* (1990) Fujii *et al.* (1991) Gillard *et al.* (1991, 1992) Quane *et al.* (1993, 1994) Keating *et al.* (1994)
		17q11.2-q24	MHS2	145600	Levitt *et al.* (1992)
		?	MHS3	145600	Sudbrak *et al.* (1993)
D. Myotonic syndromes					
Myotonic dystrophy (Steinert)	AD	19q13	**DM** (*myotonin-protein kinase*)	160900	Renwick *et al.* (1971) Friedrich *et al.* (1987) Harley *et al.* (1992) Buxton *et al.* (1992) Aslanidis *et al.* (1992) Mahadevan *et al.* (1992) Fu *et al.* (1992) Brook *et al.* (1992)

continued

Table 15-1 *continued*

Disease	Mode of inheritance [a]	Gene location [b]	Symbol [c] (gene product)	MIM [d]	Key references
E. Metabolic myopathies					
Glycogenoses					
Type II (Pompe)	AR	17q23	**GAA** (*acid maltase*)	232300	Hers (1963)
Type V (McArdle)	AR	11q13	**PYGM** (*muscle-type phosphorylase*)	232600	Mommaerts *et al.* (1959) Schmidt *et al.* (1959) Lebo *et al.* (1984) Tsujino *et al.* (1993a)
Type VII (Tarui)	AR	1cenq32	**PFKM** (*muscle-type phosphofructo-kinase*)	232800	Tarui *et al.* (1965) Vora *et al.* (1982) Nakajima *et al.* (1991)
Type IX	XR	Xq13	**PGK1** (*phosphogly-cerate kinase*)	311800	DiMauro *et al.* (1981a, 1983) Rosa *et al.* (1982)
Type X	AR	7p12-p13	**PGAMM** (*muscle phosphogly-cerate mutase*)	261670	DiMauro *et al.* (1981b) Edwards *et al.* (1989) Castella-Escola *et al.* (1990) Tsujino *et al.* (1993b)
Type XI	AR	11p15.4	**LDHA** (*lactate dehydrogenase*)	150000	Boone *et al.* (1972) Kanno *et al.* (1980) Scrable *et al.* (1990)
Disorders of lipid metabolism					
Carnitine palmitoyl-transferase deficiency	AR	1p11-p13	**CPT2** (*carnitine palmitoyl-transferase*)	255110	DiMauro and Melis-DiMauro (1973) Finocchiaro *et al.* (1991) Minoletti *et al.* (1992) Taroni *et al.* (1993)
F. Neurogenic syndromes					
Spinal muscular atrophy (SMA) Werdnig–Hoffmann (type 1)	AR	5q11-q13	SMA	253300	Gilliam *et al.* (1990) Melki *et al.* (1990b, 1994) Lefebvre *et al.* (1995) Roy *et al.* (1995)
Spinal muscular atrophy Kugelberg–Welander (type 3)	AR	5q11-q13	SMA	253400	Brzustowicz *et al.* (1990) Melki *et al.* (1990a)
Spinobulbar muscular atrophy (Kennedy disease)	XR	Xq21-22	**SBMA** (*androgen receptor*)	313200	Fischbeck *et al.* (1986) La Spada *et al.* (1991)
Familial amyotrophic lateral sclerosis (FALS)	AD	21q22	ALS **(SOD1)** (*Cu/ZN superoxide dismutase*)	105400	Siddique *et al.* (1991) Rosen *et al.* (1993)
	AR	2q33–35	ALS2	205100	Hentati *et al.* (1944)

continued

Table 15-1 *continued*

Disease	Mode of inheritance [a]	Gene location [b]	Symbol [c] (gene product)	MIM [d]	Key references
Hereditary motor and sensory neuropathies (HMSN)					
HMSN 1A	AD	17p11.2	**CMTIA** **PMP-22** (*peripheral myelin protein P22*)	118220	Vance *et al.* (1989) Matsunami *et al.* (1992) Patel *et al.* (1992) Timmerman *et al.* (1990, 1992) Valentijn *et al.* (1992) Roa *et al.* (1993)
HMSN IB	AD	1q21-23	CMT1B **PMP0** (*peripheral myelin protein P$_0$*)	118200	Bird *et al.* (1982) Guiloff *et al.* (1982) Hayasaka *et al.* (1993) Kulkens *et al.* (1993)
HMSN IC	AD	?			
HMSN (?ID)	AR	8q	CMT4A	214400	Ben Othmane *et al.* (1993b)
HMSN X-linked	XD	Xq13	CMTX (*connexin*)	302800	Gal *et al.* (1985) Bergoffen *et al.* (1993)
HMSN II (axonal)	AD	1p35-p36	CMT2A	118210	Hentati *et al.* (1992) Ben Othmane *et al.* (1993a)
HMSN III (Dejerine Sottas)	?	?			
Hereditary neuropathy with liability to pressure palsies (HNPP)	AD	17p11.2	**PMP-22** (*peripheral myelin protein P22*)	162500	Chance *et al.* (1993) Nicholson *et al.* (1994)
Hereditary ataxias					
Friedreich's ataxia	AR	9cen-q21	FA	229300	Chamberlain *et al.* (1988)
Friedreich's ataxia with selective vitamin E deficiency	AR	8q	VED	277460	Ben Hamida *et al.* (1993)
Spinal cerebellar atrophy	AD	6p23	**SCA1** (*ataxin-1*)	164400	Jackson *et al.* (1977) Zoghbi *et al.* (1991) Orr *et al.* (1993) Khati *et al.* (1993) Banfi *et al.* (1994)
Spinal cerebellar atrophy (Cuban)	AD	12q23-24.1	**SCA2**	164400	Auberger *et al.* (1990) Gispert *et al.* (1993)
Spinal cerebellar atrophy	AD	14q24.3-qter	**SCA3**	164400	Stevanin *et al.* (1994)
Spinal cerebellar atrophy	AD	?	**SCA4**	164400	Stevanin *et al.* (1994)

[a] Inheritance: XR: sex-linked recessive; AD: autosomal dominant; AR: autosomal recessive.
[b] Location: chromosomal assignment of the morbid locus, or of the gene when known.
[c] Symbol: acronym of the locus or of the gene approved by the Nomenclature Committee of the Human Gene Mapping International Workshops. Gene: when known the full name of the gene product is given in parentheses; for cloned genes the symbol is printed in **bold** type.
[d] MIM: reference number in McKusick (1992).

This table has been adapted from *Neuromuscular Disorders*, with the permission of Drs Jean-Claude Kaplan and Bertrand Fontaine and the publisher.

Table 15.2 Mitochondrial encephalomyopathies: gene mutations

Disease	Mitochondrial DNA mutation	Gene location[a]	Mode of inheritance[b]	Key references
Mitochondrial encephalomyopathies associated with mitochondrial DNA mutations: defects of mitochondrial DNA				
KSS	Single large deletion		Sporadic	Holt *et al*. (1988) Zeviani *et al*. (1988)
	Duplication		Sporadic	Poulton *et al*. (1989)
Pearson's syndrome (+ / − KSS)	Single large deletion		Sporadic	Rotig *et al*. (1989) McShane *et al*. (1991)
PEO	Single large deletion		Sporadic	Holt *et al*. (1988)
	Point mutation nt-3243 A->G	tRNA-Leu(UUR)	Maternal	Moraes *et al*. (1993c)
	Point mutation nt-5703 C->T	tRNA-Asn	Maternal	Moraes *et al*. (1993b)
Multisystem/PEO	Point mutation nt-3256 C->T	tRNA-Leu(UUR)	Maternal	Moraes *et al*. (1993b)
MELAS	Point mutation nt-3243 A->G	tRNA-Leu (UUR)	Maternal	Goto *et al*. (1990) Kobayashi *et al*. (1990)
	Point mutation nt-3252 A->G	tRNA-Leu(UUR)	Maternal	Morten *et al*. (1993)
	Point mutation nt-3271 T->C	tRNA-Leu(UUR)	Maternal	Goto *et al*. (1991)
MERRF	Point mutation nt-8344 A->G	tRNA-Lys	Maternal	Shoffner *et al*. (1990)
	Point mutation nt-8356 T->C	tRNA-Lys	Maternal	Silvestri *et al*. (1992)
MERRF/MELAS	Point mutation nt-8356 T->C	tRNA-Lys	Maternal	Zeviani *et al*. (1993)
NARP	Point mutation nt-8993 T->G	ATPase 6	Maternal	Holt *et al*. (1990)
	Point mutation nt-8993 T->C	ATPase 6	Maternal	de Vries *et al*. (1993)
MILS	Point mutation nt-8993 T->G	ATPase 6	Maternal	Tatuch *et al*. (1992) Shoffner *et al*. (1992)
Myopathy	Point mutation nt-3250 T->C	tRNA-Leu (UUR)	Maternal	Goto *et al*. (1992)
	Point mutation nt-3302 A->G	tRNA-Leu (UUR)	Maternal	Bindoff *et al*. (1993)
	Point mutation nt-15990 C->T	tRNA-Pro	Maternal	Moraes *et al*. (1993a)
	Large-scale tandem duplication		Sporadic	Manfredi *et al*. (1995)
MIMyCa	Point mutation nt-3260 A->G	tRNA-Leu(UUR)	Maternal	Zeviani *et al*. (1991)
Cardiomyopathy	Point mutation nt-3303 C->T	tRNA-Leu(UUR)	Maternal	Silvestri *et al*. (1994)
	Point mutation nt-9997 T->C	tRNA-Glycine	Maternal	Merante *et al*. (1994)
Multisystem/ cardiomyopathy	Point mutation nt-3243 A->G	tRNA-Ile	Maternal	Taniike *et al*. (1992)
Fatal congenital multisystem disorder	Point mutation nt-159233 A->G	tRNA-Thr	Maternal	Yoon *et al*. (1991)

continued

Table 15.2 *continued*

Disease	Mitochondrial DNA mutation	Gene location[a]	Mode of inheritance[b]	Key references
LHON	Point mutation nt-3394 T->C	ND1	Maternal	Brown *et al.* (1992a)
	Point mutation nt-3460 G->A	ND1	Maternal	Huoponen *et al.* (1991)
	Point mutation nt-4160 T->C	ND1	Maternal	Howell *et al.* (1991)
	Point mutation nt-4216 T->C	ND1	Maternal	Mackey and Howell (1992)
	Point mutation nt-4917 A->G	ND2	Maternal	Johns and Berman (1991)
	Point mutation nt-5244 G->A	ND2	Maternal	Brown *et al.* (1992b)
	Point mutation nt-7444 G->A	COX I	Maternal	Brown *et al.* (1992a)
	Point mutation nt-11778 G->A	ND4	Maternal	Wallce *et al.* (1988)
	Point mutation nt-13708 G->A	ND5	Maternal	Johns and Berman (1991)
	Point mutation nt-14484 T->C	ND6	Maternal	Johns *et al.* (1992)
	Point mutation nt-152570 G->A	Cyt b	Maternal	Johns and Neufeld (1991)
	Point mutation nt-15812 G->A	Cyt b	Maternal	Johns and Neufeld (1991)
LHON/dystonia	Point mutation nt-14459 G->A	ND6	Maternal	Jun *et al.* (1994)

Mitochondrial encephalomyopathies associated with mitochondrial DNA mutations: mendelian-inherited (nuclear) mitochondrial DNA defects

Disease	Mitochondrial DNA mutation	Gene location[a]	Mode of inheritance[b]	Key references
PEO	Multiple deletions	?	AD	Zeviani *et al.* (1989) Servidei *et al.* (1991)
Myopathy	Multiple deletions	?	AR	Yuzaki *et al.* (1989)
Progressive encephalomypathy	Multiple deletions	?	AD	Cormier *et al.* (1991)
Familial recurrent myoglobinuria	Multiple deletions	?	(AR?)	Ohno *et al.* (1991)
MNGIE	Multiple deletions	?	AR	Uncini *et al.* (1994)
Familial idiopathic cardiomyopathy	Multiple deletions	?	AD	Suomalainen *et al.* (1992)
Fatal infantile myopathy	Severe depletion	?		Moraes *et al.* (1991)
Myopathy of childhood	Partial depletion	?		Tritschler *et al.* (1992)
Fatal infantile hepatopathy	Severe depletion	?		Mazziotta *et al.* (1992)

KSS = Kearns-Sayres syndrome (MIM 165100); PEO = progressive external ophthalmoplegia (MIM 165130); MELAS = mitochondrial encephalomyopathy, lactic acidosis and stroke-like episodes (MIM 251910); MERRF = myoclonic epilepsy with ragged-red fibres (MIM 254775); NARP = neuropathy, ataxia, retinitis pigmentosa; MILS = maternally inherited Leigh's syndrome: LHON = Leber's hereditary optic neuropathy; MIMyCa = maternally inherited myopathy and cardiomyopathy; MNGIE = myo-neuro-gastrointestinal encephalopathy. (MIM: reference number in McKusick (1992)).
[a] Mitochondrial DNA sequence according to Anderson (1981). [b] Inheritance: AD: autosomal dominant; AR: Autosomal recessive. ?: Unknown.

This table has been adapted from *Neuromuscular Disorders*, with the permission of Dr Serenella Servidei and the publisher.

Table 15-3 Gene location, by chromosome, of genes for neuromuscular disorders, associated diseases and potentially relevant proteins

Chromosomal region	Gene/disease locus
1p11-p13	Carnitine palmitoyltransferase/deficiency
1p21-qter	Actin, alpha chains
1p13	Adenosine monophosphate deaminase 1/myopathy
1cen-q32	Muscle phosphofructokinase/glycogenosis VII
1q21-q23	Nemaline myopathy (dominant)/α-tropomyosin/α-actinin
1q21-q23	ATPase, Na$^+$/K$^+$, alpha 2 polypeptide
1q21-23	HMSN type IB/peripheral myelin protein (PMP) P$_O$
1q22-q25	ATPase, Na$^+$/K$^+$, beta polypeptide
1q31-q32	Hypokalaemic periodic paralysis/dihydropyridine-sensitive calcium channel
1p35-p36	HMSN type IIA
2p	Recessive limb girdle dystrophy
2q21-q33	Sodium channel type II, alpha polypeptide*
2q21-q32	Muscle nicotinic ACHR, alpha subunit*
2q31-q32	Nebulin
2q32-qter	Muscle nicotinic ACHR, gamma subunit
2q33-qter	Muscle nicotinic ACHR, delta subunit
2q	Desmin
3q21	Dystroglycan
4p16-q23	ATPase, Na$^+$/K$^+$, beta polypeptide-like 1
4q35	Facioscapulohumeral dystrophy
5q11-q13	Severe, intermediate and mild childhood spinal muscular atrophy
5q13	Hexosaminidase B/Sandhoff's disease
5q22-q34	Dominant limb girdle muscular dystrophy
6q	Merosin/congenital muscular dystrophy
7pter-q22	Actin, cytoskeletal*
7cen-q11.2	Myosin, heavy polypeptide 5
7p12-p13	Phosphoglycerate mutase
7q35	Muscle chloride channel/myotonia congenita
8q	Friedreich's ataxia with vitamin E deficiency
9cen-q21	Friedreich's ataxia
9q31-33	Fukuyama congenital muscular dystrophy
9q34	Torsion dystonia (some families)
10	Mitochondrial ATPase*
11q13-q13.2	Muscle phosphorylase/McArdle's disease
11p15.4	Lactate dehydrogenase
12q22-qter	Short and medium-chain acyl CoA dehydrogenase/lipid storage myopathy

continued

Table 15-3 *continued*

Chromosomal region	Gene/disease locus
13q12	Autosomal recessive limb girdle dystrophy (SCARMD)
13q21-q31	ATPase, Na$^+$/K$^+$, alpha polypeptide-like 1
14q32.3	Brain creatine kinase
15q11-q12	Angelman and Prader–Willi syndromes
15q15-q22	Recessive limb girdle dystrophy
15q22-qter	Muscle pyruvate kinase
17q12-q21	Adhalin/recessive limb girdle dystrophy
17pter-p11	Myosin, heavy chain cluster
17p12-p11	Muscle nicotinic ACHR, beta subunit*
17p11.2	HMSN type 1A (most families)/peripheral myelin protein (PMP22)
17q13.1-113.3	Na channel α-subunit/hyperkalaemic periodic paralysis/paramyotonia congenita
17q21-q22	Nerve growth factor receptor
17q23	Acid alpha-glucosidase/acid maltase deficiency
18q11.2-q12.1	Transthyretin/familial amyloid polyneuropathy, several types.
18q22-qter	Myelin base protein
19q12-q13.2	Ryanodine receptor/malignant hyperthermia/central core disease
19q13.1	Myelin-associated glycoprotein
19p13.3	Myotonic dystrophy/myotonin-protein kinase
19q13.2-q13.3	Muscle creatine kinase
21q22	Familial amyotrophic lateral sclerosis/Cu/Zn superoxide dismutase
22q13-qter	Neuroaxonal dystrophy
Xp22.2	X-linked HMSN 2
Xp21.2	Duchenne and Becker muscular dystrophies
Xq11-q13	X-linked HMSN 1
Xq13	Phosphoglycerate kinase/HMSN/connexin
Xq12-q22	X-linked spastic paraplegia*
Xq21-q22	Spinobulbar muscular atrophy/androgen receptor
Xq27-q28	Congenital myotubular myopathy
Xq28	Emery–Dreifuss muscular dystrophy

p = short arm; q = long arm; ter = end of short or long arm; c = centromere; e.g. 5q13 = band 13 on the long arm of chromosome 5 (band numbers increase moving in either direction away from the centromere), 3p21-cen = between band 21 on the short arm of chromosome 3 and the centromere, and 10 implies localized to chromosome 10, but not to any specific region.
HMSN: hereditary motor and sensory neuropathy; ACHR: acetylcholine receptor; SCARMD: severe childhood autosomal recessive muscular dystrophy.
* = provisional assignment only.

Table 15-4 Glossary of useful terms

Alternative splicing: If there are multiple exons and introns in a gene, then by choosing different splice donor/acceptor sites, different portions of the primary transcript, containing different exons, are retained in the mature transcript. By this process a single gene can give rise to multiple mature RNA transcripts, coding for proteins with variable structural elements.

Deletion: Deletions of all or part of the coding regions of the gene will delete the corresponding sequence from the protein product, or the entire product, depending on the size of the deletion. Deletions in the promotor or other non-coding regions may still impair the production of an mRNA transcript, and hence block protein production.

Exons: Exons are regions of those portions of the DNA within the gene that are transcribed into mature transcripts. They can be coding (i.e. determining a protein sequence) or non-coding (regions at either end of the RNA which regulate the translation of the transcript).

Frameshift mutation: The sequence of nucleotide triplets follows 'in frame' from the start codon (e.g. AUG,GAC,GCA). Deletion or insertion of a single nucelotide in the coding sequence alters the triplet sequence in which the codons are 'read', and shifts the reading frame (e.g. deletion of the fifth nucleotide in the above example would give AUG,GCG,CA etc.). This changes the amino acid sequence coded from this point. The shift in frame may also introduce premature 'stop' codons which will terminate the synthesis of the protein, or produce a longer protein by preventing the normal 'in-frame' stŏp codon from being recognized.

Genetic heterogeneity: Refers to the presence of more than one separate gene for an individual disease.

Introns: Introns are the regions of DNA within the gene that separate the exons. They do not (normally) code for protein sequence, but may contain regulatory elements that determine the efficiency of expression of the gene, or affect the choice of the exons included in the mature transcript.

Linkage: This expresses the association of a gene for a disease with DNA markers which are located close to it.

LOD score: This represents the logarithm of the odds for linkage and indicates the statistical support for linkage versus non-linkage between two loci. A lod score of 3 or greater, which corresponds to a p value of 0.05, has conventionally been accepted as statistical evidence for linkage and a lod score of -2 or less as evidence against linkage.

Missense mutations: These are point mutations in the coding sequence that result in the substitution of one amino acid for another in the final protein, but since the frame is unaffected, the rest of the protein sequence will be normal. The effect depends entirely on the importance of that amino acid in the protein structure, and can vary from no effect to a completely inactive protein.

Nonsense mutations: These are point mutations which produce a stop codon which terminates translation. A frameshift mutation may also introduce a stop codon downstream from the mutation site.

Point mutation: Point mutation is the alteration of a single nucleotide in the DNA to another nucleotide. Depending on the nucleotide mutated, the result may range from no effect at all, since most amino acids are coded for by more than one combination of nucleotides, to a complete block of product synthesis.

Promoter: This is a regulatory region of DNA in a gene which precedes the start of the coding sequence, and which, by interacting with a variety of protein factors, determines when, where, and how much expression of the gene should occur.

Splice mutation: A point mutation at the splice donor or acceptor sites will prevent normal splicing of the primary RNA transcript, resulting in an altered mature transcript. This may not be translatable, may be translated lacking one or more exons, or may create a new exon which includes intronic DNA, which could also be translated into protein. A point mutation may create a new alternative splice donor or acceptor site, resulting again in a defective mature transcript, or one with a different coding region.

Splicing: Splicing is the process by which the primary RNA transcript is cut, sequences corresponding to introns are removed, and the cut ends joined together so that the exons are then contiguous in the mature transcript. The places at which the splicing begins and ends are termed the splice donor and splice acceptor sites.

Transcription: Transcription is the process of copying a DNA sequence into a complementary RNA sequence, known as the primary transcript. This may then be edited by a process of splicing (see above) to form the mature mRNA used for translation into protein.

Translation: Translation is the synthesis of a protein product by assembling single amino acids into a polypeptide, the sequence of which is determined by the RNA sequence in the coding portion of the mature transcript. The amino acids are specified by triplets of nucleotides called codons.

Table 15-5 Single letter code and three-letter code for individual amino acids

Amino acid	Three letter code	One letter code
Alanine	ala	A
Cysteine	cys	C
Aspartic acid	asp	D
Glutamic acid	glu	E
Phenylalanine	phe	F
Glycine	gly	G
Histidine	his	H
Isoleucine	ile	I
Lysine	lys	K
Leucine	leu	L
Methionine	met	M
Asparagine	asn	N
Proline	pro	P
Glutamine	gln	Q
Arginine	arg	R
Serine	ser	S
Threonine	thr	T
Valine	val	V
Tryptophan	trp	W
Tyrosine	tyr	Y

Figures 15-1–15-5 Pedigree charts; patterns of inheritance. Note that roman numerals (I, II, III, IV etc) are used to designate successive generations, and arabic numerals alongside individual male or female symbols, to designate, from left to right, the individual members within the pedigree in that generation, and also the rank order within sibships. A number within a symbol e.g. ☐2, ◯4, represents the number of male or female siblings within that sibship, which are not individually designated. An oblique line through the symbol represents death, thus Ø = unaffected female who has died, ◼ affected male who has died.

Autosomal dominant

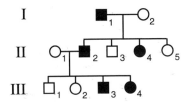

◯ ☐ Unaffected female, male
● ◼ Clinically affected female, male
Risk: One parent affected (manifesting heterozygote) (I,1 ; II,2)
50% of offspring affected (II,2 ; II,4 ; III,3 ; III,4)
50% of offspring normal (II,3 ; II,5 ; III,1 ; III,2)

Figure 15.1

Autosomal recessive

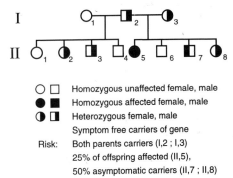

◯ ☐ Homozygous unaffected female, male
● ◼ Homozygous affected female, male
◑ ◨ Heterozygous female, male
     Symptom free carriers of gene
Risk: Both parents carriers (I,2 ; I,3)
25% of offspring affected (II,5),
50% asymptomatic carriers (II,7 ; II,8)

Figure 15.2

Homozygosity by descent
(autosomal recessive)

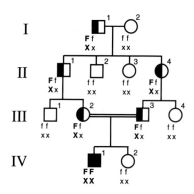

F   Gene for Fukuyama congenital muscular dystrophy

x   Gene for Xeroderma pigmentosum

■ ◐   Heterozygous for the two closely linked mutant genes, (Ff, Xx)

■   Homozygous for the two mutant genes, (FF, XX)

○–□   Consanguineous mating

Figure 15.3 Autosomal recessive: homozygosity by descent. A heterozygote carrier of two closely associated genes (I,1) will pass both genes down to next generation (II,1; II,4). If there is then consanguinity in the next generation, the two mutant genes may be carried by both partners (III,2 and III,3) and their offspring can become homozygotes for both genes (IV,1). The two genes may relate to disease (e.g. Fukuyama congenital muscular dystrophy (F) and xeroderma pigmentosum (X) on chromosome 9q (see Chapter 2)) or one may be a DNA probe with different alleles, closely linked to a gene locus (see Chapter 2).

X-linked recesssive

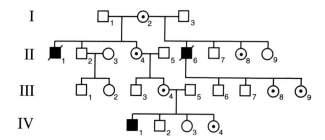

○ □   Unaffected female, male

■   Affected male

◣   Affected male, died

⊙   Carrier female, usually asymptomatic; may manifest clinical features.

Risk: 50% of sons of carrier females affected (II,1; II,6)
50% of daughters carriers (II,4 ; II,8)
All daughters of affected male carriers (III,8 ; III,9), all sons normal (III,6; III,7)

Figure 15.4

Mitochondrial / maternal inheritance

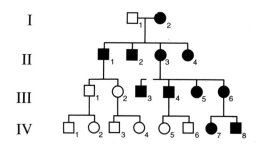

● ■   Affected female, male

○ □   Unaffected female, male

Transmission: Mother passes mutant gene to sons and daughters. Only daughters pass mutant gene to their sons and daughters, no male to male or male to female transmission.

Figure 15.5

REFERENCES

Anderson, S., Bankier, A.T., Barrel, B.G. *et al.* (1981) Sequence and organisation of the human mitochondrial genome. *Nature* 290: 457–465.

Aslanidis, C., Jansen, G., Amemiya, C. *et al.* (1992) Cloning of the essential myotonic dystrophy region and mapping of the putative defect. *Nature* 355: 548–551.

Auburger, G., Orozco Diaz, G., Ferreira, C. *et al.* (1990) Autosomal dominant ataxia: genetic evidence for locus heterogeneity from a Cuban founder-effect population. *American Journal of Human Genetics* 46: 1163–1177.

Azibi, K., Bachner, L., Beckmann, J.S. *et al.* (1993) Severe childhood autosomal recessive muscular dystrophy with the deficiency of the 50 kDa dystrophin-associated glycoprotein maps to chromosome 13q12. *Human Molecular Genetics* 2: 1423–1428.

Banfi, S., Servadio, A., Chung, M.Y. *et al.* (1994) Identification and characterization of the gene causing type 1 spinocerebellar ataxia. *Nature Genetics* 7: 513–520.

Bashir, R., Strachan, T., Keers, S. *et al.* (1994) A gene for autosomal recessive limb-girdle muscular dystrophy maps to chromosome 2. *Human Molecular Genetics* 3: 455–457.

Beckmann, J.S., Richard, I., Hillaire, D. *et al.* (1991) A gene for limb-girdle muscular dystrophy maps to chromosome 15 by linkage. *Comptes Rendus de l'Academic des Sciences (Paris)* 312: series III, 141–148.

Ben Hamida, C., Doerflinger, N., Belal, S. *et al.* (1993) Localization of Friedreich ataxia phenotype with selective vitamin E deficiency to chromosome 8q by homozygosity mapping. *Nature Genetics* 5: 195–200.

Ben Othmane, K., Ben Hamida, M., Pericak-Vance, M. *et al.* (1992) Linkage of Tunisian autosomal recessive Duchenne-like muscular dystrophy to the pericentromeric region of chromosome 13q. *Nature Genetics* 2: 315–317.

Ben Othmane, K., Middleton, L.T., Loprest, L.J. *et al.* (1993a) Localization of a gene (CMT2A) for autosomal dominant Charcot-Marie-Tooth disease type 2 to chromosome 1p and evidence of genetic heterogeneity. *Genomics* 17: 370–375.

Ben Othmane, K., Hentati, F., Lennon, F. *et al.* (1993b) Linkage of a locus (CMT4A) for autosomal recessive Charcot-Marie-Tooth disease to chromosome 8q. *Human Molecular Genetics* 2: 1625–1628.

Bergoffen, J., Scherer, S.S., Wang, S. *et al.* (1993) Connexin mutations in X-linked Charcot-Marie-Tooth disease. *Science* 262: 2039–2041.

Bindoff, L.A., Howell, N., Poulton, J. *et al.* (1993) Abnormal RNA processing associated with a novel tRNA mutation in mitochondrial DNA. A potential disease mechanism. *Journal of Biological Chemistry* 268: 19559–19564.

Bione, S., Maestrini, E., Rivella, S. *et al.* (1994) Identification of a novel X-linked gene responsible for Emery–Dreifuss muscular dystrophy. *Nature Genetics* 8: 323–327.

Bird, T.D., Ott, J. and Giblett, E.R. (1982) Evidence for linkage of Charcot-Marie-Tooth neuropathy to the Duffy locus on chromosome 1 (abstract). *American Journal of Human Genetics* 32: 99.

Boone, C.M., Chen, T.R. and Ruddle, F.H. (1972) Assignment of three human genes to chromosomes (LDH-A to 11, TK to 17, and IDH to 20) and evidence for translocation between human and mouse chromosomes in somatic cell hybrids. *Proceedings of the National Academy of Sciences of the USA* 69: 510–514.

Brook, J.D., McCurrach, M.E., Harley, H.G. *et al.* (1992) Molecular basis of myotonic dystrophy: expansion of a trinucleotide (CTG) repeat at the 3′ end of a transcript encoding a protein kinase family member. *Cell* 68: 799–808.

Brown, M.D. Volijavec, A.S., Lott, M.T., MacDonald, I., and Wallace, D.C. (1992a) Leber's hereditary optic neuropathy: a model for a mitochondrial neurodegenerative disease. *Federation Proceedings* 6: 2791–2799.

Brown, M.D., Volijavec, A.S., Lott, M.T., Torroni, A. Yang, C.-C. and Wallace, D.C. (1992b) Mitochondrial DNA complex I and III mutations associated with Leber's hereditary optic neuropathy. *Genetics* 130: 163–173.

Browne, D.L., Gancher, S.T., Nutt, J.G. *et al.* (1994) Episodic ataxia/myokymia syndrome is associated with point mutations in the human potassium channel gene, KCNA1. *Nature Genetics* 8: 136–140.

Brzustowicz, L.M., Lehner, T., Castilla, L.H. *et al.* (1990) Genetic mapping of chronic childhood-onset spinal muscular atrophy to chromosome 5q11.2-13.3 *Nature* 344: 540–541.

Burghes, A.H.M. Logan, C., Hu, X., Belfall, B., Worton, R.G. and Ray, P.N. (1987) A cDNA clone from the Duchenne/Becker muscular dystrophy gene. *Nature* 328: 434–437.

Buxton, J., Shelbourne, P., Davies, J. *et al.* (1992) Detection of an unstable fragment of DNA specific to individuals with myotonic dystrophy. *Nature* 355: 547–548.

Carrier, L., Hengstenberg, C., Beckmann, J.S. *et al.* (1993) Mapping of a novel gene for familial hypertrophic cardiomyopathy to chromosome 11. *Nature Genetics* 4: 311–313.

Castella-Escola, J., Mattei, M.G., Ojcius, D.M. *et al.* (1990) *In situ* mapping of the muscle-specific form of phosphoglycerate mutase gene to human chromosome 7p12-7p13. *Human Genetics* 84: 210–212.

Chamberlain, S., Shaw, J., Rowland, A. *et al.* (1988) Mapping of mutation causing Friedreich's ataxia to human chromosome 9. *Nature* 334: 248–250.

Chance, P.F., Alderson, M.K., Leppig, K.A. *et al.* (1993) DNA deletion associated with hereditary neuropathy with liability to pressure palsies. *Cell* 72: 143–151.

Cormier, V., Rotig, A., Tardieu, M. *et al.* (1991) Autosomal dominant deletions of the mitochondrial genome in a case of progressive encephalomyopathy. *American Journal of Human Genetics* 48: 643–648.

de Vries, D.D., van Engelen, B.G.M., Gabreels, F.J.M. *et al.* (1993) A second missense mutation in mitochondrial ATPase 6 gene in Leigh syndrome. *Annals of Neurology* 34: 410–412.

DiMauro, S. and Melis-DiMauro, P. (1973) Muscle carnitine palmityltransferase deficiency and myoglobinuria. *Science* 182: 929–931.

DiMauro, S., Dalakas, M. and Miranda, A.F. (1981a) Phosphoglycerate kinase deficiency: a new cause of recurrent myoglobinuria. *Transactions of the American Neurology Association* 106: 202–205.

DiMauro, S., Miranda, A.F., Khan, S. *et al.* (1981b) Human phosphoglycerate mutase deficiency: a newly discovered metabolic myopathy. *Science* 212: 1277–1279.

DiMauro, S., Dalakas, M. and Miranda, A.F. (1983) Phosphoglycerate kinase deficiency: another cause of recurrent myoglobinuria. *Annals of Neurology* 13: 11–19.

Dunbar, D.R., Moonie, P.A., Swingler, R.J., Davidson, D., Roberts, R. and Holt, I.J. (1993) Maternally transmitted partial direct tandem duplication of mitochondrial DNA associated diabetes mellitus. *Human Molecular Genetics* 2: 1619–1624.

Ebers, G.C., George, A.L., Barchi, R.L. *et al.* (1991) Paramyotonia congenita and hyperkalemic periodic paralysis are linked to the adult muscle sodium channel gene. *Annals of Neurology* 30: 810–816.

Edwards, Y., Sakoda, S. and Schon, E.A. (1989) The gene for human muscle-specific phosphoglycerate mutase. PGAMM, mapped to chromosome 7 by polymerase chain reaction. *Genomics* 5: 948–951.

Engle, E.C., Kunkel, I.M., Specht, L.A. *et al.* (1994) Mapping a gene for congenital fibrosis of the extraocular muscles to the centromeric region of chromosome 12. *Nature Genetics* 7: 69–75.

Finocchiaro, G., Taroni, F., Rocchi, M. *et al.* (1991) cDNA cloning, sequence analysis, and chromosome localization of the gene for human carnitine palmitoyltransferase. *Proceedings of the National Academy of Sciences of the USA* 88: 661–665.

Fischbeck, K.H., Ionasescu, V., Ritter, A.W. *et al.* (1986) Localization of the gene for X-linked spinal muscular atrophy. *Neurology* 36: 1595–1598.

Fontaine, B., Khurana, T.S., Hoffman, E.P. *et al.* (1990) Hyperkalemic periodic paralysis and the adult muscle sodium channel α-subunit gene. *Science* 250: 1000–1002.

Fontaine, B., Valesantos, J., Jurkat-Rott, K. *et al.* (1994) Mapping of the hypokalaemic periodic paralysis (HypoPP) locus to chromosome 1q31-q32 in three European families. *Nature Genetics* 6: 267–272.

Friedrich, U., Brunner, H., Smeets, D., Lambermon, E. and Ropers, H.H. (1987) Three-point linkage analysis employing C3 and 19cen markers assign the myotonic dystrophy gene to 19q. *Human Genetics* 75: 291–293.

Fu, Y.H. Pizzutti, A., Fenwick, R.G. Jr, *et al.* (1992) An unstable triplet repeat in a gene related to myotonic muscular dystrophy. *Science* 255: 1256–1260.

Fujii, J., Otsu, K., Zorzato, F. *et al.* (1991) Identification of a mutation in porcine ryanodine receptor associated with malignant hyperthermia. *Science* 253: 448–451.

Gal, A., Mucke, J., Theile, H., Wieacker, P., Ropers, H., and Wienker, T. (1985) X-linked dominant Charcot-Marie-Tooth disease: suggestion of linkage with a cloned DNA sequence from the proximal Xq. *Human Genetics* 70: 38–42.

George, A.L. Jr. Crackower, M.A., Abdalla, J.A., Hudson, A.J. and Ebers, G.C. (1993) Molecular basis of Thomsen's disease (autosomal dominant myotonia congenita). *Nature Genetics* 3: 305–310.

Gilbert, J.R., Stajich, J.M., Wall, S. *et al.* (1993) Evidence for heterogeneity in facioscapulohumeral muscular dystrophy (FSHD). *American Journal of Human Genetics* 53: 401–408.

Gillard, E., Otsu, K., Fujii, J. *et al.* (1991) A substitution of cysteine for arginine in the ryanodine receptor is potentially causative of human malignant hyperthermia. *Genomics* 11: 751–755.

Gillard, E., Otsu, K., Fujii, J. *et al.* (1992) Polymorphisms and deduced amino acid substitutions in the coding sequence of the ryanodine receptor (RYR1) gene in individuals with malignant hyperthermia. *Genomics* 13: 1247–1254.

Gilliam, T.C., Brzustowicz, L.M., Castilla, L.H. *et al.* (1990) Genetic homogeneity between acute and chronic forms of spinal muscular atrophy. *Nature* 345: 823–825.

Gispert, S., Twells, R., Orozco, G. *et al.* (1993) Chromosomal assignment of the second locus for autosomal dominant cerebellar ataxia (SCA2) to chromosome 12q23-24.1. *Nature Genetics* 4: 295–299.

Goto, Y., Nonaka, I. and Horai, S. (1990) A mutation in the tRNA$^{Leu(UUR)}$ gene associated with the MELAS subgroup of mitochondrial encephalomyopathies. *Nature* 348: 651–653.

Goto, Y., Nonaka, I. and Horai, S. (1991) A new mitochondrial DNA associated with mitochondrial myopathy, encephalopathy, lactic acidosis and stroke-like episodes (MELAS). *Biochimica et Biophysica Acta* 1097: 238–240.

Goto, Y., Tojo, M., Tohyama, J., Horai, S. and Nonaka, L. (1992) A novel point mutation in the mitochondrial tRNA$^{Leu(UUR)}$ gene in a family with mitochondrial myopathy. *Annals of Neurology* 31: 672–675.

Guiloff, R.J., Thomas, P.K., Contreras, M., Armitage, S., Schwarz, G. and Sedgwick, E.M. (1982) Evidence for linkage of type I hereditary motor and sensory neuropathy to the Duffy locus on chromosome 1. *Annals of Human Genetics* 46: 25–27.

Harley, H.G., Brook, J.D., Rundle, S.A. *et al.* (1992) Expansion of an unstable DNA region and phenotypic variation in myotonic dystrophy. *Nature* 355: 545–546.

Hattori, Y., Goto, Y., Sakuta, R. *et al.* (1994) Point mutations in mitochondrial tRNA genes: sequence analysis of chronic progressive external ophthalmoplegia (CPEO). *Journal of the Neurological Sciences* 125: 50–55.

Hayasaka, K., Himoro, M., Sato, W. *et al.* (1993) Charcot-Marie-Tooth neuropathy type 1B is associated with mutations of the myelin P_0 gene. *Nature Genetics* **5**: 31–34.

Hentati, A., Lamy, C., Melki, J. *et al.* (1992) Clinical and genetic heterogeneity of Charcot-Marie-Tooth disease. *Genomics* **12**: 155–157.

Hentati, A., Bejaoui, K., Pericak-Vance, M.A. *et al.* (1994) Linkage of recessive familial amyotrophic lateral sclerosis to chromosome 2q33–q35. *Nature Genetics* **7**: 425–428.

Hers, H. (1963) Alpha-glucosidase deficiency in generalized glycogen storage disease. *Biochemical Journal* **86**: 11–16.

Hillaire, D., Leclerc, A., Fauré S. *et al.* (1994) Localization of merosin-negative congenital muscular dystrophy to chromosome 6q2 by homozygosity mapping. *Human Molecular Genetics* **3**: 1657–1661.

Hodgson, S.V., Boswinkel, E., Walker, A. *et al.* (1986) Linkage analysis using nine DNA polymorphisms along the length of the X chromosome locates the gene for Emery–Dreifuss muscular dystrophy to distal Xq (abstract). *Journal of Medical Genetics* **23**: 169–170.

Hoffman, E.P., Brown, R.H. Jr, and Kunkel, L.M. (1987) Dystrophin: the protein product of the Duchenne muscular dystrophy locus. *Cell* **51**: 919–928.

Hoffman, E.P., Fischbeck, K.H., Brown, R.H. *et al.* (1988) Characterization of dystrophin in muscle biopsy specimens from patients with Duchenne's or Becker's muscular dystrophy. *New England Journal of Medicine* **318**: 1363–1368.

Holt, I.J., Harding, A.E. and Morgan-Hughes, J.A. (1988) Deletions of muscle mitochondrial DNA in patients with mitochondrial myopathies. *Nature* **331**: 717–719.

Holt, I.J., Harding, A.E., Petty, R.K.H. and Morgan-Hughes, J.A. (1990) A new mitochondrial disease associated with mitochondrial DNA heteroplasmy. *American Journal of Human Genetics* **46**: 428–433.

Howell, N., Kubacka, I., Xu, M. and McCullough, D. (1991) Leber's hereditary optic neuropathy: involvement of the mitochondrial ND1 gene and evidence for an intragenic suppressor mutation. *American Journal of Human Genetics* **48**: 935–942.

Huoponen, K., Vlikki, J., Aula, P., Nikoskelain, E.K. and Savontaus M.L. (1991) A new mtDNA mutation associated with Leber's hereditary optic neuroretinopathy. *American Journal of Human Genetics* **48**: 1147–1153.

Jackson, J., Currier, R., Terasaki, P., Pi, T. and Morton, N. (1977) Spinocerebellar ataxia and HLA linkage: risk prediction by HLA typing. *New England Journal of Medicine* **296**: 1138–1141.

Jarcho, J.A., McKenna, W., Pare, J.A.P. *et al.* (1989) Mapping a gene for familial hypertrophic cardiomyopathy to chromosome 14ql. *New England Journal of Medicine* **321**: 1372–1378.

Johns, D.R. and Berman, J. (1991) Alternative, simultaneous complex I mitochondrial DNA mutations in Leber's hereditary optic neuropathy. *Biochemical and Biophysical Research Communications* **174**: 1324–1339.

Johns, D.R. and Neufeld, M.J. (1991) Cytochrome b mutations in Leber's hereditary optic neuropathy. *Biochemical and Biophysical Research Communications* **181**: 1358–1364.

Johns, D.R., Neufeld, M.J. and Park, R.D. (1992) An ND-6 mitochondrial gene mutation associated with Leber hereditary optic neuropathy. *Biochemical and Biophysical Research Communications* **187**: 1551–1557.

Jun, A.S., Brown, M.D. and Wallace, D.C. (1994) A mitochondrial DNA mutation at nucleotide pair 14459 of the NADH dehydrogenase subunit 6 gene associated with maternally inherited Leber hereditary optic neuropathy and dystonia. *Proceedings of the National Academy of Sciences of the USA* **91**: 6206–6210.

Jurkat-Rott, K., Lehmann-Horn, F., Elbaz. A. *et al.* (1994) A calcium channel mutation causing hypokalaemic periodic paralysis. *Human Molecular Genetics* **3**: 1415–1419.

Kanno, T. Sudo, K., Takeuchi, I. *et al.* (1980) Hereditary deficiency of lactate dehydrogenase M-subunit. *Clinica Chimica Acta* **108**: 267–276.

Kausch, K., Lehmann-Horn, F., Janka, M., Wieringa, B., Grimm, T. and Müller, C. (1991) Evidence for linkage of the central core disease locus to the proximal long arm of human chromosome 19. *Genomics* **10**: 765–769.

Keating, K.E., Quane, K.A., Manning, B.M. *et al.* (1994) Detection of a novel RYR1 mutation in four malignant hyperthermia pedigrees. *Human Molecular Genetics* **3**: 1855–1858.

Khati, C., Stevanin, G., Durr, A. *et al.* (1993) Genetic heterogeneity of autosomal dominant cerebellar ataxia type I. Clinical and genetic analysis of ten French families. *Neurology* **43**: 1131–1137.

Kobayashi, Y., Momo, M.Y., Tominaga, K. *et al.* (1990). A point mutation in the mitochondrial $tRNA^{Leu(UUR)}$ gene in MELAS. *Biochemical and Biophysical Research Communications* **173**: 816–822.

Koch, M., Ricker, K., Otto, M. *et al.* (1992a) Linkage data suggesting allelic heterogeneity for paramyotonia congenita and hyperkalaemic periodic paralysis on chromosome 17. *Human Genetics* **88**: 71–74.

Koch, M., Steinmeyer, K., Lorenz, C. *et al.* (1992b) The skeletal muscle chloride channel in dominant and recessive human myotonia. *Science* **257**: 797–800.

Koenig, M., Hoffman, E.P., Bertelson, C.J., Monaco, A., Feener, C. and Kunkel, L. (1987) Complete cloning of the Duchenne muscular dystrophy (DMD) cDNA and preliminary genomic organization of the DMD gene in normal and affected individuals. *Cell* **50**: 509–517.

Koenig, M., Monaco, A.P. and Kunkel, L.M. (1988) The complete sequence of dystrophin predicts a rod-shaped cytoskeletal protein. *Cell* **53**: 219–228.

Kulkens, T., Bolhuis, P.A., Wolterman, R.A. *et al.* (1993) Deletion of the serine 34 codon from the major peripheral myelin protein P_0 gene in Charcot-Marie-Tooth disease type 1B. *Nature Genetics* **5**: 35–39.

La Spada, A.R., Wilson, E.M., Lubahn, D.B., Harding, A.E. and Fischbeck, K.H. (1991) Androgen receptor gene mutations in X-linked spinal and bulbar muscular atrophy. *Nature* **352**: 77.

Laing, N., Majda, B., Akkari, P. *et al.* (1992) Assignment of a gene (NEM1) for autosomal dominant nemaline myopathy to chromosome 1. *American Journal of Human Genetics* **50**: 576–583.

Laing, N.G., Wilton, S.D., Akkari, P.A. *et al.* (1995) A mutation in the α-tropomyosin gene TPM3 associated with autosomal dominant nemaline myopathy. *Nature Genetics* **9**: 75–79.

Lebo, R.V., Gorin, F., Fletterick, R.J.*et al.* (1984) High-resolution chromosome sorting and DNA spot-blot analysis assign McArdle's syndrome to chromosome 11. *Science* **225**: 57–59.

Lefebvre, S., Burglen, L., Reboullet, S. *et al.* (1995) Identification and characterization of a spinal muscular atrophy-determining gene. *Cell* **80**: 155–165.

Levitt, R.C., Olckers, Meyers, S. *et al.* (1992) Evidence of the localization of a malignant hyperthermia susceptibility locus (MSH2) to human chromosome 17q. *Genomics* **14**: 562–566.

Mackey, D. and Howell, N. (1992) A variant of Leber hereditary optic neuropathy characterized by recovery of vision and by an unusual mitochondrial genetic etiology. *American Journal of Human Genetics* **51**: 1218–1228.

MacLennan, D.H., Duff, C., Zorzato, F. *et al.* (1990) Ryanodine receptor gene is a candidate for predisposition to malignant hyperthermia. *Nature* **343**: 559–561.

Mahadevan, M., Tsilfidis, C., Sabourin, L. *et al.* (1992) Myotonic dystrophy mutation: an unstable CTG repeat in the 3′ untranslated region of the gene. *Science* **255**: 1253–1255.

Matsumura, K., Tomé, F.M.S., Collin, H. *et al.* (1992) Deficiency of the 50K dystrophin-associated glycoprotein in severe childhood autosomal recessive muscular dystrophy. *Nature* **359**: 320–322.

Matsunami, N., Smith, B., Ballard, L. *et al.* (1992) Peripheral myelin protein-22 gene maps in the duplication in chromosome 17p11.2 associated with Charcot-Marie-Tooth 1A. *Nature Genetics* **1**: 176–179.

Mazziotta, M.R.M., Ricci, E., Bertini, E. *et al.* (1992) Fatal infantile liver failure due to mitochondrial DNA depletion. *Journal of Pediatrics* **121**: 896–901.

McCarthy, T.V., Healy, J.M.S., Heffron, J.J.A. *et al.* (1990) Localization of the malignant hyperthermia susceptibility locus to human chromosome 19q12-13. *Nature* **343**: 562–564.

McClatchey, A.I., Van den Berg, P., Pericak-Vance, M.A. *et al.* (1992) Temperature-sensitive mutations in the II-IV cytoplasmic loop region of the skeletal muscle sodium channel gene in paramyotonia congenita. *Cell* **68**: 769–774.

McKusick, V.A. (1992) *Mendelian Inheritance in Man. Catalogs of Autosomal Dominant, Autosomal Recessive and X-linked Phenotypes* 10th edn. Baltimore: Johns Hopkins University Press.

McShane, M.A., Hammans, S.R., Sweeney, M. *et al.* (1991) Pearson syndrome and mitochondrial encephalopathy in a patient with a deletion of mtDNA. *American Journal of Human Genetics* **48**: 39–42.

Melki, J., Abdelhak, S., Sheth, P. *et al.* (1990a) Gene for chronic proximal spinal muscular atrophies maps to chromosome 5q. *Nature* **344**: 767–768.

Melki, J., Sheth, P., Abdelhak, S. *et al.* (1990b) Mapping of acute (type 1) spinal muscular atrophy to chromosome 5q12-q14. *Lancet* **336**: 271–273.

Melki, J., Lefebvre, S., Burglen, L. *et al.* (1994) De novo and inherited deletions of the 5q13 region in spinal muscular atrophies. *Science* **264**: 1474–1477.

Merante, F., Tein, I., Benson, L. *et al.* (1994) Maternally inherited hypertrophic cardiomyopathy due to a novel T-to-C transition at nucleotide 9997 in the mitochondrial tRNA^{glycine} gene. *American Journal of Human Genetics* **55**: 437–446.

Minoletti, F. *et al.* (1992) Localization of the human gene for carnitine palmitoyltransferase to 1p13-p11 by non-radioactive *in situ* hybridization. *Genomics* **13**: 1372–1374.

Mommaerts, W.F.H.M., Illingworth, B., Pearson, C.M., Cuillory, R.J. and Seraydarian, K. (1959) A functional disorder of muscle associated with the absence of phosphorylase. *Proceedings of the National Academy of Sciences of the USA* **45**: 791–793.

Monaco, A.P., Neve, R., Colletti-Feener, C., Berteison, C.J., Kurnit, M. and Kunkel, L.M. (1986) Isolation of candidate cDNAs for portions of the Duchenne muscular dystrophy gene. *Nature* **323**: 646–650.

Moraes, C.T., DiMauro, S., Zeviani, M. *et al.* (1989) Mitochondrial DNA deletions in progressive external ophthalmoplegia and Kearns-Sayre syndrome. *New England Journal of Medicine* **320**: 1293–1299.

Moraes, C.T., Shanske, S., Tritschler, H.J. *et al.* (1991) MtDNA depletion with variable tissue expression: a novel genetic abnormality in mitochondrial diseases. *American Journal of Human Genetics* **48**: 492–501.

Moraes, C.T. Ciacci, F., Bonilla, E., Ionasescu, V., Schon, E.A. and Di Mauro, S. (1993a) A mitochondrial tRNA anticodon swap associated with a muscle disease. *Nature Genetics* **4**: 284–288.

Moraes, C.T., Ciacci, F. Bonilla, E. *et al.* (1993b) Two novel pathogenic mitochondrial DNA mutations affecting organelle number and protein synthesis: is the tRNA$^{Leu(UUR)}$ gene an hetiologic hotspot? *Journal of Clinical Investigation* **92**: 2906–2915.

Moraes, C.T., Ciacci, F., Silvestri, G. *et al.* (1993c) Atypical clinical presentations associated with the MELAS mutation at position 3243 of human mitochondrial DNA. *Neuromuscular Disorders* **3**: 43–50.

Morten, K.J., Cooper, J.M., Brown, G.K., Lake, B.D., Pike, D. and Poulton, J. (1993) A new point mutation associated with mitochondrial encephalomyopathy. *Human Molecular Genetics* **2**: 2081–2087.

Nakajima, H., Kono, N., Yamasaki, T. *et al.* (1991) Genetic defect in muscle phosphofructokinase deficiency. *Journal of Biological Chemistry* **265**: 9292–9295.

Nicholson, G.A., Valentijn, I.J., Cherryson, A.K. *et al.* (1994) A frame shift mutation in the PMP22 gene in hereditary neuropathy with liability to pressure palsies. *Nature Genetics* **6**: 263–266.

Ohno, K., Tanaka, M., Sahashi, K. *et al.* (1991) Mitochondrial DNA deletions in inherited recurrent myoglobinuria. *Annals of Neurology* **29**: 364–369.

Orr, H.T., Chung, M.Y., Banfi, S. *et al.* (1993) Expansion of an unstable trinucleotide CAG repeat in spinocerebellar ataxia type 1. *Nature Genetics* **4**: 221–226.

Passos-Bueno, M.R., Oliveira, J.R., Bakker, E. *et al.* (1993) Genetic heterogeneity for Duchenne-like muscular dystrophy (DLMD) based on linkage and 50 DAG analysis. *Human Molecular Genetics* **2**: 1945–1947.

Patel, P., Roa, B., Welcher, A. *et al.* (1992) The gene for the peripheral myelin protein PMP-22 is a candidate for Charcot-Marie-Tooth disease type 1A. *Nature Genetics* **1**: 159–165.

Poulton, J., Deadman, M.E. and Gardiner, R.M. (1989) Duplication of mitochondrial DNA in mitochondrial myopathies. *Lancet* **1**: 236–240.

Prezant, T.R., Agapian, J.V., Bohlman, M.C. *et al.* (1993) Mitochondrial ribosomal RNA mutation associated with both antibiotic-induced and non-syndromic deafness. *Nature Genetics* **4**: 289–294.

Ptacek, L.J., George, A.L. Jr, Griggs, R. *et al.* (1991a) Identification of a mutation in the gene causing hyperkalemic periodic paralysis. *Cell* **67**: 1021–1027.

Ptacek, L.J., Trimmer, J.S., Agnew, W.S., Roberts, J., Petajan, J. and Leppert, M. (1991b) Paramyotonia congenita and hyperkalemic periodic paralysis map to the same sodium channel gene locus. *American Journal of Human Genetics* **49**: 851–854.

Ptacek, L.J., Tawill, R., Giggs, R.C. *et al.* (1994) Dihydropyridine receptor mutations cause hypokalemic periodic paralysis. *Cell* **77**: 863–868.

Quane, K.A., Healy, J.M.S., Keating, K.E. *et al.* (1993) Mutations in the ryanodine receptor gene in central core disease and malignant hyperthermia. *Nature Genetics* **5**: 51–55.

Quane, K.A., Keating, K.E., Manning, B.M. *et al.* (1994) Detection of a novel common mutation in the ryanodine receptor gene in malignant hyperthermia: implications for diagnosis and heterogeneity studies. *Human Molecular Genetics* **3**: 471–476.

Renwick, J.H., Bundey, S.E., Ferguson-Smith, M.A. and Izatt, M.M. (1971) Confirmation of linkage of the loci for myotonic dystrophy and ABH secretion. *Journal of Medical Genetics* **8**: 407–416.

Roa, B.B., Garcia, C.A., Pentao, L. *et al.* (1993) Evidence for a recessive PMP22 point mutation in Charcot-Marie-Tooth disease type 1A. *Nature Genetics* **5**: 189–194.

Roberds, S.L., Leturcq, F., Allamand, V. *et al.* (1994) Missense mutations in the adhalin gene linked to autosomal recessive muscular dystrophy. *Cell* **78**: 625–633.

Rojas, C.V., Wang, J., Schwartz, L.S. *et al.* (1991) A Met-to-Val mutation in the skeletal muscle Na channel α-subunit in hyperkalaemic periodic paralysis. *Nature* **354**: 387–389.

Romeo, G., Roncuzzi, L., Sangiorgi, S. *et al.* (1988) Mapping of the Emery-Dreifuss gene through reconstruction of crossover points in two Italian pedigrees. *Human Genetics* **80**: 59–62.

Romero, N.B., Tomé, F.M.S., Leturcq, F. *et al.* (1994) Genetic heterogeneity of severe childhood autosomal recessive muscular dystrophy with adhalin (50 kDa dystrophin-associated glycoprotein) deficiency. *Comptes Rendus de l'Academie des Sciences (Paris)* **317**: 70–76.

Rosa, R., George, C., Fardeau, M. *et al.* (1982) A new case of phosphoglycerate kinase deficiency: PGK Creteil associated with rhabdomyolysis and lacking hemolytic anemia. *Blood* **106**: 202–205.

Rosen, D.R., Siddique, T., Patterson, D. *et al.* (1993) Mutations in Cu/Zn superoxide dismutase gene are associated with familial amyotrophic lateral sclerosis. *Nature* **362**: 59–62.

Rotig, A., Colonna, M., Bonnefontt, J.P. *et al.* (1989) Mitochondrial DNA deletion in Pearson's marrow/pancreas syndrome. *Lancet* **i**: 902–903.

Rotig, A., Bessis, J.L., Romero, N. *et al.* (1992) Maternally inherited duplication of the mitochondrial genome in a syndrome of proximal tubulopathy, diabetes mellitus, and cerebellar ataxia. *American Journal of Human Genetics* **50**: 364–370.

Roy, N., Mahadevan, M.S., McLean, M. *et al.* (1995) The gene for neuronal apoptosis inhibitory protein is partially deleted in individuals with spinal muscular atrophy. *Cell* **80**: 167–178.

Schmidt, R. and Mahler, R. (1959) Chronic progressive myopathy with myoglobinuria: demonstration of a glycogenolytic defect in the muscle. *Journal of Clinical Investigation* **38**: 2044–2058.

Scrable, H.J. Johnson, D.K., Rinchik, E.M. and Cavenee, W.K. (1990) Rhabdomyosarcoma-associated locus and MYOD1 are syntenic but separate loci on the short arm of human chromosome 11. *Proceedings of the National Academy of Sciences of the USA* **87**: 2182–2186.

Servidei, S., Zeviani, M., Manfredi, G. *et al.* (1991) Dominantly inherited mitochondrial myopathy with multiple deletions of mitochondrial DNA: clinical, morphological, and biochemical studies. *Neurology* **41**: 1053–1059.

Shoffner, J.M., Lott, M.T., Lezza, A.M.S. Seibel, P., Ballinger, S.W. and Wallace, D.C. (1990) Myoclonic epilepsy and ragged-red fibres (MERRF) is associated with a mitochondrial DNA tRNAL mutation. *Cell* **348**: 651–653.

Shoffner, J.M., Fernhoff, P.M., Krawiecki, N.S. *et al.* (1992) Subacute necrotizing encephalopathy: oxidative phosphorylation defects and the ATPase 6 point mutation. *Neurology* **42**: 2168–2174.

Siddique, T., Figlewicz, D.A., Pericak-Vance, M.A. *et al.* (1991) Linkage of a gene causing familial amyotrophic lateral sclerosis to chromosome 21 and evidence of genetic-locus heterogeneity. *New England Journal of Medicine* **324**: 1381–1384.

Silvestri, G. Moraes, C.T., Shanske, S., Oh, S.J. and Di Mauro, S. (1992) A new mtDNA mutation in the tRNA^Lys gene associated with myoclonic epilepsy and ragged-red fibres (MERRF). *American Journal of Human Genetics* **51**: 1213–1217.

Silvestri, G., Santorelli, F.M., Shanske, S.N. *et al.* (1994) A new mitochondrial DNA mutation in the tRNA^Leu(UUR) gene associated with cardiomyopathy and ragged-red fibres. *Human Mutation* **3**: 37–43.

Speer, M.C., Yamaoka, L.H., Gilchrist, J.H. *et al.* (1992) Confirmation of genetic heterogeneity in limb-girdle muscular dystrophy: linkage of an autosomal dominant form to chromosome 5q. *American Journal of Human Genetics* **50**: 1211–1217.

Stevanin, G., Le Guern, E., Ravisé, N. *et al.* (1994) A third locus for autosomal dominant cerebellar ataxia (ADCA) type I maps to chromosome 14q24.3-qter: evidence for the existence of a fourth locus. *American Journal of Human Genetics* **54**: 11–20.

Sudbrak, R., Golla, A. Hogan, K. *et al.* (1993) Exclusion of malignant hyperthermia susceptibility (MHS) from a putative MHS2 locus on chromosome 17q and of the a1, b1, and g subunits of the dihydropyridine receptor calcium channel as candidates for the molecular defect. *Human Molecular Genetics* **2**: 857–862.

Suomalainen, A., Pateau, A., Leinonen, H., Majander, A., Peltonen, L. and Somer, H. (1992) Inherited idiopathic dilated cardiomyopathy with multiple deletions of mitochondrial DNA. *Lancet* **340**: 1319–1320.

Superti-Furga, A., Schoenle, E., Tuchschmid, P. *et al.* (1993) Pearson bone marrow-pancreas syndrome with insulin-dependent diabetes, progressive renal tubulopathy, organic aciduria and elevated fetal haemoglobin caused by deletion and duplication of mitochondrial DNA. *European Journal of Pediatrics* **152**: 44–50.

Sweeney, M.G., Bundey, S., Brockinton, M. *et al.* (1993) Mitochondrial myopathy associated with sudden death in young adults and a novel mutation in the mitochondrial DNA leucine transfer RNA (UUR) gene. *Quarterly Journal of Medicine* **86**: 709–713.

Taniike, M., Fukushima, H., Yanagihara, I. *et al.* (1992) Mitochondrial tRNA^Ile mutation in fatal cardiomyopathy. *Biochemical and Biophysical Research Communications* **186**: 47–53.

Taroni, F., Verderio, E., Dworzak, R. *et al.* (1993) Identification of a common mutation in the carnitine palmitoyltransferase II gene in familial recurrent myoglobinuria patients. *Nature Genetics* **4**: 314–319.

Tarui, S., Okuno, G., Ikura, Y., Tanaka, T., Suda, M. and Nishikawa, M. (1965) Phosphofructokinase deficiency in skeletal muscle; a new type of glycogenosis. *Biochemical and Biophysical Research Communications* **19**: 517–523.

Tatuch, Y., Christodoulou, J., Feigenbaum, A. *et al.* (1992) Heteroplasmic mtDNA mutation (T − >G) at 8993 can cause Leigh syndrome when the percentage of abnormal mtDNA is high. *American Journal of Human Genetics* **50**: 852–858.

Thomas, N., Sarfarazi, M., Roberts, K. *et al.* (1987) X-linked myotubular myopathy (MTM1): evidence for linkage to Xq28 DNA markers (abstract). *Cytogenetics and Cell Genetics* **46**: 704.

Timmerman, V., Raeymakers, P., De Jonghe, P. *et al.* (1990) Assignment of the Charcot-Marie-Tooth neuropathy type I (CMTIa) gene to chromosome 17p11.2. *American Journal of Human Genetics* **47**: 680–685.

Timmerman, V., Nelis, E., Van Hul, W. *et al.* (1992) The peripheral myelin protein gene PMP-22 is contained within the Charcot-Marie-Tooth disease type 1A duplication. *Nature Genetics* **1**: 171–175.

Toda, T., Segawa, M., Nomura, Y. *et al.* (1993) Localization of a gene for Fukuyama type congenital muscular dystrophy to chromosome 9q31-33. *Nature Genetics* **5**: 283–286.

Trent, R.J. (1993) *Molecular Medicine*. Edinburgh: Churchill Livingstone.

Tritschler, H.J., Andreetta, F., Moraes, C.T. *et al.* (1992) Mitochondrial myopathy of childhood associated with depletion of mitochondrial DNA. *Neurology* **42**: 209–217.

Tsujino, S., Shanske, S. and DiMauro, S. (1993a) Molecular genetic heterogeneity of myophosphorylase deficiency (McArdle's disease). *New England Journal of Medicine* **329**: 241–245.

Tsujino, S., Shanske, S., Sakoda, S. *et al.* (1993b) The molecular genetic basis of muscle phosphoglycerate mutase (PGAM) deficiency. *American Journal of Human Genetics* **52**: 472–477.

Uncini, A., Servidei, S., Silvestri, G. *et al.* (1994) Ophthalmoplegia, demyelinating neuropathy, leukoencephalopathy, myopathy, and gastrointestinal dysfunction with multiple deletions of mitochondrial DNA. *Muscle and Nerve* **17**: 667–674.

Upadhyaya, M., Lunt, P.W., Sarfarazi, M. *et al.* (1990) DNA marker applicable to presymptomatic and prenatal diagnosis of facioscapulohumeral disease. *Lancet* **336**: 1320–1321.

Upadhyaya, M., Lunt, P., Sarfarazi, M. *et al.* (1992) The mapping of chromosome 4q markers in relation to facio-scapulo-humeral muscular dystrophy (FSHD). *American Journal of Human Genetics* **51**: 404–410.

Valentijn, L., Bolhuis, P., Zorn, I. *et al.* (1992) The peripheral myelin gene PMP-22/GAS-3 is duplicated in Charcot-Marie-Tooth disease type 1A. *Nature Genetics* **1**: 166–170.

Van den Ouweland, J.M.W., Lemkes, H.H.P.J., Ruitenbeek, W. *et al.* (1992) Mutation in mitochondrial gene in a large pedigree with maternally transmitted type II diabetes mellitus and deafness. *Nature Genetics* **1**: 368–371.

Vance, J., Nicholson, G., Yamaoka, L. *et al.* (1989) Linkage of Charcot-Marie-Tooth neuropathy type 1a to chromosome 17. *Experimental Neurology* **104**: 186–189.

Vora, S., Durham, S., de Martinville, B. *et al.* (1982) Assignment of the human gene for muscle-type phosphofructokinase (PFKM) to chromosome 1 (region cen-q32) using somatic cell hybrids and monoclonal anti-M antibody. *Somatic Cell Genetics* **8**: 95–104.

Wallace, D.C., Singh, G., Lott, M.T. *et al.* (1988) Mitochondrial DNA mutation associated with Leber's hereditary optic neuropathy. *Science* **242**: 1427–1430.

Wijmenga, C., Frants, R.R., Brouwer, O.F., Moerer, P., Weber, J. and Padberg, G. (1990) Location of facioscapulohumeral muscular dystrophy gene on chromosome 4. *Lancet* **336**: 651–653.

Wijmenga, C., Padberg, G., Moerer, P. *et al.* (1991) Mapping of facioscapulohumeral muscular dystrophy gene to chromosome 4q35-qter by multipoint linkage analysis and *in situ* hybridization. *Genomics* **9**: 570–575.

Wijmenga, C., Hewitt, J., Sandkuijl, L. *et al.* (1992) Chromosome 4q DNA rearrangements associated with facio-scapulohumeral muscular dystrophy. *Nature Genetics* **2**: 26–30.

Wijmenga, C., Wright, T.J., Baan, M.J. *et al.* (1993) Physical mapping and YAC-cloning connects four genetically distinct 4qter loci (D4S163, D4S139, D4F35S1 and D4F104S1) in the FSHD gene-region. *Human Molecular Genetics* **2**: 1667–1672.

Wright, T.J., Wijmenga, C., Clark, L.N. *et al.* (1993) Fine mapping of the FSHD gene region orientates the rearranged fragment detected by the probe p13E-11. *Human Molecular Genetics* **2**:. 1673–1678.

Yoon, K.L., Aprille, J.R. and Ernst, S.G., (1991) Mitochondrial tRNA[Thr] mutation in fatal infantile respiratory enzyme deficiency. *Biochemical and Biophysical Research Communications* **176**: 1112–1115.

Young, K., Foroud, T., Williams, P. *et al.* (1992) Confirmation of linkage of limb-girdle muscular dys-trophy, type 2, to chromosome 15. *Genomics* **13**: 1370.

Yuzaki, M., Ohkoshi, N., Kanazawa, I. *et al.* (1989) Multiple deletions in mitochondrial DNA at direct repeats of non-D-loop regions in cases of familiar mitochondrial myopathy. *Biochemical and Biophysical Research Communications* **164**: 1352–1357.

Zeviani, M., Moraes, C.T., DiMauro, S. *et al.* (1988) Deletions of mitochondrial DNA in Kearns-Sayre syndrome. *Neurology* **38**: 1339–1346.

Zeviani, M., Servidei, S., Gellera, C., Bertini, E., Di Mauro, S. and Di Donato, S. (1989) An autosomal dominant disorder with multiple deletions of mitochondrial DNA starting at the D-loop region. *Nature* **339**: 309–311.

Zeviani, M., Gellera, C., Antozzi, C. *et al.* (1991) Maternally inherited myopathy and cardiomyopathy; association with mutation in mitochondrial DNA tRNA[Leu(UUR)]. *Lancet* **338**: 143–147.

Zeviani, M., Muntoni, F., Savarese, N. *et al.* (1993) A MERRF/MELAS overlap syndrome with a new point mutation in the mitochondrial tRNA[Lys] gene. *European Journal of Human Genetics* **1**: 80–87.

Zhang, Y., Chen, H.S., Khanna, V.K. *et al.* (1993) A mutation in the human ryanodine receptor gene associated with central core disease. *Nature Genetics* **5**: 46–50.

Zoghbi, H., Jodice, C., Sandkuijl, L. *et al.* (1991) The gene for autosomal dominant spinocerebellar ataxia (SCA1) maps telomeric to the HLA complex and is closely linked to the D6S89 locus in three large kindreds. *American Journal of Human Genetics* **49**: 23–30.

Index

α-actinin, in nemaline myopathy, 147, 148
acetazolamide, ion channels disorders, 272, 283
acetylcholinesterase (AChE) inhibitors, 409, 418
acetylcholine receptor (AChR), structure, 399
AChR, structure, 399
AChR antibodies, 398, 413
    circulating, 407
    pathophysiology of myasthenia, 399, 413
    and severity of myasthenia, 400
acid maltase deficiency (type II glycogenosis), 180–8
    animal model, 188
    case histories, 182–7
    enzyme replacement therapy, 181
    mild forms, 180–1
acidaemias, hypotonia, 471
acyl–CoA dehydrogenase deficiency
    short, medium and long-chain forms, 215
    therapy, 216
Addison's disease, 320
adhalin (50kD DAG), 82
adrenal disorders, 320
adynamia episodica hereditaria, 277
alpha-glucosidase deficiency, 180–8
    enzyme replacement, 181
alpha-2 laminin see merosin
amino acids, codes for, 519
aminotransferases, 11–12
AMP deaminase deficiency, 203
amylo-1,6-glucosidase (debranching enzyme), 188
amylopectinosis (branching enzyme deficiency), 191–2
'amyoplasia congenita', 473
'amyotonia congenita', 457
amyotrophic lateral sclerosis, 390
    familial form, 390
Andersen's syndrome, 281
animal models
    acid maltase deficiency, 188
    CMT1A, Trembler mouse, 381
    lipid disorders, 216
    malignant hyperthermia, 300
    of MD
        dy/dy mouse, 104–5

gene therapy, 72–3
    myoblast transfer, 71
    Xp21 muscular dystrophies, 68–70
    phosphofructokinase deficiency, 198
    phosphorylase b kinase deficiency, 199–200
anterior horn cell disease
    with arthrogryposis, 366, 476
    with congenital fractures, 364
    with congenital heart defects, 364–5
    with pontocerebellar hypoplasia, 364
anticholinesterase compounds, management of
        myasthenia gravis, 409, 418
apoptosis, programmed cell death, 357–8
arthrochalasis multiplex congenita, 464
arthrogryposis, 97
    animal model, 481–2
    with anterior horn cell disease, 366
    clinical syndromes, 476–81
    management, 482
    neonatal myasthenic, 413
    and oligohydramnios, 480
    pathogenesis, 473–6
    terminology, 473
ataxia, molecular genetics, 513
ATP synthase deficiency, 250
ATPase reaction, type 1 and 2A–C fibres, 30
ATPase-6 mutation syndrome (NARP), 252, 256
azathioprine
    for dermatomyositis, 445, 448
    in myasthenia gravis, 409

bacterial myositis, 452
Becker muscular dystrophy, 73–82
    clinical features, 73–7
        atypical presentations, 79
    course and prognosis, cardiac involvement, 77
    differentiation from spinal muscular atrophy, 18
    immunocytochemistry, 54–5
    inheritance, molecular genetics, 77–9
    investigations, serum enzymes (CK), 77
    preclinical, 74–5
    see also Duchenne muscular dystrophy; muscular
        dystrophies

'benign congenital hypotonia', 457
benign infantile myopathy, 249
Bethlem myopathy, 35, 91, 92
botulism, 418
branching enzyme deficiency (type IV glycogenosis), 191–2
Brody's disease (Ca-ATPase deficiency in cytoplasmic reticulum), 299
bulbar paralysis
    progressive, 366
    X-linked, 366–7

calcinosis, dermatomyositis, 429, 436, 438
callipers *see* orthoses
cardiac glycogenosis, 180
cardiac involvement
    in dermatomyositis, 429
    nemaline myopathy, 147
cardiomyopathy
    BMD, 79
    complex III deficiency, 249
    DMD, 47–8
carnitine
    biochemistry, 211
    deficiency, 212–13
        myopathic, 212
        systemic, 213
        therapy, 216
carnitine palmitoyl transferase
    biochemistry, 212
    deficiency, 169, 213–14
        mixed forms, 214
Ca²⁺ channels, disorders, list, 267
Ca²⁺-ATPase deficiency in cytoplasmic reticulum, 299
cell death (apoptosis), 357–8
cell transplantation, myoblast transfer, 68–71
central core disease
    case histories, 138–41
    clinical features, 135–7
    genetics, 142
    histopathology, 137–8
    historical aspects, 135
    and malignant hyperthermia, 138
    see also mini-core disease
centronuclear myopathy, 156
Charcot–Marie–Tooth disease
    historical aspects, 370
    X-linked CMT, 382
    see also hereditary motor and sensory neuropathies
chloride channels
    disorders
        cystic fibrosis, 266
        list, 267
        myotonia congenita, 282
cholinergic crisis, 409
chondrodystrophic myotonia, 278–9
chromosomes, gene locations, 516–17
classification, clinical, 2
clinical assessment
    clinical examination, 4–11
    history, 3–4
    questionnaire, 31

Clostridium botulinum, contamination, honey, 418
club foot, 482
CNS disorders, hypotonia without weakness, 459, 460
Cockayne syndrome, 392
coeliac disease, 322
coenzyme Q₁₀ deficiency (complex II deficiency), 248, 259
    in KSS, 259
complex I–V deficiencies, mitochondrial disorders, 247–50
computed tomography, 14, 16–18
congenital club foot, 482
congenital familial external ophthalmoplegia, 120
congenital fibre type disproportion, 164–7
congenital fibrosis of extraocular muscles, 120
congenital fractures, with anterior horn cell disease, 364
congenital heart defects, with anterior horn cell disease, 364–5
congenital hypomyelination neuropathy, 366, 476
congenital muscular dystrophy, 93–101
    animal model (*dy/dy*)
    CNS involvement, 102–3
    differential involvement, 100
    Fukuyama type, 101, 103
    historical aspects, 98–9
    investigations, 99–101
    management, 101
    molecular genetics, 35, 103–5
        animal model (*dy/dy*) mouse, 104
        gene location for FCMD, 104
        gene location and 'pure' CMD, 104
    merosin and, 104
    muscle-eye-brain disease, 101–2
    'pure', 102
    Walker–Warburg syndrome, 102, 103
    see also muscular dystrophies
congenital myopathies, 134–76
    classification, structural, list, 135
    clinical features, 134
    investigations, 134–5
    molecular genetics, 510
    see also metabolic myopathies; myopathies; *specific disorders*
congenital myotonic dystrophy, 289–99
    see also myotonic dystrophy
congenital torticollis, 483–4
connective tissue disorders, 459, 460–5
    fibrodysplasia ossificans progressiva, 492–4
    see also Ehlers–Danlos syndrome
connexin 32, in CMTX, 382
constipation, myotonic dystrophy, 287
conversion disorders
    case histories, 502–6
    clinical features, 502
    management, 502–6
Cori's disease (debranching enzyme deficiency), 188–91
corticosteroids, in mitochondrial myopathy, 259
COX *see* cytochrome oxidase deficiency
Coxsackie virus infection, 443, 452
cramps, 4, 193, 200, 211, 212
creatine kinase
    assay, 11–12

Becker muscle dystrophy, 77
  Duchenne muscular dystrophy, 49–50
    carriers, 61
  Emery–Dreifuss muscular dystrophy, 108
  glycogenosis type II, 180
  malignant hyperthermia, 304
  rigid spine syndrome, 485
  spinal muscular atrophy, 346
cretinism, 316
curare
  contraindications in MG, 410
  pregnancy, 480
cushingoid facies, steroid toxicity, 433
Cushing's syndrome, 320
cyclophosphamide, for dermatomyositis, 443, 445, 447
cyclosporin
  for dermatomyositis, 445, 447
  Duchenne muscular dystrophy, 61
  in myasthenia gravis, 409
cystic fibrosis
  chloride channel, 266
  transmembrane conductance regulator (CFTR), 267
cysticercosis, 453
cytochrome *b* deficiency, 249
cytochrome *c* deficiency, 258
cytochrome *c* reductase, defects, 258
cytochrome oxidase, 28–9
  deficiency (COX)
    complex V deficiency, 249–50
    correlation with mtDNA depletion, 258
  partial deficiency, 230
cytoplasmic body myopathy, 168

DAGs *see* dystrophin-associated glycoproteins
dantrolene, malignant hyperthermia, 301
debendox, in pregnancy, 480
debranching enzyme deficiency (type III glycogenosis), 188–91
deflazocort, in DMD, 61
Dejerine–Sottas disease, 379
  historical aspects, 370–1
  point mutations, 383
  see also hereditary motor and sensory neuropathies
deletions, definition, 518
demyelinating neuropathies, investigations, nerve
    conduction velocity, 15
denervation
  histology, 29
  investigations, 19, 23
  in SMA, 353
dermatomyositis/polymyositis, 422–49
  case histories, 429–42
    calcinosis, 429, 438
    Coxsackie virus infection, 443
    overlap syndrome, 440
    polymyositis, 441
    'terminal' myositis, 434–5
    vasculitis, 442–54
  classification, 422
  clinical features, 425–9
    acute dermatomyositis, 423–5
    chronic dermatomyositis, 429

course and prognosis, 444
  diagnosis, 429–32
  graft-vs-host disease, 444, 448
  historical aspects, 422
  investigations, 432
  isolated 'polymyositis', 425
  treatment, 444–9
    efficacy and order of preference, 447
    azathioprine, 445, 447
    plasma exchange, 445
    steroids, 444, 447
    other immunosuppressive therapy, 444, 445, 447
DeToni–Fanconi–Debré syndrome, 257
development, motor milestones, 5–6
diagnosis and classification, 1–33
3,4-diaminopyridine, 418
dihydropyridine receptor
  calcium channels, 267, 282
  hypokalaemic periodic paralysis, 282
distal muscular dystrophy, 92–3
  autosomal dominant (Welander form), 92
  autosomal recessive (Miyoshi), 92–3
Duchenne muscular dystrophy
  antenatal diagnosis, 50
  carrier detection, *see* inheritance
  classification, functional activity, 121
  clinical features
    deformities, 44
    motor milestones, 41–2
    onset, 39–41
    presenting symptoms, 41
    tendon reflexes, 10
    toe-gait, 10
  course and prognosis, 44–9
    cardiac involvement, 47–8
    intellectual impairment, 48–9
    respiratory deficit/failure, 46–7
    smooth muscle involvement, 48
  histology, 29
  incidence, 39
  inheritance, 39
    carrier detection, 61, 62, 66–7
    female patients, 63, 67
    molecular genetics, 62–73
  investigations
    EMG, 50–1
    immunocytochemistry, 54–5
    molecular genetic, 62–3
    muscle biopsy, 51–4, 66–8, 77
    serum enzymes (CK), 49–50
    ultrasound imaging, 51
  management, 55–61
    drug therapy, 59–61
    gene therapy, 70–3
    loss of ambulation, 55–7
    scoliosis, 57–8
  screening, 50
Duffy blood group, chromosome 1q, 380–1
dy/dy mouse, animal model of MD, 104–5
dysautonomia, familial, 392
dysphonia, 428

dystonia
  dopa response, 500
  hereditary progressive, with diurnal fluctuation,
      499–500
dystonia musculorum deformans, 497–9
dystroglycan, 83
dystrophin
  dystrophin-associated glycoproteins (DAG), 82–9
    43kD DAG, 104
    50kD DAG, 82–9
  dystrophin-related protein (DRP), 83
  immunocytochemistry, 54–5, 67
  interactions, 64
  in muscle biopsy, 66–7
  types, 62, 64
  Western blot, 66
dystrophin gene, 62, 64
  animal models, 68–70
  frameshift mutations, 79
  size of deletion, 64

early-onset, benign autosomal dominant limb girdle
      myopathy with contractures, 92
edrophonium, 405–7, 411
Ehlers–Danlos syndrome
  case histories, 460–4
  classification, subtypes, 462
  see also connective tissue disorders
electromyography, 15–16, 22–3
  concentric needle electromyography, 22
electrophysiological investigations, 15–19
emerin, 485
Emery-Dreifuss muscular dystrophy
  carriers, 108
  clinical features, 105–8
  differentiation from type II glycogenosis, 187
  investigations, 108
  molecular genetics, 108–9
  rigid spine in, 485
endocrine myopathies, 315–24
  adrenal disorders, 320
  parathyroid disorders, 317–18
  pituitary disorders, 320
  renal rickets, 318
  thyroid disorders, 315–17
enzymes
  assays in special investigations, 11–12
  replacement, in α-1,4-glucosidase deficiency, 181
  see also creatine kinase; *investigations, under specific
      conditions*
epidemiology of muscle disorders, 2–3
epilepsy *see* myoclonus epilepsy
episodic weakness, 4
Eulenberg's disease, 275–6
exercise-induced muscle stiffness, 299
exons, 518
exophthalmic ophthalmoplegia, and thyrotoxicosis,
      315–16

facioscapulohumeral muscular dystrophy
  clinical features, 111–15
  investigations, 115–18

management, 118
  molecular genetics, 35, 118
facioscapuloperoneal muscular atrophy, 385
facioscapuloperoneal syndrome, 119
family history, 4
faradism, 36
fasciculations, 10
  potentials, 19, 23
fatal infantile multisystem disorders, 247
fatal infantile myopathy, 249
Fazio–Londe disease, 366
fibrodysplasia ossificans progressiva, 492–4
fibronectin abnormality, 462
fingerprint myopathy, 168
floppy infant syndrome, 457–72
  clinical features, 11
  diagnosis, 457, 458
  terminology, 457
  see also hypotonia; spinal muscle atrophy, severe type
Forbes' disease (debranching enzyme deficiency), 188–91
frameshift mutations, 79, 518
Friedreich's ataxia, 384
Fukuyama type congenital muscular dystrophy, 101, 103
  gene location, 35, 104
  laminin, 104
fumarase deficiency, 241

gallamine, contraindications in MG, 410
gammaglobulin
  for dermatomyositis, 445, 447
  for myasthenia gravis, 409–10
gas gangrene, 452
gastrointestinal involvement, in dermatomyositis, 429
gene therapy
  animal models, 72–3
  DMD, 70–3
genetics, 509–27
  amino acid codes, 519
  gene locations, 516–17
  glossary of terms, 518
  mitochondrial encephalomyopathies, 514–15
  neuromuscular disorders, 510–13
    gene locations, 516–17
  pedigrees, 519–20
  see also specific conditions (under *genetics* and
      molecular genetics)
globoid cell leucodystrophy, 392
glossary, genetics terms, 518
α-1,4-glucosidase deficiency, 180–8
  enzyme replacement, 181
glutaric aciduria type II, 215
glycogenoses, 177–210
  classification, list, 178–9
  clinical features, 178
  enzyme deficiency types:
    II, 180–8
    III, 188–91
    IV; 191–2
    V, 192–7
    VII, 197–8
    VIII, 198–200
    IX, 200

X, 201
XI, 201–2
gene locations, 178
lysosomal glycogen storage with cardiomyopathy,
    mental retardation and vacuolar myopathy,
    202
glycolysis, enzyme deficiencies, 179–80
Gotron's nodules, 429
Gowers' manoeuvre, 37, 42, 146
Gowers, W R, *quoted*, 36
graft-vs-host disease, 444, 448
GTP cytohydrolase-I, 500
Guillain–Barré syndrome, 386–7

Hammersmith myometer, muscle power, 9
Harrington procedure, 360
hepatomegaly, in type III glycogenosis, 189–90
hereditary motor neuropathies, 370–97
    historical aspects, 370–1
hereditary motor and sensory neuropathies
    autosomal recessive demyelinating, 384
    classification, HMSN types I-V, 371
        type I (hypertrophic neuropathy), 372–4, 380–2
        type II (neuronal type of peroneal muscular
            atrophy, 375–9, 383
        type III (hypertrophic neuropathy of infancy), 379,
            383
        type IV (hypertrophic neuropathy with excess
            phytanic acid), 380
        type V (peripheral neuropathy with spastic
            paraplegia), 380
    molecular genetics, 380–4, 513
    other types, 384–6
    X-linked, 382
    see also Charcot–Marie–Tooth disease; Dejerine–
        Sottas disease
histidine, excretion, 60
histological staining, 28–30
HIV myositis, 453
HLA class I antigens, inflammatory myopathy, 432
HMSN *see* hereditary motor and sensory neuropathies
Hoffmann's syndrome, 316–17
homozygosity by descent, 103
hyaline body myopathy, 169
hyperaldosteronism, 320
hyperkalaemic periodic paralysis, 269–70
    molecular genetics, 280–1
    pathophysiology, 279–80
hypermetabolic myopathy, 232–3
hyperthermia *see* malignant hyperthermia
hypertonia, generalized, 501
hypertonic muscular dystrophy, 501
hypertrophic neuropathy
    with excess phytanic acid (HMSN IV), 380
    HMSN type I, 372–4
    of infancy (HMSN III), 379
hypokalaemic periodic paralysis, 267–9
    molecular genetics, 281–2
hypomyelination neuropathy, congenital, 476
hypotonia
    associated with non-neuromuscular disorders, 460–71
    incidental, in paralytic conditions, 458

investigations, 458–9
with lactic acidosis, 248
metabolic disorders, 471
of neuromuscular origin, 458–9
non-paralytic conditions, 459
see also floppy infant syndrome
hysterical disorders of movement *see* conversion
    disorders

immunocytochemistry, 30
incidence, defined, 3
inclusion body myositis, 449
    familial, 449
inflammatory myoglobinuria, 305
inflammatory myopathies, 422–56
inheritance, pedigree charts, 519–20
intellectual impairment, DMD, 48–9
introns, 518
ion channel disorders, 266–314
    channels and receptors, 267
    classification, 267
    molecular genetics, 511
Isaacs' syndrome, 399, 500
isaxonine, 59

joint fixation *see* muscle contractures; rigid spine
    syndrome
joint laxity, 462–5

K-walker, 364
Kearns–Sayre syndrome
    case-histories, 235–9
    coenzyme Q_{10} deficiency, 259
    distiguishing features, 240, 242
    molecular genetics, 251
    prognosis, 251
    see also mitochondrial disorders
α-ketoglutarate dehydrogenase deficiency, 241
King–Deborough syndrome, 302–3
Kocher–Debré–Semelaigne syndrome, 316
Krabbe's disease, 392
Krebs cycle
    defects, deficiencies, 247
    overview, 241
kwashiorkor, 320

lactate dehydrogenase deficiency (type XI glycogenosis),
    201–2
lactic acidosis
    cytochrome oxidase deficiency, 249
    with hypotonia, 248
    mitochondrial disorders, 240
    see also mitochondrial encephalomyopathy, lactic
        acidosis, stroke-like episodes
Lambert–Eaton myasthenic syndrome, 399, 411
laminin (merosin)
    complex, 88
    Fukuyama type congenital muscular dystrophy, 104
Leber's hereditary optic neuropathy (LHON), 242, 243
    point mutation of mtDNA, 246
Leigh's syndrome, 392
    cytochrome oxidase deficiency, 249–50

leucodystrophy
  globoid cell, 392
  metachromatic leucodystrophy, 391–2
Leyden–Möbius muscular dystrophy, 37; *see also* limb
      girdle muscular dystrophy
limb girdle muscular dystrophy, 79–90
  clinical features, 80–2
  differential diagnosis, 80–2
  differentiation from glycogenosis type II, 181
  historical aspects, 37
  investigations, 82–3
  50kD DAG deficiency, 82
  molecular genetics, 82, 510
  see also dominant limb girdle dystrophy; mild
      autosomal recessive muscular dystrophy;
      severe autosomal recessive muscular
      dystrophy
limit dextrinosis (debranching enzyme deficiency),
      188–91
lipid disorders, 211–18
  acyl–CoA dehydrogenase deficiency, 215
  animal models, 216
  carnitine deficiency, 211, 212–13
  carnitine palmitoyl transferase deficiency, 169, 213–14
  clinical features, 212
  glutaric aciduria type II, 215
  investigations, 216
  long-chain 3-hydroxyl-CoA dehydrogenase deficiency,
      215
  sulphatide lipidosis, 391–2
  treatment, 216
LOD score, 518
long-chain 3-hydroxyl-CoA dehydrogenase deficiency,
      215–16
long-chain acyl–CoA dehydrogenase deficiency, 215
lower motor neurone disorders, 325–69
  classification, 2, 325
    anatomical approach, 2
    nomenclature, 325
  see also motor neuropathies; spinal muscular atrophies
Lowe's (oculo–cerebro–renal) syndrome, 318–19
luciferase reaction, 50
Luft's syndrome, 241
Luque procedure, 342, 360
lysosomal autophagic vacuoles, 169
lysosomal glycogen storage with cardiomyopathy,
      mental retardation and vacuolar myopathy, 202

McArdle's disease (type V glycogenosis), 192–7
  case histories, 194, 196
magnetic resonance imaging, 14–15
Mahgrebian muscular dystrophy, 82
malignant hyperthermia
  animal model, 300
  associated diseases, 302–6
  and central core disease, 138
  characteristics, 299–300
  diagnosis, 301–2
  Duchenne and Becker dystrophy, 303
  King-Deborough syndrome, 302
  molecular genetics, 300–1
  pathophysiology, 301
  treatment, 301

march myoglobinuria, 305
marrow–pancreas (Pearson) syndrome, 242, 250, 251–2
maternal inheritance, 242
  mitochondrial genome, 244
  pedigree charts, 520
maternally inherited disorder with adult-onset myopathy
      and cardiomyopathy, 242, 243, 256
mdx mouse, 68
medium-chain acyl–CoA dehydrogenase deficiency, 215
MELAS *see* mitochondrial encephalomyopathy, lactic
      acidosis, stroke-like episodes
Mendelian inheritance, pedigree charts, 519–20
meningitis, pneumococcal, muscle contractures, 483
MERFF *see* myoclonus epilepsy with ragged-red fibres
merosin, 104, 510
  see also laminin
Meryon, *quoted* on muscular dystrophy, 37
metabolic myoglobinuria, 305
metabolic myopathies
  molecular genetics, 512
metachromatic leucodystrophy, 391–2
methotrexate, for dermatomyositis, 444, 447
3-methyl histidine, excretion, 60
mexiletine, ion channels disorders, 272, 275, 283
mild autosomal recessive muscular dystrophy, 90
MIMyCa (maternally inherited disorder with adult-onset
      myopathy and cardiomyopathy), 242, 243, 256
mini-core disease
  case histories, 143–6
  clinical features, 142–6
  histopathology, 145
  historical aspects, 142
minicore(s)
  coexistence with whorled fibres, 152
  and nemaline myopathy, 153
minimal change myopathy, 169–72
  case histories, 170–2
  with rigid spine syndrome, 490–1
minipolymyoclonus, 147
mitochondrial disorders, 217–65
  (*see also* mitochondrial DNA)
  biochemical aspects, 240–1
    Krebs cycle, 241
  case histories, 219–39
    see also specific disorders
  classification by biochemical abnormalities, 241
  classification by genetic abnormalities
    communication defects, nuclear and mitochondrial
        genomes, 256–8
    defects of mitochondrial DNA, 250–2
    defects of nuclear DNA, 247–50
    point mutations, 242, 252–6
  classification of mtDNA-associated syndromes, 242
  clinical syndromes, 226, 239
    distinguishing features (comparative study), 240
    hypermetabolic myopathy, 232–3
  complex I-V deficiencies, 247–50
    cardiopathy, 249
    CoQ$_{10}$ deficiency, 248
    cytochrome oxidase deficiency, 249–50
    fatal infantile multisystem disorders, 247

mitochondrial encephalomyopathies, 248
  myopathies, 247, 248
genetics and molecular genetics, 242–8
  deletions of mtDNA, 252
  point mutations, 252–6
histological diagnosis, 218
historical aspects, 217–18
investigations
  magnetic resonance spectroscopy, 247
  physiological measurements, 246
protein transport defects, 250
respiratory chain defects
  combined defects, 250
  complex I-V deficiencies, 247–50
treatment, 258–9
see also KSS; LHON; MELAS; MERFF; MIMyCa;
    MNGIE; NARP
mitochondrial DNA
  characteristics, 244
  communication with nuclear genome, 246
  defects of genome, 246
  deletions and duplications, 250–2
    multiple deletions, 256–7
  depletion, 257–8
  mitotic separation, 245
  mutations, list, 514–15
  mutations of nuclear genes, 246
  in oocyte, 244–6
  point mutations, 252–6
  schema, 243
  threshold effect, 245
  see also mitochondrial disorders
mitochondrial encephalomyopathy, 248
  biochemical classification, 241
  gene mutations, 514–15
mitochondrial encephalomyopathy, lactic acidosis,
    stroke-like episodes
  case history, 255
  clinical features, 254–5
  distiguishing features, 240
mitochondrial genome, 514–15
mitochondrial lipid glycogen storage myopathy, case
    histories, 218–25
mixed myopathies, 152
Miyoshi myopathy, 92–3
  genetics, 35
MNGIE syndrome (myoneurogastrointestinal disorder
    and encephalopathy), 249, 256
morphine, contraindications in myasthenia gravis, 410
motor abilities, assessment, 8
motor milestones, 5–6
motor neurone disease, 390
motor neuropathies *see* hereditary motor neuropathies
movement disorders, 497–508
  see also conversion disorders
MRC scale and score, muscle power, 7–8
multi-core disease *see* mini-core disease
multiple deletion syndrome, 242
muscle atrophy, 10
  denervation, fibre group atrophy, 29
  see also spinal muscular atrophy

muscle biopsy, 19–30
  carrier detection, 61
  needle biopsy, 25–26
    concurrent needle biopsy, 81
  preparation of specimen, 26–7
    histological staining, 28–30
  see also specific disorders (*under* investigations)
muscle contractures, 473–96
  animal models, 481–2
  clinical syndromes, 476–81
    benign congenital, 483
    congenital torticollis, 483–4
    dermatomyositis, 432
    rigid spine syndrome, 484–91
  management, 482
  see also arthrogryposis
muscle cramps, 4, 193
muscle–eye–brain disease (Santavuori), 35, 101, 103
muscle enlargement
  focal hypertrophy, 9–10
  pseudohypertrophy, 9–10
muscle fibres, biology of normal muscle
  histology, 29
muscle fibres, pathological reactions
  central cores, 137–8
  congenital fibre type disproportion, 164–7
  continuous muscle fibre activity, 500
  histology, progression in DMD, 29, 52–3
  rippling muscle disease, 500
  type 1 fibre hypotrophy, 156–61
muscle histology
  histological staining, 28–30
  normal vs dystrophic muscle, 28–30
muscle imaging, 12–15
muscle power
  MRC scale, 7
  myometry, 8–9
muscular dystrophies, 34–133
  classification, 35
  genetics
    gene locations and symbols, 35
    molecular genetics, 510
  historical aspects, 36–8
  nomenclature, 38
  severe autosomal recessive, 82–9
  see also Becker muscular dystrophy; Duchenne
      muscular dystrophy; other *specific conditions*
mutations, *glossary of terms*, 518
myasthenia gravis, 398–421
  associated diseases, 405
  case histories, 400–6
  classification of congenital syndromes, 414–16
  clinical features, 400–1, 405
    congenital syndromes, 416
  diagnosis, 405–7
  forms, 398
    autoimmune, 400–10
    congenital syndromes, 413–18
    Lambert–Eaton myasthenic syndrome, 411
    limb-girdle, 406, 418
    myasthenia with facial malformation, 418
    other syndromes, 418
    transient neonatal, 411–12

historical aspects, 398–9
investigations, 418
  electromyography, 22
management, 407–10
  anticholinesterase compounds, 409
  drugs to be avoided, 410
  flow diagram, 408
  plasma exchange, 410
  steroids, 409
  thymectomy, 410
myasthenic crisis, 409
neonatal, 476
pathophysiology, 399
and thyrotoxicosis, 315
myasthenic arthrogryposis, 413
myelin protein
  peripheral (PMP-22), 381–2, 384
    point mutations, 382
  protein zero, 381
myelination disorders
  amyelination neuropathy, 383
  congenital hypomyelination neuropathy, 476
  hypomyelination neuropathy, 383
  investigations, nerve conduction velocity, 15
myoadenylate deaminase deficiency, 203
myoblast transfer
  lacZ labelling, 73
  mdx mouse model, 71
myoclonus epilepsy with ragged-red fibres
  clinical features, 252–4
  defect, association with genotype and phenotype, 253
  distiguishing features, 240
  molecular genetics, 254
  muscle biopsy, 254
'myodystrophica congenita', 473
myoglobinuria
  aetiology, 305
  inflammatory, 305
  metabolic, 305
  paroxysmal, 305
  in rhabdomyolysis, 304–6
  toxic, 305
myometer, muscle power, 9
myoneurogastrointestinal disorder and encephalopathy
    (MNGIE syndrome), 249
myopathies
  with abnormality of subcellular organelles (non-
      mitochondrial), 168–9
  centronuclear myopathy, 156
  congenital
    classification of structural myopathies, list, 135
    clinical features, 134
    molecular genetics, 510
    non-specific, 169–72
  cytoplasmic body myopathy, 168
  fingerprint myopathy, 168
  focal myopathy, 79
  hyaline body myopathy, 169
  inflammatory, 422–56
  investigations, 134
  minimal change myopathy, 169–72
  molecular genetics, 512

myotubular myopathy, 156
  with type 1 fibre hypotrophy, 156–61
oculopharyngeal myopathy, 120–1
reducing-body myopathy, 168, 449–50
sarcotubular myopathy, 168
severe X-linked myotubular myopathy, 161–3
T-cell-mediated attack, 60
vacuolar, 202
X-linked myopathy with autophagic vacuoles, 169
zebra-body myopathy, 168
see also glycogenoses; inflammatory-; metabolic-;
    mitochondrial-; muscular dystrophies;
    specific disorders
myositis
  bacterial, 452
  focal, 449
  inclusion body, 449
    familial form, 459
  known aetiology, 452–3
  parasitic, 453
  viral, 452–3
  see also dermatomyositis/polymyositis
myositis ossificans, 492–4
myotonia
  see also myotonia congenita; myotonic dystrophy;
      paramyotonia congenita
  animal models, 267, 272, 280
  chemically-induced, 272
  clinical forms, 271–2
  defined, 270–1
  electromyography, 19
  eliciting, 271
  investigations, 19
  molecular genetics, 280–2, 280–3
  pathophysiology, 279–80
  pseudomyotonia, 19
myotonia congenita
  Becker form, 273
  chloride channel, 282
  clinical features, 273
    compared with paramyotonia and periodic
        paralyses, 272
  depolarization hypothesis, 280
  genetics, 273
  historical aspects, 272–3
  investigations, 273
  molecular genetics, 282
  sodium channel biophysics, 282–3
  Thomsen's form, 273
  treatment, 273–5
myotonic dystrophy, 283–9
  anaesthetic risk, 289
  case histories, 285–8
  classification, 283
  clinical features, 284–9
    cardiac involvement, 287–9
    constipation, 287
    smooth muscle involvement, 286–7
  congenital form, 289–99
    case histories, 290–6
    clinical features and course, 289–92
    genetic counselling, 297–8

intellectual impairment, 291
    investigations, 292, 297
    management, 297
    molecular genetics and clinical applications, 298–9
    prenatal diagnosis, 299
    historical aspects, 283–4
    molecular genetics, 511
myotonic syndromes, 270–99
myotubular myopathy, 156
    case histories, 157–60
    genetics, 161
    severe X-linked, 161–3
    with type 1 fibre hypotrophy, 156–61

NADH-CoQ reductase deficiency (complex I deficiency), 247–8
NADH-cytochrome *c* reductase, 248
NADH-TR, histochemistry, 28–9
NARP (ATPase-6 mutation syndrome), 242, 243, 252, 256, 514
nemaline myopathy
    case histories, 148–51
    clinical features and prognosis, 147–51
        cardiac involvement, 147
        hypotonia in, 150–1
    histopathology, 147–150
        plus minicores, 153
        severe congenital, with intranuclear rods, 152
        whorled fibre myopathy, 154–5
    mixed myopathies, 152
neonatal examination, 5–6
neonatal myasthenic arthrogryposis, 413
neostigmine, in management of myasthenia gravis, 407, 409
Nernst potential, 279
nerve biopsy, HMSN, 375
nerve conduction velocity
    clinical investigations, 15, 22–3
    motor potentials, latency, 22
neuraxonal dystrophy, 392
neurogenic syndromes, molecular genetics, 512–13
neuromuscular disorders
    chromosomes, gene locations, 516–17
    molecular genetics, 510–13
    prevalence, 3
neuronal neuropathy, 384
neuropathies
    congenital hypomyelination, 476
    demyelinating *see* hereditary motor and sensory neuropathies, type I
    hereditary, with liability to pressure palsies (HNPP), 386
    neuronal, 384
    tomaculous, 386
    see also hereditary motor and sensory neuropathies; peripheral neuropathies
neuropathy, ataxia and retinitis pigmentosa (NARP), 242, 243, 252, 256
nitrofurantoin, pregnancy, 480
Nonaka muscular dystrophy, 35
normal development, motor milestones, 5–6
nutritional myopathies, 320, 322

obesity, Prader–Willi syndrome, 467–71
ocular syndromes, 120
oculo–cerebro–renal (Lowe's) syndrome, 318–19
oculopharyngeal myopathy, 120–1
oligohydramnios, and arthrogryposis, 480
ophthalmoplegia
    congenital familial external, 120
    progressive external (PEO), 246, 256
        sporadic PEO with ragged-red fibres (RRF), 251
orthoses, 55–7, 359–64
    knee-ankle-foot (KAFOs), 361
osteomalacia, 317–18
overlap syndrome (dermatomyositis), 440
oxaline derivatives, in DMD, 61
oxidative phosphorylation, alterations, physiological measurements, 246
oximetry studies, 47
OXPHOS defect *see* cytochrome oxidase deficiency

parachute response, 7
paramyotonia, clinical features, compared with myotonia congenita and periodic paralyses, 272
paramyotonia congenita (Eulenberg's disease), 275–7
    clinical features, 275–7
    molecular genetics, 280–1
    pathophysiology, 279–80
parasitic myositis, 453
parathyroid disorders, 317–18
paroxysmal myoglobinuria, 305
Pearson marrow-pancreas syndrome, 242, 250, 251–2
pedigree charts, 519–20
Pena-Shokeir syndrome, 480
PEO *see* ophthalmoplegia, progressive external
peptic ulcers, dermatomyositis, 443
periodic paralyses
    clinical features, compared with myotonia congenita and paramyotonia, 272
    historical aspects, 266
    hyperkalaemic, 269–70
    hypokalaemic, 267–9
    normokalaemic, 270
    thyrotoxic, 269, 315
peripheral neuropathies
    acute inflammatory demyelinating polyradiculoneuropathy, 386–7
    arthrogryposis in, 476, 479
    chronic inflammatory demyelinating polyradiculoneuropathy, 387–8
peroneal muscular atrophy
    (HMSN I), 372–4
    neuronal type (HMSN II), 375–9
PGAM *see* phosphoglycerate mutase deficiency
phenytoin, in myotonia, 274–5
phosphofructokinase deficiency (type VII glycogenosis), 197–8
phosphoglycerate kinase deficiency (type IX glycogenosis), 200
phosphoglycerate mutase deficiency (type X glycogenosis), 201
phosphorylase
    cloning and sequencing of gene, 195
    deficiency (type V glycogenosis), 192–7

case histories, 194, 196
  severe infantile form, 197
heterogeneity, 195
phosphorylase *b* kinase deficiency (type VIII
      glycogenosis), 198–200
phytanic acid, storage disease (HMSN IV) (Refsum's
      syndrome), 371, 380
pituitary disorders, 320
plasma exchange, treatment for dermatomyositis, 449
point mutations, 518
poliomyelitis, 390
POLIP (polyneuropthy, ophthalmoplegia,
      leucoencephalopathy and intestinal pseudo-
      obstruction), 249
polymicrogyria, central, arthrogryposis in, 476–9
polymyositis *see* dermatomyositis/polymyositis
polyneuropthy, chronic relapsing, 388–9
polyphasic potentials, 23
polyradiculoneuropathy
  acute inflammatory demyelinating, 386–7
  chronic inflammatory demyelinating, 387
  see also HSMN
Pompe's disease (acid maltase deficiency), 180–8
pontocerebellar hypoplasia, with anterior horn cell
      disease, 364
potassium channels, antibodies, 399
Potter's syndrome, 480
Prader–Willi syndrome, 467–71
prednisolone, prednisone *see* steroids
pregnancy, medication, and arthrogryposis, 480
pressure palsies in HNPP, 386
prevalence, defined, 3
procainamide, myotonia, 275
progressive bulbar paralysis, 366
progressive degenerative disorders of CNS, 390–2
progressive torsion spasms, 497
protein–calorie malnutrition, 320, 322
ptosis, congenital, 120
pyomyositis, 452
pyridostigmine, myasthenia, 411
pyruvate carboxylase deficiency, 241
pyruvate dehydrogenase complex (PDHC), 247
  deficiency, 241

quadriceps, 'congenital' contracture, 482–3
questionnaire, history, 31
quinine, myotonia, 274–5

ragged-red fibres
  myoclonus epilepsy with, 240, 252–4
  occurrence in mitochondrial syndromes, 242
  with PEO, 251
reducing body myopathy, 168, 452
Refsum's syndrome, historical aspects, 371
renal involvement, in dermatomyositis, 429
renal rickets, 318
renal tubular acidosis, 317–18
respiratory chain defects
  combined defects, 250
  complex I-V deficiency, 247–50
  see also mitochondrial disorders

respiratory deficit/failure, DMD, 46–7
  see also under specific neuromuscular disorders
respiratory involvement, in dermatomyositis, 429
reticuloendothelial involvement, in dermatomyositis,
      429
Reunion Island, mild autosomal recessive muscular
      dystrophy, 90
rhabdomyolysis, 304–6
riboflavin, multiple acyl–CoA dehydrogenase
      deficiency, therapy, 216
rickets, 321–2
Rieske protein, 250
rigid spine syndrome, 109, 484–91
  management, 485–91
  with minimal change myopathy, 490–1
rippling muscle disease, 500
Roussy–Lévy syndrome, 373
  historical aspects, 370
ryanodine receptor, 142

sarcoidosis, 452
sarcosporidiosis, 453
sarcotubular myopathy, 168
scapulohumeral muscular dystrophy, 109–10
  genetics, 35
scapuloperoneal muscular atrophy, 197–8, 385–6
SCARMD *see* severe autosomal recessive muscular
      dystrophy
Schwartz–Jampel syndrome, 278–9
scoliosis, 11
  in DMD, 57–8
  in SMA, 330, 359–60
SDH *see* succinic dehydrogenase
Segawa syndrome, 499–500
sensory conduction velocity, 15
serum enzymes *see* creatine kinase; enzymes;
          investigations, under specific conditions
severe autosomal recessive muscular dystrophy, 82–9
  genetic counselling, 88
  management, 88
  molecular genetics, 82–3
  prognosis, 88
  see also limb girdle muscular dystrophy
severe spinal muscular atrophy *see* spinal muscular
      atrophy
severe X-linked (congenital) myotubular myopathy,
      161–3
short-chain acyl–CoA dehydrogenase deficiency, 215
sideroblastic anaemia, Pearson marrow–pancreas
      syndrome, 242, 250, 251–2
smooth muscle, involvement in DMD, 48
sodium channels
  270 kD α-subunit, 282
    and malignant hyperpyrexia, 301
  biophysics, 282–3
  disorders, list, 267
  link to hyperkalaemic periodic paralysis, 280–2
  mutations and domains, 281
  Nernst potential, 279
  paramyotonia congenita, 280
  pathophysiology of myotonia, 279
  schema, 282

sodium-channel myotonia, 281
spastic paraparesis, 501
spastic paraplegia, with peripheral neuropathy, 380
spectrin antibodies, 67
spheroid body myopathy, 168
spinal muscular atrophies, 325–69
    aetiology, 357–8
    clinical picture, 327–8
    genetics, 353–7
        molecular genetics, 356–7
    historical aspects, 326
    investigations, 346–53
        creatine kinase, 346
        ECG, 335
        EMG, 346
        fasciculations, 23
        muscle biopsy, 346–53
        ultrasound imaging, 346
    management, 358–64
    mimicking syndromes, 364–6
        differentiation from muscular dystrophy, 18
        differentiation from Pompe's disease, 180
    neuropathology, 353
    pathogenesis, 353, 357–8
spinal muscular atrophies, types
    classification
        numerical, 337
        types 1–3, 327
    intermediate severity forms
        case histories, 331–4
        clinical features, 330
        prognosis and management, 359–64
    mild form (Kugelberg–Welander)
        case histories, 335–7
        clinical features and prognosis, 335
    severe form (Werdnig–Hoffmann)
        case histories, 328–34
        clinical features, 328–30
        prognosis and management, 358–9
    severe/intermediate (borderline) cases, 337–340
    X-linked (Kennedy disease), 366–7
Steinert's disease *see* myotonic dystrophy
'sternomastoid tumour', 484
steroids
    for dermatomyositis, 444–5, 447
    for Duchenne muscular dystrophy, 59–61
    for myasthenia gravis, 409
    steroid myopathy, 320
    toxicity, dermatomyositis, 433
stiff man syndrome, 501
succinic dehydrogenase, 29, 248
    27.7 kD Fe-S protein, 250
    ATPase reaction, 30
    muscle biopsy, 248, 250
sudden infant death syndrome, and MH, 304
sulphatide lipidosis, 391–2

T-cell(s), in DMD, 60
T-cell-mediated attack, muscle pathology, 60
talipes equinovarus, 482
target fibres, defined, 138
Tarui's disease (phosphofructokinase deficiency), 197–8

tendon reflexes, 10
tenotomy
    and orthoses, management of DMD, 55–7
    see also muscle contractures
tensilon (edrophonium), myasthenia, 405–7, 411
tetrahydrobiopterin-synthesizing enzymes, 500
thiopentone, risk in myotonic dystrophy, 289
Thomsen's disease *see* myotonia congenita
thyroid disorders, 315–17
thyrotoxic periodic paralysis, 269, 315
thyrotoxicosis, 315–16
tibial muscular dystrophy, 35, 93
tocainide, myotonia, 274–5
toe-gait, 10
tomaculous neuropathy, 386
torsion dystonia, 497–9
    genetics, 499
    treatment, 499
torticollis
    congenital, 483–4
        treatment, 484
    in torsion dystonia, 498
toxoplasmosis, 453
transaminases, 11–12
Trembler mouse, model of CMT1A, 381
tremor, 10
trichinosis, 453
trisomy-18, 480
tuberculosis, 452
twins, monozygotic, carriers of Duchenne gene, 61

ulcers, dermatomyositis, 427–8, 430, 443
ultrasound imaging, 12–15
    central core disease, 138, 140
    congenital muscular dystrophy, 99
    dermatomyositis, 432
    DMD, 51
    SMA, 346
'universal muscular hypoplasia', 457
uterine constraint, arthrogryposis, 475–6
utrophin (dystrophin related protein), 83
    in DMD, 90

vacuolar myopathy
    in acid maltase deficiency, 182, 185, 186, 187
    in lysosomal glycogen storage with cardiomyopathy, 202
    in periodic paralysis, 268, 270
vasculitic ulcers, dermatomyositis, 427–8, 430, 443
vastus lateralis pathology, ultrasound vs biopsy, 14, 100
viral myositis, 452–3
vocal cord paralysis, 439

Walker–Warburg syndrome, 102, 103
    genetics, 35
Welander myopathy, 35, 92
Werdnig–Hoffmann disease *see* spinal muscular atrophy
Western blot, dystrophin, 54–5
wheelbarrow posture, 7
whorled fibre myopathy, 154, 154–5

X-linkage, pedigrees, 519–20
X-linked myopathy
  with autophagic vacuoles, 169
  myotubular myopathy, 161–3
X-linked spinal muscular atrophies (Kennedy disease),
    366–7
xeroderma pigmentosum, and Fukuyama type congenital
    muscular dystrophy, 104
XMD animal models of muscular dystrophy, 68–70
Xp21 muscular dystrophies
  animal models, 68–70

Becker muscular dystrophy, 77–9
  discovery, 62
Xq28 region
  EDM, 109
  severe myotubular myopathy, 161

Z discs (lines), 147
  rods in nemaline myopathy, 152
zebra-body myopathy, 168